Hearing
and Deafness

Contributors

Donald R. Calvert, Ph.D., Director, Central Institute for the Deaf; Professor of Audiology, Washington University

Hallowell Davis, M.D., Sc.D., Research Associate and Director Emeritus of Research, Central Institute for the Deaf; Professor Emeritus of Physiology and Research Professor Emeritus of Otolaryngology, Washington University

Norman P. Erber, Ph.D., Research Associate, Central Institute for the Deaf: Assistant Professor of Audiology, Washington University

Robert Frisina, Ph.D., Director, National Technical Institute for the Deaf, Rochester, New York

Ira J. Hirsh, Ph.D., Director of Research, Central Institute for the Deaf; Professor of Psychology, Washington University

Helen S. Lane, PhD., Psychologist, Central Institute for the Deaf; Professor of Education, Department of Speech and Hearing, Washington University

Rachel I. Mayberry, M.S.., Assistant Professor, Program of Audiology and Hearing Impairment, Northwestern University

Arthur F. Niemoeller, Sc.D., Research Associate, Central Institute for the Deaf; Associate Professor of Electrical Engineering, Washington University

Michael M. Paparella, M.D., Chairman, Department of Otolaryngology, University of Minnesota

David P. Pascoe, Ph.D., Coordinator of Audiology Services, Central Institute for the Deaf; Assistant Professor of Audiology, Washington University

Ann L. Perry, M.S., Aural Rehabilitation Therapist, Central Institute for the Deaf; Instructor in Speech and Hearing, Washington University

Donald A. Ramsdell, Ph.D., late Chief, Clinical Psychology Section, Veterans Administration, Boston

Jerome D. Schein, Ph.D., Director, Deafness Research and Training Center, and Professor of Deafness Rehabilitation, New York University

S. Richard Silverman, Ph.D., D. Litt, D.H.L., LL.D., Director Emeritus, Central Institute for the Deaf; Professor of Audiology, Washington University

Hearing and Deafness

FOURTH EDITION

Hallowell Davis, M.D.

S. Richard Silverman, Ph.D.

Central Institute for the Deaf

HOLT, RINEHART AND WINSTON
New York   Chicago   San Francisco   Atlanta   Dallas
Montreal   Toronto   London   Sydney

Library of Congress Cataloging in Publication Data

Davis, Hallowell, ed.
  Hearing and deafness.

  Includes bibliographies and indexes.
  1. Deafness. 2. Hearing I. Silverman,
S. Richard, joint ed. II. Title
[DNLM: 1. Deafness 2. Hearing. WV270 D262h]
RF290.D38 1978   617.8   77-22533

ISBN 0-03-089980-X

Cover design by: Arthur Ritter

Preface

What really is deafness? Is it a number on a decibel scale that describes the severity of hearing impairment? Is it a disease like mumps or measles or meningitis? Is it an ankylosed stapes? Is it a piece of tissue in the auditory system that would be judged to be abnormal if viewed under a microscope? Is it an affliction to be conquered by the ingenious scientist? Is it the burden of a child whose parent hopes persistently and fervently that the scientist will be successful, and soon? Is it a special mode of communication? Is it something that is encountered occasionally in the man or woman whose fingers fly and whose utterances are arrhythmic and strident? Is it a cause to which diligent, skillful, and patient teachers have committed themselves for generations? Is it the agony of isolation from a piece of the real world? Is it the joy of accomplishment that mocks the handicap? Is it the bright mind and the potentially capable hands for which the economy has no use because they are uncultivated? Is it a crystallization of attitudes of a distinctive group whose deafness, modes of communication, and other associated attributes (such as previous education) that they have in common cause them to band together to achieve social and economic self-realization? Of course, it is all of these and more, depending on who asks the question and why.

In seeking the answer to the question, we all have our own motives, our own purposes, and our own responsibilities. Public officials are concerned with the magnitude and severity of the problem, ways of organizing to solve it, legislative needs, and costs; physicians and investigators study causes and pathology of deafness, its "psychology," and its management; educators consider the physical plant, personnel requirements, and methods of instruction and communication; rehabilitators are sensitive to training and job opportunities; and deaf people themselves and those close to them seek the opportunity to be all they can and want to be. As in the legend of the three blind men, it is difficult to perceive and comprehend the whole elephant.

This fourth edition of *Hearing and Deafness* is intended to be a comprehensive textbook for those who wish to explore the needs of the deaf and possible remedies for deafness, that is, for students of audiology who are preparing to be audiologists or to work in closely related fields. For others it may be useful as a reference book or as a summary of the present status and state-of-the-art of audiology. It emphasizes principles. It does not go into fine details of anatomy, surgical technique, the administration of particular tests of hearing, or methods of instruction or counseling of the deaf. It provides a guide to the literature in the form of lists of suggested readings at the end of each chapter. These lists consist chiefly of other books and summary or survey articles in addition to a few specific citations of original sources. Brief characterizations of these other books or articles should assist students in their search for further information.

We have tried not to burden the book with unnecessary mathematical or electronic detail or unnecessary medical terminology, although more of these have been introduced in this revision. Students must certainly learn the meanings of the more common professional and technical terms. To help them identify and understand the technical terms more readily, we have freely used italics and quotation marks to tag such words when they first appear and when their meaning can easily be understood from the context. A glossary systematically presents some definitions that are scattered in the text, particularly those that are relatively new or recently standardized.

Hearing and Deafness originated as a "guide for laymen"—laymen who were personally interested in impairments of hearing. Dr. Hallowell Davis edited the first edition, (1947), but most of the chapters were prepared by specialists in various fields—surgery, psychology, electronics, speechreading, education of the deaf, and others. The various authors read and criticized one another's chapters, and Dr. Davis wrote several chapters and gave some unity to the whole. The first edition served its purpose well, but it unexpectedly served another purpose equally well: it became a textbook for students in the new academic and professional fields of audiology. The second edition was revised to improve and update the book as a text, with less emphasis on the needs of individuals who are trying to understand their own handicap or to use a hearing aid and more emphasis on the basic sciences. Military audiology was replaced by industrial audiology, and so on. In the third edition and in the present one this development has continued, with considerable expansion of the treatment of acoustics, psychoacoustics, neurophysiology, genetics,

audiometry, the handicaps of hearing, and the education of deaf children and a new emphasis on social problems and government involvement with education and the handicapped. Some of the less relevant material has been condensed or eliminated to allow for the expansions.

In the present revision of the chapters on conservation of hearing, audiometry, special auditory tests, and standards and medicolegal rules, we have included rather extensive direct quotations from certain authoritative statements or reviews that have been published so far only in technical journals or pamphlets. The presentation, which is more detailed and technical than that of the more familiar material, was chosen for the benefit of those who are professionally engaged in some branch of audiology. We hope that these more technical chapters will be interesting to casual readers also, but the difference in treatment represents more than the personal caprice of their authors. It reflects the difference in the availability elsewhere of information on these particular topics.

It is inevitable and even desirable that there be some overlap in a book dealing with so broad a field as audiology, especially when chapters are written by different authors. Such overlap emphasizes both the points that are repeated and the interrelationships among the topics. Examples will be found in the chapters on speechreading and auditory training, hearing handicap in the adult and in the child, and educational and rehabilitative procedures.

In the table of contents the chapters have been grouped as before into six parts. From the titles of the sections it is obvious that the general sequence of the book is from physics, psychophysics, biology, medicine, and surgery to modern studies of impaired hearing and hearing aids and thence to special education and rehabilitation of adults with impaired hearing. The emphasis then shifts to the problems of the education of deaf and hard-of-hearing children and finally to employment and adjustment of adults. In general, the sequence is from inanimate nature to the individual human being to complex social problems.

The sequence is probably as familiar as it is arbitrary. It has a disadvantage in that it places some of the more difficult technical chapters first. Readers with educational and social interests may skip boldly to their own territory at once. After all, something has to come first, and the present arrangement has the advantage of explaining basic terms and ideas, such as the decibel and hearing loss, before they are used in other contexts.

In spite of the shift from physical to biological to social, there is one theme that runs evenly throughout the book. It could not be concentrated in any one place, and nearly every chapter must be read to learn all we have to say about it. That theme is *psychology*. Hearing, our main topic, is certainly a province of psychology. Communication may use physical tools and have social aspects, but it is basically a psychological process. Tests of hearing are also squarely in the province of the psychologist. The reaction of the individual to deafness and the basic problems of self-adjustment, education, and vocational guidance are clearly psychological. At first glance it may seem that psychology has been slighted and that only one chapter deals with a single and rather special aspect of psychology. On the contrary, the entire book is permeated with it. In fact, the psychological aspects of the various sections give our book its unity.

This might be a good place to point out that our use of the masculine generic pronouns throughout the book is not automatic. We use these pronouns merely to avoid distracting complexities of wording, and they should always be understood to mean either sex. We trust the activist in the "role of the sexes" movement will not treat our decision too harshly.

SURVEY BY CHAPTERS

The following survey of this fourth edition by chapters is intended to give the reader a brief topical summary of the substance of each chapter and thus supplement the table of contents as a guide to selective reading. For those who are historically minded it may be interesting to compare this survey with the corresponding surveys in the first three editions. The transformation of the book from a guide for laymen to a textbook for professionals will be very evident. At the same time the great changes in some chapters, in contrast with the very minor changes in others, reflect the usual uneven rate of progress in any technical or professional field. In some areas there are breakthroughs and periods of rapid advance. Elsewhere, particularly if advance was rapid in a previous decade, the picture is much the same as it was seven or even thirty years ago. We should emphasize, however, that even the most static of our chapters have been reviewed carefully.

1. Audiology

Audiology is now well established as an area of scientific interest and also of service to the public. A professional organization, the American Speech and Hearing Association, sets examinations and issues certificates of qualification. Audiology ranges from audiology as a paramedical specialty closely related to otology to an independent profession related to handicaps, resulting from impaired hearing, in learning or utilizing language skills. At the present time the audiologist performs services in a variety of organization frameworks.

2. Acoustics and Psychoacoustics

This chapter, rewritten for the third edition, stands almost unchanged except for the emergence of the dBA scale of the sound level meter as the preferred scale for the measurement of noise levels and of 20 μPa (pascals) as the designation of the reference level for acoustic pressure levels. It reviews the necessary fundamentals of acoustic measurements and also of psychoacoustics. Particular attention is given to the abilities of human listeners and the concepts of psycho-acoustics that do or might form the basis of audiometric tests of hearing.

3. Anatomy and Physiology of the Auditory System

Our knowledge of the gross anatomy of the ear has not changed much in thirty years and the drawings prepared for the first edition of *this book* still rank with the best. The microscopic anatomy of the sense organ and how the sense organ acts as a mechanical analyzer of sound and a transducer of sound energy to nerve impulses are discussed in some detail. In particular Dr. Davis describes the "auditory sensory unit" and its "tuning curve." These concepts are the basis of his later interpretations of sensorineural hearing loss. There is also a discussion of the organization of the central auditory system, its development, and some principles of central nervous activity in general. New material relates to the innervation of the organ of Corti and the great difficulties of reconciling these and other new findings in anatomy and bioacoustics and neurophysiology with one another.

Dr. Davis writes with authority in this chapter, as he has investigated the biophysics and neurophysiology of the auditory nervous system for nearly fifty years.

4. Abnormal Hearing and Deafness

This chapter, originally written by Dr. Davis and the late Dr. Edmund P. Fowler, Jr., for the second edition, was expanded considerably for the third edition by Dr. Davis with the advice and assistance of many able medical colleagues. Both conductive and sensorineural hearing loss are analyzed in terms of biophysics and physiology. Two new sections discuss genetics and congenital defects such as those arising from maternal rubella. A theory is presented that attributes difficulty in learning language ("dyslogomathia") to early sensory deprivation. The section on func-

tional deafness has been revised, but Dr. Davis's original account of psychogenic deafness is retained.

5. Conservation of Hearing or Prevention of Hearing Loss

In a complete rewriting of this and the following chapter the prevention of hearing loss has been made a unifying theme. It begins with the prevention or treatment of several diseases such as rubella and jaundice of the newborn and also considers the problem of hereditary deafness. The prevention of otitis media in children comes next, with an evaluation of the rather disappointing contribution of audiometric screening for this purpose. Ototoxic drugs are another hazard to hearing, and next is excessive noise exposure. In this context, monitoring audiometry and the regulations of the Occupational Safety and Health Act (1970) and the Environmental Protection Agency (1973) are considered in some detail, including the various possible risks from noise and the difficulties of setting acceptable criteria for the protection of hearing. Later sections deal with the possible risks in the use of hearing aids and conservation of hearing in elderly people.

6. Medical and Surgical Treatment of Hearing Loss

Dr. Michael M. Paparella is a new collaborator. He is an otologic surgeon with a major interest in medical treatment of disease of the ear and an active investigator of these problems. (He replaces the late Dr. E. P. Fowler, Jr., and the late Dr. T. E. Walsh.) He has combined the medical and surgical treatments of hearing loss in a single chapter and has critically reviewed both of the two preceding chapters.

Dr. Paparella explains in some detail how infection reaches the ear canal and particularly the middle ear, the principles of aural hygiene to prevent it, the effectiveness of tonsillectomy for this purpose, the proper use of drugs, and particularly the timely intervention by surgery to check the progress of the disease. Next he considers chronic otitis media and the various forms of mastoid surgery to relieve it and the rebuilding of a damaged middle ear to improve hearing. For otosclerosis, the fenestration operation has been almost completely replaced by stapes surgery, which introduces an artificial stapes as a substitute, with great success.

The medical treatment of disorders of the inner ear, notably Menière's disease, is less satisfactory than for the middle ear and surgery has only a little to offer, but Dr. Paparella explains in some detail just how much can be expected, what some of the limitations are, and where some of the hopes for the future lie. Finally the authors give a careful evaluation of the present status and the prospects of the so-called "cochlear implant" for electrical stimulation of the auditory nerve to restore hearing to adults who have become totally deaf.

7. Audiometry: Pure Tone and Simple Speech Tests

The standard tuning fork tests, effectively used by otologists but often neglected by audiologists, are described quite fully. The electric pure-tone audiometer is discussed in terms of a new ANSI (American National Standards Institute) standard which at the present writing is practically assured of early adoption. The previous national standard, issued in 1969 by the USA Standards Institute, had already adopted the international (ISO) reference levels for pure tone audiometers. This fourth edition of *Hearing and Deafness*, like the third, uses the new (ISO-ANSI) reference levels exclusively, but it is not so much concerned with the problems of transition. A full historical account is included, nevertheless.

Speech audiometry, with its word tests and articulation scores, is described and evaluated. In 1947 and 1960 we had great hopes for speech audiometry, but now our assessment is more sober. Speech audiometry seems to be firmly established and it makes a real contribution to audiological practice, but the difficulties in the way of standardization and precise measurements are formidable. Nearly all of the word and sentence lists in current use are given in the Appendix with brief statements on the character and particular usefulness of each. Their use in general is directed toward the phonemic study of language and to articulation testing of speech-communication systems quite as much as to clinical audiometry.

8. Audiometry: Other Auditory Tests

Here we consider various additional audiometric tests that are in current use, including loudness balance, the SISI test, and fast-tone decay. They are all useful aids to otologic or neurologic diagnosis, the detection of feigning (malingering), and the educational assessment of children. Our emphasis is on principles; for details of technique we rely on other books to which references are given.

In this fourth edition the discussion of impedance-admittance measurements as an audiological tool has been considerably expanded. Under "electric response audiometry" (ERA), the newer brainstem response audiometry and the electrocochleogram have largely replaced not only electrodermal but also cortical electric response audiometry as the methods of choice for testing the peripheral auditory system in young or uncooperative children. They may be helpful in problems of otoneurology also.

9. Hearing Handicap, Standards for Hearing, and Medicolegal Rules

The present revision of this chapter reviews systematically the use of audiometry to assess the fitness or the handicap of an individual with respect to his hearing. The general criterion of handicap, endorsed by several important medically oriented groups including the American Medical Association, is "one's personal efficiency in every day living, particularly in the hearing of speech." Numerical values for this criterion are given in extensive verbatim quotations from the "Guide for the Classification and Evaluation of Hearing Handicap" published by the American Academy of Ophthalmology and Otolaryngology. These values are then compared with information on the prevalence of hearing handicap, taken from reports on the 1960–1963 National Health Survey. For standards of hearing and screening levels the current U.S. Army regulation (AR 40-501) serves as an illustration.

Various medicolegal rules for calculating the compensation appropriate for various degrees of hearing impairment are summarized, and an extensive list of pertinent references is given. Dr. Davis introduces his concept of "actuarial hearing thresholds," meaning the expected median threshold for a given age and sex. He also discusses the delicate problems of "normal hearing" and multiple causation of a hearing impairment.

10. Hearing Aids

The basic design objectives for hearing aids remain essentially the same in 1977 as they were in 1969, but light weight, small size, and inconspicuousness have been more fully realized, thanks to hybrid and integrated circuits. Recent trends in hearing-aid design indicate the increased use of electret condenser microphones, with both directional and nondirectional polar responses, and compression amplification. Therefore we have included discussions of these features in this chapter.

Dr. Arthur F. Niemoeller is Associate Professor of Electrical Engineering and also Research Associate at Central Institute for the Deaf. He writes from firsthand experience of the principles of operation of a hearing aid, the advantages and disadvantages of group aids for school children, and ear-level hearing.

11. Counseling About Hearing Aids

Dr. David P. Pascoe, who replaces Dr. Davis as co-author of this chapter, is Assistant Professor of Audiology and Coordinator of Audiology Services and Training at Central Institute for the Deaf. He writes as an investigator and clinical audiologist concerned with hearing-aid selection. He and Dr. Silverman consider the many practical questions that arise concerning who should wear a hearing aid, on which ear, whether it should be a body-worn or an ear-level instrument, and so on. They incorporate the information developed in the previous chapter into a set of directions and suggestions addressed to the prospective user. This material also constitutes advice to an audiologist on how to compare instruments with one another while using a minimum of equipment.

12. Auditory Training

A new chapter under the old title has been written by Dr. Norman P. Erber, an audiologist, and Dr. Ira J. Hirsh, a psychologist. The authors discuss various aspects of hearing and auditory perception as they relate to speech, and they intro-

duce a simple model to help the reader organize the variety of stimuli and the types of response tasks that are involved in speech perception. They consider the rehabilitation of the adult who has lost part of his hearing and related auditory training in the use of a hearing aid. They also discuss the steps in the auditory eduction of the deaf child and examine the question whether one's instructional methods should stress unisensory or multisensory modes.

13. Speechreading

Ann L. Perry is joined by Dr. Silverman in the revision of Dr. Miriam Pauls Hardy's chapter on speechreading from the previous edition. The principles remain as they were in 1947, but current investigations enable us to elaborate them. The process is called speechreading, not lipreading, because so much information is obtained from gestures, facial expression, and attention to the entire situation. The authors point out that speechreading and a hearing aid supplement one another beautifully if the deaf person has any residual hearing. They close with a series of very practical suggestions for all who are hard of hearing.

14. Conservation and Development of Speech

Dr. Silverman and Dr. Donald R. Calvert, who is Professor of Audiology, Washington University, and Director of Central Institute for the Deaf, present a fundamental description of speech production and those factors that influence its intelligibility and its conservation and development in hearing-impaired individuals.

15. Manual Communication

This chapter by Rachel I. Mayberry, Assistant Professor, Program of Audiology and Hearing Impairment, Northwestern University, is new. Its inclusion recognizes the growing scientific and professional interest in manual modes of communication. Ms. Mayberry is well qualified to write this chapter and to suggest the kinds of questions that need to be addressed to increase our understanding of manual communication. She combines experience as the daughter of deaf parents, a registered interpreter, and an instructor of teachers with investigations in linguistic aspects of manual communication.

The remaining chapters of the book deal with problems rather than with techniques. The problems differ according to the age at which the impairment occurs and its severity. The second and third editions reflected the shift of problems from a wartime to a peacetime basis.

16. *From Aristotle to Bell—and Beyond*

Dr. Silverman surveys the gradual development of our present social attitude toward the deaf: the deaf are no longer regarded as imbeciles; deaf children are considered to be handicapped children in need of special education. The author recounts the parts played by the pioneers in the education of the deaf. He also notes the important increasing involvement of the United States government in this and related problems. Here he writes from the vantage point of one who has advised about and also participated in implementing some of these developments.

17. *Early and Elementary Education*

For this edition Dr. Silverman and Dr. Helen S. Lane are joined by Dr. Donald R. Calvert in substantial revision of the chapter on deaf children in the third edition. They have combined treatment of educational problems of both deaf and hard-of-hearing children in one chapter: Much material from Dr. Silverman's chapter in the *Handbook of Speech Pathology* edited by Dr. Lee Travis is retained. Once again we are indebted to Dr. Travis and to the publishers, Prentice-Hall, for their courtesy in allowing reuse of the substance and often entire sections of Dr. Silverman's chapter in the revised edition of their *Handbook*.

The chapter reviews several historic controversies between different schools of thought and should provide a starting point for any future discussions of the methods of education of hearing-impaired children, whether by the auditory, oral, or total communication method.

18. *Postsecondary Education*

This chapter by Dr. Robert Frisina, Director of National Technical Institute for the Deaf, is new. It traces the development of postsecondary education in the United States and its role in increasing and improving career choices for hearing-impaired individuals in a changing occupational world. The problems as well as the opportunities associated with higher education for the hearing impaired are discussed.

19. *The Psychology of the Hard-of-Hearing and the Deafened Adult*

Dr. Donald A. Ramsdell wrote this chapter in 1946 on the basis of his experiences as psychologist at the Army Rehabilitation Center at Deshon General Hospital. He took his cue from the oft-repeated statement by deafened soldiers that "the world has gone dead," and he proceeded with a thoughtful and original psychological analysis. Nothing has appeared since 1947 to amplify or to controvert his observations and interpretations. The present chapter is basically unchanged from the third edition but includes a brief discussion of the application of Dr. Ramsdell's views to the work on cochlear implants. The chapter constitutes a fitting memorial to Dr. Ramsdell, who died in 1965.

20. *The Deaf Community*

In this new chapter Dr. Jerome D. Schein, Director, Deafness Research and Training Center, and Professor of Deafness Rehabilitation, New York University, describes the concept and documents the reality of the "deaf community." He discusses the cohesive forces that give it identity and acquaints us with its economic, social, and cultural characteristics.

The source of data used in our graphs and tables is usually noted in the accompanying legend or in an occasional footnote.

We have already noted that we have tried to confine our Suggested Readings at the end of each chapter to secondary sources of a general or survey character. Also we have named in the text only a few of the distinguished workers in the cause of the deaf and the hard of hearing, chiefly workers of previous generations. Nevertheless, since many chapters in the fourth edition have been expanded to include more and more new technical detail, we have mentioned the names of more investigators and have therefore included their writings in our reading lists. Many of these investigators are still active. Here the purpose is not to single out a few for special honor but to enable the student to identify the appropriate citation in the list of suggested readings or to serve as a guide for those who wish to go directly to the scientific literature. Actually, the serious student of audiology must learn who are or recently have been important contributors to the development of the science and profession of audiology, including many whose names do not appear in our citations or text.

In this revision some of the original authors are no longer represented. Three of them, Dr. Edmund P. Fowler, Jr., Dr. Donald A. Ramsdell, and Dr. T. E. Walsh, have died, but much of what they wrote is retained. Eight authors are newcomers: Dr. Michael M. Paparella, Chairman, Department of Otolaryngology, University of Minnesota; Dr. David P. Pascoe, Coordinator of Audiological Services, Central Institute for the Deaf, and Assistant Professor of Audiology, Washington University (St. Louis); Dr. Norman P. Erber, Research Associate, Central Institute for the Deaf, and Assistant Professor of Audiology, Washington University; Ann L. Perry, Aural Rehabilitation Therapist, Central Institute for the Deaf, and Instructor in Speech and Hearing, Washington University; Dr. Donald R. Calvert, Director, Central Institute for the Deaf, and Professor of Audiology, Washington University; Rachel I. Mayberry, Assistant Professor, Program of Audiology and Hearing Impairment, Northwestern University; Dr. Robert Frisina, Director, National Technical Institute for the Deaf; and Dr. Jerome D. Schein, Director, Deafness Research and Training Center, and Professor of Deafness Rehabilitation, New York University.

Dr. S. Richard Silverman, Director Emeritus of Central Institute for the Deaf and co-editor of the second and third editions, has continued as co-editor. He has edited or rewritten Chapters 10–20. Dr. Hallowell Davis has written the expansions of Chapters 1–9.

We thank our colleagues in other institutions for their contributions, both old and new. Among the new contributions for which we are grateful are thoughtful and helpful critiques of the manuscript of this edition provided by Dr. John F. Brandt, University of Kansas, and Dr. Cornelius P. Goetzinger, University of Kansas Medical Center.

By and large, however, this fourth edition is a product of Central Institute for the Deaf. We hope that our point of view is not too one-sided; it has the advantage of being unified.

HALLOWELL DAVIS
S. RICHARD SILVERMAN

St. Louis, Missouri
August 1977

Foreword to the First Edition

Granted that the first handicap of deafness lies in communication, it has often seemed to me that a close second might be the attitude of hearing people toward it and that the former would be considerably lessened if we could do something to improve the latter.

Man's need for communication with his fellow man is possibly his greatest need and the fulfillment of his other needs and desires is largely dependent upon, or at the last greatly facilitated by, his ability to satisfy this basic one. The development of language, both spoken and written, as a means of communication is one of mankind's greatest achievements. Yet, because from birth we hearing people effortlessly, almost unconsciously, have *absorbed* this magnificent tool simply because we are lucky enough to hear, we take it very much for granted and tend to belittle, to shun, or to look somewhat askance at anyone who has had to fashion, bit by bit, word by word, sound by sound, a workable, even though imperfect, language tool for himself.

By turns I have been amused, annoyed, angry, and frustrated by this attitude and its various manifestations. However, I have tried to remind myself that people are like this because they don't know any better. Some thought and perhaps a little effort often *are* required to understand the speech and to follow the language of a deaf or severely hard-of-hearing person. It often *does* entail more attention than we usually give to our casual conversations to enable the deaf or hard-of-hearing person, who must depend mainly upon our lip movements, to understand what we are saying. I find very few people who are willing to give this attention or make this effort. Perhaps most people's impatience, even their rudeness, is partly due to this too swiftly paced, this tabloid, he-who-runs-may-read age and partly to a natural laziness of mind. However, I believe a great deal of it is due to almost complete lack of understanding of the problems faced by those with a hearing loss and to the narrowness and fear and insecurity bred of ignorance.

There is no other subject that vitally affects the lives of so many people on which there is so little positive information and so much fuzzy and widespread misinformation and misunderstanding. I doubt if over 5 percent of our population has ever read anything authentic on the deaf or the hard of hearing. And yet the impression that the deaf have no vocal cords and so cannot speak is widespread. It might surprise you to know how many people ask if the deaf learn to read Braille.

A great many of the misconception concerning the deaf undoubtedly can be traced to that inaccurate and unfortuante term "deaf and dumb." The implications it has given rise to in the minds of generations of hearing children and the attitudes it has engendered, not to mention the devastation it has caused in the hearts of parents, are incalculable. Fortified with those words alone, many people are almost determined in their belief that the totally deaf cannot possibly speak.

Education for the deaf, speech reading, and speech are not new. Speech has been taught in this country for close to a century. And yet, accurate, not to mention easy-to-read, articles or books for the layman, this fellow whom we must reach, whose attitudes we must change, are so few as to be almost nonexistent. I often have said that educators of the deaf talk to other educators of the deaf, write for other educators of the deaf in magazines for educators of the deaf and nothing reaches the layman—the layman who one day may be the totally unprepared mother or father of a little deaf baby, the layman who himself may become deaf or hard of hearing.

So my spirits leapt when I read the title of this book, *Hearing and Deafness: A Guide for Laymen*. Here at last is information, correct, easy to read, covering nearly every phase of the problem in a manner suited to that numerically large and needy group of people—laymen.

Hearing and Deafness should do much to change an attitude and, in consequence, be the means of greatly lessening the handicap of deafness.

I feel very honored and happy to be able to have even such a small finger in this notable work.

LOUISE TRACY

The John Tracy Clinic
Los Angeles, California
August 1947

Introduction to the First Edition

If there is another book which fulfills the aims and purposes of this one, I have not seen it. In my opinion the resolution of the editor

... to answer the thousand and one questions that are continually being asked by all sorts of people about the nature of hearing and the problem of deafness, ...

has been most effectually carried out.

When one desires to read something concerning his own problem, he turns naturally to pertinent articles that are easy to get and simple to understand. A large number of such writings on the treatment of deafness has recently appeared in some of our popular magazines. These commentaries, written ostensibly in an informative vein but produced plainly for "reader appeal," were composed by professional lay writers who have constantly before them two cardinal questions in journalism: (1) Is it new or unusual? and (2) Does it have human or dramatic appeal?

These articles, semi-scientific in character but produced in journalistic style and given extensive circulation, seem to have aroused in an untold number of persons an interest in their deafness that long had remained dormant, and that never would have been so completely stimulated, had it not been for the journalist and his manner of writing.

Similarly, new interests in the problems of deafness, new operations to restore hearing, new electrical apparatus to give more perfec

sound reception to improperly functioning ears, new methods of ensuring the preservation of speech, and a new understanding of the mental attributes of the hard of hearing have made almost mandatory the publication of an up-to-date, authoritative, and comprehensible reference work that covers the field of *audiology* both as a textbook and as a guide.

Hearing and Deafness: A Guide for Laymen is just such a text. Not without a dash of the "new and unusual" and not without its human appeal, this "guide" contains factual and instructive discussions of various phases of audiology. In the early pages we are informed that the sequence of chapters is "from inanimate nature to the individual human to complex social problems" and that in spite of this shift "there is one theme that runs evenly throughout the book." That theme, we are told, is *psychology*. Unquestionably, this topic reaches its climax when we are enlightened concerning the importance of "auditory backgrounds" which are responsible for that "comfortable sense-of-being-a-part-of-a-living-active-world," and also when we recognize the significance of the *three psychological levels of hearing.* Furthermore, suspicion, so characteristic a feature of the hard of hearing, is admirably discussed and is a matter that should be thoroughly understood by all deafened persons who retain it.

Every otologist, every teacher of the deaf, every social worker, every chapter of the

American Hearing Society, and every other person "concerned with auditory rehabilitation or with the conservation of hearing" should welcome the publication of this book, for in what other compact form can one find reliable answers to such questions as (1) "Why did I lose my hearing?" (2) "Is my deafness bad enough to require the use of a hearing aid?" (3) "Should I buy a bone or air conduction instrument?" and (4) "In which ear should I wear the 'aid'?"

Or if the problem involves a congenitally deaf child, we have replies to such queries as (1) "Why doesn't my child talk?" (2) "Will he be able to talk?" and (3) "What about his education?"

Among the other "thousand and one questions that are continually being asked" and that have received such impressive answers are (1) "Why do I hear a buzzer when I cannot hear a doorbell or telephone?" (2) "Will the fenestration operation cure my deafness?" (3) "Does industry discriminate against the hard of hearing?" (4) "Why do people stop talking when I come into the room?" and (5) "Why does the intense stillness so depress me?"

Further perusing the pages of this work, we become interested in the variations of normal hearing, and in finding out just what Miss Brown, Mr. Jones, and Mrs. Smith can expect from the use of a hearing aid. And while the mechanically minded inquirers are running their fingers up and down the "Cause, Test and Remedy" columns of the "Troubleshooting Chart," and as the speechreading class is memorizing the twelve suggestions for "ease of communication," the daring among us are venturing to trespass upon that special preserve where the more erudite disquisitions are lurking.

Surely this work, so extensive in scope, so practical in application and so expert in composition will serve a real need. Conceived, as it is, in the spirit of altruism and occupying, as it does, a niche not held by any other work, it deserves highest commendation and should be in the hands of all the thousands upon thousands of those who ask the questions and want to get the correct answers.

C. STEWART NASH
President
American Hearing Society

Rochester, New York
September 1947

Contents

Part IV
REHABILITATION FOR HEARING LOSS

Appendix
TESTS OF HEARING 525

Hearing
and Deafness

Part I
AUDIOLOGY AND HEARING

Hallowell Davis, M.D.

1
Audiology

You who read this book may be deaf yourself or perhaps your hearing is not as keen as it used to be. You may have a parent or a friend whose hearing is failing. Possibly your child is deaf and needs special teaching so that he[1] may understand and be understood. Imperfect hearing is so common that sooner or later it comes close to everyone. Perhaps you are beginning your training to become a professional audiologist. Whatever your motive—whether you want to help yourself or want to help others or are merely curious—you want to know what can go wrong with hearing and what can be done about it.

Seven hundred years ago you might have consulted for guidance the writings of Saint Albertus Magnus, teacher of Saint Thomas Aquinas and the dominant figure in Latin learning and natural science of the thirteenth century, who wrote: "Lion's brain, if eaten, causes madness; but remedies deafness, if inserted in the ear with some strong oil."[2] A century earlier, another widely respected authority, Saint Hildegard of Bingen, held that "deafness may be remedied by cutting off a lion's right ear and holding it over the patient's ear just long enough to say, 'Hear, *adimacus*, by the living God and the keen virtue of a lion's hearing,' " and that "the heart of a weasel, dried and placed with wax in the ear, benefits headache or deafness."[3]

Well-meaning though these learned saints of centuries ago were, their remedies merely reflected the best knowledge of their time. Nor did people know

[1] For simplicity only, we use the masculine generic pronouns in this book to mean either sex. See Preface.

[2] Lynn Thorndike, *A History of Magic and Experimental Science* (New York: Columbia University Press, 1923), II, 561.

[3] Ibid., pp. 145–146.

3

much more about hearing and deafness for many hundreds of years after them. Only in the last few decades has the body of knowledge relating to hearing and the treatment of deafness grown to a point where it can offer a great deal of guidance, help—and hope. That is the purpose of this book.

This book not only attempts to guide the student in problems relating to hearing and deafness; it also gives a survey of a general field of knowledge and of social endeavors centering around hearing. *Audiology*, meaning the science of hearing, seems to be a useful name for this field.[4] We shall use "audiology" in a very broad sense. For some purposes it may be helpful to speak more specifically of "medical audiology" when medical aspects of impaired hearing are our primary concern. The government use of the term (as in the title "Consultant in Audiology") is in a definitely medical context. The word is particularly useful here, however, because it indicates an interest in the *function* of the ear, not just in *diseases* of the ear. The diseases of the ear, the recognized province of *otology*, may be a threat to life, and hearing then becomes secondary. *Audiology* considers the ear as an *aid* to life.

Since 1946 audiology has become a profession as well as an area of knowledge. Numerous "clinical audiologists" are engaged in testing hearing in hospitals, in special clinics and other institutions, and in private offices. Many of these men and women are members of the American Speech and Hearing Association. This association has established a Committee on Clinical Certification, which sets examinations in hearing and issues certificates of qualification both in speech and in hearing.

Clinical audiologists test hearing and may

---

[4] Linguistic purists may object, pointing out that "audiology" consists of a Greek suffix added to a Latin root, but the word is here to stay, partly because it fills a need.

make recommendations concerning the use and choice of hearing aids and aural rehabilitation. The business of distribution and sale of hearing aids is generally handled by hearing-aid dealers. Some otologists and audiologists are now dispensing hearing aids as a part of rehabilitation.

The development of audiology and specifically of clinical audiology has led to many serious discussions of the relation of audiology to otology. How far do the rights and responsibilities of the clinical audiologist, with his special training and experience, go —particularly in the directions of making a diagnosis, recommending the use of a hearing aid, and planning a course of education or rehabilitation? In the medical area he is clearly dependent on and subordinate to the physician, but other areas are his own. Where is the boundary?

Probably the best statement of a point of view that seems to be more and more widely accepted was drafted in 1955 by a committee, under the cochairmanship of Dr. Gordon Hoople and Dr. Raymond Carhart and including Dr. Silverman, that was concerned with this problem. The report of this committee has never been published in full, but permission has been granted to reproduce from it the following:

A STATEMENT OF ORIENTATION

We have learned a great deal during the past quarter century about (1) how to measure sound; (2) how to assess hearing; (3) how to study the physiology, biophysics, and psychophysics of the auditory system; (4) how to deal with hearing impairments by surgical or medical means; and (5) how to educate and to rehabilitate persons with impaired hearing. Representatives from many disciplines are now concerned with the facts of hearing and the problems of hearing loss. Their various activities have come to carry the label "audiology."

Audiology is the science of hearing. In other

words, audiology is undergirded by the competences and methods of many fields. Among the contributing fields are (1) physics, which studies acoustic events as one manifestation of matter and motion; (2) medicine, which is concerned with the human organism in sickness and health; (3) psychology, which deals with responses of the organism to stimuli; (4) education, which seeks to modify and guide the behavior of the organism; and (5) sociology, which attacks the problems of fitting the individual into his culture. Audiology, then, is not a particular academic discipline or professional activity. It is the mobilizing of professional skills to cope with the phenomena of hearing. Thus, when an individual concentrates his training, his competence, and his experience on problems of auditory communication, he is working in the field of audiology. His interest may be to investigate auditory phenomena, his chosen task may be to train others to work in the field, or his goal may be to serve clinically and educationally those persons who suffer impaired hearing.

Current emphasis among those who use the term "audiology" is heavily clinical. Consequently, important problems of interprofessional relationships have arisen. Among these is the question of how to achieve optimal interaction between otologists and clinical audiologists, as we shall in this report designate specialists in managing nonmedical aspects of auditory impairment.

The two committees agreed that otology and clinical audiology have distinctive yet related tasks. These tasks may be described as follows:

1. Otology has basic responsibility for the biological function of hearing. *It alone rightfully undertakes the work of diagnosing diseases of the ear, of specifying the causation of hearing impairment, and of treating pathologies of the auditory mechanism.*

2. Clinical audiology deals with hearing as a foundation to the learning and the utilizing of language skills. *The emphasis is upon understanding the social functions of hearing and upon increasing the ability of handicapped individuals to cope with the communicational demands of everyday life.*

3. The two fields share responsibility for jointly planning the proper sequence in management of the individual patient. Information on the patient should be exchanged freely. Moreover, decisions regarding otological management of the patient should always precede decisions on audiological management, since maximal social efficiency can be achieved only after biological function has been restored as fully as possible.

Audiology in relation to otology is concerned with diagnostic tests of hearing and the evaluation of the results of medical or surgical efforts to improve hearing. Actually the otologist himself may perform many simple diagnostic tests. He becomes an audiologist the moment he picks up a tuning fork. The more complicated tests, however, and particularly those that require electronic equipment and soundproof booths, the otologist usually delegates to a professional specialist. This audiologist is usually not himself a physician, but he is one of an increasing number of "paramedical specialists" who have special training and competence in particular complex chemical or physical diagnostic procedures. He shares with the otologist a biological orientation toward hearing, and it is important for him to understand the anatomy and physiology of the ear and the nature of the various diseases and disorders of the ear in order to adapt his tests intelligently to the needs of a particular patient and to help the otologist evaluate the results of the tests. The final responsibilities of diagnosis and of treatment, however, still rest with the physician.

Another orientation of the audiologist, however, is toward assessing the hearing handicap of his client and assisting him to overcome the handicap by means other than medicine or surgery—once the medical management of the case has been established. He gives advice concerning hearing aids and evaluates their effectiveness and, from special knowledge of the possibilities of special education or rehabilitative training, he participates in decisions concerning education and the improved utilization of language skills. Just as the otologist may perform simple audiological diagnostic tests so the educator, the clinical psychologist, the speech pathologist, and even the hearing-aid dealer may perform simple audiological tests to evaluate a hearing handicap. The audiologist, however, is equipped and trained to perform more accurate and extensive tests. If he knows the fundamental principles of hearing aids, of special education for the deaf, and of the rehabilitation of the deaf and hard of hearing, he can also perform the very important service of evaluating his patient's handicap and guiding the appropriate audiological management.

The relations of otology and other specialties with audiology are clear enough in principle, although they have been obscured by the variety of organizations under which audiological services have been made available. There is nevertheless a fundamental unity in audiology because its tests are nearly all psychological tests. They are based squarely on the branch of psychology known as psychophysics, and more particularly on psychoacoustics. Thus a firm foundation in psychoacoustics, including familiarity with the principles of acoustics and with the electronic equipment appropriate to psychoacoustics, is essential for all audiologists, whatever their orientation may be.

CONTRIBUTIONS OF AUDIOLOGY

The contributions of audiology are not trivial. Recent developments in medicine, in electronics, in our social point of view, and in education have greatly increased its importance. Surgery can now improve hearing in otosclerosis and other middle-ear condi-

tions, but the conditions must be correctly diagnosed and evaluated. Auditory tests now assist the neurologist as well as the otologist. Hearing aids are efficient electroacoustic instruments and with increasing miniaturization are becoming more and more acceptable to potential users; but candidates for hearing aids still need advice. Deaf children apparently suffer from a specific handicap, not from a general mental inferiority, and even profoundly deaf children can be taught to speak and to read speech. This is most effectively done if special instruction is begun early, and the audiologist plays a very important part in the early identification and assessment of deaf babies and preschool children. Of course, older children and adults also benefit from improved opportunities for rehabilitation. Identification and assessment are both easier than with babies, but the assessment must be correct. Actually the identification of children with hearing handicaps requires a cooperative effort of physicians, audiologists, educators, and an informed public.

THE ADMINISTRATIVE PATTERNS OF AUDIOLOGY

Within the past 30 years there have been significant changes of attitude toward the handicaps of hearing. It is now recognized that with special education the deaf can and do become or remain fully responsible members of society. The federal government of the United States is becoming increasingly involved in problems of prevention, medical care, education, and rehabilitation, including those of the hearing-handicapped.

The establishment of new federal agencies discussed in Chapter 16 has added to the diversity in the administrative framework through which audiological services are offered. Audiological activities have quite often been conducted as part of the program of a university department of speech, department of education, or department of psychology. Again these activities have frequently been organized as a subdivision of a department of otolaryngology. Under these circumstances audiology has been included within the services of departments of rehabilitation or of public health, or within programs for crippled children, within the services of a hospital, within the private practice of the otolaryngologist, within schools for the deaf, or in community speech and hearing centers. Finally, clinical audiology has been made an independent enterprise in a few instances.

In view of the many ways in which audiological services are being made available, it is probably unwise to specify any particular organizational or administrative pattern as the only proper one. The contemporary situation is furnishing a trial of the effectiveness of the various patterns. We may expect the most desirable organizational practices to evolve only if we avoid premature opinions and encourage sympathetic insight among all those who have a part in the development and administration of programs in audiology.

Hallowell Davis, M.D.

2

Acoustics and Psychoacoustics

"Sound is what we hear." So says the man just in from the street.

"No," says a physicist, "sound is a form of energy, It is an organized movement of molecules; it is a series of waves of pressure in the air or water or whatever medium is transmitting the sound."

"Yes," says a psychologist, "but you should add that sound is a sensation, something that exists only within ourselves. The sensation is aroused when sound waves tickle our ears and send nerve impulses running to the brain along the auditory nerve. We all know what sound is like in experience. It is real but intangible. We can't weigh it on a pair of scales, measure it with a meter, or even take it out and look at it."

And while the physicist glares at the psychologist, the man from the street raises the old question: If a bomb explodes in the midst of the Sahara Desert or at the South Pole with no man or other living creature there to hear, will there be any sound?

"Of course there will," says the physicist.

"Impossible," says the psychologist. "Didn't I tell you. . . ." And so it goes.

WHAT IS SOUND?

The sort of argument recorded above was once taken quite seriously, until it was realized that words and their meanings are not created in Heaven but are consciously or unconsciously made by man for his own use. And how clumsy, foggy, and ambiguous he often makes them! The word "sound" is used, and we shall so use it, to mean *both* the physicist's pressure waves and moving molecules and the psychologist's subjective sensation in the mind of the listener. And now that we realize that the word has a double meaning, there need actually be no confusion. Which meaning is intended is usually quite clear. The physicist's sound can be measured by apparatus, and it can do work; it can push small objects back and forth or generate heat. The other kind of sound is all in our minds. It may be high-pitched or low-pitched, loud or faint, pleasant or unpleasant. These attributes cannot be measured by thermometers or voltmeters, but they can be appreciated by a listener; and a listener can tell us a lot about his sensations and about the relations among them: which of two sounds is louder, which is higher in pitch, and so on.

Between the physical sound of pressure waves and our insubstantial but intensely real sensations lie our ears, our nerves, and our brains. The physiologist, who thinks of sound in the physical sense, studies how the sound waves are gathered by the external ear, conducted by the middle ear, and concentrated and analyzed in the inner ear, as well as how they set up nerve impulses in the auditory nerve. He follows the nerve impulses up to the gray matter of the brain and can tell us something of how their pattern in time (and in distribution among the thousands of nerve fibers in the auditory pathways) corresponds to the original pattern of the physicist's sound waves. But no one can say how the patterns of nerve impulses generate our subjective sensations.

The psychologist who wants to relate sensations to objects and events in the physical world gets little help from the physiologist. He must go back to the beginning and compare the loudness, the pitch, or the unpleasantness of the sensations as reported by his subjects with the intensity, the frequency, the waveform, the temporal pattern, or other measurable attribute of the physical sound. This sort of study is known as psychophysics, and much of what we shall have to say about sound and hearing will be statements of just these relationships between the objective and the subjective aspects of sound. The relationships are properties not of physical sound but of the connection between physical sound and the properties of human beings, particularly of their ears and their brains.

The physicist's sound is a form of energy. It can be "created" only by transformation from another form of energy, and it in turn can do work and be transformed into still other forms. Specifically, it is an organized movement to and fro of the molecules of a gas, liquid, or solid. Small solid objects, such as particles of dust in the air, move bodily with the air molecules and help us visualize the organized movement of the molecules.

Solid objects may "vibrate," one part moving back and forth in relation to other parts. The to-and-fro motion of the vibrating part is much the same as the motion of the air molecules in sound waves except that the molecules of the bell, the tuning fork, or the violin string are stuck together and must move as a mass. The branch of physics that deals with this vibratory form of energy, whether in air, in water, or in solid objects, is known as *acoustics*.

The Physical Nature of Sound

The commonest source of sound waves in the air is a vibrating solid body. As the air molecules fly about and collide with one another in their random dance, they are pushed back by the solid body when it starts to vibrate, just as a jostling crowd of spectators awaiting a parade is pushed back by a cordon of police. The molecules, or spectators, in the front ranks collide more powerfully with their neighbors and push them back; and so the wave spreads through the crowd. Then each molecule (or spectator), bumping and jostling, takes advantage of the reverse movement of the solid body (or a relaxation of the cordon), and surges back to or beyond the original position, only to be pushed away once more. Among the molecules, as in the crowd, there are zones of denser pressure that move away from the source of the disturbance. These are the *sound waves*. The waves of pressure travel slowly in a New Year's Eve crowd, but they go at about a thousand feet a second in air. ("Mach 1," the velocity of sound in air, is about 760 miles per hour at sea level. The Mach number is now familiar as a unit of speed of jet planes and rockets.) Each molecule moves only a very short distance, however, and then returns to or beyond its original position. The air movement does not become a wind. The crowd is still in Times Square, not charging down Broadway. And anyone who has been a "molecule" in a large crowd will recall the "pressure waves" that made him surge back and forth.

Most solid objects vibrate when they are suddenly set in motion or suddenly stopped. Their *inertia* keeps them from starting all at once. Their *momentum* keeps parts moving even after one portion has met an obstacle. The momentum makes the wood, metal, or whatever it may be stretch until the attractions that hold the molecules together finally stop the forward movement. Now if the object has only stretched out of shape and not shattered to bits, the elastic forces restore it to shape. Usually they restore the shape so rapidly, however, that it overshoots in the opposite direction, like the swing of a pendulum, and it may take many swings before the energy of vibration is dissipated and

the vibration ceases. Each movement pushes out a sound wave in the surrounding air. The vibration may be kept going by some continuing force, like wind flapping a flag; or the original event may be repeated, like a clock striking twelve. Air itself becomes turbulent when it moves rapidly, and its eddies and surges generate the sound waves that we hear as the wind whistles through a crack, around an airplane, or in our own ears.

Nature is as full of sound as it is of wind, of splashing water, and of hard, vibrating objects. It is a rarity to find a really silent event, except for those that take place so slowly that we can hardly even see them happen. Few objects are so soft and spongy as to be noiseless, although skin, flesh, and fur qualify as well as any. Nature, particularly inanimate nature, is noisy.

Waveform and Frequency: Pure and Complex Tones

The simplest form of acoustic, vibratory, or electromagnetic wave is the *sine wave*, or sinusoid (see Figure 2-1). It is a smooth wave that has the interesting mathematical property that its first derivative (or slope or rate of change) follows a cosine curve that has the same form as the sine wave but is a quarter of a cycle in advance of it. The sinusoid is also related to circular motion. Imagine a rotating cam shaft that carries a circular eccentric cam. A vertical rod like the valve shaft of an automobile engine is moved up and down by the cam. On it is mounted a pen that writes on a vertical sheet of paper beside it. The sheet of paper moves horizontally at a constant speed. The pen on the valve shaft writes a sine wave on the paper.

It is a fundamental fact of physics that many natural free oscillations, such as electromagnetic oscillations, the swing of pendulums, mechanical oscillation of loaded springs (like watch springs) or tuning forks,

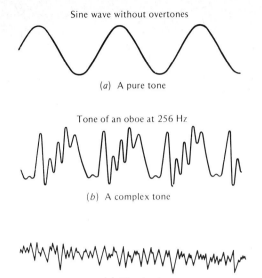

Sine wave without overtones

(a) A pure tone

Tone of an oboe at 256 Hz

(b) A complex tone

(c) Street noise

Figure 2-1 See text for explanation. Curve *b* is redrawn after D. C. Miller, *The Science of Musical Sounds (by permission Macmillan Company).* Curve *c* is a draftsman's copy of an original illustration by Fletcher. The fine detail of the original is not reproduced. The drawing serves, by contrast with *a* and *b* above, to show the mixed, irregular, random, and nonrepetitive character of noise. *(After Fletcher, Speech and Hearing, D. Van Nostrand Company)*

and certain simple acoustic oscillations are sinusoidal. A simple sinusoidal acoustic signal is known as a *pure tone.*

Two kinds of measurement are enough to define a pure tone completely. One is *frequency,* usually measured in cycles (complete swings or double vibrations) per second. In these days of radio we should all be accustomed to the idea of frequency. The other measurement is *magnitude,* or *intensity,* and may be measured as the alternating *pressure* of sound waves or as the *velocity* with which air particles move to and fro. We may also think of an alternating rate of *flow of energy* in horsepower or watts.

Frequency refers to the recurrence of similar events per unit of time. Usually the recurrence is regular, and each of the equal intervals of time is known as a cycle. The course of events within each cycle, whether the

simple swing of a pendulum to and fro or the sequence of puffs from the exhaust during one turn of the crankshaft of a motor, is similar. For sound waves and mechanical vibrations the second is the most convenient unit of time, and for many years acoustic frequencies have been expressed in *cycles per second* (abbreviated as cps or c/s) or for higher frequencies as *kilocycles per second* or kc.

In 1960, however, the Eleventh General Conference on Weights and Measures, held in Paris, recommended that this unit of frequency, one cycle per second, be known as a *hertz,* abbreviated Hz, in honor of the German physicist, Heinrich Hertz, who studied electromagnetic radiation and discovered the hertzian waves. This usage, established for many years in Germany, has now been adopted internationally. The hertz is the exact equivalent of cycles per second and a 1000-cps tone becomes a 1000-Hz tone. Similarly, the kilohertz (kHz) has replaced the kilocycle per second. It has been suggested that when two different cycles of different events are both involved simultaneously, it will reduce ambiguity if "cycles per second" is retained for the slower sequence. Thus we may have a signal that consists of periodic bursts of a 100-Hz tone at the frequency of three bursts per second. One burst and the silent period that follows it constitutes one cycle of the signal, and there are three such cycles per second. We prefer here to speak of 1000-Hz tone bursts at a repetition rate of 3 per second.

Many acoustic and mechanical systems, including most musical instruments, vibrate in more complicated although recurring patterns (see Figure 2-1). Such a *complex tone* can be analyzed by acoustic (or electric) filters into a set of component pure tones, each with a definite frequency and intensity. The waveform of the complex tone depends also on the time relations, technically known as the *phase relations,* among the component pure tones. The graphic record of a complex tone can be resolved into its sinusoidal components by a mathematical procedure known as *Fourier Analysis*. The application of the Fourier analysis in practice usually fails to preserve information on phase relations.

In a complex musical tone the various additional higher frequencies are known as *overtones* or *harmonics*, and their frequencies are simple, integral multiples of the frequency of the lowest tone, or *fundamental*. The frequencies and intensities of the harmonics are represented in the form of a *line spectrum* of the sound, as in Figure 2-2. It is called a line spectrum because the graphic representation of this distribution of energy is a series of vertical lines, not a continuous curve. The higher harmonics give a *quality* to the tone that is characteristic of the particular instrument. For the human voice the relative strengths of the components of higher frequency formants are responsible for the differences between the different vowel sounds that allow us to distinguish them.

Noise Most of the sounds we hear are neither pure, single-frequency tones nor even musical tones containing only one fundamental frequency and its higher harmonics. Instead, they are a scramble of many frequencies that may or may not stand in any simple numerical relation to one another. In fact, one very familiar noise, the hiss of an air jet or escaping steam, is completely random in its waveform. If we analyze such a random noise, we find equal amounts of energy in a given bandwidth (range of frequencies) regardless of the part of the spectrum we examine. High, low, and middle frequencies are equally represented. The spectrum is continuous, with equal intensity per cycle of bandwidth. Since there is here an obvious analogy to white light, such a noise is often called *white noise*. It is a useful tool for the acoustical physicist, and for-

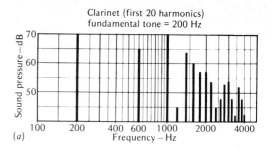

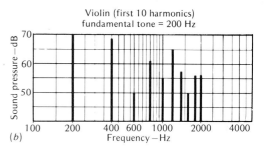

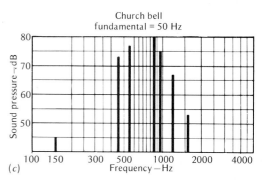

Figure 2-2 Line spectra. In the clarinet spectrum *(a)* the second and fourth harmonics (400 and 800 Hz) are more than 30 dB below the intensity of the fundamental tone. The sixth harmonic is also very weak. In the violin spectrum *(b)* the second, fourth, and sixth harmonics are the strongest and the odd-numbered harmonics are weak. The "overtone structure" gives the characteristic quality of each instrument. The strength of each harmonic is easily measured with the help of electric filters that allow only a very narrow band of frequencies (a constant number of hertz) to pass through. The sound of a bell also has a line spectrum *(c)*, but the energy is very irregularly distributed among a few of the higher harmonics. In the sounds of many bells, inharmonic frequencies are also strongly present. *(All from H. Fletcher,* American Journal of Physics, *14:215–225; 1946; by permission)*

tunately it is easily generated by merely amplifying the background hiss produced in certain electronic devices. Other noises have a predominance of high or low frequencies, and, although their pitches may be very vague, we can recognize that one such noise is pitched higher than another. The noises may be thought of as more or less "colored." The pure tone, with its spectrum consisting of a single line, corresponds to a pure color. A noise may be a mixture of a line spectrum, like the hum of an airplane motor, and a more or less uniform band spectrum, like the wind noise around the wings of the plane. Of course, unless the line spectrum (of the motor or from any other source) is more intense than the band spectrum at that particular frequency, the pure tone will be submerged in the noise, and the ear will be unable to detect it. The pure tone is then said to be "masked" by the noise. The masking of speech by traffic noise is very familiar to all of us.

Measure of Sound: Intensity

We are all accustomed to steady pressure, such as 30 pounds per square inch in a tire, and to steady velocities, such as 1000 feet per second, approximately the velocity of sound in air. Alternating pressures and velocities are less familiar. They bear the same relation to steady pressures and velocities that an alternating electric current bears to direct current. Both kinds can do work, but the alternating current is continually reversing its direction. The concept of power, illustrated by the horsepower of our automobiles or the watts of electric power consumed by our electric light bulbs, is familiar to us. Acoustic power, although the quantities are extremely small, can be measured in the same units. Thus the physicist says that the acoustic power of the faintest 1000-Hz tone that can be heard by a good ear is about 0.000 000 000 000 000 1 watt per square centimeter or, in a more familiar unit,

0.000 000 000 000 000 000 000 13 horsepower per square centimeter. Noise becomes uncomfortable, as in a boiler shop, at 0.0001 watt and sharply painful at 0.01 watt per square centimeter.

Numbers of this sort, consisting chiefly of a decimal point followed by a string of nothingness, are more impressive than convenient. Moreover, the range that is covered between the faintest audible and the sharply painful sounds is tremendous. The latter are 10 million times as powerful as the former. It helps a little, but only a little, if we talk about the pressure (which is what the acoustical engineer actually measures with his sound-level meter) instead of the power, because the pressure is proportional to the square root of the power, and fewer zeros are required. (The faintest audible 1000-Hz tone has an acoustic pressure of about 0.0002 dynes per square centimeter; the painful tone, 2000 dynes per square centimeter.) Even so, our calculations consist chiefly of locating the decimal point correctly.

To deal conveniently with such an unwieldy range of values, a logarithmic system has been universally adopted in acoustics and in electrical engineering. The system has no fixed unit, like the pound or the centimeter, but deals only in ratios, like double, tenfold, or hundredfold. One logarithmic unit (to the base 10) of the ratio (of one acoustic power to another) is known as a *bel*, in honor of Alexander Graham Bell, who invented the telephone. Thus 1 bel means tenfold the power, 2 bels means tenfold and tenfold again, that is, a hundredfold the power. The bels count the number of steps the decimal point takes along the chain of zeros.

To avoid inconvenient fractional values of the bel, the *decibel*, which is one-tenth of a bel, is usually employed instead. It is abbreviated dB. (The capital B follows the rule of capitalizing abbreviations that are derived from proper names, such as Bell or Hertz.)

Unfortunately there is the slight additional

complication that we usually deal with *pressures*, whereas the decibel is defined as a ratio of two *energies* or powers. Acoustic pressures are proportional to the square root of the corresponding power. The ratio of the *squares* of the acoustic pressures corresponds to the simple ratio of the acoustic powers, and therefore the logarithm of the pressure ratio is *double* the logarithm of the power ratio. Thus tenfold (for acoustic pressures) is 20 dB, a hundredfold is 40 dB, and double pressure turns out to be almost 6 dB.

The decibel scale is logarithmic. This means, among other things, that when we add decibels we *multiply*. If we wish to add sound pressures, as when sounds from two sources are present at the same time, we must first translate the decibels to actual intensities in watts per square centimeter. We then add the watts arithmetically and translate back into decibels relative to the reference level. For example, suppose that two different sounds measure 74 and 77 dB (relative to 0.0002 dyne per square centimeter), respectively. Their combined sound pressure is *not* 151 dB. As shown by the scales in Figure 2-4, 74 dB correspond to 1 dyne per square centimeter or 2.5×10^{-9} watt per square centimeter; 77 dB correspond to 5.0×10^{-9} watt per square centimeter. On the decibel scale this is about 78.8 dB relative to 0.0002 dyne per square centimeter. (Such calculations are readily made with the help of tables that resemble the familiar tables of logarithms.)

A decibel has no fixed absolute value or any units. It is simply a ratio, telling by what proportion one value is greater or less than another. To give the decibel scale an anchor, so to speak, we conventionally assume certain reference levels that are understood unless otherwise specified. For acoustic pressures the *standard reference level* is 0.0002 dyne per square centimeter, or 2×10^{-5} newtons per square meter (N/m²). One newton per square meter is a *pascal* (Pa) and the standard reference level is now usually writ-

ten as 20 μPa. This value is conveniently close to the intensity of the faintest sound that is heard on the average by normal young ears under the best listening conditions. Sound that is painful, at 140 dB, exerts a pressure $10^{14 \div 2} = 10^7 = 10,000,000$ times as great. And the increase in absolute pressure from 140 to 141 dB is 10 million times as great as the increase from 0 to 1 dB (see Figure 2-4).

It might seem inconvenient to have the absolute value of the decibel change as we go up and down the intensity scale, but actually it is a convenience because the just noticeable difference that the ear can detect in the intensity of a sound has been found to be a nearly constant ratio or percentage, and thus an approximately constant number of decibels. The just noticeable difference varies only from 3 or 4 dB for very faint sounds to about 0.3 dB for very intense sounds. We can easily hear a pin drop if the room is almost quiet; but if an airplane engine is warming up nearby, a 10-pound box of pins might fall unheard. But the ability of an additional decibel of sound intensity to attract our attention varies only a little. There is also another way in which the logarithmic decibel scale corresponds approximately to the way in which the ear hears sounds. A sound that is 10 dB more intense than another sound of the same frequency sounds about twice as loud. Thus if a sound 40 dB above the standard reference level is increased to 70 dB, it sounds $2 \times 2 \times 2$, or eight times as loud. This is a very convenient approximate rule. However, if two sounds are of different frequencies, the rules for predicting their combined loudness when they are sounded simultaneously are much more complicated, as we shall see.

The Sound-Level Meter

We have mentioned the *sound-level meter*. This is a basic tool for the acoustical engineer. The sound is converted into a corresponding electric signal, which is then amplified and measured with a meter. The meter is calibrated to give directly the *sound-pressure level* (SPL) in decibels relative to the standard reference level. The ear, as we shall see, is more sensitive to sounds of some frequencies than to others; but the sound-level meter is so constructed as to be almost equally sensitive to all frequencies from 20 to 10,000 Hz. It is strictly "flat" from 100 to 2000 Hz and "rolls off" gradually to 6 dB less sensitive at 21 Hz and at 11 kHz.[1] This frequency characteristic is designated as the "C scale" of the meter.

For special purposes two "weighting networks" are provided to give the "A scale" and the "B scale," respectively. These scales and their use will be described near the end of this chapter. When more than one frequency is present, the meter reads the total acoustic pressure as an *overall sound level*. This overall sound level is understood when we say, for example, that the noise in a weaving room is 100 dB and on a busy street is 70 dB (see Figure 2-3), but it is helpful to be explicit and write 100 dBC because the A scale is rapidly coming into widespread use (dBA).

Another basic acoustic instrument is the electric filter, which rejects signals that are above or below a desired *passband*. If desired, the passband can be made very narrow, only a few hertz in width. The filter is then said to be sharply "tuned" to a desired frequency. With such a filter the engineer can measure separately the components of a complex tone such as a musical chord. (The line spectra illustrated in Figure 2-2 were obtained in this way.) Or the passband can be made wider, say a third of an octave or half an octave or a full octave in width. With such an *octave-band filter* the sound-pressure level of each octave of a complex noise, such as street noise or airplane noise, can be measured separately. In this way the *band*

spectra illustrated in Figure 2-3 were obtained. The band spectrum is a very useful way of describing a complex noise and gives the acoustical engineer part of his fundamental data if he needs to design, for example, an audiometric booth to exclude the noise in question. High frequencies are, in general, easier to exclude than low frequencies; hence it is important for him to know not only the overall level, but also how much energy is present in each octave band.

In Figure 2-3 the frequencies that divide one octave band from the next are 75, 150, 300, 600, 1200, 2400 and 4800 Hz. These and the corresponding series of half-octave and third-octave bands were for many years the conventional bands for acoustical measurements. In 1967, however, the USA Standards Institute (now the American National Standards Institute) issued a standard for preferred frequencies and band numbers (ANSI S1.6-1967). The entire series of frequencies is based on 1000 Hz as its central point and is symmetrical with respect to it; 1000 Hz is the geometric midfrequency of one of the bands. The dividing cutoff frequencies for the octave bands in the preferred system are 45, 90, 180, 355, 710, 1400, 2800, and 5600 Hz. The corresponding midfrequencies are 63, 125, 250, 500, 1000, 2000, and 4000 Hz. The preferred values are gradually replacing the original values that appear in Figure 2-3.

Sound Power

The acoustical engineer finds it very convenient to calculate the total acoustic power output of sound sources, such as jet engines, automobiles on the highway, ventilating fans, or the human voice. The sound power is expressed in watts, but here again it is convenient to use the decibel scale and to talk about the "power level" (PWL). Unfortunately, this additional use of the decibel leads to' much confusion. The *power levels* are, of course, always much higher than the *intensity levels* (IL) that the same sources

[1] IEC Recommendation 179 (1965).

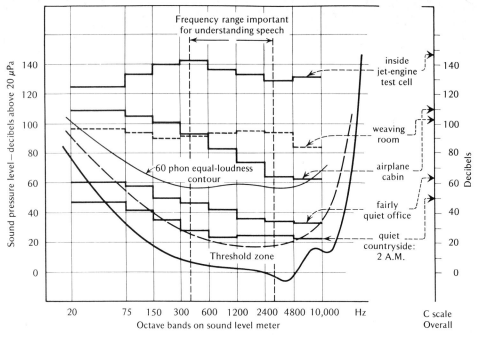

Figure 2-3 The auditory area and octave band spectra of five steady background noises. The threshold zone is the same as in Figure 2-4. It is not strictly logical to plot data based on pure tones, such as thresholds and equal-loudness contours, on the same scale of sound-pressure levels that is used for octave-band analyses. The error is not large, however, in relation to the large dynamic range of the sounds represented here, and it does not affect the comparisons of one noise with another. The 60-phon equal-loudness contour is at a comfortable listening level. It lies entirely above the spectrum of the quiet office but below the spectrum in the airplane cabin.

The top spectrum was measured inside a typical jet engine test cell, with the engine operating at military power. The peak of acoustic energy is in the 300- to 600-Hz band. The weaving room had mechanical looms; the floor was wooden. These two spectra are fairly "flat." The airplane spectrum was taken at the last window seat while the piston-engine plane was climbing. It is a sharply sloping spectrum. Notice that its overall sound pressure level (right) is higher than that for the weaving room because of the large contribution of the lowest, 20- to 75-Hz, band. Speech is better understood in the airplane noise, however, because in the 600- to 1200-Hz and 1200- to 2400-Hz bands the sound levels are lower than those in the weaving room. (The levels are nearly equal in the 300- to 600-Hz band.)

In the "fairly quiet office" there were no business machines. Its overall sound level of 64 dB is deceptively high because of the sloping spectrum. The "C scale" of the sound-level meter, used for these measurements, was "flat" from 100 to 2000 Hz and only 6 dB less sensitive at 40 and 10,000 Hz. The spectrum of the quiet countryside at 2 A.M. lies almost entirely within the threshold zone; that is, some people with hearing within the range of normal would hear only a very faint rustle (600 to 4800 Hz), although the overall sound level is 50 dB. It is now customary to measure such faint noises on the A scale (dBA). The noise in the jet engine test cell is above the threshold for pain. *(Adapted from a figure by J. R. Cox, Jr., in* Industrial Hygiene and Toxicology, Vol. I. New York: Interscience Publishers, 1958)

produce at the ears of the listeners. The power level is a measure of all of the watts of acoustic energy radiated in all directions by the source. The intensity level is only the number of watts that flows through 1 square centimeter at the position of the sound-level meter. Thus a full symphony orchestra may generate 140 dB PWL (relative to 10^{-12} watt), but the listener may receive only 90 dB IL

(relative to 10^{-16} watt per square centimeter) at his seat in the balcony.

The usual reference for power level is the same as for sound level. For power it is usually expressed as 10^{-12} watt per square *meter*, which is the same physically as 10^{-16} watt per square *centimeter*. The sound-power level is conceived as a flow of acoustic energy through an area of 1 square meter that forms the surface of an imaginary spherical source. Only a tiny fraction of this power reaches a distant listener. Our principal present concern with sound power is to avoid being misled when we encounter this other use of the decibel scale.

Resonance

In describing the electric filter, we referred to "tuning" the filter to a desired frequency. This idea of a tuned circuit should be familiar to everyone who "tunes" his radio or television circuit to a desired broadcast frequency or who tunes acoustical devices such as musical instruments. We know that a violin or piano string vibrates at a higher frequency when it is pulled tighter as in "tuning up," or when, on the violin, the vibrating part is shortened by the player's finger. And we have probably noticed that the bass strings of these instruments are thicker and heavier than those in the treble.

In general, any mechanical system that is free to vibrate tends to vibrate at a *natural frequency* that is determined by the mass of the vibrating parts and their stiffness. It is easier to set the system vibrating or *oscillating* at this frequency than at any other, in the sense that at a given amount of alternating pressure the vibrating system will build up a greater amplitude of movement. The system tends to move of itself or "oscillate" exactly in step with the driving force and does not tend to either lag behind or creep ahead. This relation of tending to move exactly in step with the driving force and to fall off in amplitude if the driving frequency is either increased or diminished is called *resonance*.

Energy tends to be stored in a resonant system, whether it be acoustic or electric. This energy is continually being changed back and forth from kinetic energy to potential energy. In a typical mechanical system these forms of energy are represented by the momentum of a moving mass and the elonga-

tion of a spring, respectively. Energy is removed from the system by doing work elsewhere or by being dissipated into heat by friction. Acoustic radiation of energy is a step toward frictional loss. Frictional dissipation of energy is called *damping*. "Damping" means to reduce the amplitude of mechanical vibration, and should not be confused with "dampening," meaning to moisten. It is better to "damp" the oscillation of a tuning fork than to "dampen" it, even though some dictionaries sanction the latter usage. If a system is too heavily damped it will not vibrate at all, but when displaced will simply creep back slowly to its position of rest without overshoot. Imagine a violin string vibrating in molasses!

For our purposes it is important to recognize that air in a container that has one or more openings is a resonant system. Air has mass, and it acquires momentum as it moves in and out of the container. The air is also compressible, so it acts as both the mass and the spring. The natural frequency or frequencies of an air-filled system depend on the volume of the container, on the size of the openings, and, in more complicated ways, on the shape of the cavity. We know that the trombone player lengthens his "pipe" to reach a low note and that if we blow across the mouth of an empty bottle, it resonates at a lower frequency (lower pitch) than if it is half full, and so on. We shall see that the resonances of air-filled cavities enable them to store energy at certain frequencies and also to transmit these frequencies more effectively than others from one end to the other. This principle was utilized in the construction of nonelectrical hearing aids. The same principle in electric circuits is the basis of most electric filters.

The Time Pattern of Sounds

To describe music or speech, the physicist tells how the frequencies and the corresponding intensities vary from moment to moment. The rhythm (*stress pattern*) and the tempo, whether regular or irregular, are essential features that we learn to recognize as well as we do the sequence of different pitches. Speech and music are not static but are patterns that change from moment to moment.

Biological and Psychological Aspects of Hearing

Sound is produced incidentally by almost all events in nature that involve the rapid motion of air or water or even moderate movement, particularly the impacts of solid objects. It is very difficult to make any sort of machine run without some noise. Sound is one of nature's surest signs of activity, and therein lies its primitive biological significance. Hearing keeps us *informed* of activities going on at some distance from us and *gives us warning* if that activity becomes more powerful or approaches very close. The important psychological consequences of loss of the primitive awareness and warnings of hearing are discussed in detail in a later chapter. Sight, to be sure, also informs us of distant events, but hearing is the true "watchdog" of the senses. (A watchdog should really be called a "harkdog," for he hears the stranger approach by night before he sees him.) The sun never sets for hearing, and sound waves come to us around corners and reach our ears whichever way our heads are turned. No "earlid" covers the ear in sleep. Experiments on the electrical activity of the brain show that the sleeping brain is at least partially aroused by sounds, even by rather faint sounds if they are unusual or if we have learned that they are warning signals for us.

When we recognize a warning sound, we usually also have some sense of the direction whence it comes. The sense of direction, *au-ditory localization*, is usually good enough to cause us to look in more or less the right direction. Both ears are necessary for this localization (or better lateralization) or *stereophonic effect*, and we must admit that we are often misled by the curved path of sound around corners and by its reflection as an echo from any large flat surface. It is interesting, however, that bats, dolphins, and some other birds and animals have developed to an extraordinary degree the power of locating distant objects by the reflection of high-pitched chirps that they themselves emit. Nature developed this sonar principle (like radar, but using sound) long before World War II! The blind can learn to make practical use of it, just as the deaf learn speechreading to replace a lost auditory function.

The highest level of audition lies in the recognition of the nature of distant activity. We know what is going on when we hear footsteps, traffic noise, barking dogs, and the like. And, above all, man, by his ability to distinguish and recognize the meaning of sounds, together with his ability to produce a great variety of them with his voice, has developed a system of communication with his fellows that far outdoes the communication between any other animals. The practical and social importance of speech and the hearing of speech need no elaboration. Two of man's greatest biological endowments are, first, his erect posture and his opposable thumb, which give him hands suited to the use of tools, and, second, the capacity and organization of a brain suitable for the development of *language*. Language gave man not only the ability to share experience but a tool for abstract thinking.

Frequency Limits of Audible Sound

The range of audible frequencies extends from about 20 to 20,000 Hz. Neither limit is at all precise. Both the frequency and the intensity of a sound determine whether or not we can hear it (see Figure 2-4). The ear is limited, like a radio receiver, to a band of frequencies. For the ear the most sensitive range is from 500 to 5000 Hz, approximately the same range of frequencies that is most important for understanding speech. Above 5000 Hz the sensitivity of the ear declines more and more rapidly, but the tones can still be heard at moderate intensities by most young ears. An uncertainty about the limits arises from individual differences in ears, particularly with increasing age. The child may be able to hear the "inaudible" dog whistle at about 20,000 Hz, whereas the old man may no longer hear even the overtones of the human voice at about 5000 Hz. These changes with age will be considered in detail in a later section (Chapter 4). We begin to *feel* very low tones through the nerves of touch as well as to *hear* them through the auditory nerve, but the smooth tonal character of the sound is lost and is replaced by a "flutter" at about 18 Hz (see Figure 2-5).

Below and above the range of frequencies that the ear can detect lie the *subsonic* (vibration) and the *ultrasonic* frequencies, respectively. The ultrasonic frequencies used to be called *supersonic*, but present usage is to speak of "ultrasonic frequencies" (by analogy with ultraviolet light) and "supersonic speeds." The ultrasonic waves can be compared to short-wave radio broadcasts, which cannot be picked up by an ordinary radio receiver. The physicist with his instruments cares little for the arbitrary limits imposed by human ears. The limits of hearing are certainly higher for dogs, cats, rats, and probably all small mammals. The physicist's instruments carry him on up into the ultrasonic region of high frequencies, where blasts of air, crackling of twigs, the chirping of many insects, and the cries of bats all produce pressure waves in air of the same kind as ordinary sound, but they are inaudible to

us because of their high frequency. Actually, these ultrasonics in nature are rarely very intense and would probably not be very important to animals of our size, even if we could hear them. They do give fairly accurate information of the direction of their sources, for they travel in straighter lines, bend less around corners, and consequently cast deeper "sound shadows" than do the lower frequencies. However, as a general rule, ultrasonics are generated by *small* objects and are not transmitted so well through the air as are the longer wavelengths. The air is partially opaque to the ultrasonics, and, even if fairly intense at their source, they can be detected only at relatively short distances. The near ultrasonics in the first octave or so above the human limit may be important for small animals, but not for us. We need not fear them as possibly injurious, as has been sometimes suggested, for they are feeble. Theory and experience agree that they are practically quite harmless.

The Sensitivity of the Ear

When we said in a previous section that nature is noisy, we did not mean that nature's sounds are unpleasantly loud; we merely meant that they are audible. The sound waves have enough energy to stimulate the ear, and if nature is noisy, it is partly because our ears are so sensitive within the frequency range of best hearing. The human ear is actually so sensitive that at its best it can almost hear the individual air molecules bump against the eardrum in their random thermal flight. The distance that the eardrum moves in and out with each wave when we just hear the faintest audible tone at the most favorable frequency is far too small to be resolved under an ordinary microscope. It is of molecular dimensions.

The extraordinary sensitivity of the ear is due to its highly specialized structure. The inner ear, protected in a special chamber within the hardest bone of the body, is actually just about as sensitive as it could usefully be. If the cells were stimulated by the random thermal motion of molecules we would hear a continuous meaningless rattle or hiss. Nature has apparently approached this limit rather closely, if we can accept inferences from the energy levels that are involved.

Intense sounds can be felt, either as a single blast or as vibration, by the sense of touch. Our hairs may be set in vibration by the sound waves of the air and tickle the *touch corpuscles* at their roots. (A hair and its touch corpuscle, as we shall see, can be thought of as a crude large-scale model of the actual sense organ in the inner ear.) Or with the tips of our fingers we may feel a piano case vibrate. We may even distinguish with our fingers, though crudely, whether the piano is vibrating rapidly (when a medium or high note is struck) or slowly (when one of the lowest notes is sounded). The sense of vibration, which is one aspect of the sense of touch, and the sense of hearing merge into one another in two ways.

From the point of view of evolutionary development, the inner sense organ of hearing is a highly specialized organ of touch, specialized to be "touched" only by vibrations of the air and never by a solid object. Second, when we "hear" the very lowest notes of a pipe organ, we are probably *feeling* the vibration quite as much as we are *hearing* it. As tones get lower and lower in frequency, the ear is less and less sensitive to them, and the tones must be stronger, with larger vibrations, in order to be heard. Finally, the point is reached at which the pressure waves begin to stimulate the skin of our hands, the linings of our noses and throats, the hairs of our heads, and even our bones, joints, and inner organs. The sense of hearing and touch merge as imperceptibly as do smell and taste. But touch, like taste, cannot distinguish the fine differences for which hearing (like smell) is specialized. Therefore, although we may, for example, perceive the *rhythm* of a piece of music as accurately by touch as by ear, we cannot feel the *tune*, because touch is so poor at discriminating the frequencies that give us our sense of musical pitch. Likewise, the tempo and stress of very loud speech can be felt, but only in the most favorable *context* can words ever be understood through touch alone.

Minimum Audible Field

The psychophysicist is interested in the relations between our sensations and the dimensions and magnitudes of the changes in the external world (the stimuli) that arouse them. We know that the dimensions of physical sound are frequency and intensity, measured, respectively, in hertz and in decibels. On a chart scaled off in these two dimensions we can map the *area of audible tones* (Figure 2-4). It is bounded at the bottom by the *threshold of hearing*. The "threshold" is the faintest sound of a given frequency that a person can detect on 50 percent of a number of trials. The threshold curve expresses the *acuity* of human hearing, although the term "acuity" is ambiguous and is sometimes understood as referring instead to the ability to *discriminate* between two tones that are nearly the same. It is, therefore, safer to say that the curve in question represents the *threshold of sensitivity* of human hearing or the "threshold of detectability" of pure tones. Tones above threshold are audible, those below are inaudible.

In Figures 2-4 and 2-5 we have represented the threshold by a heavy solid line and four other lighter lines nearly parallel to it. We have done so because, in addition to differences related to age, people have different thresholds. Furthermore, one person's

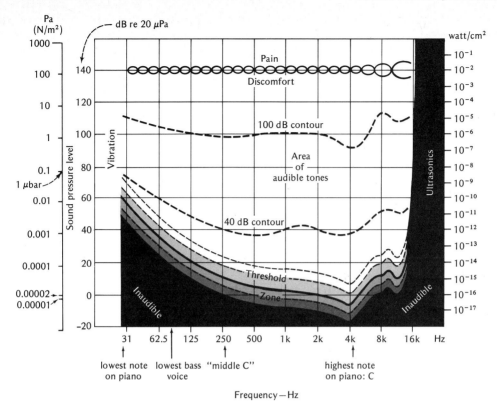

Figure 2-4   The area of audible tones was determined for a group of otologically normal men listening with both ears, facing the source, in a free acoustic field. The heavy lower contour represents their median hearing thresholds: the shaded zones show one and two standard deviations (σ) above and below it. Dips at 4000 and 12,000 Hz are due largely to resonance in the ear canal and diffraction patterns around the head. The area of audibility at low frequencies merges into vibration. On the high-frequency side lie the inaudible ultrasonics. The practical upper limit is the threshold for pain, at about 140 dB SPL.

Two equal-loudness contours are shown for tones judged to sound as loud as 1000-Hz tones at 40 dB and at 100 dB SPL., respectively. *(Adapted from D. W. Robinson and R. S. Dadson, Journal of the Acoustical Society of America, 29:1284–1288; 1957; and British Journal of Applied Physics, 7:166–181; 1956; by permission)*

threshold varies somewhat from day to day and even from trial to trial. We must therefore think of a *threshold zone* rather than a sharp fixed boundary. Fortunately, for a given class of persons, such as males between 18 and 25 years of age whose ears show no abnormality when examined with an otoscope, the distribution of threshold turns out to be a random scatter above and below a median value with a strong "central tendency." The heavy "threshold" line in Figure 2-3 actually represents the median val-

ues for such an 18- to 25-year-old group tested at the National Physical Laboratory in England. These men were healthy and otherwise average individuals. The lighter flanking lines show the dispersion of the thresholds. The lines are one and two standard deviations, respectively, above and below the median. The heavy line, the median, is, of course, the 50 percentile contour. The zone between the two one-standard-deviation lines includes about 68 percent of the total group and the two-standard-deviation

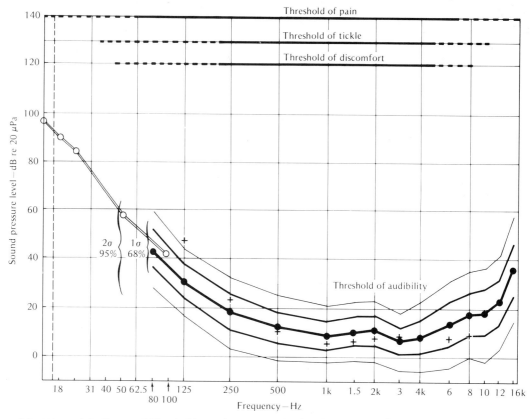

Figure 2.5 "Area of Audiometry." Threshold sound-pressure levels under an earphone, or minimum audible pressure (MAP), as determined at the National Physical Laboratory (British). The heavy solid line and filled circles show the median values for 99 men (198 ears) otologically normal and 18 to 25 years of age. The distributions of the thresholds are normal, and the modes, the medians, and the means are almost identical. The lighter lines show one and two standard deviations (σ) above and below the medians.

The pressures were measured with a probe-tube microphone "at the entrance to the ear canal," the average of two positions: one 7 mm outside, the other 3 mm inside the meatus. (The values at the latter position are slightly modified above 1 kHz by resonance effects of the ear canal.)

Coupler measurements were made for the same earphone (4026-A) using a British standard coupler (B.S.2042). At 250 Hz and above they all lie within 1σ of the probe-tube data plotted in the figure. These coupler measurements entered into the calculation of the ISO reference zero levels for pure-tone audiometers. (These are also the ANSI values.) The ISO values, for the U.S. earphone and coupler (WE 705-A and NAS 9A, respectively), are shown in the figure by the crosses (+). *(Adapted from R. S. Dadson and J. H. King, Journal of Laryngology and Otology, 66:366–378; 1952; by permission)*

The thresholds for the very low frequencies (open circles and double lines) and the fusion frequency were deter-

mined in a separate study on ten subjects, using different, specially designed equipment. *(N. S. Yeowart, M. E. Bryan, and W. Tempest, Journal of Sound and Vibration, 6:335–342; 1967; by permission)* They are included here to extend the area of audiometry to its logical limit at the "fusion frequency" of 18 Hz, below which the smooth tonal quality is lost. Actually, audiometric measurements are rarely made below 125 Hz.

The thresholds of pain, tickle, and discomfort shown here were measured at Central Institute for the Deaf in 1945–1946. *(S. R. Silverman, Annals of Otology, Rhinology, and Laryngology, 56:658–677; 1947; by permission)* They are coupler pressures (PDR-10 earphone and NBS 9-A coupler), comparable to the ISO reference levels. They were determined by increasing the sound-pressure level, starting at 100 dB, by 1 or 2 dB every 1.5 seconds until the subjects reported first discomfort, then tickle, then pain. This method allowed some habituation to the high-level sound and ensured that the intra-aural reflex was active throughout the test. Sounds of sudden onset from a low background level show somewhat lower thresholds of pain, tickle, and discomfort. These three upper thresholds were the same for subjects with normal hearing and for those hard of hearing. They are the approximate median values for the group. The dashed portions of the lines are extrapolations beyond the experimental data.

zone includes about 95 percent of the group.

This sort of scatter is perfectly normal. Individuals differ with respect to their sensitivity of hearing just as they do with respect to other measurable characteristics such as height and weight. To avoid confusion at this point we do not speak of a standard of normal hearing but instead of a *range of normal hearing*.

It is not easy to determine the threshold of hearing of normal listeners because great care must be taken to exclude all echoes and all unwanted background noises from both the environment and the source of the test sounds. Also, the subjects must be well motivated to listen carefully and consistently. Only under the best listening conditions can these extremely low thresholds be measured. The data obtained at the National Physical Laboratory actually agree well with data from earlier but less extensive studies performed at the Bell Telephone Laboratories.

The intensity of the sound field in such tests as these is measured, before the listener enters it, at the position corresponding to the center of the listener's head. The listener faces the source of the sound and listens with both ears. The threshold of hearing, measured under these conditions is called the *minimum audible field* (MAF). The dips in the threshold curve at 4000 and 12,000 hertz (Figure 2-3) are due partly to the acoustic resonance of the ear canals of the listeners and even more to the pattern of reflection and refraction of sound waves around their heads and ears. The thresholds vary, depending on the angle of direction (azimuth) of the source of sound with respect to the listener's head. and are different for a so-called "plane wave" advancing from a single direction as opposed to random incidence from all directions.

As we have noted, the frequency at which sounds become inaudible depends not only on the intensity of the sound but on the age of the listener. For low frequencies the threshold rises more gradually, and age is not a factor. The difficulties for very low frequencies are, first, to distinguish hearing from feeling and, second, to generate really pure low tones. The higher harmonics can be heard easily even though they may have less than one ten-thousandth of the acoustic energy of the fundamental.

The auditory area is bounded at its upper edge, for practical purposes, by the thresholds of discomfort, of tickle, and, finally, of pain. These thresholds vary from person to person and with the attitude of the listener toward these very loud sounds and toward the tests. There are also problems of just what the words "discomfort," "tickle," and "pain" mean. Many listeners are likely at first to report pain for a sensation that they later call merely "tickle" after they have once felt the sharp stab of true auditory pain. If prolonged, such very intense sounds are dangerous to hearing as well as painful, so the practical upper limit of the auditory area at about 135 dB sound pressure level is real. As it happens, these thresholds of discomfort, tickle, and pain are pretty nearly constant, regardless of frequency. Only the first unpleasantness, the *discomfort*, is a truly auditory sensation. Actually the *loudness* of the sounds keeps on increasing as the intensity is increased, regardless of discomfort, tickle in the ear, or pain.

Minimum Audible Pressure and Hearing–Threshold Level

Some tests for impaired hearing are conducted binaurally in a free acoustic field, particularly with young children (as described in Chapter 8), but in most tests the two ears are studied separately, using a pair of earphones. The earphones have the great practical advantage of fitting snugly against the side of the head and excluding much of the ambient background noise. It is far easier and cheaper to build a booth that is quiet enough for such audiometry than a room that is quiet enough and adequately sound-treated for measuring minimum audible field. Less sound exclusion is needed for the conventional audiometric booth and, although some internal sound absorption is desirable, it is not necessary to prevent echoes entirely. Details of audiometric booths, audiometers, and the calibration of audiometers are given in Chapter 7, but the relations between monaural and binaural listening and between field listening and earphone listening will be examined here. These relations are important because we use our ears chiefly as a pair in an open auditory field, but our ears are usually tested separately, using the acoustic pressure developed in the very restricted volume of air under an earphone. These two situations are quite different.

The difference between hearing with one ear instead of two is not difficult to state if we are concerned only with the measurement of thresholds. Careful tests, both in an acoustic field and with earphones, have shown that two ears are more sensitive than one. The gain is about 3 dB. This gain in sensitivity is, however, a very minor advantage for binaural hearing compared with other major advantages, namely, the ability to recognize the direction of the source of a sound, the better detection of signals, and better discrimination of speech in the presence of noise. These three other advantages will be considered later, and we do not need to be concerned here with the way in which the greater sensitivity of hearing is achieved. It is not, as was once supposed, simply a matter of scooping up twice as much acoustic energy. It involves complicated interactions between the inputs from the two ears within the central nervous system.

The matter of measuring the acoustic pressure developed under the earphone is more difficult. It is possible to make such measurements by means of a probe-tube microphone. The plastic tube attached to the microphone is long and flexible enough to pass under the cushion of the earphone to almost any desired position except one. It is not practical to measure acoustic pressure deep in the ear canal, just in front of the drum membrane, while the subject is wearing earphones, although this can be done readily enough in an acoustic field. The usual choice is to measure the acoustic pressure just at the outer entrance of the ear canal. This position must be closely specified on account of acoustic resonances within the ear canal and in the small airspace under the earphone.

In addition to the problem of defining the standard position at which to measure the pressure, it now appears that the efficiency of the ear in detecting a faint sound is modified by the volume of air contained under the earphone and also, if this volume is small, on certain acoustic characteristics known technically as the "acoustic impedance" of the source of the sound. Even worse, the interaction between the ear and the source depends, in turn, on the anatomy and on the acoustic impedance of the ear that is under the earphone. The impedance and the resonances vary significantly from one ear to another. One way out of this difficulty is to make the volume of air under the earphone very large, of the order of a liter or so. Unfortunately, such an audiometer is clumsy. Its large ear chambers, too heavy for a headband, require firm independent support. It has never been popular in the United States as a clinical instrument.

The differences and uncertainties that we are discussing are not large enough to be of great practical significance, but they make very difficult the standardization and calibration of audiometers. Nevertheless, it would seem that if we could measure the acoustic pressure in the field and also at the entrance to the ear canal under the earphone, the threshold pressures should be the same.

Unfortunately there is still a rather large discrepancy, about 6 dB, for which there is still no complete and satisfactory explanation. It probably involves effects such as resonances, acoustic impedances, directional effects, and perhaps others. The discrepancy is known as "the missing 6 dB."

This unexplained discrepancy was pointed out by Fletcher and his collaborators at the Bell Telephone Laboratories more than 40 years ago. It was confirmed 20 years later by the studies at the National Physical Laboratory in England to which we have already referred. The curve for minimum audible pressure (monaural earphone listening) lies about 6 dB above the minimum audible field (monaural listening) and does not have such large peaks and troughs above 3000 Hz (compare Figures 2-4 and 2-5).

For completeness we should also mention here the standard of pressure used for the calibration of audiometers. This is the acoustic pressure measured in a carefully standardized *coupler* or *artificial ear* when the earphone that is placed on it is driven by a voltage that corresponds to the hearing threshold of an appropriate sample of otologically normal ears. Details are given in Chapter 7. The point here is that the standard artificial ear has a volume (6 cubic centimeters) corresponding to the airspace under an ordinary audiometric earphone, including the external and middle ear, but it has its own set of resonances and its own acoustic impedance. Its advantage lies in its simplicity and its reproducibility. The coupler pressures are of the same order of magnitude as the minimum audible pressures, but they are not identical with them. They differ slightly for different models of earphone. In particular, these standard threshold coupler pressures must not be confused with the sound pressure of the minimum audible field.

A set of standard reference levels for pure-tone audiometers has been recommended by the International Organization for Standardization (ISO) on the basis of a number of studies of the hearing of healthy young adults. (Details will be given in Chapter 7.) These reference zero levels are given as coupler pressures. They represent median values for many listeners. In this respect they are similar to the median minimum audible field, which is also based on the hearing of a similar population of young adults. The minimum audible pressure, from 500 to 8000 Hz, is of the same order of magnitude as the physicist's reference level of 20 μPa, but it lies a few decibels above the physicist's level because of (1) the binaural advantage (about 3 dB), (2) the missing 6 dB, and (3) an arbitrary decision that put the physical reference level at the level of "good" rather than "average" hearing. This last difference is about 3 or 4 dB, according to Robinson and Dadson.

The upshot of all this is that an ear that is, for example, 10 dB less sensitive than the median will require a level 10 dB above the reference level (ISO) of the audiometer to reach threshold. In an open auditory field the threshold (binaural) for a man with two such ears will likewise lie 10 dB above the median minimum audible field. Across the range frequencies from 500 to 3000 Hz this median minimum audible field is approximately 4 dB above 20 μPa. The man in question should therefore be able to hear a tone in this frequency range at about $10 + 4 = 14$ dB sound-pressure level (SPL).

The Audiogram

Figure 2-5 shows the minimum audible pressure measured under an earphone, as determined at the National Physical Laboratory. The corresponding coupler pressures were determined also, and later they entered into the averages that constitute the international reference zero levels for audiometers. The crosses represent the international reference zero values, now given as coupler pressures for the WE 705-A earphone in MX-41 cushions measured in a National Bureau of Standards (USA) NBS-9A coupler. The thresholds of pain, tickle, and discomfort at the top of the figure were also measured under nearly similar earphones and are also given as coupler pressures. The three upper thresholds are therefore directly comparable to the crosses representing the zero of the audiometer.

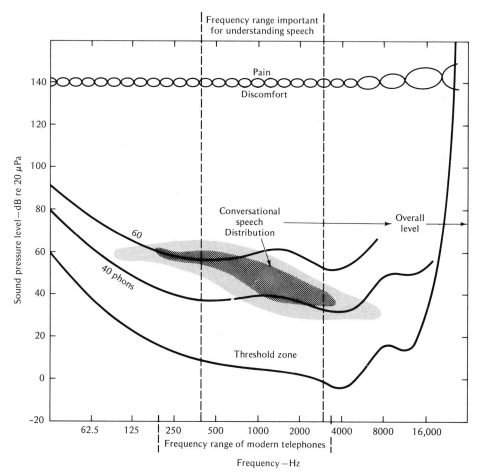

Figure 2-6 The speech area. Speech is a mixture of complex tones, wide-band noise, and transients. Both the intensities and the frequencies of speech sounds change continually and rapidly. It is difficult to measure them and logically impossible to plot them precisely in terms of sound-pressure levels at particular frequencies. This figure shows the approximate distribution of sound-pressure levels with respect to frequency that would occur if brief but characteristic bits of phonemes of conversational speech were actually sustained like pure tones. The density of the shaded area represents roughly the probability of finding in a sample of speech the particular combinations of intensity and frequency. Individual voices differ, however, and obviously the boundaries of the speech area are not sharp.

The overall sound-pressure level of the stronger vowels in conversational speech at 1 meter is about 72 dB. The fundamental frequency of a deep bass voice is about 100 Hz, but the fundamental frequencies of most women's and children's voices are about 250 Hz. The strongest individual sounds in the frequency range below 100 Hz are louder than 60 phons, and the weakest significant elements are about 30 dB below the strongest. The weaker elements are very often masked by background noises. For good understanding of everyday speech the range from 400 to 3000 Hz is sufficient. This range includes almost all of the "formant" frequency bands of speech, which distinguish the vowels and many consonants. (See *Man's World of Sound* by Pierce and David for a good acoustic description of speech.)

A pure-tone audiometer is calibrated so that its zero reading at each frequency corresponds to the median hearing level for healthy young adults (the international standard). The average reference value is different for different frequencies. The audiometer measures the number of decibels that the threshold of the subject lies above each median value. The difference is the *hearing-threshold level*. The graph of hearing-threshold levels, illustrated in Figures 7-6 and 7-7, is known as the *audiogram*. Here the reference zero levels are drawn as a straight horizontal line across frequencies. Positive hearing-threshold levels, representing additional pressure needed to be heard by ears less sensitive than the average, are conventionally plotted *downward* to express the idea of reduced sensitivity of the ear. This convention was established by otologists who thought in terms of the sensitivity of the ear. It is opposite to that of the physicist who plots sound pressures as increasing upward (as in the figures in Chapter 4). The physicist thinks in terms of the *sound* that is the *stimulus* to the ear. The measuring instrument for the physicist is the sound-level meter, but for the audiologist it is the hearing-level meter or audiometer.

The Speech Area

A particularly important part of the auditory area is the range of frequencies most important for the understanding of speech. This range extends roughly from 400 to 3000 Hz. Speech contains frequencies above 3000 Hz and below 400 Hz, but they are not necessary for almost perfect intelligibility of everyday conversational speech. The importance of the speech range will appear later in relation to the design of hearing aids and to the problem of auditory handicap. The part of the auditory area that is important for speech is bounded at the top by the thresholds of tolerance and, at the bottom, for practical purposes, by the background sound level against which we are likely to hear faint everyday speech. Practically, this is at an octave-band level of approximately 30 to 40 dB SPL in this part of the frequency spectrum. Figure 2-6 shows the range of frequencies most important for good understanding of everyday speech. It also shows the approximate distribution with respect to frequency and intensity of the actual sounds of conversational speech.

The extent to which a background noise will interfere with ordinary conversational speech depends on the relations of the spectrum of the noise (see Figure 2-3) and its intensity. An index for noise, known as the *speech interference level* (SIL), consists of the arithmetic average of the three octave-band levels 600 to 1200 Hz, 1200 to 2400 Hz, and 2400 to 4800 Hz. This index is very useful to the acoustical engineer in predicting whether speech will be intelligible in certain noisy situations.

Psychoacoustics

Psychoacoustics is concerned with what we hear. It describes the relations of our auditory sensations to the physical properties of the acoustic stimulus, such as its frequency spectrum, its wave form, its intensity, and its temporal relations. Psychoacoustics deals with attributes of sensation such as pitch and loudness and the apparent location of the source and also with judgments as to how loud a noise is, either relative to another noise or on an absolute scale. It is concerned with the ability of listeners to distinguish differences between stimuli. It is not concerned directly with the physiological mechanisms that underlie the detection or the differentiation of sounds but with the judgments and reports of human listeners. Most tests of hearing used to describe and measure impairments of hearing are actually psychoacoustic tests.

We shall not undertake a complete exploration of psychoacoustics, but we shall mention some of its important principles and define a few terms that may be encountered in relation to some of the more elaborate tests of hearing, particularly those designed to assess central rather than peripheral impairments. In the next chapter we shall examine the intermediate anatomical and physiological mechanisms and consider how anatomy, biophysics, and neurophysiology set certain limits on the psychoacoustic performance of human listeners.

Pitch

Pitch is a quality of the sensation of sound that is most clearly recognized for pure tones. It is a quality by which we can arrange sounds on a scale from *low* or bass to *high* or treble. It is the quality that enables us to recognize a tune. The musical pitch of a note depends chiefly on the physical frequency of the sound waves and also, to a very limited extent, on their intensity. The positions of the lowest and the highest notes of the piano and its middle C (261.6 Hz) are shown in Figure 2-4. The relation of the *musical scale* to simple numerical ratios of the frequencies of the sound waves should be familiar. There is a particularly close musical relation between two frequencies that are an octave apart. The higher frequency is exactly double the lower frequency. The musical scale is thus related simply and directly to the *logarithm* of frequency.

The higher harmonics of musical tones, the human voice, and many other sounds are related in frequency to the fundamental and to one another in simple numerical ratios, such as 3 to 2, 5 to 3, and so on. These relations are implicit in the line spectra shown in Figure 2-2. The overtones are said to be *harmonically related* to one another. These simple relations are the basis of musical harmony and of musical scales.

Individuals differ considerably in their ability to recognize, remember, and reproduce musical *intervals*, either in sequence (melody) or in combination (harmony). Training and practice improve performance. Some people can "carry a tune" easily and accurately after only one or two hearings, and the ability to recognize and to mimic dialects in speech is closely related. Other people have very poor *musical memories*. A few gifted individuals have the faculty of *absolute pitch* and can identify a note (on the musical scale) as A or C sharp or E flat, for example, or sing such a note on demand. The relative contributions of endowment and training to absolute pitch are still debated.

The mel scale   In addition to the musical scale, there is another *psychological scale* of pitch. It is demonstrated (and defined operationally) by asking listeners to find, by adjusting an oscillator, a tone whose pitch is "half as high" or perhaps "twice as high" as that of a standard tone, without regard to musical interval. Or we may present a tone of medium pitch, say at 500 Hz, and tell the listener that it stands at 10 on the pitch scale. Then we present other tones of various frequencies in random order and ask the listener to give to the pitch of each tone an appropriate number of the pitch scale. Variations of these methods are to ask the subject to bisect the pitch interval between two tones or to judge whether intervals between two pairs of tones are the same or different. These various psychophysical methods agree in producing a subjective scale of pitch that is quite different from the musical scale. Octaves in different parts of the scale have different subjective magnitudes. They are much smaller below 500 Hz than above it. For this subjective scale, a unit has been defined: the *mel*. The pitch of a tone of 1000 Hz at 40 dB above threshold is 1000 mels. The pitch curve is shown in Figure 2-7 as a solid line. The dashed line shows how it would be if each semitone, or each octave, were equal in subjective magnitude.

The smallest difference in pitch that a listener can detect on 50 percent of a series of trials is known as his *differential threshold* or *difference limen* (DL) for pitch. ("Limen" is the Latin word for threshold.) We usually present a random series of pairs of successive tones that differ only slightly in frequency and ask the subject to tell us whether the members of each pair sounded the same or different. With these data we construct the *psychophysical curve* that relates percentage correct to the frequency difference between the tones. The curve is typically an "ogive," rising slowly, then steeply, then slowly to 100 percent correct. The difference limen, at 50 percent correct, is about 2 or 3 Hz for 1000 Hz at moderate intensities. The DL turns out to be very nearly constant with frequency if it is expressed in mels. *One just noticeable difference (j.n.d.) turns out, quite by coincidence, to be about one mel. This is*

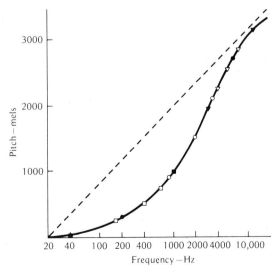

Figure 2-7 The solid curve shows the pitch scale in mels as a function of frequency. The dashed line shows the relation that would apply if all octaves were equal in subjective magnitude. *(Data from S. S. Stevens and J. Volkmann,* American Journal of Psychology, *53:329–353; 1940; by permission)*

not an exact rule because the size of the DL (or j.n.d.) depends significantly on just how the tones are presented to the listener and also on individual differences among listeners in their ability to discriminate pitch differences.

A corollary of the approximate equivalence of the mel and the j.n.d. is that all j.n.d.s for pitch are of the same subjective magnitude. This is not surprising, and for many years this equality was simply assumed without proof. We mention it, however, because we shall soon see that for loudness the just noticeable differences are *not* all subjectively equal.

The pitch of complex sounds The pitch of a continuing pure tone is clear and definite. The situation is more complicated when the tone is very brief or when more than one tone reaches the ear at once. Let us consider the second case first. The simplest and most common combination of frequencies is a fundamental and its series of higher harmonics (Figure 2-2). We hear the pitch as the same as that of the fundamental, although its musical quality is different. This is true even when the fundamental is very weak and most of the loudness is carried by the higher harmonics. It is still true when the fundamental itself is eliminated, leaving only the equally spaced overtones. This is known as "the case of the missing fundamental," and it explains why the bass notes of music are heard as well as they are through hearing aids and many small loudspeakers.

A musical chord does not, in general, have the simple harmonic series of frequencies, and modern music may contain almost any combination of frequencies, consonant or dissonant. The pitch of chords may be hard to specify. Sometimes they sound single, with a pitch somewhere between the extremes of the tones that are combined. Sometimes the components are heard separately, each with its own pitch and loudness. Even noises with continuous spectra, if they have a large part of their energy concentrated in one part of the spectrum, have more or less pitch.

Ohm's law and periodicity pitch   If two tones have frequencies that are not harmonically related, that is, in simple numerical ratio to one another, or if their frequencies are very different, it is usually easy to distinguish them and "hear them out" separately. The ability of the ear to analyze such a mixture, like a set of physical acoustic filters, is known as *Ohm's acoustical law*. (This law must not be confused with Ohm's electrical law, which relates the voltage, the current, and the resistance in an electric circuit.) Ohm's law is one of the classical laws of psychoacoustics, but it is only a first-order approximation. What we hear in a complex mixture depends significantly on whether we try, by an effort of attention, to separate the components or whether we accept the mixture as a single auditory sensation. However, the ear is more than a simple set of acoustic filters. It is sensitive to the periodic recurrence of peaks of acoustic pressure that may be produced by the interaction of tones that are not harmonically related, or perhaps by a series of clicks or brief bursts of high-frequency noise. In other words, the ear can hear certain pitches that are *not* detected as acoustic frequencies by a set of physical acoustic filters. Unlike the acoustic filters, the ear is sensitive, to a limited extent, to wave form as such and thus to the phase relations in a mixture of pure tones. We shall return to this phenomenon of *periodicity pitch* in connection with the temporal pattern of nerve impulses in the auditory nerve.

It is of practical significance for the possibility of hearing by direct electrical stimulation of the auditory nerve by the so-called "cochlear implant" (see Chapter 6). If only a single electrode is employed, the subject is unable to detect pitch according to Ohm's law but only by periodicity pitch. His frequency discrimination is poor and it extends upward only to about 1 kHz. The patients are frustrated because speech can be made almost intelligible, but not quite.

The pitch of brief tones: transients   The tonality or definiteness of pitch of a sound depends also on the abruptness of onset and on the duration of the tone. A sinusoidal electric signal can be started or stopped instantaneously and at any phase of its cycle, but such an abrupt onset must contain, mathematically and physically, other frequencies than that of the continuing pure sinusoid. Acoustic energy is "scattered," as we say, into other parts of the acoustical spectrum. This energy at other frequencies is known as the *starting transient*. Mathematically a tone is pure and has a single frequency only if it is of infinite duration. In addition, any physical transducer, such as a loudspeaker that has inertia, will be "excited" to vibrate or "ring," as we say, at its own resonant frequency unless it is sufficiently (critically) damped. The ear itself is one such transducer, and it is not critically damped. For all of these reasons, a spurious click is heard at the sudden onset (or termination) of an otherwise pure tone. To avoid such starting and stopping transients, we must make the onset and offset of a tone gradual over several cycles at least. Only then will we hear the tone as pure. Incidentally, such a gradual onset is required in standard pure-tone audiometers (see Chapter 7).

Quite apart from the starting and stopping transients, a tone must last for an appreciable time if it is to have a completely definite pitch. Some pitch quality is present even for stimuli of only one or two cycles, but the subjective pitch is not clear unless the tone lasts for something like a twentieth or even a tenth of a second. The necessary duration depends greatly on just how we define *clear* pitch. One reason that impulsive sounds like knocking on wood are indefinite in pitch is that they start abruptly and die out very rapidly, and they may also ring at more than one frequency simultaneously. A knock on wood may seem to have no pitch at all, but if it is followed by another knock on a different piece of wood, the pitch difference is easily recognized. We can play a tune with a set of well-chosen sticks of wood.

Very brief acoustic stimuli with a single dominant frequency may be produced by ringing an electric filter with a brief electric pulse. Such "filtered clicks" or "tone pips" are useful tools in psychoacoustic and physiological research, and as stimuli in electric response audiometry (Chapter 8), but their pitch is rather vague, like clicks, knocks, or thumps. "Pitchness" grades without boundries from the definite pitch of a pure tone to the indeterminate pitch of unfiltered clicks or white noise.

We may comment here that, although some listeners have more "acute" hearing than others in the sense that their difference limens for pitch are smaller, we never encounter a person with any useful degree of hearing who is completely *tone deaf*. This term should be avoided. If it means anything, it should mean inability to distinguish differences in pitch. It is often misused in popular language to mean poor musical memory or poor ability to identify the components of a complex tone.

Beats, aural harmonics, and combination tones
Let us return to the question of how we hear two tones of approximately the same intensity but with frequencies that are very nearly the same. If the tones differ by only one cycle per second, the peaks of the waves will coincide and physically reenforce one another at one moment, but half a second later the slower will lag behind the other by

half a cycle, and the two waves will cancel one another more or less completely. After another half second, they will be in phase again and again reenforce one another. This periodic waxing and waning or "amplitude modulation" will be heard as a waxing and waning of loudness at a frequency of 1 per second. These changes in loudness are known as "beats." They are the basis of a delicate method, used by piano tuners, to determine when two sound sources are exactly in tune. If the beats are slow, less than about 6 or 7 per second, the effect is not unpleasant. A little faster and the effect becomes a "vibrato." If the difference in frequency is more than 20 per second or thereabouts, the sound is rough and unpleasant. Two such piano strings would be definitely out of tune. This detection of beats is another way in which the ear differs from a set of perfect acoustic filters. The two frequencies "overlap" and affect some of the same detector elements.

If the difference in frequency is made wider still, we can begin to hear the sound as a mixture of two tones. The necessary difference for separate identification is one way of defining a *critical band* of frequency within which the sensation is fused or single. We shall return to this important property of the ear and define it more carefully in relation to loudness and to the phenomenon of the "masking" of one sound by another.

A final aspect of pitch is the phenomenon of combination tones and of "aural harmonics," which refers to our hearing of new frequencies that correspond to the sums or the differences of the frequencies of two clearly separated tones that are presented simultaneously. Suffice it to say that these effects are produced physically in the inner or middle ear because the ear is not a perfect linear transmitting system. In fact we shall see in the next chapter that the mechanical nonlinearity of the ear begins at about the middle of the area of audible tones (Figure 2-4). There are increasing protective restraints of an elastic sort on the amplitude of movement in the inner ear as those movements tend to become large. Asymmetries and nonlinearity of the system introduce higher harmonics and also the sum and difference tones, including interaction among the higher harmonics of the two original tones. The same effect is produced in nonlinear or "overloaded" physical systems, and is the basis of troublesome harmonic distortion in hearing aids that are working near the limit of their capacity.

Other Qualities of Sounds

We have discussed the pitch of pure tones and the different quality that is introduced by the presence of strong higher harmonics. We have mentioned also the quality of roughness that results from rapid beats or amplitude modulation. Several other psychological attributes of sound such as "timbre," "brightness," "brilliance," "density," and "volume" have been described. They seem to depend on various combinations of frequencies and intensities in the physical pattern of the stimulating sound. With one exception the details need not concern us in the present survey.

The exception is the particular and characteristic quality of a musical instrument or the human voice that is given by the reinforcement, by the principle of resonance, of all frequencies, whether fundamental or harmonics, that fall within a certain broad band or bands of frequency. The range of frequencies that is reinforced is called a *formant*, and it gives a very distinctive character or quality to the sound. The pitches of the tones may change, but those of the formants remain fixed. The vowels of speech differ from one another in the formants that are imposed by the resonant cavities of the mouth and pharynx. The formants change with different positions of lips, tongue, and jaw; but they are independent of the fundamental frequency of the voice. The latter is determined by the vibration of the vocal bands that periodically interrupt the stream of air through the larynx.

Binaural hearing of pitch   A sound of a given frequency does not, in general, have exactly the same pitch when heard in the right ear as it does in the left ear, yet most people are not aware of such differences between their ears. The discrepancies pass unnoticed for several reasons. First, the differences are usually small. The frequency in the right ear need be changed by only 1 or 2 percent to make the pitches equal. Second, the differences are not systematic. A difference of as much as 1 percent may extend over only a fraction of an octave, and the right ear may hear some tones sharper, others flatter, than the left; but systematic search almost always reveals noticeable differences at some frequencies. Third, we usually hear the same external sound in both ears simultaneously and do not make the necessary successive comparisons. When the pitches and the loudnesses are nearly the same, we hear a single pitch that is the average of the right pitch and the left pitch. Only when the difference exceeds some critical amount do we hear two discordant pitches and complain of *diplacusis* or double hearing (see Chapter 4). When the sound is much louder in one ear, the pitch of that ear is dominant.

Loudness   Loudness is the aspect of auditory sensation that relates most directly to the physical intensity or energy of the sound waves. It extends from "barely audible" through "comfortably loud" to "uncomfortably loud" and finally to "barely tolerable" and painful, as indicated in Figure 2-4. It happens that all audible sounds become intolerably loud at about the same physical intensity, about 135 dB sound-pressure level, regardless of their frequency. At low physical intensities, say 30 dB SPL, some frequencies are inaudible, others are barely audible, and still others, in the range from 1000 to 4000 Hz, are clearly audible.

It is not difficult, with a little practice, for listeners to match quite reliably tones or noises of different frequencies or frequency spectra with respect to their loudness. In fact, as we shall see in Chapter 7, such *loudness balances* between tones of different frequency presented alternately are an important clinical diagnostic test of hearing. On the basis of a series of such loudness balances, we can construct a series of *equal-loudness contours* such as those shown in Figures 2-3, 2-4, and 2-6. Each of these contours is identified by the physical intensity of the 1000-Hz tone through which it passes. The 100-dB and the 40-dB contours for free-field binaural listening are shown in Figure 2-4.

Phon   The loudness of a 1000-Hz tone defines a *loudness level*. The name of the unit of loudness level is the *phon*. Thus if a tone or a noise of any freqency spectrum is judged to be just as loud as a reference tone of 1000 Hz at 40 dB SPL (binaural field listening facing the source), it has a loudness level of 40 phons. The phon scale is a decibel scale that corresponds to the sound-pressure level of the reference tone. It helps to describe the stimulus. It is not, however, a unit of subjective loudness. To generate a loudness scale we must go to the methods of magnitude estimation, half-loudness, double-loudness, and so on, exactly as we did for the pitch scale of mels.

Loudness difference limens   The difference limen (DL) for loudness is approximately 1 dB. It has sometimes been stated, quite

wrongly, that this is the basis for the choice of the decibel as a unit of measurement in acoustics. Actually, the difference limen varies from about 4 dB near threshold to less than 0.5 dB at high intensities, and it is larger for very high and very low tones than for tones in the middle range.

An old and familiar law of psychophysics, Weber's law, states that the just noticeable difference in sensation (the difference limen) is a constant fraction of the total stimulus. This law would require that the DL for loudness should be a constant number of decibels. Weber's law is, therefore, only an approximation, and it breaks down rather badly at the ends of the scales of both frequency and intensity.

Weber's law was extended by Fechner to the question of psychological magnitudes. Fechner's "law" states that the psychological magnitude grows as the logarithm of the magnitude of the stimulus. But in spite of the nearly universal acceptance of this law for a hundred years, it is actually, like Weber's law, only a first approximation to the facts. Furthermore, it is founded on the *assumption* that all just noticeable differences are equal in subjective magnitude. This proposition, as we have noted, is true for pitch, but it is definitely false for loudness.

During the last 20 years, much attention has been given to loudness and loudness scales and more recently to other scales of subjective magnitudes also. One of the foremost investigators has been S. S. Stevens at Harvard University. Let us quote from a semipopular article written by him in 1957. He discusses loudness level and the phon, much as we have done above, and then emphasizes that "loudness level and loudness are really quite different concepts." He elaborates as follows:

Loudness level in phons is an arbitrary yardstick, and one that is nonlinearly related to loudness. What we need to know is how loudness itself depends upon loudness level. By this we mean: What do people say when they try to describe loudness in quantitative terms? In asking this question we are merely looking for the empirical answer to a very empirical question: How do people describe the apparent strength of a 1000-Hz tone when we present it at different levels and the listener describes its loudness in a numerical language instead of adjectives.

The practical side of this question had its origin in the fact that after the decibel scale was adopted, the acoustical engineers noted that equal steps on the decibel scale do not *sound* like equal steps and that a level of 50 dB does not sound like half of 100 dB. Since the engineer often faces the problem of communicating with a customer, it was soon realized that there was a need for a loudness scale whose numbers would make more sense to the customer than do the numbers of the decibel scale.

The generation of a loudness scale is in principle quite simple. All we need to do is produce an array of sounds and ask a group of listeners to assign numbers to them in such a way that the numbers reflect the perceived loudness of the sounds. In practice, of course, it turns out that many alternative techniques are possible and that subtle differences in experimental procedure sometimes influence what the listener says or does. The measurement of a subjective experience like loudness is difficult—so much so that many have argued that it is impossible. But results obtained in several laboratories in at least four different countries make it plain that people can make quantitative estimates of loudness.

Four classes of methods have been used. They all concur in showing that loudness, as estimated by the median listener, approximates a power function of the intensity of 1000-Hz tone. *Loudness is proportional to the 0.3 power of the intensity (energy flux density).* Or, if we define a unit of loudness, the sone, as the loudness heard by the typical listener confronted with 1000-Hz tone at an SPL of 40 dB (40 phons), we can write the equation as

$$\log_{10} S = 0.03P - 1.2$$

where S is loudness in sones and P is loudness level in phons. . . . Since people's judgments are

variable, an equation of this sort must be regarded as only a first-order approximation. What the formula tells us is that in order to produce a 2:1 change in loudness we must change the stimulus by about 10 dB.

The power law The power law for loudness as stated in the foregoing quotation relates loudness to the acoustic "energy flux density." The data fall close to a straight line in a log-log plot, and the slope of this line is about 0.3. We encounter here an unfortunate ambiguity that turns on the double meaning of "power." Stevens employed the term in its mathematical sense in the phrase "loudness is proportional to the 0.3 power of the intensity." That is why he refers to "the power law." But sound intensity, the basis of the acoustic decibel scale, is closely related to sound "power" (explained above). So far there is no real confusion, but it is often more convenient to express the relation of loudness to sound pressure rather than to sound intensity. The pressure is proportional to the square root of the intensity, and therefore the slope of the line, which is the exponent in the "power law" equation, is twice as large, about 0.6. To avoid this possible ambiguity we shall call this relation the "sound-pressure law" or the power law (sound pressure). The full relation between loudness (L) and sound pressure (p) is given by the equation

$$L = k(p - p_0)^{0.6}$$

where k is a constant that depends on units and p_0 is the threshold value.

The mathematical relation expressed by the power law has applications far wider than merely loudness. It appears to be the general "psychophysical law" for all "sensory continua" that relate to subjective intensity such as loudness, brightness, lifted weights, and so on: that is *equal stimulus ratios produce equal sensation ratios.*

The various sensations, when studied by the methods of fractionation or direct estimation of magnitude, all yield power functions, but the value of the exponent (the slope of the line in a log-log plot) is characteristic of the particular sensation. The steepest that has been measured is electric shock (4.5), and brightness is the most gradual (0.33). Several sensations, such as temperature (cold on the arm), duration (of a white noise), and pressure (on the palm) have exponents very close to 1.0. The exponent for the apparent force of handgrip is 1.7.

Since the intensity of each sensation is described by a power law, it follows mathematically that when one sensation is compared directly with another, the relation will be another power law with its exponent equal to the difference between the two original exponents. A subject can match intensity across different sense modalities, just as he can match the loudness of two tones of different pitch, and he can squeeze a dynamometer in his hand and thus express his judgment of the loudness of a sound. This procedure generates a power law without requiring the subject to make a numerical judgment. This point has some theoretical significance. Also the instructions to the subject and the procedure are simple. It lends itself to possible clinical application in tests of hearing in which the rate of increase of loudness is abnormal (see Chapter 8).

The exponent of the power law is not completely fixed and definite, however. Even for a single modality, such as hearing, individuals differ rather widely from one another. In one experiment, for example, the average increase in sound pressure for 11 subjects required to double the loudness was 8.2 dB. One subject, however, was satisfied by 5.5 dB, although another, at the other extreme, required 15 dB. These subjects also produced rather different slopes in the second session as compared with the first. It is important, however, that the power law does

apply to individuals and is not merely an artifact of averaging.

Binaural loudness It was assumed for many years that a sound heard with both ears sounds twice as loud as it does with one ear alone. This statement, like several others we have mentioned, is only approximately true. It is true at one particular loudness level, namely at 90 dB. The threshold for binaural listening is, as we have noted, some 3 dB lower than for monaural listening, and loudness increases a little more rapidly for binaural hearing. The exponent of the sound-pressure law is about 0.60 for binaural and 0.54 for monaural. The power law is a very convenient way in which to describe these differences between monaural and binaural listening. The differences also emphasize the important part played by the central nervous system in integrating the input from the two ears and in determining the power law itself.

Loudness at different frequencies We have described the equal-loudness contours in an earlier section. We now call attention to the narrowing of the auditory area in the low-tone and in the very high-tone range in which the threshold zone rises to meet a nearly horizontal threshold of discomfort (Figure 2-4). In these ranges the equal-loudness contours are spaced more closely, and the power law for sound pressure has larger exponents. It is in the middle of the frequency range, in which the dynamic range of hearing is greatest, that the exponent for loudness averages 0.6 or perhaps 0.66.

Masking The loudness of a sound heard in the presence of another (background) sound is a matter of special interest. We all know from personal experience that faint sounds cannot be heard in the presence of background ("ambient") noise. The faint sound is said to be *masked*. The extent of the masking depends on the frequency and intensity of the test tone and the spectrum and intensity of the masker. We can determine the *masked threshold* for our test tones in a noise just as we determine the *absolute threshold* in quiet.

If the masking sound is a pure tone, its masking effect is greatest for tones near it in frequency, although the beats between test tone and masker when they are at nearly the same frequency confuse the issue. If a narrow band of noise is used, the beats are eliminated, and we find that masking is greatest in the frequency band of the masker. The elevation of threshold of the test tone becomes less and less as the frequency of the test tone recedes from that of the masker, but the curve of masked threshold is not symmetrical, except perhaps at very low sensation levels. At high levels it falls off rather sharply toward the lower frequencies and much less rapidly toward frequencies higher than that of the masker.

The phenomena of masking have been explored in great detail. Complications arise when high intensity levels are tested, due in part to physical nonlinear effects and harmonic distortion within the ear. The shape of the masked threshold curves is of theoretical interest in relation to the mechanism of the inner ear. So is the problem of the signal-to-noise ratio between test tone and masker, and the ability of the ear to "dig the signal out of the noise" as compared with acoustic or electrical filters, but we shall be content here with this bare outline.

When a tone is just heard in a background of masking noise, it sounds, of course, very faint. A small increase in its intensity increases its loudness considerably. Finally, a tone 30 dB above its masked threshold sounds as loud as if the masking noise were absent. The power law applies in this situation in which the noise partially masks the test tone (see Figure 2-8). For the first 30 dB above threshold the slope (exponent) is greater than for a free unmasked or, as Stevens puts it, "uninhibited" tone in the quiet. (The concept of inhibition is very useful here, as we shall see when we consider, in Chapter 3, the neural mechanisms that are involved in these interactions.) In vision there is an analogous inhibition of brightness of a test light by the glare of the background, and here too the slope of the power law for brightness is increased.

In more detail Stevens and his co-workers tell us that the slope of the power law for an inhibited tone is constant from the masked threshold up to a level 30 dB above the masked threshold. Beyond this level the loudness increases more slowly, following the same function as a free, uninhibited tone. The complete function is a broken line with a "knee" in it. If the masking noise is fairly narrow in bandwidth, about two critical bands (see below) or less, and the tone lies within its frequency range, then the noise and the tone have about the same sound pressure level at the "knee," and they sound about equally loud. Probably at this point the noise and the tone are each inhibiting the other equally. If the tone is made less intense, it becomes more inhibited by the noise. If it is made more intense, it begins to inhibit the noise more than the noise inhibits the tone.

There are many second-order effects that have been described, related to the band width of the noise, to matching inhibited tones to free tones, to the increasing steepness of slope as the SPL of the noise is increased, and so on. The relation that we wish to emphasize is the emergence of the tone from "inhibition," as schematically diagramed in Figure 2-8.

Recruitment A phenomenon very similar to the masking or inhibition of a tone by a surrounding band of noise is encountered in ears with certain types of sense-organ im-

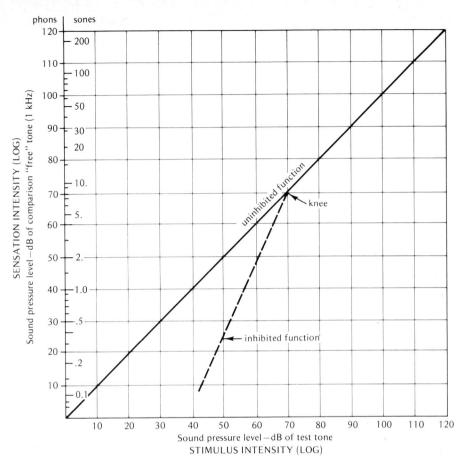

Figure 2-8 Schematic diagram to show the power law function for loudness (solid line) and how masking increases the scope (exponent) of the lower portion of this function (dashed line). A given inhibiting sound (masker) affects only sounds weaker than itself. The overall psychophysical function consists of two straight lines that intersect to form a "knee." The knee is usually 30 dB above the masked threshold. *(After S. S. Stevens and M. Guirao, "Loudness Functions Under Inhibition," Perception and Psychophysiology, 2:459–465; 1967; by permission)*

The scale of stimulus intensity is logarithmic, in decibels.

The scale of sensation magnitude (sones), based on magnitude estimation, is also logarithmic. An alternate scale is the physical intensity of another equally strong sensation such as loudness, brightness, strength of handgrip, and so on, also on a logarithmic scale. The particular alternate scale in this figure is phons, that is, the sound-pressure level of a comparison free tone of 1000 Hz. The relation between sones and phons was determined experimentally. The relation between sones and sound pressure of other tones or bands of noise differs, depending on frequency and bandwidth.

pairment that involve an elevation of threshold. The loudness of a tone grows more rapidly with increase in physical intensity than it does in the normal ear. This corresponds to the steeper slope of the power law for the partially masked tone, but in this case there is no masking noise to provide the "inhibition." This effect, first described by E. P. Fowler, Sr., is known as *recruitment of loudness*, and it will be discussed at greater length in Chapter 4. It is not yet clear how accurately the power law holds for these abnormal ears, and the variability from one individual to another is considerable.

Addition of loudness When two tones or noises are heard at the same time, the combination sounds louder than either one alone. The laws of addition or "integration" of loudness have been studied intensively, but full agreement has not yet been reached on the rule or formula that is most satisfactory. The question is more important for the evaluation of loud noises that are disturbing or annoying than it is for the analysis of impairments of hearing, and for this reason we shall not go into detail but shall merely state a few useful generalizations that have emerged and that give us some idea of how the auditory system deals with complex sounds. The question is difficult because individuals differ in their judgments when matching the loudness of sounds that differ widely in their frequency spectra. Also, when two quite different sounds are heard at the same time, some subjects, according to their own statements, tend to hear them separately and judge the loudness of one or the other; but other subjects "integrate" them and hear the combined loudness as greater than that of either component.

There is no doubt, however, that sounds of nearly the same frequency or relatively narrow bands of noise are heard singly, and one of the basic concepts is that of a *critical band* of frequencies within which interaction or integration of loudness is quite complete for everyone. The overall sound-pressure level within the critical band is all that really matters for loudness or for masking. The width of this band is related also to the pitch or mel scale. One rule is that the critical band for loudness is about 100 mels wide (over most of the frequency range), which is a very convenient coincidence. A critical band is approximately one third of an octave in the middle frequency range, and it does not vary greatly with loudness level, except perhaps near threshold or at very high intensities. The bandwidth in hertz varies from about 90

Hz at the low end to 2000 Hz near 10,000 Hz. The range from 20 to 9300 Hz comprises 22 critical bands.

The concept of the critical band was introduced by Fletcher in 1940, but Fletcher was forced to make one plausible assumption in order to calculate the widths of his bands. Fletcher's bands, now often called "critical ratios," were narrower than our present bands by a factor of two and a half, but they were similarly related to frequency and to the pitch scale.

The critical band for loudness can be measured in several ways. One way is to sound several tones, equally spaced, at nearly the same frequency and then to increase the spacing between them. Listeners compare the loudness of the complex mixture to that of a single tone at the center frequency of the complex. When the overall spacing of the tones exceeds a certain amount, the complex begins to sound louder. (The complex may also be a band of noise of variable bandwidth.)

Another method is to measure the threshold, either the absolute threshold or the masked threshold, for two closely spaced tones or for a band of noise of variable width. The threshold for two such tones is lower than for a single tone, but as more tones are added or as the band of noise is made wider, a critical bandwidth is reached, beyond which the threshold remains constant.

Another test is to determine the masked threshold for a narrow band of noise centered between two pure tones. As the separation of the tones is increased, the masked threshold of the noise remains constant until the separation reaches a critical value, after which the masked threshold decreases rather abruptly. Still another rather similar test is based on the sensitivity of the ear to phase differences.

These various measures of the critical band may not all yield quite the same numerical values, but they are all of the same order of magnitude, and all of them bear very much the same relation to frequency and to the mel scale. The critical band for masking is of practical importance in audiology in relation to the masking of a tone in one ear when testing the threshold of the opposite ear, as in tests of the bone-conduction threshold. Masking is fully efficient, and the loudness of the masker is the least when a critical band of noise, centered on the tone to be masked, is employed. The critical band is also of theoretical importance in the relation to the action of the inner ear in the detection and analysis of sounds and of the central auditory system also.

Formulas for Addition of Loudness

If two or more sounds of rather different frequencies are heard simultaneously, they do not seem as loud as the total sum of the loudness of each of them heard separately. On the other hand, the total loudness is greater than that of the loudest single component. Several empirical formulas have been proposed for calculating the total loudness. In general, we are more concerned with the loudness of noises with continuous spectra, like traffic noise or aircraft noise, and not with a collection of pure tones, like a symphony orchestra, and it is convenient to measure the sound pressure of the noise in octave bands (as in Figure 2-2), or perhaps in third-octave bands. Tabulations are available of the loudness (in sones) of each of the octave bands at various loudness levels (in phons). The simplest formula, that of Stevens, states that

$$S_t = S_m + 0.3 \, (\Sigma S - S_m).$$

That is to say, the over-all loudness (S_t) is equal to the loudness of the loudest octave band (S_m) plus three-tenths of the sum of the loudnesses of all the remaining bands. The

factor of three-tenths is strictly empirical. If third-octave bands are used, the factor is 0.15.

Various tabulations, charts, and nomograms to facilitate the calculations by this (and by other) methods have been published, but we shall not go into detail. For us it is enough to know that the loudness of a noise with a complex spectrum is dominated by, but not wholly determined by, the loudest part of its spectrum, and that addition is nonlinear in that the whole is less than the sum of the parts. There are interactions, probably of the nature of mutual inhibition or something analogous to partial masking, among the different octave bands of a noise.

Examples of loudness When the sound-level meter was first devised it was called a noise-level meter, and its designers tried to make it deal with sounds in approximately the same way the ear does, so that its readings (in decibels) would correspond to the loudness (sones) that we hear. Two sets of filters (the so-called A network and the B network) were provided. Their passbands corresponded roughly to the shapes of the human equal-loudness contours for faint and for moderate sounds, respectively. For example, the ear is much less sensitive to the 60-Hz hum that is usually present to some extent in the music that comes from our radios than it is to frequencies from 800 to 4000 Hz in the upper part of the musical range. If the music is soft, we may hear only the music, even though the hum is physically more intense than the music. If this is the case, the overall level in decibels measured by the sound-level meter with the "flat" or "C" setting (no filter) will be determined chiefly by the hum. In this situation there is simply no practical relation between the loudness that we hear and the decibel reading on the meter.

For loud sounds like factory noise or heavy traffic, the C setting was to be used.

For a number of years the meter was used consistently according to the original rules, and many characteristic "noise levels" in decibels were published. But after 1940, when octave-band filters came into general use, the A and B networks were used less and less, and the early noise levels measured with them were often confused with overall sound levels measured with the "flat" C setting. About 1960, however, the use of the A setting was suddenly revived, for three reasons: (1) It corresponds much better to what we actually hear at low levels. (2) Coincidentally, long exposure to the dBA values correspond quite well to the risk of injury to hearing from long exposure to loud noises of different spectral composition (see Chapter 4). (3) The dBA values also correspond fairly well to the amount of interference with speech communication caused by moderate sounds. Specifications for maximum allowable noises are written almost exclusively in terms of dBA (see Chapters 9 and 16). Some approximate A-weighted sound levels are shown in Figure 2-9.

Figure 2-9 includes some numbers on the sound level of speech, but this introduces a new difficulty. The sound-pressure level of speech varies from instant to instant, from one word to the next, and from sound to sound within the word. The momentary instantaneous peaks of pressure are 10 to as much as 20 dB above the overall long-time average. The needle of the sound-level meter dances up and down, and we must be content to settle for its "average maximum swing." A rather vague rule indeed! Abrupt brief sounds like a pistol shot or a hammer blow give particular difficulty. Certain special meters called "impact meters" deal with them better than does the simpler sound-level meter, but even these are not yet fully satisfactory, and the measurements made with them are not easy to interpret. For all of these reasons it requires some special in-

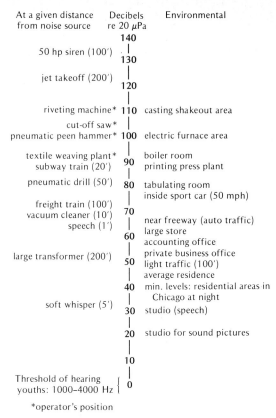

Figure 2-9 Typical A-weighted sound levels measured with a sound-level meter. *(From A. P. G. Peterson and E. E. Gross, Jr.,* Handbook of Noise Measurement, *7th ed., General Radio, Concord, Mass.; by permission)*

struction and training to use even the ordinary sound-level meter properly and to interpret the measurements made with it.

Short-term summation of loudness In the previous section we have referred to brief sounds like those of speech and also transients like pistol shots, hammer blows, and other "impulsive" sounds. The reading of a meter in response to an impulsive sound depends largely on the ballistic characteristics of the meter, including its damping and overshoot. The human ear, somewhat like a meter, integrates the energy of brief sounds to some extent. For example, as faint tones are made very brief, less than a fifth of a second, their thresholds rise. If they last for only a few cycles, the threshold may be 10 dB or more higher than for a prolonged tone of the same sound-pressure level. It requires about 200 milliseconds (abbreviated ms) for a steady tone to reach its full loudness. The ear actually behaves as though some quantity that we can call "excitation" is produced in proportion to the intensity of the sound and decays exponentially with a characteristic time constant. Such situations are familiar in neurophysiology. The integration and decay probably occur in the central nervous system and not in the ear.

Threshold Shift, Fatigue, and Adaptation

There are several quite distinct changes in the sensitivity of the ear that are produced by exposure to sound and can be detected either during the exposure or after it ends. The nature of the effect and the time it lasts depend greatly on the intensity of the exposure tone or noise. Because of the variety of conditions and effects, many terms have been employed, including *adaptation*, which implies a simple physiological adjustment, like dark adaptation in vision; *fatigue*, which implies a temporary exhaustion of a reserve of some sort; *residual masking*, which is confusing; and *acoustic trauma*, which clearly implies injury. A more neutral and less confusing term is *threshold shift*. We shall have more to say about threshold shifts, both permanent and temporary, in Chapter 4 when we consider the effects of exposure to high-intensity industrial noises.

To emphasize the complexity of the situation, we point out that at least three or four quite different mechanisms have been identified that can, and presumably do, contribute to the reduced sensitivity or reduced output of the ear. Unfortunately, the part played

by each in various situations is not clear. One of these mechanisms is a reflex contraction of the muscles of the middle ear (the intra-aural or stapedius reflex), rather like the constriction of the pupil or an eyeblink. Another is the action of efferent nerve fibers from the brain to the inner ear. Another is the physiological decrease in rate of discharge (the "adaptation") of nerve fibers to steady levels of stimulation. Another is an unspecified change, either physical, chemical, or both, in the sensory cells of the ear. Another is outright physical rupture and destruction of nerves, sensory cells, or supporting structures. Another is adaptation or "habituation" in the central nervous system.

"Per-stimulatory adaptation" refers to a diminution in loudness that occurs rather rapidly after the onset of a tone. It is demonstrated by making loudness balances between a stimulated ear and the opposite unstimulated ear. (This experiment is not quite as simple as it sounds.) The reduction in loudness level is rather considerable for a tone of moderate intensity.

The temporary threshold shift in certain pathological conditions may be so great that the tone simply becomes inaudible with an exposure of less than 30 seconds. In normal ears a short-lasting elevation of threshold for a test pulse usually develops rapidly, and recovery also takes place rapidly. Sometimes, however, the complete recovery takes place in two or three phases. The elevated threshold falls, then it rises or "bounces" to a second maximum at about 2 minutes after the end of the exposure tone, and then settles down to its stable level.

In general, threshold shifts following moderate exposures are rather quick adjustments, not always clearly related in extent to the strength and duration of exposure. The effect is greatest at the frequency of the exposure tone. At sound-pressure levels of about 90 dB and higher, however, a curious effect occurs. Threshold shift develops more rapidly, with increasing intensity and duration of exposure, as we would expect; but the frequency at which the shift is greatest is no longer than that of the exposure tone but now lies about half an octave above it. Lesser amounts of shift occur far into the frequency range above the exposure frequency, but little or no shift occurs more than about half an octave below it. This unexplained distribution in frequency and a slower rate of recovery should help us to distinguish this high-intensity variety of threshold shift from the quick shifts and adaptations that occur at lower sound-pressure levels. The former is more suggestive of a severe fatigue in the usual sense and possibly the beginning of injury, although followed by repair.

Backward Masking

Another effect in the time domain is known as "backward masking." A brief test tone is followed after a short interval by a louder and longer burst of noise. Even though it may start as much as 50 to 100 ms later, the louder sound makes the earlier fainter sound inaudible. Clearly this effect takes place in the central nervous system where the excitation from the strong stimulus somehow overtakes and masks the earlier input. Masking involves much more than the basic physical interaction of sound waves at the physical level.

Binaural Hearing: Directionality

We have already noted that two ears are better than one in detecting faint signals, either in a background of noise or in quiet, and that sounds are heard louder with two ears than with one. But by far the most important contribution of binaural hearing is to allow us to hear sounds from different sources as coming from different directions. Of course we are sometimes confused by echoes, and our sense of direction is confined to the horizontal plane, assuming the head to be upright; but in the primitive biological function of warning and identification, the sense of direction of the source is very important information.

We can learn something about the direction of a sound source with only one ear, if we search, and scan, and notice at which orientation of our head the sound is loudest. In this case we take advantage of the directionality of the ear, set as it is in the large acoustic baffle formed by the side of the head. But stereophonic hearing is far better than this. The sense of direction is immediate, and two sound sources are heard as clearly separate in space.

Two sets of clues provide the directionality. One of these is the relative intensity of corresponding sound waves entering the two ears. The differences in intensity, due to the "sound shadow" of the head, are considerable for high frequencies, and for frequencies above 2000 or 3000 Hz this loudness difference is the chief clue. At very low frequencies, however, the intensity differences are small, and the other clue, difference in time of arrival of corresponding sound waves, becomes dominant. The length of acoustic path around the head is great enough to provide for something approaching a millisecond of time delay. The two ears are sensitive to time differences of the order of a hundredth of a millisecond, enough to determine the direction (azimuth) within a few degrees of arc. The time differences are less effective above 1000 Hz, partly because at 1000 Hz the time difference between waves is 1 ms, and one sine wave is just like the one before and the one following. Thus the time differences above 1000 Hz become ambiguous.

Time differences and intensity differences usually reinforce one another, but if we present the sounds through earphones we can manipulate them independently. Time differences can be traded for decibels in the task of keeping the apparent source of the sound "centered." A curious effect occurs with earphones, however. The sound does not seem to come from straight ahead, even when timing and intensity are both equal, but to be *inside* the head at the midline. A little imbalance shifts the apparent source to right or to left, and if the difference is considerable, the source seems to be at one ear canal or the other. (Sometimes the sound seems to move around the back of the head or neck, but usually it stays inside.)

The centering of the image of a sound source in the midline of the head when the sound waves are simultaneous and equally intense in the two ears has been used as a delicate test for equal loudness. Centering the sound image is an easier, quicker, and more reliable judgment than listening to two tones alternately and adjusting them to equal loudness. Unfortunately, however, the processes in the central nervous system that lead to the sensation of "center image"are not the same as those for "equal loudness." Both are related to the intensity of the inputs of the two ears, but in different ways. This has led to difficulties in certain audiological tests in which it was assumed that the operations were identical.

LISTENING IN NOISE

When a sound from a discrete nearby source, such as a friend talking to us, is heard in a background of noise such as traffic noise or many other voices competing loudly in the "cocktail-party effect," we have some difficulty understanding our friend's words, and we hear them much more clearly with two ears than with one. One of our ears is likely to have some relative advantage of being turned more or less toward him, but in addition we notice that the sound to which are are listening comes from one place, and the noise comes from some other place or

from many places. Somehow this makes the voice easier to "track," and the noise less confusing. These advantages of binaural hearing become very important in relation to the use of hearing aids, wherein the inability to hear voices clearly in noisy places is a major complaint. We shall return to this problem and the use of binaural hearing aids in Chapters 10 and 11.

In general a listener can detect signals in noise, and can understand speech in the presence of a background noise, better when he uses two ears than when he uses only one. A person can easily demonstrate this to himself in a roomful of talking people when he wishes to understand the conversation of only one. If he finds himself just barely understanding that speech, he will observe a marked decrease in its intelligibility and sometimes its detectability if he simply puts a finger in one ear.

An exception to this general case has also been reported under somewhat artificial conditions provided by binaural earphones. If the phones are wired in such a way that both the noise and the signal to be detected are in phase at the two ears, the detectability of the signal is no better than, and sometimes worse than, if listening were with one ear only. If, however, the circuits are so arranged that the noise is in phase at the two ears and the signal is out of phase, or vice versa, the detectability is much better than in the binaural homophasic case or the monaural case. This release from masking provided by changing one, but not both, of the interaural phase relations has sometimes been called *binaural unmasking*. The difference between the two binaural cases, one in which the noise and signal phases are both the same as opposed to the condition in which they are opposite to each other, is referred to as the *masking level difference* (MLD).

Much attention has been given recently to the problem of detecting signals that are very nearly masked in noise. Noise is a random affair and is best described in statistical terms. It appears that the performance of an observer should be described in the same way, perhaps because his nervous system is full of "physiological noise." His "threshold" varies at random from moment to moment. Typically, he is asked to state whether he did or did not detect a signal in a given interval of time during which it might or might not have been presented. For a given signal-to-noise ratio, he will correctly report the signal as present in a certain percentage of trials and as absent in others. He will also, however, give a few "false alarms," stating that he heard the signal when it was not there, and he will make some "misses" in failing to report some signals that were present. The listener can deliberately change or be induced by proper instruction to change his criterion from a cautious conservative attitude to a liberal take-a-chance point of view, or vice versa. The instructions and the basis of reward or "payoff" are important. With a liberal attitude, the observer will score many more hits but at the expense of more false alarms. Forty years ago we argued

about the "maybe-maybe" threshold of the psychologist and the "honest-to-goodness" threshold of the engineer. Now we know that the relation among hits, misses, and false positives is quite lawful. A graphic representation of the relation is known as the *receiver operating characteristic* (ROC) curve. We shall not go into detail, but merely emphasize that here another variable in psychophysics, namely the attitude of the listener, has been brought under experimental control and mathematical description. The analysis allows us to measure separately two elements that determine the response of the listener. One is his *strategy*, liberal or conservative; the other is his basic *sensitivity*.

It is also possible to record and make use of the degree of confidence that the observer feels with respect to each particular judgment. The "detection theory" has already made significant contributions to our theoretical understanding of the nature of the psychophysical threshold and the processes of detection and discrimination, and it influences the design and conduct of many audiological tests.

SUGGESTED READINGS AND REFERENCES

American National Standards Institute, Inc., 1430 Broadway, New York, N.Y. 10018:
ANSI S1.4—1971. *Specification for Sound Level Meters.*
ANSI S1.6—1967 (R1971). *Preferred Frequencies and Band Numbers for Acoustical Measurements.*
ANSI S1.8—1969 (R1974). *Preferred Reference Quantities for Acoustical Levels.*
ANSI S1.11—1966 (R1971). *Specifications for Octave, Half-Octave, and Third-Octave Band Filter Sets.*
ANSI S1.13—1971. *Methods for the Measurement of Sound Pressure Levels.*
Bergeijk, W. A. van, J. R. Pierce, and E. E. David, Jr. *Waves and the Ear.* New York: Doubleday, 1960.
A very readable little paperback.
Fletcher, H. *Speech and Hearing.* New York: D. Van Nostrand Company, 1929.
A classic, now out of print.

————. *Speech and Hearing in Communication*. New York: D. Van Nostrand Company, 1953.
A rather extensive revision of his earlier monograph.

Peterson, A. P. G., and E. E. Gross. *Handbook of Noise Measurement*. Concord, Mass.: General Radio Company, 1972.
Clear, practical, and up to date.

Pierce, J. R., and E. E. David, Jr. *Man's World of Sound*. New York: Doubleday, 1958.
A very readable and informative introductory treatment.

Stevens, S. S. (ed.). *Handbook of Experimental Psychology*. New York: John Wiley & Sons, 1951.
Chapter 25 ("Basic Correlates of the Auditory Stimulus," by J. C. R. Licklider) and Chapter 26 ("The Perception of Speech," by J. C. R. Licklider and G. A. Miller) are especially pertinent.

Stevens, S. S. "Calculating Loudness," *Noise Control*, 3:11–22 (1957).
A semipopular article with useful graphs.

————. *Psychophysics: Introduction to Its Perceptual, Neural and Social Prospects*. G. Stevens (ed.). New York: John Wiley & Sons, 1975.
The posthumous publication of Dr. Stevens' final, wide-ranging discussion of his "power law."

————. "The Psychophysics of Sensory Function," Chap. 1 in *Sensory Communication*, Walter A. Rosenblith (ed.). Cambridge: M.I.T. Press, and New York: John Wiley & Sons, 1961.
An authoritative discussion.

————, and H. Davis. *Hearing: Its Psychology and Physiology*. New York: John Wiley & Sons, 1938.
This monograph for advanced students is now out of print. The second part, physiology, is now chiefly of historical interest.

————, F. Warshofsky, and the Editors of LIFE. *Sound and Hearing*. New York: Time, Inc., 1965.
A wide popular survey, beautifully illustrated.

Yost, W. A., and D. W. Nielsen. *Fundamentals of Hearing: An Introduction*. New York: Holt, Rinehart and Winston, 1977.
A beautifully illustrated, well-written presentation of the basics of audition at an introductory level. An excellent supplement to Chapters 2 and 3.

Hallowell Davis, M.D.

3

Anatomy and Physiology of the Auditory System

The structure of the ear and how it gathers sound waves and brings them to the sensory cells are subjects about which we can be rather definite. Some study of both the structure and the function of the various parts of the ear is needed if we are to understand the different types of deafness and the means of preventing or circumventing them.

THE OUTER EAR AND THE CANAL

The external ear, the *pinna* or *auricle*, is not very important acoustically. Man has lost or never acquired the three main functions of the external ear of most animals: (1) to collect and focus the energy of a large cross section of sound waves from a particular direction; (2) to make possible precise judgments of the direction of sound by turning the ears (instead of the whole head) until the sound becomes loudest; and (3) to keep water and dirt out of the ear canal, as seals and moles do, by special valvelike movements of some of the external parts that for us are rudimentary rigid structures.

The human pinna does, however, contribute a few decibels to the sensitivity for high frequencies, due mostly to the acoustic resonance of the concha (see Figure 3-1). In addition, its complicated shape and its partial flexibility favor the making and holding of a good acoustic seal with individually fitted earmolds for hearing aids (see Chapter 10).

The human ear canal is irregularly oval in cross section and varies from in-

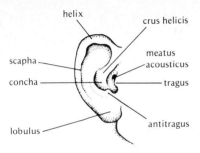

Figure 3-1   The outer ear.

dividual to individual in details of size and shape quite as much as does the external ear —to the distress of those whose task it was during World War II to devise a simple earplug for all ears for protection against the blasts of heavy artillery and antiaircraft batteries. In some cases the canal is nearly round; in others it is little more than a vertical slit. The canal runs nearly horizontally toward the center of the head for a little less than an inch (2.5 cm) as shown in Figure 3-2, and there it dead-ends at the drum membrane or *tympanic membrane.* The skin of the outer portion of the canal bears stiff hairs and secretes a dark, bitter-tasting wax (cerumen) that as a rule discourages the entry of insects and keeps the skin of the canal and drum membrane from drying out.

THE MIDDLE EAR

The middle ear (see Figures 3-3 and 3-4) includes the tympanic membrane and the air-filled cavity behind it, as well as its contents, including the set of tiny bones, the *ossicles.* The entire structure is known as the eardrum from its resemblance to the familiar musical instrument. In popular usage the drum membrane that terminates the external canal is called the "eardrum" but it is only one surface of a three-dimensional structure. It is more accurate to call it the *drumhead* or *drum membrane.*

With proper illumination and when the

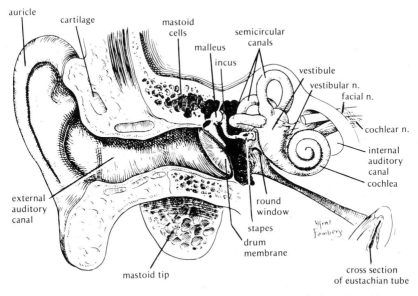

Figure 3-2   In this semidiagrammatic drawing of the ear, the inner ear is shown with the temporal bone cut away to reveal the semicircular canals, the vestibule, and the cochlea. The cochlea has been turned slightly from its normal orientation to show its coils more clearly. The opening for nerves through the bone to the brain cavity of the skull is quite diagrammatic. The eustachian tube actually runs forward as well as downward and inward. The muscles of the middle ear, shown in Figures 3-3 and 3-4, are omitted.

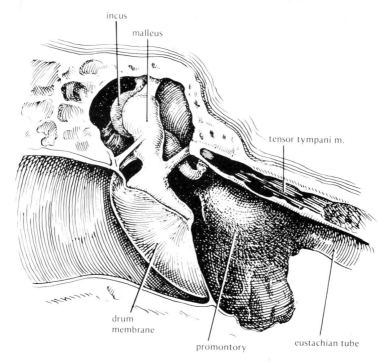

Figure 3-3 This view of the drum membrane (partly cut away) and the middle ear is from a slightly more lateral angle than that in Figure 3-2. The tensor tympani muscle lies in a separate canal (partly cut away) just above the eustachian tube. Its tendon turns at nearly a right angle in the tendonous sheath from which it emerges.

canal is straightened by pulling the pinna gently backward and upward, the drumhead can be seen as a pearl-gray wall at the end of the canal. The thin, tough, flexible fibrous membrane is attached to the bony wall of the canal by a tough ring of fibrous tissue, the *annulus*, and forms a diagonal partition as shown in the diagram in Figure 3-3. It is not stretched flat across but is conical in shape like the cone of a loudspeaker. It points upward and inward into the middle-ear cavity behind it. The angle of the cone, about 135 degrees, is very favorable for stiffness.

The stiff central portion moves as a whole when driven by waves of sound pressure, except for frequencies above 2000 Hz. It can do so because the outer edge is slack or folded, again like the cone of a loudspeaker (see Figures 3-3 and 3-6). Its area is about 0.67 cm² (or a tenth of a square inch) on the average. Through the translucent membrane can sometimes be seen, like the hour hand of a clock at 11 o'clock (in the right ear), the "handle" of the hammer, the *malleus*, the first of the chain of ossicles that transmit the vibrations of the drumhead to the inner ear. The malleus serves also to keep the membrane stretched tight and cone-shaped under the influence of a small muscle, the *tensor tympani*, that attaches to it near the base of the handle.

The enlarged round head of the malleus nestles into a well-fitting socket in the anvil or *incus*, the second of the ossicles, and for sounds of ordinary intensities the two move together as a single unit. They execute a rocking motion as the drumhead vibrates, turning around a horizontal axis just behind the upper edge of the drumhead and perpendicular to the external canal (see Figure 3-5). The axis on which they turn is formed by a short, axlelike projection of the malleus and another from the incus. The projections are attached by firm but flexible ligaments to the walls of the middle-ear cavity. The bony mass of the ossicles is delicately balanced around the axis so that the inertia (or, more accurately, the *turning moment*) of the system is small, and thus the ossicles do not tend to strain and rattle when they vibrate. The incus ends in a long, slender, curved tip near the center of the middle-ear cavity and in contact with the tiny head of the stirrup (*stapes*), the last of the three ossicles.

The stirrup is well named from its shape,

and its oval footplate is sealed by the *annular ligament* into the *oval window* that looks into the inner ear. The stapes moves in and out like a piston at low and moderate amplitudes of movement. At high amplitudes, such as those reached by really loud low-frequency sounds, the movement of the stapes is restrained by the annular ligament. The ligament is thicker and narrower at the posterior than at the anterior end of the oval window, and as a consequence the footplate of the stapes swings like a door, with its hinge at the posterior end. The classical descriptions of the movements of the ossicles are based on observations of movements of sufficient amplitude to be clearly visible. These movements are nonlinear, but the

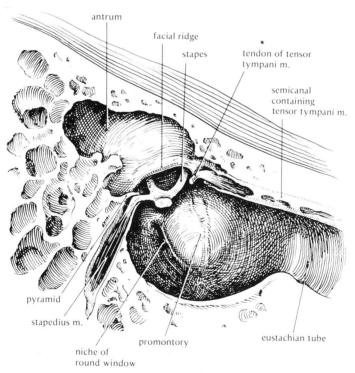

Figure 3-4   The middle ear is here viewed from the external canal, with the drum membrane, the malleus, the incus, and some of the surrounding temporal bone cut away. The tendon of the stapedius muscle turns at an angle as it emerges from the tip of the "pyramid." When the stapedius contracts, the stapes rocks on the posterior (left in this figure) end of its footplate so that the footplate swings outward like a door into the cavity of the middle ear. The facial nerve runs in a bony canal in the facial ridge just above the stapes.

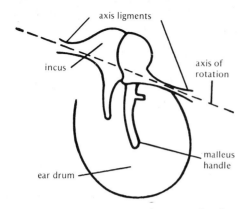

Figure 3-5 Diagram of the axis of rotation of malleus and incus. *(From von Békésy and Rosenblith, in S. S. Stevens, ed.,* Handbook of Experimental Psychology, *John Wiley & Sons, 1951; by permission)*

smaller linear oscillations are actually more typical. The restraint of movement by the annular ligament is one of a series of mechanical restraints in the middle and inner ear that protect the sense organ from rupture at high amplitudes. They do this at the expense of more or less harmonic distortion.

The tendon of another tiny muscle, the *stapedius*, attaches to the neck of the stapes. It pulls the stapes outward and backward, thus counteracting the opposite pull of the tensor tympani. The two muscles work together to take up any slack in the ossicular chain and to stiffen the whole system. The balance between them is so good that the drum membrane itself scarcely moves at all when they contract.

The middle-ear cavity is a narrow cleft between the slanting eardrum and the irregular bony wall opposite it and is nearly filled by the ossicles. Its capacity varies from 1 to 2 cm³. However, it opens directly into the air cells of the temporal bone behind, and the *eustachian tube* opens into its anterior wall about midway between floor and roof. The two muscles that we have mentioned are not located in the middle-ear cavity itself. The tensor tympani lies alongside the eustachian

tube, and the stapedius in a little bony tunnel all its own. The longest dimension of the middle ear—the vertical dimension—is about 1.25 cm or half an inch, and a magnifying glass is required to appreciate the fine mechanical architecture of the ossicles with balanced suspension and their adjusting muscles.

Another opening between the middle ear and the inner ear is the *round window*, located just under the oval window. It is closed by an elastic membrane rather like the tympanic membrane, but thinner, much smaller, and stretched flat. This opening serves as an elastic termination of the acoustic pathway in the inner ear, as shown in Figure 3-6. If the walls of the inner ear were completely rigid, the stapes could not move in the oval window, because the fluid within is practically incompressible. Pressure could be transmitted, but the mechanical movements would be negligible, and it is mechanical movement that ultimately stimulates the sensory cells.

The air-filled cavity of the middle ear and the mastoid air cells that lead from it as a blind alley are ventilated periodically through the eustachian tube. The tube connects the middle ear with the back of the nasal cavity, called the *nasopharynx*. The first portion runs through the temporal bone. It is permanently open, like a funnel, in contrast to the longer, wider portion toward the pharynx, whose walls are composed of cartilage and flexible membrane, and which is normally collapsed. The eustachian tube enters the nasopharynx diagonally under a valve-like flap of tissue that closes the orifice except during certain movements, such as swallowing and yawning. The tube sometimes also opens during a sneeze or a cough or when the air pressure is increased by blowing the nose.

The function of the eustachian tube in equalizing the air pressure inside and outside the eardrum is described more fully later. Immediate equalization of small changes, such as those caused by contraction of the tensor tympani muscle, is provided by a small, slack segment of the eardrum itself at its top and above the axis of rotation of the malleus. Equalization for a longer term is needed, however, because any air bubbles left in the tissues of the body are gradually dissolved and absorbed by the blood: first the oxygen and then, slowly, the nitrogen. The air in the middle ear must therefore be replenished periodically.

The middle ear, with its drum and ossicles, increases the sensitivity of hearing for airborne sound. The drum receives energy

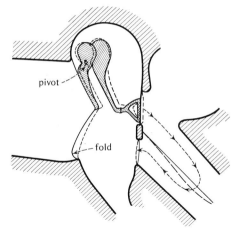

Figure 3-6 Schematic diagram of the tympanic membrane, the ossicles, and the basilar membrane. The solid figures of the ossicles and the solid lines for the tympanic, the basilar, and the round-window membranes show the positions of these structures at rest. The broken outlines of the ossicles and the broken lines for the membranes show their directions of movement during inward displacement of the tympanic membrane by a sound wave. The cross shows the axis around which the ossicles rotate. The dot shows their center of gravity. The stapes is drawn at right angles to its true position in order to show its motion clearly. At high intensities it rocks around an axis through the posterior edge of the round window. The movement of the stapes, for moderate tones, is almost certainly like a piston, not a door. The "fold" in the tympanic membrane and the amplitude of movement are exaggerated. *(Modified from Stevens and Davis,* Hearing: Its Psychology and Physiology, *John Wiley & Sons, 1938)*

from a relatively large cross section of light, tenuous, highly compressible air. The energy is delivered through the ossicles to the smaller footplate of the stapes, about one-thirtieth the area of the drum. This reduction of area favors the efficient transfer of the energy to the dense, watery, almost incompressible fluid that fills the inner ear. From a technical point of view the membrane and ossicles represent a very efficient impedance-matching device between the two media: air and water. The total force is the same, the pressure is increased, and the volume displacement is reduced. The drum and ossicles, thereby increase the sensitivity of the ear appreciably. Loss of drum and ossicles causes some hearing loss, but not a very serious one. Simple interruption of the train of ossicles reduces the sensitivity of about 25 dB. A simple hole in the drum may cause only a 5- or 10-dB loss.

The ear and its drum membrane and ossicles probably serve also to protect the inner ear from injury by loud sounds. The air enclosed in the rather small middle ear must exert some cushioning effect for low tones because loud tones of low frequency have a very appreciable amplitude of movement. Just how important this effect may be has not yet been determined. The joint between the malleus and the incus also yields elastically when the sound waves become very powerful, and at very high amplitudes the stapes begins to rock in a different and less efficient direction, sideways instead of lengthwise of the footplate.

INTRA-AURAL REFLEXES

The contractions of the muscles of the middle ear stiffen the drum membrane and the ossicular chain and thereby reduce the transmission of low tones. Contraction in response to loud sound is set off by reflex action from the lower centers of the brain a few hundredths of a second after a loud sound first reaches the eardrum. The increased tension of the membrane also raises the "natural period" of vibration of drum and ossicles. The net result is a rather considerable loss of sensitivity for low and for high tones and a rather slight loss for the middle range. The most important practical result is probably the protection the intra-aural muscles give to both the middle and the inner ear against possible damage by large amplitudes of movement. We have used the general term *intra-aural reflex* for the reflex contraction of one or both of the intra-aural muscles in response to sound. It is sometimes called the *acoustic reflex*. Also, because the stapedius muscle reacts much more vigorously to sound, it is known as the *stapedius reflex*. The stapedius reflex is bilateral even if only one ear is stimulated.

Contractions of the tensor tympani muscle are evoked by tickling the skin near the entrance to the ear canal or by a tiny puff of air directed into the corner of the eye.

The stapedius reflex has been studied extensively by detecting changes in the *acoustic impedance* of the ear (see Chapter 8). The method depends on measuring the proportion of the energy of a test tone that is reflected back from the drumhead. The changes in impedance can be analyzed into changes in stiffness and in resistance, respectively. When a tone of 90 dB or so is first turned on, the reflex contraction is brisk, but apparently it is not well maintained. It is much better maintained if the stimulating sound is an irregular noise. The threshold of the reflex is well above the threshold for hearing, somewhere in the middle range of intensities. The measurements of acoustic impedance and the intra-aural reflexes are useful tools for several audiological tests, which are described in Chapter 8.

Another method for study of the action of the stapedius and tensor tympani muscles is to implant electrodes in them in chronic animal experiments. The electrical output of each muscle (its electromyogram) signals each contraction and its relative intensity. Apparently these muscles are very active, at least in cats, and participate in almost all patterns of movement that involve much of the musculature of the head and neck.

In human psychoacoustics it is still a question how much in the way of adaptation or other changes of threshold (or loudness) should be attributed to the activity of the intra-aural muscles. They are certainly involved more or less directly and probably significantly in all experiments at 90 dB SPL and above—and perhaps below as well.

THE INNER EAR

The inner ear is a series of channels and chambers in the temporal bone that are so complicated in shape that they are known as the labyrinth (Figure 3-7). In these bony canals, filled with clear watery fluid, lie a corresponding series of delicate membranous tubes and sacs, filled also with a watery fluid and containing sensory cells and their supporting structures. The central portion, the *vestibule*, of the labyrinth joins the snail-like coil of the organ of hearing, the *cochlea*, and the loops of the three *semicircular canals* that form the sense organ for turning in space. In the vestibule itself lie the *utricle*, sensitive to the pull of gravity and to acceleration (as in an elevator or automobile), and the *saccule*. The latter apparently shares the functions of the utricle, although in fishes, which have no cochlea, it seems to be the sense organ for vibration and whatever true hearing a fish may have.

These different mechanical senses, responsive to sound and to acceleration, have very similar sensory cells that are special-

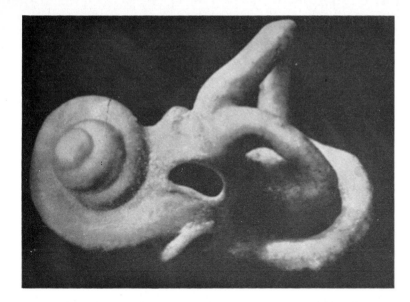

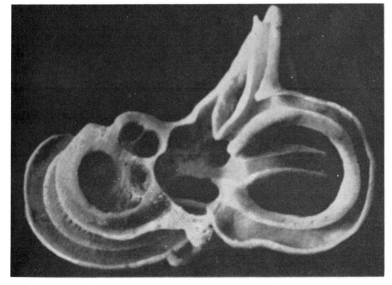

Figure 3-7 *Above:* The left bony labyrinth of an infant, removed from the substance of the temporal bone. The oval window appears clearly in the center. Below it, seen obliquely, is the protruding rim of bone around the opening of the round window.

Below: The right bony labyrinth, viewed from within the head, opened to show the hollow vestibule and canals. Note the spiral shelf of bone that partly subdivides the canal of the cochlea (lower left). The hollow central core of the cochlea, through which the nerve emerges, is clearly shown. The round window (lower center), with rim partly cut away, opening into the canal of the cochlea, also is clearly shown. *(Rudinger)*

ized organs of touch. The cochlea "feels" the alternating mechanical movements caused by sound waves. Gravity is felt by the utricle as it pulls on tiny grains of calcium carbonate attached to microscopic hairlike extensions of the sensory cells. The cells at the enlarged ends of the semicircular canals feel the pressure of the fluid within the canals, since it tends to lag behind, because of its inertia, when we turn our heads.

Two practical consequences of the close anatomical association between the nonauditory labyrinthine sense organs and the cochlea are: (1) the symptom of dizziness (vertigo) is often associated with certain forms of deafness; (2) tests of the function of the nonauditory labyrinth are very helpful in the differential diagnosis of certain forms of hearing loss. Other details of this part of the labyrinth need not concern us here.

The cochlea is coiled like a snail in a flat spiral of two and a half turns (Figure 3-8). The canal within is a little over an inch (35 mm) long and ends blindly at the apex. The canal is partly divided into upper (*vestibular*) and lower (*tympanic*) galleries (scalae) by a spiral shelf of bone protruding outward from the inner wall of the passage like a shelf along the inner wall of a circular staircase. The division of the two galleries is completed by a fibrous flexible membrane, the *basilar membrane*, that stretches across from the lower edge of the bony shelf to the spiral ligament that attaches it to the outer wall. The basilar membrane and the shelf both terminate a millimeter or two short of the end of the galleries so that the two galleries join at the apex of the cochlea. On the vestibular surface of the basilar membrane lies the membranous tube that contains the sensory cells and their supporting structures, known as the *organ of Corti*. The basilar membrane is just over an inch (32 mm) long and tapers in width from about 0.5 mm near the apex down to 0.05 mm at the base of the cochlea near the oval window. The oval window opens into the vestibule near the end of the vestibular gallery, and the round window opens into the tympanic gallery at the base of the cochlea.

We have mentioned the membranous tube that contains the sensory cells of the cochlea. This is part of the *membranous labyrinth* that follows the general pattern of the channels of the *bony labyrinth* (Figure 3-7) and encloses all of the sense organs. The membranous labyrinth is a closed system. It contains a watery fluid, *endolymph*, that differs significantly in chemical composition from the *perilymph* that surrounds it and fills the remainder of the bony labyrinth. The peri-

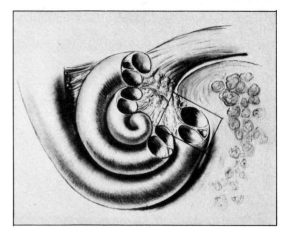

Figure 3-8 The cochlea, opened to show cross sections of its turns and also the distribution of the nerve to the turns. The area in the rectangle is shown enlarged in Figure 4-10.

lymph has very nearly the same composition as the cerebrospinal fluid that bathes the brain and spinal cord, and in fact there is a small channel, the *perilymphatic duct*, that connects the perilymphatic space with the cranial cavity.

The endolymph of the cochlea is apparently secreted and perhaps reabsorbed also by a very vascular glandular structure, the *stria vascularis*, that lies along the outer wall of the endolymphatic space or *scala media*. The scala media is triangular in cross section. Its bottom, in the conventional view of Figure 3-9, is the basilar membrane and the special structures of the organ of Corti attached to it; the outer wall is largely the stria vascularis; and the third side is a very thin membrane, *Reissner's membrane*, that separates the endolymph of scala media from the perilymph of scala vestibuli. The basilar membrane and the structures attached to it plus Reissner's membrane are sometimes called the "cochlear partition" because, with the bony spiral lamina, they divide scala vestibuli from scala tympani. This overall term is a convenient simplification when we are talking about mechanical movements and acoustic properties. We shall simplify even further and usually speak only of the basilar membrane. This is legitimate because the basilar membrane provides nearly all the stiffness, mass, and acoustic resistance of the partition and thus determines its acoustic properties. Reissner's membrane is acoustically "transparent," although it is a good chemical and electrical barrier.

The organ of Corti, which contains and supports the sensory cells, is rather complicated in structure. It is stiff mechanically, and it protects the sensory cells from movement and deformation except at the precise place on their upper surface where the minute acoustic vibrations cause the first step in the physiological excitation that leads to setting up nerve impulses. Figure 3-9 shows a typical cross section of the organ of Corti in a guinea pig.

The heavy *pillars of Corti,* which are cells stiffened by intracellular filaments, join at

their tops to form a series of triangular arches. The basilar membrane forms the base. The space within is the *tunnel of Corti.* The knobs or plates at the upper ends of the pillars form part of a stiff upper surface of the organ of Corti, the *reticular lamina.* This surface includes also the platelike upper ends of specialized supporting cells, *Deiters' cells,* and of the sensory cells. The latter are set into the reticular lamina much like rows of small manhole covers in a tile pavement. The supporting structure is completed by the somewhat softer outer wall of *Hensen's cells* and the inner supporting cells near the inner pillars of Corti. A solid ridge of fibrous tissue, the *limbus,* is firmly attached to the upper surface of the bony spiral lamina. The limbus provides attachment for one edge of Reissner's membrane and also for the *tectorial membrane.* The tectorial membrane lies on the reticular lamina and is attached at its outer edge to Hensen's cells.

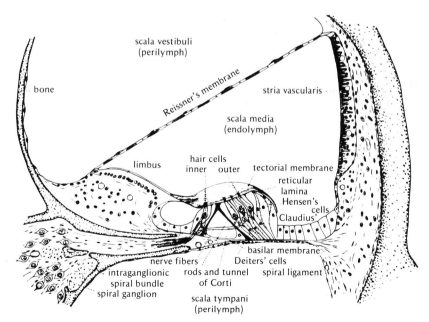

Figure 3-9   Cross-sectional drawing of the canal in the second turn of a guinea pig's cochlea. The human cochlea is very similar to this. The position corresponding to this section can be identified in Figure 3-8 by the triangular cross section of the scala media within the guide rectangle. Note the nerve cell bodies in the spiral ganglion at the left.

The tectorial membrane is a viscous, slow-flowing jelly stiffened by a system of fibers that arise from the outer edge of the limbus. The tectorial membrane is thus a long ribbon attached firmly along one edge to the limbus and more flexibly at its outer edge to the organ of Corti. The tectorial membrane can swing up and down, rather stiffly, like the cover of a book. Within the restriction of its double attachment to the organ of Corti, it can also slide across the reticular lamina as the two structures move up and down together, as illustrated in Figure 3-11. This sliding, shearing action stimulates the sensory cells by bending the fine hairs or *cilia,* which project up from the sensory cells or *hair cells* and are embedded in or attached to the lower surface of the tectorial membrane. Perhaps the final action is a tilting or bending of the surface from which the cilia arise.

Many of the older descriptions and pictures of the tectorial membrane show it floating free from the organ of Corti, waving like a leaf on a stem attached to the limbus. The reason is that the chemical fixation necessary to preserve tissue for the usual microscopic study shrinks the tectorial membrane very badly and pulls loose its attachments to Hensen's cells, the inner supporting cells, and the hair cells. Our description is based on studies of fresh specimens seen under the dissecting microscope. The relation between the tectorial membrane and the hair cells is similar to the relation in the utricle, saccule, and semicircular canals where the cilia of hair cells are embedded in gelatinous accessory structures that are acted upon by fluid pressure, gravity, or inertial forces.

Under the dissecting microscope the physical properties of the basilar membrane have been explored by probing, pulling, and cutting. The organ of Corti and the tectorial membrane tend to move together as a single, relatively stiff section of the cochlear parti-tion. Most of the bending takes place in the remaining flexible portion of the basilar membrane, as shown in Figure 3-10. The basilar membrane is not under lateral tension, as was once supposed. If it is cut, the edges do not draw apart. The narrow portion in the basal turn is much stiffer than the broader portion near the apex by a factor of at least 100 when measured in terms of the volume displacement of fluid that is produced by a given force.

From observations such as these it is practically certain that when the organ of Corti is moved up and down by sound waves, as described in the next section, the tectorial membrane must slide past the reticular lamina as shown in Figure 3-11. This is a mechanical necessity because these two rather stiff structures have different hinge points on limbus and bony lamina, respectively. Thus the final mechanical action of which we are sure is a lateral bending or shearing of the cilia, in and out with each sound wave.

Before considering the fine anatomy of the sensory cells and the nerve fibers that innervate them, let us consider in more detail and movement of the cochlear partition as a whole when driven by sound.

Analysis of Sound by the Ear

When the stapes is forced like a piston into the oval window, it presses on the perilymph in the vestibule. The perilymph is nearly incompressible, like water, and the walls of the bony labyrinth are rigid except for the flexible round-window membrane. The pressure wave spreads very rapidly throughout the labyrinth, and the round window bulges outward into the air-filled middle ear. This allows the stapes to move inward more freely, and fluid is displaced toward the round window. The cochlear partition is in the path of this movement of fluid and, being flexible, is displaced toward

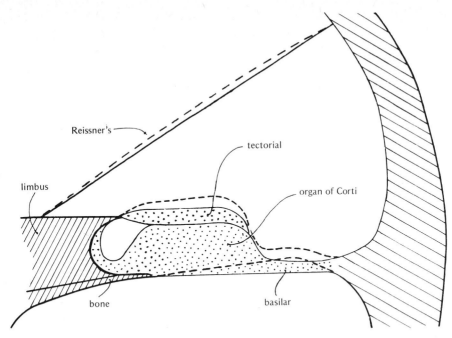

Figure 3-10 The organ of Corti and the tectorial membrane form a relatively stiff section of the cochlea partition. Most of the bending takes place in the more flexible portion of the basilar membrane between the organ of Corti and the spiral ligament. *(After von Békésy)*

the round window, as shown in Figure 3-6. If the movement is slow, or if the position is maintained, there is time for fluid to flow up the scala vestibuli, through the helicotrema, and down the scala tympani. For sounds of more than about 60 Hz, the basilar membrane is flexible enough and the inertia of the fluid great enough for the fluid near the helicotrema to remain stationary while the cochlear partition and also the round-window membrane bulge back and forth.

The basilar membrane has some stiffness, as we have mentioned. It is elastic enough to return to its original shape and position after

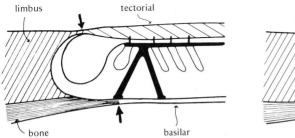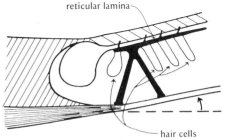

Figure 3-11 *Left:* The organ of Corti and tectorial membrane are in the position of rest. Their respective "hinge points" where they attach to the limbus and the bony lamina are shown by the heavy arrows. *Right:* The partition has moved "upward." Because of its different hinge point the tectorial membrane must slide past the reticular lamina and bend the hairs. *(After von Békésy and also ter Kuile)*

it has been deformed or displaced, and it has appreciable mass. It therefore has a natural period or resonant frequency at which it will move most easily and at greatest amplitude when driven by an alternating force like a sound wave. The basilar membrane is graded in width, widest at the apex and narrowest at the base of the cochlea. The stiffness is closely related to the width. Thus the membrane is stiffest at the base and most flexible at the apex. The resonant frequency is highest in the basal turn and lowest at the apex. In accordance with the principles of resonance, the basilar membrane does, indeed, show maximum amplitude of vibration for high tones near the base, for medium tones in the second turn, and for low tones near the apex.

This relation was proposed as a hypothesis by Helmholtz, but we are indebted to Georg von Békésy for the most complete experimental analysis of the acoustics of the ear and the details of how it acts as a frequency analyzer. Georg von Békésy was a physicist by training, and his methods primarily acoustical and optical. The experiments were difficult to perform and are rather complicated in detail. He actually measured, under the microscope, the amplitudes of movement at different positions along the membrane in relation to different frequencies and intensities of driving sound. For these and other studies of the ear, extending over 25 years, he was awarded the Nobel Prize in Physiology and Medicine in 1961.

The pattern of mechanical activity described by von Békésy has been confirmed by other workers and in other ways. The electrical output of the hair cells, for example, has been used to detect and measure movements of the organ of Corti instead of direct observation of these movements under a microscope. And it is gratifying that the map relating frequency to position along the basilar membrane, as derived from direct physiological experiments, agrees with inferences drawn from psychoacoustics, notably the relation of the mel scale to frequency (see Chapter 2). In Figure 3-12 the approximate positions of maximum movement are given, as compiled by Stuhlman in 1943. This map is still satisfactory. We now feel justified in speaking of the *place principle* of frequency analysis in the cochlea to denote this well-established relation between frequency of sound waves and position of maximum mechanical movement.

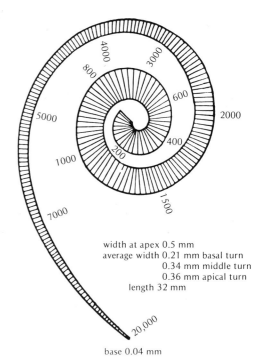

width at apex 0.5 mm
average width 0.21 mm basal turn
0.34 mm middle turn
0.36 mm apical turn
length 32 mm

base 0.04 mm

Figure 3-12 In this diagram the width of the basilar membrane is exaggerated relative to its length to show more clearly its progressive widening as it approaches the apex. The approximate positions of maximum amplitude of vibration in response to tones of different frequency are also indicated. *(From O. Stuhlman, Jr.,* An Introduction to Biophysics, *John Wiley & Sons, 1943; by permission)*

Place Principle, Cochlear Map, and Psychoacoustic Correlates

Several features of the cochlea map are worth noting. First, the highest audible frequency, about 20,000 Hz, is associated with the extreme basal end of the membrane just behind the round window. The frequency of 2000 Hz lies at the midpoint along the basilar membrane between base and apex. From the upper limit down to 1000 Hz, or perhaps 500 Hz, each octave occupies about the same distance along the membrane, approximately 5 mm. Below 1000 Hz the spacing is equal distance for equal bandwidth instead of equal distance for equal ratio of frequencies. This results in a progressive compression of the lower musical octaves into shorter and shorter distances. The apical end of the membrane at the helicotrema is reached at about 60 Hz. A curious result of the compression of the lower octaves is the position of middle C of the piano (262 Hz), which is much nearer to 90 percent than to 50 percent of the distance between the two ends. We should recall from Chapter 2, however, that the mel scale of pitch shows a very similar compression of subjective pitch in the low frequencies, and so do the difference limens, each of which is equal to about 1 mel. From this correspondence we arrive at the generalization that one just noticeable difference in pitch corresponds to a constant difference in position of maximum amplitude of about 0.02 mm. The relation of critical bandwidth to frequency follows a similar trend, and we find a rough equivalence of one critical band to 1 mm of length and to about 100 mels.

The reader is reminded that a certain amount of pitch information seems to be carried, for low frequencies, by the periodicity of waveform, whether sinusoidal or complex. We shall return to this point, but the *periodicity principle* of pitch should be mentioned here as an important supplement to the basic place principle outlined above.

Damping and Frequency Discrimination

The frequency analysis in the cochlea depends directly on the principle of resonance (see Chapter 2). If a system such as a portion of the basilar membrane is to be selective with respect to frequency, it must be free to continue vibrating for at least one or two oscillations after the driving force ceases. In other words, the system must be less than critically damped and not "dead beat." For the finest discrimination it should be only lightly damped. On the other hand, a lightly damped system builds up only slowly to its maximum amplitude and is a poor instrument for detecting time differences between signals. The ear actually combines the properties of good frequency resolution and good time resolution. At large amplitudes of movement the ear is a little less than critically damped (von Békésy). On the other hand, at small amplitudes within 40 dB of threshold, the system behaves like a set of lightly damped resonators. The mechanism responsible for such different behaviors is not clear at the present time. We shall return to this problem in connection with the "tuning curves" and "response areas" of single auditory units.

The Traveling-Wave Pattern of the Basilar Membrane

The time pattern of the movement of the basilar membrane when driven by a continuous tone is quite complicated. The various parts do not move in step (in phase) with one another. The natural periods of different segments differ, as we have noted, and, according to the principles of resonance, the portions of the membrane that are tuned to frequencies higher than the driving force tend to move ahead of the force while the parts with lower natural periods tend to lag behind. But the membrane is a continuous structure, not a set of independent resonators. No segment can get very far head of or lag far behind the adjacent portion. The final pattern of movement in any system in which the stiffness, and consequently the tuning, is graded continuously, as they are in the basilar membrane, is a series of *traveling waves*. The waves arise at the stiffer end and travel toward the more flexible region. At the stiff end the movement is very nearly in phase with the driving force. As the waves travel, they increase in amplitude but lag more and more behind the driving force. At the position of maximum aplitude they lag by nearly a full cycle. The details of the pattern are shown in Figure 3-13.

The behavior of the membrane in response to a single wave, pulse, or transient is quite similar. A traveling wave starts at the basal end and moves up the cochlea. The point at which it reaches its maximum amplitude depends on the duration of the original (unidirectional) pulse. If the wave arrives at the apical turn, it does so only after a delay (travel time) of more than a millisecond. The mechanism of transmission of such a pulse is *not* like the travel of a wave down a rope when we shake one end, in which the energy is passed from segment to segment along the rope. The pressure wave in the fluids spreads very rapidly throughout the cochlea. The movement of the membrane under the influence of the pressure differences across it requires time, more in the apical than in the basal turn, although, as we have noted, the movement of each segment is modified by its coupling to its neighbors.

In recent years much attention has been given to the exact form of the *Békésy* enve-

lope. The very flat plateau shown in Figure 3-13 does not agree with the very sharp tuning of single auditory units, to be described below. Some improvement is made by relating the amplitude of movement of the cochlear partition to the velocity of the stapes instead of to sound-pressure level. This gives a sharper cutoff toward the apex. Measurements of the movement by refined methods such as laser beams or the Mössbauer effect give still sharper cutoffs, particularly for the lower basal turn (high frequencies), but the physical problem of good frequency discrimination in the cochlea has not yet been solved.

In summary, the *envelope* of the traveling wave pattern is located at a position that depends on frequency, as shown in Figure 3-13. The envelope is not symmetrical. All of the membrane basal to the position of the maximum moves somewhat. At a short distance apical to the maximum there is no movement. At the maximum there is a considerable phase lag in the instantaneous displacement, but at low and middle frequencies the basal region moves nearly in phase with itself and also with the driving force. The basal region is therefore capable of giving accurate time information both for steady tones and for transients.

Bone Conduction

Any vibration of the basilar membrane will stimulate the sensory cells and give rise to the sensation of sound. It makes no difference how the vibrations in the cochlea may have been set going. Ordinarily the pathway for sound is through the external ear and across the chain of ossicles, but sound waves may also be transmitted directly through the bones of the skull. A vibrating tuning fork may be heard by air conduction if it is held opposite the open ear or by bone conduction if its stem is applied to the top of the head,

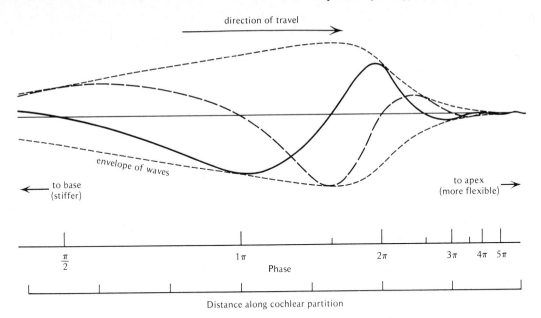

direction of travel

envelope of waves

to base
(stiffer)

to apex
(more flexible)

$\frac{\pi}{2}$ 1π 2π 3π 4π 5π

Phase

Distance along cochlear partition

Figure 3-13 The waves in the basilar membrane move from base toward apex. Their velocity becomes progressively slower and their wavelength shorter. The solid curve shows the pattern of displacement at the instant that the upward displacement at the basal end is maximal. The dashed curve shows the pattern a quarter of a cycle ($\pi/2$) later. The phase differences are relative to the extreme basal end. The dotted lines are the envelopes of the displacement patterns. The envelope increases slowly, goes through a maximum between $3\pi/2$ and 2π and then falls off rapidly. The position of the maximum along the membrane is a function of frequency, as shown in Figure 3-11, but the relation of maximum to phase lag is constant. The small short waves beyond about 3π are probably of no physiological importance. In this diagram the vertical dimension of displacement is exaggerated to show the patterns more clearly. The formation of traveling waves depends on the gradient of stiffness along the cochlear partition. *(After von Békésy)*

to a tooth, or to the mastoid bone behind the ear. Transmission is not so efficient across the skin and through the bone as it is by the normal route, but if the normal route is obstructed, as in certain forms of deafness, bone conduction may be put to great practical use. Its diagnostic importance will also be discussed in later chapters.

The sound waves traveling in the skull probably set up mechanical movement of the fluid relative to the bone in several ways. For one thing, the membrane of the round window is more flexible and yielding than is the footplate of the stapes, and thus when the labyrinth as a whole is compressed by a sound wave reaching it through the bone, the round window is the most yielding of the various outlets. The fluid from the vestibule and the semicircular canals, as well as that within the cochlea, is therefore driven toward the round window. This fluid movement is exactly like that normally set up by the vibrations of the footplate of the stapes and is analyzed by the cochlea and heard in the brain exactly like airborne sound. For another thing, the head is vibrated as a whole by sounds below about 800 Hz. The ossicles tend to lag behind because of their inertia. The resulting relative movement of skull and ossicles is exactly equivalent to vibrations set up by airborne sound. Fortunately this effect is minimized by the dynamic balance of the malleus and incus around their axis of rotation described earlier in this chapter.

These are two of the most important, but by no means all, of the mechanisms and

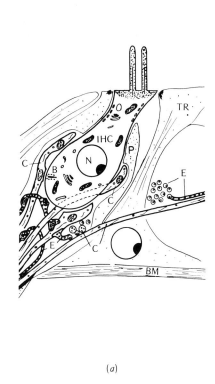

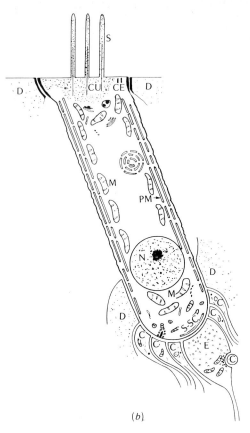

(a)

(b)

Figure 3-14 (a) Diagram of an inner hair cell (IHC) and its innervation. B, synaptic bar; BM, basilar membrane; C, afferent cochlear nerve fibers; E, efferent nerve fibers of the olivocochlear bundle; N, nucleus; P, phalangeal supporting cell; TR, tunnel rod. Note the nerve fibers cut in cross section, forming the inner spiral bundle and the tunnel bundle. Note how the efferent fibers to the inner hair cells form synaptic junctions on the afferent nerve fibers and endings.

(b) Diagram of an outer hair cell, at a higher magnification than (a). B, synaptic bar; C, afferent cochlear nerve fiber; CE, centriole; CU, cuticular plate; D, Deiters' cells; E, efferent nerve terminal; M, mitochondria; N, nucleus; S, stereocilia; S-SC, subsynaptic cisterna. *(Courtesy of C. A. Smith. Reproduced from* Advancement of Science, *Vol. 24, No. 122; June 1968; by permission)*

pathways of bone conduction. Of course, any very intense sound in the air will set the skull vibrating to some extent; a telephone receiver held tightly against the ear may do so even more effectively. Our own voices generated inside our heads reach our ears by bone conduction as well as by air conduction. But it is air conduction that gives the ear its great sensitivity, particularly for the higher audible frequencies.

The Hair Cells and Their Nerves

In the description of the organ of Corti we mentioned briefly the sensory cells, known as hair cells, and their orderly arrangement in one row of "inner" or internal hair cells on the side of the tunnel of Corti nearer to the modiolus and three rows (with sometimes parts of a fourth row) of "outer" or external hair cells on the opposite side. The inner and outer cells differ somewhat in shape and size, as shown in Figure 3-14, and also in the shapes of the nerve endings that attach to their lower ends, and in their relations to their supporting cells. Inner and outer are alike, however, in the set of "hairs" or *cilia* (stereocilia) that project from their cuticular surfaces into the endolymphatic space. There are as many as 80 cilia on each hair cell, and they are arranged in rows in the same overall patterns. On an inner hair cell they form nearly a straight line; on an outer hair cell the shape is like a W, with its narrow, double-pointed base turned away from the modiolus, as shown in Figure 3-15.

An electron microscope is needed to see the hairs clearly. They are about a micron (0.001 mm) in diameter and perhaps ten times as long. A "root" can be traced well

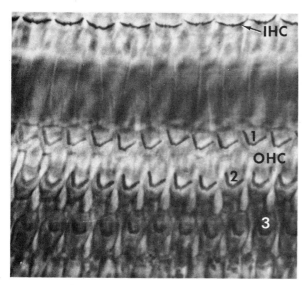

Figure 3-15 Photomicrograph of a surface preparation of a section of the organ of Corti of a chinchilla, viewed from the scala vestibuli. There are one row of inner hair cells (IHC) and three rows of outer hair cells (OHC 1, 2, 3). The mosaic arrangement of cells is evident. On each IHC the stereocilia form a nearly straight line; on each OHC they form a W. The focus was adjusted for a clear image of the stereocilia. *(Courtesy of Dr. B. Bohne)*

down into the cuticular layer, but the electron microscope does not tell us whether the cilia are primarily chemical, electrical, or mechanical devices. They are of different lengths and the outer ends of the longer ones are embedded in, or at least attached to, the tectorial membrane. Apparently in the cochlea, as well as in other related organs, when the cilia are bent toward the base of the W, nerve impulses are triggered off in the nerve fiber that connects with the hair cell. When they are bent the other way, the nerve impulses are inhibited. When bent sideways, there is no effect.

The inner hair cells are snugly packed among the supporting cells. The "upper" cuticular surfaces of both inner and outer hair cells form part of the stiff reticular lamina. The lower end of each outer hair cell rests in a cup provided by a specialized supporting cell (Deiters'). The remainder of the hair cell is bathed by a fluid, probably much like perilymph, that fills the tunnel of Corti and other intracellular spaces in the organ of Corti. Many nerve endings, in intimate contact with one another as well as with the hair cells, cover the end of the cell opposite to the hair-bearing end (see Figure 3-14).

The electron microscope shows two different types of nerve endings. Some are large and contain many vesicles; others are smaller and clearer. Each nerve fiber usually branches, some of them very extensively, but all of the endings on any one nerve fiber are always the same type. The nerve fibers in the auditory nerve and out to the habenula perforata have myelin sheaths, but as they enter the organ of Corti the sheaths are lost and the peripheral portions of the fibers are nonmyelinated. The cell bodies of the *afferent* neurons, which carry nerve impulses from the hair cells to the brain, are located in the spiral ganglion in the modiolus of the cochlea, close to the hair cells that they innervate.

The cell bodies contain the nucleus and other vital structures. The nerve endings of the afferent fibers are the small ones mentioned above.

The *efferent* fibers are far fewer in number than the afferent group, but they have large nerve endings with many vesicles. They bring nerve impulses from the brain to the organ of Corti. Their cell bodies are located in the brain stem in the superior olivary nucleus. About three-quarters of the efferent fibers cross the midline within the brain stem and run to the contralateral cochlea. The efferent fibers run in the *olivocochlear bundle* through the internal auditory meatus as part of the auditory nerve. Most of them innervate the outer hair cells, but some make contact with afferent nerve fibers near the inner hair cells, though not with the inner hair cells themselves. The function of the efferent nerve supply to the cochlea is not clear. In animal experiments strong stimulation of the efferent tract in the brain stem causes a slight elevation of the threshold of the afferent system, but only by about 20 dB at most. We shall disregard the efferent system in our interpretations of cochlear function.

Number of Hair Cells and Their Innervation

The total number of hair cells in a human ear is about 12,000. About 3000 of them are inner hair cells; the remainder are outer cells. Each inner hair cell is about 10 microns in diameter; the outer hair cells, about 8 microns. The basilar membrane is about 32 mm long. There are, therefore, about 400 hair cells per millimeter. Another approximate relation is that one octave in the middle range of frequencies occupies some 5 mm, and one just noticeable difference in pitch corresponds to about 10 microns or the diameter of a single inner hair cell.

The number of nerve fibers is about double the total number of hair cells. There are about 25,000 to 30,000 cell bodies in the spiral ganglion of Corti (see Figure 3-9) within the modiolus. Each cell body sends a short receptor fiber to the organ of Corti and a long nerve trunk, an axon, to the cochlear nucleus. There are, in addition, about 500 efferent fibers.

The efferent fibers run up and down the cochlea in the intraganglionic bundle (Figure 3-9), or as the internal spiral fibers beneath the inner hair cells or the external spiral fibers among the external hair cells. They branch freely, as they obviously must, since there are about 20 times as many hair cells as there are efferent fibers.

The afferent fibers are divided very unequally between inner and outer hair cells. The inner hair cells receive about 95 percent of the total. Even without branching there are many more nerve fibers than inner hair cells. In the cat a hair cell may be innervated by as many as 20 afferent nerve fibers. On the other hand, the outer hair cells are more numerous than the available afferent nerve fibers. Each fiber runs for a short distance toward the basal end and then branches to innervate a fairly compact group of hair cells. These rather surprising relations, summarized in Figure 3-16, have been well established by Spoendlin for the cat, and are now generally accepted as the probable pattern for humans as well. Their physiological significance is not yet entirely clear.

Nerve Impulses: The All-or-None Law

We have described the organs of the inner ear, their physical properties, and how they move under the influence of sound waves. The movements are graded continuously in amplitude, and they all occur in a single sound-conducting system or "channel," whether it be the air of the external canal, the ossicles in the middle ear, the fluids, or the

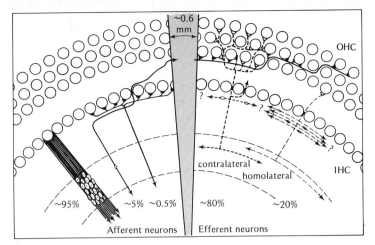

Figure 3-16 Horizontal innervation schema of the organ of Corti. The different types of afferent neurons and efferent neurons are at left and right, with their corresponding approximate percentages. *(From H. Spoendlin. Reproduced from* Audiology, *14:402; 1975; by permission)*

cochlear partition. At the cochlear partition the single channel begins to subdivide. The frequency analysis performed by the basilar membrane means that some sensory cells are moved more than others according to their position and the frequency of the sound.

At the sensory cell a very different kind of action occurs. The input to the cell is a bending of its "hairs," or cilia. The final result is an output of nerve impulses in the sensory nerve that innervates it. The relation of this output to the mechanical input is highly nonlinear; it is discontinuous in both intensity and time, and it involves the contribution of energy by both the sensory cell and the nerve fiber to support this new form of activity. We often refer to the "triggering" of nerve impulses. The action is analogous to pulling the trigger of a machine gun and thereby firing one or a series of shots. We shall consider first the action of a typical nerve cell or neuron and then the process of excitation in a sensory cell.

The nerve impulse is the unit of action in a nerve fiber. It is a wave of electrochemical activity that travels in the auditory nerve fibers at about 25 meters per second (m/s). (Some nerve fibers of larger diameter conduct more rapidly, about 100 m/s, whereas small nonmyelinated fibers in the autonomic nervous system conduct at about 1 m/s.) The nerve impulse can be compared to the burning of a fuse of gunpowder. The heat of the burning ignites the next adjoining section of the fuse, which ignites the next one, and so on in a chain reaction. The energy of the nerve impulse, like the heat of the burning fuse, comes from the fiber itself, not from the initial stimulus (the match) that triggers it off. The impulse is not graded in intensity according to the strength of the stimulus. Its strength depends only on the state of the fiber at that particular point. The fuse burns or its does not burn. The impulse, like the burning, is "all or none."

There is an important difference between the nerve impulse and the fuse. The nerve automatically recharges itself after each impulse and is ready to conduct another impulse after an interval of about 1 to 3 ms. This recharging interval is known as the *refractory period.* Another difference is that the excitation of the impulse from segment to segment of nerve is electrical—not thermal, as in the fuse. We can place an electrode on the nerve fiber and record the electrical change or "action potential" (see Figure 3-19). This allows us to *measure the activity of a nerve fiber in terms of the number of impulses per second.*

The typical *neuron* consists of four major parts. One is the *cell body*, which contains the nucleus and other vital structures necessary for the continued life of the cell. Special chemical substances are formed here and are distributed down the nerve fibers by a slow outward flow of protoplasm. The second part of a neuron is its receptor, or *dendritic portion*, which receives stimuli, usually chemical, from other neurons or sensory cells. It responds, as we shall see, by generating a local, graded electric current. A third part is a set of effector *terminals*, which form synapses with other neurons and secrete a particular *chemical mediator*. These junctional or synaptic actions will be described in more detail in the next section. The fourth major part of most neurons is absent in some small nerve cells in the central nervous system, but it constitutes most of what we know as a peripheral "nerve." It is the nerve fiber or *axon*. It is long and threadlike, and it connects the input (dendritic) with the output (secretory) endings. The larger axons, including those of the auditory nerve, are covered with a thin insulating sheath of a white fatty substance known as *myelin*. The axon is specialized for rapid, economical, and reliable transmission of very simple all-or-none messages, the *nerve impulses.*

The discontinuous all-or-none activity is carried out very economically. It provides very reliable transmission of signals over long lengths of nerve, as from the foot or hand to the brain, and the transmission is very rapid. On the other hand, the code of the nerve fiber is very limited. The impulses are not graded in intensity like electric currents in a telephone wire. They are merely dots in a very simple telegraphic code, more like those of a digital computer. The only significant gradations are (1) the average number of impulses per second and (2) the time relations between impulses in the same and in neighboring fibers. Each fiber is effectively insulated from its neighbors. The maximum frequency of impulses is 1000 per second for the first two or three impulses, falling rapidly to an average maximum rate of about 200 per second.

A major problem of auditory neurophysiology is to understand how all of the auditory information that reaches the brain passes through the bottleneck of the auditory nerve. How is it coded in sequences of dot-dot-dot impulses in the individual nerve fibers? We may add that the same problem appears again and again in the central nervous system wherever information is coded for transmission by the axons that make up the "tracts" of white matter.

Synapses and Synaptic Action

Within the neurons and hair cells we shall not be concerned with the nucleus, the mitochondria, and many other details of internal structure that are revealed by the electron microscope. With the exception of the cilia of the hair cells, they are common to most cells throughout the body. The surfaces of contact between cells themselves are of special interest to us, however. These specialized junctional structures are known as the *synaptic junctions* or *synapses*. Nearly all synapses are chemical mechanisms. By this we mean that a particular "neurohumor," or *chemical transmitter*, is liberated from a ready state and diffuses rapidly across the very narrow "synaptic cleft" and reacts with a specialized receptor surface on the receiving neuron.

Under the influence of the transmitter substance certain charged particles (ions) become free to move, and an electric current begins to flow in the receiving neuron. In many nerve cells we can, with very fine intracellular electrodes, detect and measure the associated "postsynaptic potentials." The postsynaptic potentials from many nerve endings combine with one another. The excitatory effect is related to the total number of excitatory impulses reaching a particular neuron. When an adequate integrated postsynaptic potential is reached at the origin of the axon it triggers off a nerve impulse. (Only the axon, not the dendrites, is electrically excitable and can conduct impulses.)

There are a number of different chemical transmitters. Acetylocholine and norepinephrine are two of the best known, but the transmitters in the cochlea have not yet been identified. Not all synaptic action is excitatory. Some nerve fibers and their terminals are specialized to secrete *inhibitory transmitters*. Inhibition in this context means a process that opposes or makes more difficult the triggering of nerve impulses in a neuron. This is the action of the efferent fibers to the cochlea. There are several mechanisms of inhibition, but the most common is a change in the electrochemical properties of the postsynaptic surface of the "receiving" neuron, specifically to reduce the electrical impedance so that the excitatory postsynaptic potentials are short-circuited and do not combine so effectively with one another or spread so far.

From Sound Waves to Nerve Impulses

One of the steps in the chain of transmission of auditory signals to the brain that is not fully understood is how the mechanical bending of the cilia of the hair cells controls the release of the chemical transmitter at the opposite end of the hair cell. We do know that in various sense organs the receptor cells are specialized to be extremely and selectively sensitive to one particular form of incoming energy, whether it be chemical (taste and smell), thermal (temperature sense), light (vision), electrical (electrical organs in certain fish), or mechanical (touch, acceleration, and hearing). The hair cells of the ear with their cilia are the most sensitive of the *mechanoreceptors*. They are sensitive to deformations of atomic dimensions and at energy levels only just above that of thermal agitation of molecules. Because of this extreme sensitivity we can be quite sure that at the critical point of deformation, whether it be in the cilia or in the cuticular plate in which they are embedded, there must be a release of energy by the hair cell like the first step in the triggering of a nerve impulse—in other words, an amplifying or "booster" action.

The hair cells do actually respond with an electrical output. The response is not an explosive all-or-none reaction like a nerve impulse, but instead it is graded, like a local postsynaptic potential, according to the amplitude of the mechanical displacement. At low and moderate intensities it follows the waveform faithfully without discontinuities or refractory periods. It can be detected readily by placing a pair of electrodes, either one on the round window and another elsewhere near the cochlea, or, better, both within the cochlea, one on each side of the cochlear partition. The electrical response recorded in this way is generated chiefly by the outer hair cells. It has been used extensively to study the action of both normal and injured ears. It is known as the *cochlear microphonic* because the transduction of the signal from an acoustical to an electrical form resembles the action of a microphone. The cochlear microphonic is an alternating-current electrical response to stimulation. There is also a set of direct-current responses, known as the *summating potentials.* One variety appears, like the cochlear microphonic, across the organ of Corti. Another appears as an overall difference between one segment of the cochlear duct and a remote reference point. These potentials may be of either polarity, depending on where the electrodes are placed in relation to the crest of the Békésy envelope. The mechanism of their generation is quite uncertain, and they are mentioned here chiefly because at least one of them may be involved in the excitatory processes in the hair cells or the nerve endings, as noted in a later section.

As to the cochlear microphonic, its generation is not a passive piezoelectric effect as in a crystal microphone. It resembles more closely a resistance microphone in which the mechanical movement modulates or valves the flow of electric current from a battery. The battery in this case is the hair cell itself, which maintains an electric potential between its inner and outer surface in the same way that a nerve fiber recharges itself after transmitting an impulse. This concept of the action of the hair cell is somewhat theoretical, but it seems to be our best working hypothesis at present. It is illustrated in Figure 3-17.

The second step in the action of the hair cell is the liberation of its chemical transmitter. The liberation of chemical transmitter is presumably controlled by the current flow of the cochlear microphonic through the cell, just as the liberation of transmitter from axon terminals at synapses is controlled by the action potentials of the nerve impulses arriving over the axons. The hair cell is rather like a neuron without any axon.

In this summary account we have bypassed certain interesting specializations in the cochlea, such as the unique high potassium content of the endolymph and the strong electrical polarization of the endolymphatic space of scala media. The polarization and presumably the chemical composition also are maintained by the stria vascularis (see Figure 3-17). These specializations probably make the cochlea more sensitive or more efficient, but one or both are absent in other simpler mechanoreceptors.

This hypothesis of mechanoelectrical excitation meets the requirement of providing a "biological amplifier" in the receptor cell, and it is in harmony with both experimental observations of the cochlear microphonic and analogous electrical action in other receptor organs. Fortunately our overall understanding of the action of the ear does not rest on this particular model of the excitatory action of the hair cells. We know that some excitatory process does operate, even at threshold levels of input, and we can study the output of nerve impulses in the fibers of the auditory nerve and relate this output directly to the acoustic input to the ear.

The Sensory Unit and Its Response Area

At this point we introduce the concept of the *auditory sensory unit,* meaning *one afferent auditory neuron and the hair cell or cells that excite it.* This concept is very helpful in understanding many forms of auditory impairment. The cells innervated by any one afferent fiber form a reasonably compact group, and we disregard the overlap that results from the innervation of one hair cell by two or more afferent neurons.

The definition of the auditory unit centers on the afferent nerve fiber and its responses to auditory stimuli. This is realistic because in animal experiments we can place a very fine electrode on or in a single fiber in the auditory nerve and both count and time the nerve impulses of the particular sensory unit. We can determine its threshold of response at various frequencies and thus de-

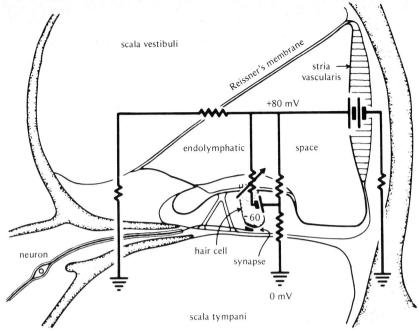

Figure 3-17   Model for mechanoelectrical excitation in the cochlea. Only one (external) hair cell is shown, to represent all hair cells. The endolymph in scala media is polarized 80 mV positive, and the interior of the hair cells 60 mV negative relative to scala tympani. These polarizations are maintained by biological "batteries" shown in the stria vascularis and the (lateral) cell membrane of the hair cell, respectively. The electrical pathways through Hensen's cells and basilar membrane and through Reissner's membrane and limbus represent all of the shunting pathways from scala media to scala tympani. A variable resistance, sensitive to mechanical deformation, is represented at the cuticular surface of the hair cell. It may be located near the centriole (see Figure 3-14). Changes in the resistance modulate the leakage current through the hair cell and thus the level of polarization at the synaptic surface at the lower end of the hair cell. The level of polarization here controls the rate of liberation of the chemical mediator which excites the afferent nerve ending. The cochlear microphonic, that is, the potential difference between scala media and scala tympani, is the result of the IR drop across the variable resistance in the cuticular layer. (Ohm's law states: E = IR; i.e., the potential difference, E, is equal to the product of current, I, multiplied by resistance, R.)

scribe its "tuning." We find, as a matter of fact, that each unit is sensitive to only a limited band of frequencies. The band is broader for intense than for weak tones. Each unit is most sensitive for one particular frequency, which is called its *characteristic frequency* or "best frequency."

The *response area* refers to the entire group of tones to which the unit responds. Plotted in the dimensions of frequency and intensity, as in Figure 3-18, the response area is a triangle pointing downward, with its vertex at the best frequency. In general the response areas are very steep on their high-frequency side, but they extend rather widely toward the lower frequencies at high intensities. Without going into detail we can say that this asymmetrical shape is what would be expected from the asymmetrical shape of the envelope of the traveling waves (see Figure 3-13).

Several features of single-unit activity and the response areas are surprising, however, and are difficult to reconcile with one another and with the innervation of the hair cells. First, all auditory units tested in animal preparations show *spontaneous activity* in the absence of acoustic stimulation. The

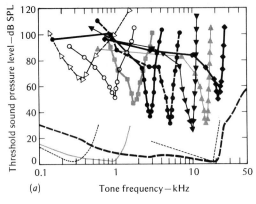

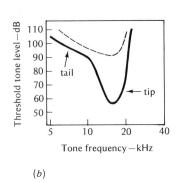

(a)   Tone frequency—kHz   (b)

Figure 3-18 *(a)* Response areas (tuning curves) of 8 auditory sensory units from 6 guinea pigs in dB SPL measured at the tympanic membrane and corrected to closed bulla condition. The curves below are analogous curves derived from the measurements of the vibration amplitude of the guinea pig basilar membrane by von Békésy *(1944)* (curves at 0.27 and 0.9 kHz); Johnstone et al. *(1970)* (curve at 18 kHz); Wilson and Johnstone *(1972)* (dashed curve at 20 kHz). These curves are corrected for the guinea pig middle-ear frequency response to relate them to the sound pressure at the tympanic membrane and are positioned arbitrarily on the intensity scale. *(b)* Effect of hypoxia on the (smoothed) frequency-threshold curve of a single cochlear fiber (cat). Solid line = control, before hypoxia; dashed line = during hypoxia (5% O$_2$). Note loss or elevation of the tip while the tail is very little affected. *(From E. F. Evans. Redrawn from Audiology, 14:419–442; 1975; by permission)*

average rate is rather low, usually less than 25 impulses per second, and the timing is not regular. The impulses in different units are not synchronized, and gross electrodes applied to the whole nerve do not detect the spontaneous activity. Because of the spontaneous activity the *threshold of response* of a single unit is usually defined as a clear increase, by 20 percent or nearly, in the rate of discharge or by the appearance of volleys of nerve impulses such as those that determine the threshold in electrocochleography, as described in Chapter 8. Above threshold the rate of discharge in each single unit increases with growing intensity to a maximum of about 200 per second (for a sustained tone). This increase occurs quite abruptly, mostly within a range of only about 20 dB. Thus most auditory units are either discharging at a slow, spontaneous rate or at their saturation rate. The saturation rate depends on the degree of "adaptation."

A second feature is the great sensitivity of all of the auditory units at their characteristic frequencies. Careful acoustic calibrations and determinations of thresholds show that the best thresholds lie within a few decibels of the behavioral threshold curve for that species. The surprise here is that there is *only one "population"* of units. Formerly it was assumed that the outer hair cells were more sensitive than the inner hair cells by some 30 or 40 dB; but no second population of high-threshold units has ever been demonstrated in normal ears. Here we must remember the very different innervation ratios of inner and outer hair cells (Figure 3-16). It is clear from this that the *inner* hair cell units are very sensitive. But it is hard to believe that the smaller population (5%) of the outer hair cell units have never been encountered in the random sampling of nerve fibers by the microelectrodes.

The sharpness of "tuning" of the auditory units is not uniform. It is much sharper ("higher *Q*") for units with characteristic frequencies above 2 kHz than below (see Figure 3-18) but the gradation is gradual. We have mentioned the steeper slope of the response areas toward the high frequencies. Some investigators hope that this steepness can be explained by the sharp termination of the Békésy envelope, but the slopes toward the lower frequencies are still much too steep to be explained in this way (see Figure 3-18). More and more it appears that response areas, particularly the high-frequency response areas, are *composite*. They consist of a sensitive, sharply tuned "tip" and a flat, less sensitive "tail" that extends to the very lowest audible tones. The long tail is obviously due to stimulation of high-frequency units by the traveling wave as it traverses the basal turn.

The most surprising feature of the response areas is that *their sensitive tips can be suppressed or greatly modified* by anoxia or by certain drugs without affecting the tails, and this detuning or elevation of threshold (or both) of the tips is *reversible*. The response areas are clearly composite, with a relatively insensitive, broadly tuned tail to which is added a very sensitive, sharply tuned "tip."

The existence of tips and tails has been verified in several laboratories, but the anatomical and physiological mechanisms are entirely speculative. Evans speaks of a "second filter" that provides the tip, but he suggests no anatomical basis for it. Zwislocki postulates an inhibitory action of outer on inner hair cells to account for the sharp tuning, but he postulates a neural (synaptic) connection between the two sets of neurons. The anatomists of the ear (Spoendlin, Smith, and others) have sought carefully for synaptic connections within the organ of Corti and firmly deny their existence. Dallos and others postulate a "sensitization" of the inner by the outer hair cells. If there is a trend of opinion at the present time (1977), it is toward some sort of interaction between outer and inner hair cells, probably by way of the

cochlear microphonic or the negative summating potential or both. Both excitatory and inhibitory (Eldredge) interactions have been suggested. It is worth recalling that the cochlear microphonic and probably the negative summating potential are generated chiefly by the outer hair cells.

The situation should be clarified within the next decade. In the meantime, audiologists who employ electrical responses of the cochlea or brain stem (Chapter 8) must proceed on an empirical basis and always be aware of the paradoxes that surround the response areas of the auditory units. Mechanisms remain unknown, but at least two substantial principles do emerge. First, the triangular shape of the response areas provides for the gradation of neural activity as a function of intensity in spite of the abrupt increase in the rate of discharge in each unit. At each frequency the units with that characteristic frequency will respond at the lowest sound level; however, as the level increases, other units, particularly those with higher characteristic frequencies, will also respond. Finally the "tails" of units that are quite remotely tuned will also be stimulated.

Loudness is presumably related to the total overall activity. Moreover, frequency discrimination is obviously based on the steep upper-frequency boundaries of the response areas, but we note here that discrimination is materially improved by inhibitory interactions in the cochlear nucleus that tend to sharpen the gradients of activity along the frequency dimension. Finally, the differential suppression of the tips of the response areas offers a perfect model for the phenomenon of recruitment (see Chapters 2, 4, and 8). The threshold is elevated because of the suppression of tips, but with stronger stimulation the tails are encountered. They are packed into a relatively restricted dynamic range, but the units can all still be excited by strong stimuli.

Summary of Peripheral Auditory Physiology

A diagram in the next chapter, Figure 4-1, summarizes the sequence of actions in the ear from the external air to the axon terminals of the sensory units in the cochlear nucleus. It shows how the transition from sound conduction and frequency analysis to nerve impulses is located in the cochlea. There the excitation of the sensory units occurs, and the auditory nerve transmits all-or-none impulses to the brain stem. The diagram also illustrates how the bone-conduction pathway through the skull bypasses the middle ear, with its drum membrane and ossicular chain, but joins the primary air-conduction pathway in the fluids of the inner ear before the frequency analysis is performed by the basilar membrane. The arrangement of the hair cells in the figure is completely diagrammatic. Each cell in the diagram represents a group of cells in a short segment of the organ of Corti corresponding perhaps to a critical band. The arrangement of units lengthwise of the organ of Corti expresses the tuning of the units, each with its best frequency. The gradation of thresholds among sensory units with slightly different tuning is also indicated.

The general pattern represented here is very useful in helping to understand the various forms of auditory impairment that will be described in Chapter 4, notably the distinction between conductive impairment, sense organ or sensory impairment (referring to the organ of Corti), neural impairment (referring to the neurons of the auditory nerve), and central impairment in and beyond the cochlear nucleus. Each sensory unit is represented as dividing to terminate in three different regions in the cochlear nucleus. (Three is probably a minimum number.) The different areas probably initiate different forms of "information processing." In and beyond the cochlear nucleus the connections and processes become very complicated, and we refer to them as neurological and, in another frame of reference, psychological, as we will explain shortly.

The Volley Principle and Periodicity Pitch

If the ear is stimulated by a low-frequency tone, say 500 Hz or less, the nerve impulses in the sensory units that respond are grouped together in successive bursts or "volleys." There is a preferred phase or portion of the cycle in which impulses tend to be excited, and actually they are more or less *inhibited* during the opposite half of the cycle. Each axon does not fire at exactly the same phase of every cycle, and it may skip one or several cycles. When it does fire, there is a random distribution in the timing, sometimes earlier, sometimes later, as shown in Figure 3-19. Impulses in different sensory

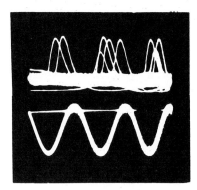

Figure 3-19 Action potentials (upper tracing) recorded from a microelectrode in a nerve fiber of the auditory nerve of a guinea pig. The lower trace shows the sound stimulus, a 1000 Hz pure tone, recorded by a microphone. Approximately 170 sweeps were superimposed. Ten nerve impulses appeared. The action potentials are all-or-none transients, but three of them appear smaller here because of the electrical background noise, shown by the broad baseline. Note that the action potentials all are approximately, but not exactly, in the same time relation to the sound waves. *(From I. Tasaki, J. Neurophysiol., 16:97–122; 1954; by permission)*

units that are excited by the same sound wave thus differ a little in their times of arrival. Nevertheless, in animal experiments, when we record from the auditory nerve as a whole, the grouping of nerve impulses is very clear at 500 Hz. Volleys are definite at 1000 Hz and clearly detectable at 2000 Hz, but barely demonstrable at 4000 Hz. Above 5000 Hz the timing of the impulses is truly random. Below 1500 Hz, however, the grouping represents a signficant mechanism by which frequency information is conveyed to the brain.

This information is the basis of the psychoacoustic phenomenon of periodicity pitch described in Chapter 2, but the frequency principle makes only a limited contribution, for low frequencies only, and it is not the major or sole mechanism for conveying frequency information as Rutherford originally (1886) and Wever and Bray later (1930) suggested.

Electrical Stimulation of Hearing

If an alternating electric current of a frequency in the audible range is passed through the head in the neighborhood of the inner ear and adjusted to a suitable intensity, it is sometimes possible to hear a tone or at least a noise. This is known as the "electrophonic effect." The current is most effectively applied by filling the external ear canal with salt solution and immersing the end of one wire in it. The circuit is completed through a metal plate on the forearm. The strength of the current must be carefully adjusted because at only a few decibels above the threshold of hearing the current may begin to be felt as a tickling, burning, prickling, and, finally, painful sensation. The effect may also be obtained when an amplitude-modulated carrier wave in the ultrasonic frequency range is applied with both electrodes on skin outside the ear canal.

There are several different mechanisms of the electrophonic effect. Most of them depend on the conversion of the alternating electric current into mechanical movement of the tympanic membrane, the ossicles, or the skin. It is in this way that pure tones can be heard, either corresponding to the frequency of the electric current or one octave above it. The fundamental action is like that of a condenser microphone operated in reverse as a loudspeaker. It takes advantage of the alternating attractions between two oppositely charged conducting structures, such as the tympanic membrane and the bony wall of the middle ear, separated by a dielectric, such as the air in the middle ear. When a high-frequency carrier is used, a rectifying action in the tissues precedes the transduction into mechanical movement, and the movement, usually of the skin, may be carried to the cochlea by bone conduction.

These mechanisms are all basically electrostatic effects of one sort or another, even though they have been mistaken for electrical stimulation of the ear or even of the brain itself! If a pure tone is heard, we can be quite sure that some cochlear function remains.

A quite different form of the electrophonic effect is the actual electrical stimulation of the auditory nerve. Sometimes this can be achieved before muscular twitching or pain, or both, become intolerable. Electrodes have actually been introduced experimentally into (damaged) human cochleas to stimulate the nerve or parts of the nerve selectively and to test the possibility of developing a hearing aid on this principle. (See Chapter 6.)

Unfortunately the sensation produced by such direct electrical stimulation of the auditory nerve is not a pure tone. It is either a noise or at best a sort of buzz. The sensation corresponds to the periodicity pitch discussed in the previous section and in Chapter 2, and, as might be expected, the buzzlike "tone" is heard at only rather low frequencies.

The efforts to develop a wearable "cochlear implant," the difficulties encountered, and the degree of success are described in some detail in Chapter 6. It seems clear that stimulation of a single segment of the cochlea can give some sense of pitch for low tones but that useful communication by speech cannot be expected. The reason is that the normal frequency analysis of the cochlea is lost, and pure periodicity pitch is not adequate alone.

Psychophysiological Relations

The physical and physiological properties of the ear help us to understand the boundaries of the auditory area. The behavioral threshold is at roughly the same level as the threshold of physiological stimulation of the auditory units, at their best frequencies. Discomfort and pain occur when the mechanical restraints on amplitude of movement become severe and injury is imminent. The upper frequency limits in behavioral animal experiments correspond roughly to the highest frequencies for which good electrical responses are obtained from the cochlea. In pitch discrimination the difference limen seems to correspond to about the same distance on the basilar membrane as the width of a hair cell. These order-of-magnitude agreements somehow give a comfortable feeling of confidence that we "understand" the detection of faint sounds, the discrimination of pitch, and so on. But this feeling is legitimate only as long as we remember that we have only a bare outline and an order-of-magnitude approximation of a few aspects of the auditory mechanism. For other aspects, such as loudness and particularly the auditory qualities and the ability to pick a particular signal or voice out of a confused mixture

of sound, we have only very poor models or, in the anatomical or physiological sense, no model or "understanding" at all.

THE CENTRAL AUDITORY SYSTEM

As we proceed inward from the sense organ into the central nervous system, both the anatomy and the physiology suddenly become much more complicated. The system is composed of nerve cells, or *neurons,* and a special supporting tissue, the *glial* cells. Most of the neurons have axons, many of them covered with myelin sheaths as in peripheral nerves, which conduct the familiar all-or-none nerve impulses. In many places these myelinated axons are grouped together, as in peripheral nerves, and form definite *tracts* (white matter) that connect one area of the brain with another. But there are other areas (gray matter) where the cell bodies and the dendrites of the neurons are concentrated in vaguely defined masses, or *nuclei.*

The gray matter is where specialized axon terminations make contact (*synapses*) with the widely branching *dendrites* or with the cell bodies of other neurons. We can study the cell bodies with fine microelectrodes. Their all-or-none discharges resemble those of their axons, but they also show graded modifications of their resting electrical polarization that are produced by synaptic action (*postsynaptic potentials*). Another feature not seen in peripheral nerves is a tendency to synchronized electrical activity. The resulting slow waves can be detected by large electrodes placed in or near the areas of gray matter. Another difference in the gray matter is a very much higher rate of metabolism, which in turn requires a much richer blood supply. Chemical events, including chemical transmission from axon to dendrite at the synapses, become very important, and the action of nuclei or "nerve centers" can easily be modified by anesthetics, stimulants, or other drugs. Many of these synaptic properties are represented in the periphery in the junctions between sensory cells and nerve fibers or between axon terminations and muscle cells, but in the gray matter they are dominant. The greatest complexity of the central nervous system, however, arises from the sheer number of neurons (billions) and the extraordinary richness of their branching, their distribution, and their interconnections. The interconnections include many feedback loops.

In a general way the central nervous system is organized around four major sensory input systems and two major motor output systems. The major sensory systems are: (1) the chemical senses of smell and taste, (2) the somatosensory system from skin and skeletal muscles, (3) the visual system, and (4) the auditory system. In addition, there is the vestibular system for orientation to gravity and for acceleration, but this is closely integrated with the feedback kinesthetic system from the muscles and also with the visual system. The control system for the skeletal muscles is one of the motor outputs. It is sometimes called the "voluntary" muscle system, but a better term is *somatic*. The other motor system is the "involuntary" or *autonomic* system. With the endocrine glands of internal secretion, the autonomic nervous system is concerned with the internal regulation of the body.

The structure of nervous tissue, from the various classes of neurons and glia down to the microstructure revealed by the electron microscope, is still under study. The larger anatomical tracts and nuclei that constitute each of the sensory and motor systems are well known, but additional subdivisions and also numerous cross connections among the various systems are continually being discovered. In addition there are large areas of gray matter, with interconnecting tracts of white matter, that are not clearly related to any one of the primary sensory or motor systems. They form a large part of the *cerebral cortex* (see Figure 3-20) and are usually known as the "association areas."

Much is known about the function of the nervous system in terms of reflex motor responses to well-defined sensory stimuli and to combinations or sequences of stimuli. Behavior is related to bodily needs and their associated "drives" and to physiological states such as waking and sleeping.

Electrical "evoked responses" from particular areas within the brain help to relate neurophysiology to neuroanatomy. Still more is learned by direct stimulation, usually electrical but sometimes chemical, of central nervous structures and from simply observing the patterns of spontaneous electrical activity (the "electroencephalogram") in various physiological states such as waking and sleeping. The disruptive effects of lesions, either as they occur naturally by disease or accident, or deliberately as in experimental investigations in animals, or as they relieve symptoms of disease in humans, are also very informative.

The purpose of this topical review is to emphasize the complexity of the central nervous system and the variety of different kinds of information that contribute to our knowledge of it. One of the difficulties in the study of the central nervous system is to integrate these different classes of information.

The integration of neuroanatomy, neurochemistry, and neurophysiology is fairly satisfactory, although it is by no means complete. We do *not* understand, for example, the forces that guide growth and development or the intimate relations at the molecu-

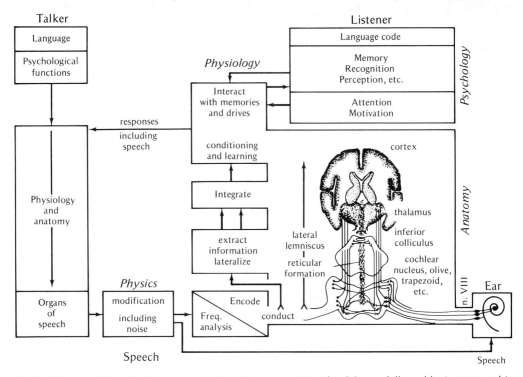

Figure 3-20 Diagram of the physical, anatomical, physiological, and psychological aspects of speech communication, from talker (left) to listener (right). The simplified anatomical diagram shows the ear, the eighth nerve, the major auditory tracts and nuclei of the medulla, the inferior colliculus of the midbrane, the medical geniculate body in the thalamus, and the primary auditory projection area in the superior convolution of the temporal lobe of the cortex. The centrally located reticular formation is also indicated. The cerebral hemispheres and the thalamus are cut in frontal section, the medulla and midbrain in cross section. Note the crossing of many but not all of the auditory pathways to the opposite side of the medulla and brain stem, and input to the reticular formation. Many other connections, for example, to the cerebellum, and the efferent pathways, are omitted.

The physiological processes that correspond very roughly to the successive anatomical levels appear in the central column. The psychological processes (at the top) are not assigned to any particular level, but in general they require the participation of the cerebral cortex. *(Modified from H. Davis in* International Audiology, *3:209–215; 1964; by permission)*

lar level among chemistry, microstructure, and physiological activity. We have no conception of the physical substrate of memory or learning. There is no need for a longer catalog of our ignorance.

On the positive side a rough parallelism has been established between successive anatomical areas or "levels" along the sensory input pathways. This relation is outlined for the auditory system in Figure 3-20. In this diagram the assignment of particular functions to particular "levels" or nuclei in the midbrain is purposely vague. The functions undoubtedly overlap greatly. The diagram does not include the efferent or feedback relations from the "higher" levels, remote from the sense organ, to the "lower" or more peripheral levels. In fact, one of the problems of sensory neurophysiology is to determine the contribution made by each tract and nucleus to the overall function of the whole system, both when the system is intact and when it is modified, either by lesions or by drugs.

In the diagram the physiological functions are arranged in sequence from bottom upward in order of their apparent complexity. So too the anatomical structures increase in complexity, both in terms of the absolute number of neurons and in terms of interconnections, as we go from auditory nerve to cerebral cortex. The psychological functions, such as perception, memory and motivation, abstract ideas, and the language code, are located in the diagram at the very top of the scale of complexity and are vaguely assigned by inference to the thalamocortical anatomical area. In fact it can be argued plausibly that such very complex activities as speech, language, abstract thinking, and planning for the future require a certain minimum gross amount of available nervous tissue available for the task. As a matter of comparative anatomy, only the larger whales and some dolphins have brains that are as large as, or larger than, the human brain.

An "understanding" of the anatomical and physiological substrate of perception, memory, thinking, and so on, is a difficult but fascinating long-term goal. It bridges the chasm between the subjective (and strictly psychological) inner world of each of us and the objective physiological, anatomical, chemical, and physical world of our bodies and their environment. The two worlds coexist in *time*, but the only thing that is able to cross the bridge between them is information. Both worlds are real, but the methods of observation and the concepts derived from them are different, and logically we must keep them separate.

Psychology studies behavior of the whole animal or person without concern for anatomy or physiological mechanisms and constructs its own laws of learning, memory, drives, and so forth. Psychology also studies the modification of behavior by lesions, disease, and drugs. Physiology and psychology meet, so to speak, in that they study the same man or animal, and often they use the same words, such as memory, learning, and drive. But the physiologist and the psychologist cannot "explain" one another's observations or concepts. They can only seek parallelisms that may suggest further experiments and observations, each in its proper frame of reference. And when the physiologist talks and thinks about psychology, he is usually guilty of outrageous oversimplification, and vice versa.

A useful aphorism concerning the central nervous system is: *Remember that everything is more complicated than you think.* Perhaps this is an understatement, and we should say "Everything is very much more complicated that we can readily conceive."

As implied in the foregoing discussion, the neurophysiology and the neurology of the auditory system are far too complex to be summarized usefully in this textbook of audiology. The point of view of audiology is fundamentally that of psychology, with special emphasis on psychophysics. It might even be misleading to present here an oversimplified systematic outline of neuroanatomy and neurophysiology. We shall therefore present only a few generalizations that this writer has found useful in his teaching.

Excitation, Inhibition, and Summation: Integration

In the central nervous system, *inhibition*, meaning reduction of ongoing activity or raising the threshold for new activity, is as important and widespread as excitation. Many neurons secrete an inhibitory instead of an excitatory chemical transmitter at their axonal synaptic endings. The inhibitory transmitter increases the electrical conductance of the surface membrane of the dendrite or cell body and thus short-circuits and makes ineffective the excitatory postsynaptic potentials. The dendrites and the neuronal cell bodies sum algebraically the simultaneous inhibitory and excitatory inputs that reach them from different sources. This is known as *spatial summation*. The neuron discharges all-or-none impulses along its axon when a critical level of electrical depolarization is reached at a particular region, usually the "axon hillock," where the axon originates. The frequency of discharge depends on the degree of depolarization. A slow "spontaneous" or "tonic" discharge may continue indefinitely. The postsynaptic electric potentials that are summed outlast the individual incoming nerve impulses, so *temporal summation* takes place over times up to a tenth of a second. This amounts to a very short-term memory. In general either temporal or spatial summation or both are required to modify the output of a neuron.

The summation of excitatory and inhibitory inputs, over space and time, are characteristic of the dendrites of neurons and thus of the gray matter in the nervous system. They are called neural "integration." Only through the balancing of excitation and inhibition, combined with negative feedback, are close motor control and coordination possible. In sensory systems inhibition is essential for fine discrimination. The principle of organization here is a *mutual inhibitory action*, based on anatomical cross connections between neighboring sensory units or between the second-order neurons that they activate. The interaction is strongest between the units that are closest to one another. The result is that a unit that is more strongly stimulated tends to inhibit its neighbors and thereby to be released from their inhibitory influence. This is a sort of positive (or double negative) feedback that serves to enhance contrast at boundaries. The mechanism is often called "lateral inhibition" because it was first described in the visual system between sensory units that lie side by side. "Mutal inhibition" is a more general term. In the mammalian auditory system this mutual inhibition is very clear in the first synaptic integrating area, namely the cochlear nucleus in the medulla oblongata, and clearly assists in sharpening the response areas of its second-order neurons.

Successive Integrating Stations, Multiple Pathways, and Parallel Processing

Various nuclei in the brain stem that are linked by clear tracts or "bundles" of white matter constitute the auditory system. The more important of them are indicated in Figure 3-20. The system branches repeatedly, first in the cochlear nucleus where the incoming sensory neurons divide and distribute to two major subdivisions (see also Figure 4-1). There are several output pathways from this nucleus.

There is always a delay of the order of a millisecond between the arrival of a volley (a nearly synchronous group) of impulses in incoming fibers and the appearance of a corresponding output volley. The cumulative delay measured at successive stations gives an estimate of the minimum number of synapses that must have been crossed. The term "second-order neuron" in the previous section means a neuron that lies beyond at least one synapse, not counting the junction, if any, between specialized receptor and the first or primary neuron. The minimum number of synapses between the primary neuron and the cerebral cortex is probably three. This minimum number, and also the minimum delay along the shortest route to the cortex, can be established by observing the evoked responses at various points along the pathway. The first volley, which is the easiest to observe, has probably been overemphasized in the past. The later volleys of impulses (or asynchronous impulses) in the same or other pathways are equally important. There is at least one major pathway to the cortex in addition to the one shown in Figure 3-20, probably through the reticular formation. Other pathways may be anatomically quite diffuse.

The classical term "relay station" for the successive nuclei misses a most important point. *Integrating station (or area)* is much better. Output to motor mechanisms, to other sensory systems, or feedback to more peripheral parts of the auditory system occur at all anatomical levels. The auditory cortex is only one of many final "destinations" of the incoming information. Auditory input is distributed widely. Different aspects of information contained in it are extracted in different ways (for example, by mutual inhibition as opposed to spatial summation), in different places, and for different purposes. We must think of simultaneous multiple and parallel processing of information.

Tonotopic Organization

In the auditory pathways, as in other sensory systems, the spatial relations within the original sensory surface, whether organ of Corti, retina, skin, or somatic musculature, tend to be retained. This orderly arrangement is clear in each of the two major divisions of the cochlear nucleus. Since position along the organ of Corti is related to acoustic frequency, the arrangement is said to be "tonotopic." The tonotopic organization becomes less clear in successive integrating areas, and may be almost absent in the auditory cortex of many animals, including the cat.

Electrical activity in response to the onset of a pure tone is very widespread throughout the auditory area. Furthermore, the primary auditory area, defined by the distribution of fibers from the medial geniculate body in the thalamus, is probably not the only auditory gateway to the cortex.

In the human brain the "primary projection area" of the medial geniculate body is located in the temporal lobe, on its superior surface deep in the Sylvian fissure. It is oriented perpendicular to the surface of the skull, and its electrical activity is not effectively recorded by a scalp electrode placed over the Sylvian fissure. Other neighboring areas, called secondary auditory areas, seem also to be part of the auditory system, both in man and animals, but the difference in function of these secondary areas, which are present in all of the sensory systems, is not known. Between the major sensory or motor areas lie the less clearly assigned "association areas," which are essential for certain very complex functions such as language, the meaning of visual symbols, memory of spatial relations, or the ability to plan effectively for the future.

Homolateral versus Contralateral Representation: Dominance

In the somatosensory system (skin and somatic muscles) the topological representation is clear and systematic. The representation of each organ (hand, foot, mouth, torso, and so on) is roughly proportional to its sensory use in exploring the environment. (The manual skills of man and monkey are probably an outgrowth of this exploratory use of the hand as opposed to locomotion.) The right side of the body is represented in the left thalamus and cortex, and vice versa; that is, representation is contralateral.

In the motor control and the somatosensory representation of the limbs, the separation of right and left is complete and representation is strictly contralateral. In man, one side or the other, usually the right hand and its left cortex, are preferred or "dominant" for the learning and execution of motor skills. The visual system is organized in man with the left half of each retina projecting to the left cortex and the right half to the right cortex. Lateral dominance or preference of right or left eye as a whole may be demonstrable, but it is not particularly important. In the auditory system both ears seem to share each auditory cortex to a large extent, although the contralateral ear is more strongly represented. The extent of the homolateral representation is uncertain.

The partial crossing of the afferent auditory pathways to the opposite side takes place in the medulla in the tracts from the cochlear nucleus to the trapezoid bodies and to the superior olivary complex and the other midbrain auditory integrating areas (Figure 3-20). Each area receives some innervation from each cochlear nucleus. The first area, in time sequence and anatomical directness, in which interaction between right and left input occurs is apparently the superior olivary complex. Here some sort of priority or dominance is established in favor of the *earlier* or the *stronger* auditory input, right or left. The subjective counterpart is a perception of the sound in a spatial frame of reference, usually external, but under conditions of receiver listening inside or at the surface of the head. Another integrating area, the inferior colliculi, where there are clear pathways across the midline, seems to be related to reflex turning of head, eyes, or both toward the source of a new sound. There are feedback connections to the cochlear nuclei from anatomically "higher" centers and also from the superior olivary complex to the cochlea (bundle of Rasmussen).

The relative simplicity and directness of the first interaction between right and left suggests that its function is both primitive and important biologically. Apparently it is the orientation of ears (or head) to the direction of the source. This response appears early in human infancy.

There are very few indications of a dominant ear if neither one is impaired. There is, however, a strong dominance of one cerebral

cortex, usually the left, for the learning of speech, both its receptive and its motor aspects. (The hemisphere not dominant for speech is probably dominant for learning spatial relations.) The dominant hemisphere for speech is not necessarily the dominant hemisphere for manual skill. Dominance for any of these functions may be altered, or develop differently, if there is early injury (before 2 years of age). The uninjured side becomes dominant. This so-called "plasticity" in the developing human brain wears off gradually after 2 years of age. Sensory input certainly and probably some sort of motor feedback also seem to be involved in establishing the initial patterns of sensory organization and motor skill, which later appear as dominance.

Much attention is currently being given to the proposition that language, mathematics, and analytic reasoning are based in the left hemisphere, whereas spatial relations, music, and other nonlanguage sounds and the "holistic" aspects of sensory information are dealt with by the right hemisphere. The possiblity of independent learning in the two hemispheres when the connection between them (corpus callosum) is cut provides dramatic examples of differences in the normal functions.

Midbrain Functions and Cortical Functions

Contrary to earlier opinion, the basic auditory discriminations of pitch and loudness, and perhaps other qualities as well, *can be* relearned or even learned originally by an animal that has been completely deprived of its auditory cortex. Original learning in the normal animal does involve the cortex, as shown by loss of the learned response following removal. The ablation must be complete, primary and secondary areas bilaterally. Any small part of the auditory area is sufficient for retention of the learned discrimination. This is evidence of a broad type of cortical "localization" or organization and also of an extraordinary degree of "equipotentiality" within the major area. In the cortically deprived animal, however, there are limitations of another sort. Broadly, the animal cannot use auditory information effectively in either the temporal or the spatial frame of reference. It can learn to discriminate tones but not to recognize *sequences* of tones, that is, even the simplest of tunes. Also it is handicapped in correct *lateralization of the source* on the basis of the cues of relative loudness or temporal precedence. The human loses his ability to understand speech after injury to certain "speech areas." One interpretation of these deficiencies related to cortical injury is that a short-term auditory memory, which is necessary for the recognition of temporal patterns, has been lost.

when we ask where memories are stored. The answer seems to be "everywhere and therefore nowhere." Somehow it seems to be the wrong question. The memory file in the nervous system is not item by item, spatially organized as in a filing cabinet. Memory seems to be diffuse. The clearest handicap that is related in general to the loss of central nervous tissue, either locally or diffusely (if it is less than an entire auditory or motor or somatosensory area), is a loss of speed. The job can be done but more slowly. Also learning is more difficult. It is as if a certain number of neuron-microseconds are required for complicated tasks of pattern recognition, and so on, but that a considerable amount of trading of neurons for microseconds is possible. Perhaps some neural operations that formerly could be performed in parallel must now be carried out serially by the remaining available neurons.

Anatomical Equipotentiality and Speed of Execution

The principle of equipotentiality, meaning that any part can perform the function of the whole, apparently operates within large subdivisions of the brain. This power of "substitution," or "alternate pathways," or "cortical reserve" may extend beyond the cortex, although it is less and less clear as we approach the periphery, either on the sensory or the motor side. Certainly the nervous system is extremely adaptable in many ways. Equipotentiality is very puzzling, however,

Other Aspects of Neurophysiology

These disjointed comments do little more than sample the complexities of the nervous system and how it operates. For example, we will not even comment on the effects of electrical stimulation of the cerebral cortex. Further detail on some topics will be provided in appropriate contexts in other chapters, notably in Chapter 4 in relation to central dysacusis, and in Chapter 8 in relation to some of the more complicated audiometric tests.

SUGGESTED READINGS AND REFERENCES

Békésy, G. von. *Experiments in Hearing*, E. G. Wever, (ed.). New York: McGraw-Hill Book Company, 1960.
   A collection of all of von Békésy's papers on the ear, beautifully edited, arranged, and indexed. The earlier papers, written in German, have been translated into English.

Békésy Commemorative Issue of the *Journal of the Acoustical Society of America*, Vol. 34, No. 9—part 2, 1962.

Twenty-five papers dealing with auditory anatomy, physiology, or psychophysics. Some are reviews, others are original contributions. They include electron microscopy, the efferent olivocochlear bundle, the impedance of the middle ear, and the acoustic reflex.

Dallos, P. *The Auditory Periphery, Biophysics and Physiology*. New York and London: Academic Press, 1973.

A unified authoritative account of cochlear function, including the electric potentials.

Davis, H. "A Model for Transducer Action in the Cochlea," *Sympos. Quant. Biol.* (Sensory Receptors), 30: 181–190 (1965). Cold Spring Harbor, N.Y.: Cold Spring Laboratory of Quantitative Biology.

This is the author's most recent discussion of his model for cochlear excitation.

Field, J., H. W. Magoun, and V. E. Hall (eds.). *Handbook of Physiology, Section 1: Neurophysiology*. Washington, D.C.: American Physiological Society, 1959.

See, especially, Chapter 23 ("Excitation of Auditory Receptors," by H. Davis) and Chapter 24 ("Central Auditory Mechanisms," by H. W. Ades). This is a standard reference book for neurophysiologists.

House, W. F. "Cochlear Implants." *Ann. Otol.* (Suppl. 27), 85:1–93, 1976.

The history of the development of the cochlear implant at the Ear Research Institute (Los Angeles), and an assessment of its present status and prospects. Case histories of 16 patients are included.

Keidel, W. D., and W. D. Neff (eds.). *Handbook of Sensory Physiology*. Vols. V(1), V(2), V(3) (Auditory System). New York: Springer-Verlag 1974, 1975, 1976.

Extensive and exhaustive treatment (three volumes) of the auditory system in many separate chapters by leading investigators.

Kiang, N. Y-S. *Discharge Patterns of Single Fibers in the Cat's Auditory Nerve*, Research Monograph No. 35. Cambridge, Mass.: M.I.T. Press, 1965.

A landmark volume in auditory neurophysiology.

Møller, A. R. (ed.). *Basic Mechanisms in Hearing*. New York: Academic Press, 1973.

This multidisciplinary symposium was sponsored by the Swedish Medical Research Council, the Natural Science Research Council, and the Royal Swedish Academy of Sciences.

Polyak, S. L., G. McHugh, and D. K. Judd. *The Human Ear in Anatomical Transparencies*. Elmsford, N.Y.: Sonotone Corporation, 1946. (Distributed by T. H. McKenna, Inc., New York.)

A unique and very effective presentation of the anatomy of the ear, accompanied by an excellent text.

"Proceedings of the International Conference on Audiology, St. Louis, May 1957." *Laryngoscope*, 68:209–682 (1958).

*This volume contains a planned symposium on the physiology of the audi-
tory system and also many contributed papers. It is probably the best summary of several aspects of audiology in the English language as of 1957.*

Rasmussen, G. L., and W. W. Windle (eds.). *Neural Mechanisms of the Audi-
tory and Vestibular Systems.* Springfield, Ill.: Charles C. Thomas, 1960.
*This volume is based on the proceedings of a conference sponsored by the
National Institute for Neurological Diseases and Blindness in 1959.*

Simmons, F. B. "Electrical Stimulation of the Auditory Nerve in Man," *Arch.
Otolaryng. (Chicago)*, 84:2–54 (1966).
*An excellent review and a full account of the operation, and also the results
of an 18-month study of a single case.*

Stevens, S. S. (ed.), *Handbook of Experimental Psychology.* New York: John
Wiley & Sons, 1951.
*Chapter 27 ("The Mechanical Properties of the Ear," by G. von Békésy and
W. A. Rosenblith) and Chapter 28 ("Psychophysiology of Hearing and
Deafness," by H. Davis) are particularly pertinent.*

Wever, E. G., and M. Lawrence. *Physiological Acoustics.* Princeton, N.J.:
Princeton University Press, 1954.
This book deals authoritatively with sound conduction in the middle ear.

Zwislocki, J. J., H. Spoendlin, P. Dallos and E. F. Evans. "A Symposium on
Cochlear Function, at the 12th International Congress of Audiology (Paris),"
Audiology, 14 (5–6): 381–455 (1975).
*A very informative review of the innervation, the biophysics, the electrical
activity, and the frequency selectivity of the cochlea.*

Part II

ABNORMAL HEARING: PREVENTION AND TREATMENT

Hallowell Davis, M.D.

4

Abnormal Hearing and Deafness

DEFINITIONS AND DISTINCTIONS

The word "deafness" has been used to mean either partial or total loss of hearing. In French the word *surdité* and in Spanish the word *sordera* have just this broad meaning. In English, however, the term "hard of hearing" has been introduced to replace the phrase "partially deaf." Unfortunately we have no corresponding noun, "hardness of hearing," equivalent to the German *Schwerhörigkeit*, to replace "partial deafness." Our nearest equivalents are "impairment of hearing" and "hearing loss."

The medical and social problems of hard-of-hearing patients are quite different from those of the totally deaf, and therefore the two should not be grouped together indiscriminately. The psychological value of this point is discussed at some length in later chapters, but there is still some confusion resulting from old habits of speech and from the necessity of distinguishing between two or three terms.

The introduction of new terms and the change in the meaning of old ones depend on the gathering of new information, the development of new insights, and the formulation of new purposes. We therefore repeat some old definitions, carefully worded and phrased, and introduce certain new or nearly new additional terms. A change in terminology involves, of course, the rejection of some old terms and the restriction of the meaning of others.

Deafness, Hearing Loss, and Dysacusis

The simple, everyday concept of "deafness" is a total or severe impairment of hearing, and in this book we shall continue to use "deafness" to include total loss of hearing, whatever the cause. Impairment of hearing of the sort that simply requires the other person to talk louder we shall call a "hearing loss," and we shall avoid the term "partial deafness." Hearing loss and deafness both imply a loss of sensitivity of hearing, presumably in the peripheral hearing mechanisms. Both lie along the same dimension, and the question is where to draw the line between hard of hearing and deaf.

The usefulness of a criterion depends on our purposes, and the important purposes for which these terms are useful are social, educational, and medical. We shall adopt a *social criterion for deafness,* namely, that *everyday auditory communication is impossible or very nearly so.* In terms of hearing levels we find a zone of uncertainty from 70 to 90 dB (ANSI) averaged over the frequencies 500, 1000, and 2000 Hz. Within this zone some individuals are socially deaf, but more of them are merely very hard of hearing. The frequent successful use of hearing aids makes it undesirable to include this "gray area" automatically under the term "deaf," as has often been the custom in the past. *We propose to confine the term deafness to hearing-threshold levels for speech greater than 92 dB.* A good reason for selecting this particular boundary is that the most authoritative medical rule for estimating the handicap imposed by hearing loss (see Chapter 9) reads "if the average hearing-threshold level at 500, 1000, and 2000 Hz is over 92 dB (ANSI), the handicap for hearing everyday speech should be considered total." Our criterion thus has a medical sanction in a social and economic context.

We do not here propose any educational criterion for deafness. Whether a child is judged to be "educable" or not may involve his visual skills, his intelligence, his emotional stability, and so on, perhaps in addition to handicaps other than deafness. Most deaf children, as well as hard-of-hearing children, can be educated, although the methods may differ, as we shall see in Chapter 17.

The successful use of a hearing aid may make the difference between being socially deaf or being merely hard of hearing even for some persons whose hearing-threshold levels for speech are 93 dB or higher. For them, "hard of hearing" is a better practical designation than "deaf." This is true even though in the context of accidental injury or industrial hearing loss their handicap for hearing everyday speech is considered total. In assessment of handicap for purposes of compensation the evaluation is made without the use of a hearing aid.

So far we have considered only the dimension of sensitivity of hearing. On this dimension the zone of normal includes hearing-threshold levels for speech from 0 to 25 dB. The condition known as hard of hearing begins at 27 dB and that for deaf begins at 93 dB (see Chapters 2 and 9). There is, however, another dimension—or, rather, there are several other dimensions of hearing—that may be impaired. For example, a person may say, "Don't shout, I hear you, but I can't make out the words." Then it is his "discrimination for speech" that is faulty. Or he may be unable to attach meaning to auditory signals because of a failure of understanding of the type we call "auditory agnosia." And there are other kinds of impairment, which we shall consider in more detail later in this chapter. All of these other types of impairment of hearing have one feature in common that makes it desirable to have a single term to include all of them. The common feature is that *they are not simple losses of sensitiv-*

ity of hearing. These impairments cannot be measured properly in decibels. *The inclusive term that we shall use for all of these other impairments of hearing is dysacusis.*

Dysacusis is not a new word in the medical vocabulary, but it is not yet widely used. It means, however, just what we want to say: "faulty hearing." "Acusis" (or acousis) refers to hearing, as in the more familiar terms "presbycusis," "diplacusis." "Dys-" as a prefix may mean "ill" or "painful," but it also means "difficult," "faulty," "impaired," or "abnormal."

Dysacusis (also spelled "dysacusia" and "dysacousia") may be due to malfunction of the sense organ, or it may be due to abnormal function of the brain. Thus certain forms of diplacusis, presbycusis, and discrimination loss we will call "peripheral dysacusis," and we will use the term "central dysacusis" for such conditions as psychogenic or hysterical block of hearing, auditory agnosia, phonemic regression, and so on.

A point that must be emphasized immediately is that *deafness or hearing loss* on the one hand and *dysacusis*, both peripheral and central, on the other hand, *are not mutually exclusive.* A patient may have both a hearing loss, measurable in decibels, and also a dysacusis in the form of a loss of discrimination, some phonemic regression, or the like. In case of doubt, dysacusis should be considered the broader term equivalent to impairment of hearing of all kinds, two or three of which may be present at the same time. Hard of hearing *implies specifically one kind of impairment*, the one that is best understood and most readily measured, namely *simple loss of sensitivity*, presumably in the ear itself or in its nerve. Deafness will remain the general term for the symptom of total or nearly total loss of hearing, but we shall avoid the term "central deafness." Of course, before a diagnosis is made we may use the terms "deaf" and "dysacu-

sic," or "hard of hearing" and "dysacusic" pretty much interchangeably. Dysacusis is the word to use when we wish to emphasize either (1) that the symptom is not merely reduced sensitivity of hearing, or (2) that the trouble may lie in the central nervous system rather than in the ear.

For those who enjoy complete, well-rounded systems of nomenclature there are the terms *anacusia* (or "anacousia") and *hypoacusia* (or "hypoacousia"), which can be used as exact synonyms for deafness and hearing loss, respectively.

Varieties of Auditory Impairment

From the medical and anatomical point of view there are three major types of impairment of hearing: poor conduction of sound to the sense organ, abnormality of the sense organ or its nerve, and impairments that result from some injury to or failure of function in the central nervous system (CNS). These broad divisions are illustrated in Figure 4-1. One problem of otological and audiological diagnosis is to assess correctly the part played by each *type of impairment* for each particular patient. Another is to determine just *where* the impairment is located, whether in the external ear, the middle ear, the cochlea, the organ of Corti, the auditory nerve, or within the central nervous system. Another problem, of course, is to determine the probable *cause* of the difficulty. The emphasis is different in each case, but the problems overlap, and this has led to considerable difficulty in the choice and consistent use of appropriate terms.

The common mild or moderate impairments that are due to failure of normal physical conduction of sound to the cochlea are hearing losses, and the people who suffer from them are hard of hearing. If it is only physical conduction that is impaired, the hearing threshold level cannot be worse than

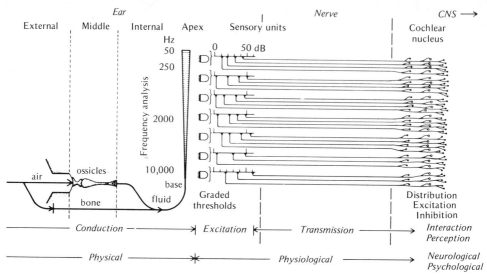

Figure 4-1 This summary diagram of the peripheral auditory mechanism is semianatomical. The air-conduction pathway shows the ossicles simplified to a subdivided columella, disregarding their lever action. The single bone-conduction pathway combines all of the pathways that bypass the ossicular chain. The air and bone pathways unite beyond the ossicles in the fluids of the inner ear. The tapering basilar membrane is represented as straight. Here acoustic frequency analysis takes place, as indicated. All of this is part of the physical process of sound conduction.

   The sensory units are represented by nerve fibers (with cell bodies omitted), running from the hair cells arranged along the basilar membrane to the cochlear nucleus where they branch to several (here three) distinct regions, each of which preserves the tonotopic organization of the basilar membrane. Each of the hair cells shown in the diagram represents the group of cells in a short segment of the organ of Corti. The sensory units from any small segment, represented arbitrarily here by groups of 3 or 4, have different thresholds for any given tone. The gradation of thresholds is represented here by an arbitrary scale of decibels, 0 to 50, for each small segment. The actual range of gradation is not known, nor is its relation to anatomical distribution, such as inner versus outer hair cells. (Further discussion in text in Chapter 3.) The efferent auditory nerves are omitted from this diagram.

about 70 dB because at this level bone conduction takes over and the sound is heard, provided that the sense organ is still intact. Really loud speech can still be understood, and the successful use of a hearing aid is relatively easy. We shall therefore speak of *conductive hearing loss* and give up the old term "conductive deafness." As we shall see, conductive hearing loss includes but is not quite equivalent to "middle-ear impairment."

   Auditory agnosia, phonemic regression, and hysterical or psychogenic dysacusis are very clearly the result of some abnormal functioning of the central nervous system. The patient may or may not respond to a test with an audiometer, and he may give very different results on different trials. He is,

however, unable to understand speech, or does so only in a very limited way, even though he may "hear" something on the audiometer.

   Greater difficulties of definition appear when the trouble lies anatomically within the cochlea or in the central auditory connections, or both. For this group of disorders we shall use either dysacusis or hearing loss, depending on whether we wish to emphasize loss of discrimination or loss of sensitivity. We shall lean toward the medical tradition in our basic classification and usually speak of sensorineural hearing loss. Sometimes we want to distinguish between disorders of the sense organ and impairment of the auditory nerve. Modern diagnostic tests are making this distinction possible, and, as we shall see, the accurate diagnosis of the site and type of the trouble is of great importance for prognosis and, above all, for treatment. We shall then speak of "sense-organ dysacusis" or "sense-organ hearing loss" on the one hand and "neural hearing loss" (or sometimes "neural dysacusis") on the other. We shall avoid the familiar but less grammatical form "nerve deafness," and particularly the pernicious term "perceptive deafness." The latter is a wastebasket term once much used by otologists to catch everything that is not conductive. This usage disregards the prior use of the terms "perception" and "perceptive" by psychologists. If the term ever had a proper logical meaning, it should have meant approximately what we now call "auditory agnosia" or "central perceptive dysacusis," but for a long time it was a synonym for "nerve deafness."

Still another term is necessary to describe the common combination of conductive and sensorineural hearing losses. For this we shall use the familiar term "mixed hearing loss," but it will not include impairments that lie central to the auditory nerve.

When, as also may happen, a person has some conductive, or sensorineural, or mixed hearing loss, and also some *central* difficulties of the central perceptive or of the psychogenic variety, we shall speak of a "combined dysacusis" or perhaps of a "peripheral hearing loss with a psychogenic (or central or agnosic) overlay."

The proper antonym for "central" is "peripheral." "Peripheral" hearing loss means "conductive, or sensorineural, or mixed" hearing loss. The otologist may sometimes use the word "retrocochlear" to cover the anatomical areas beyond the cochlea—that is, auditory nerve, brain stem and beyond, or, practically speaking, everything outside the primary domain and responsibility of otology. "Retrocochlear" or "retrolabyrinthine"

includes tumors of the auditory nerve but excludes sense-organ impairment.

A pair of contrasting terms in common use are "organic" and "functional." Organic implies that the difficulty is caused by an anatomical injury or abnormality that a pathologist could identify if he looked in the right place. Functional may mean either "nonorganic" or "physiological" or "with no visible pathology" or "better understood on a psychological than on an anatomical basis." An objection to these terms, in addition to the vagueness of functional, is the implication that they usually carry that a difficulty is exclusively organic *or* functional, whereas, more often than not, anatomical, physiological, and psychological factors are all significant.

Hearing loss and hearing level   The term "hearing loss" has carried a heavy burden for the last three decades. In the medical and social senses in which we have used it here it has served to mean "an impairment of hearing that does not entirely prevent practical communication by speech." But hearing loss has also been used to mean the number of decibels by which the threshold of hearing is elevated above the zero level to which an audiometer is calibrated. Hearing loss has also been used to mean a change for the worse or shift of threshold from one level to another. Thus, the term can be very confusing, as in the following statement, which might have been made in a court or before an industrial commission.

This employee suffered a hearing loss of 40 dB from exposure to noise. He had a hearing loss of 25 dB before employment, which, however, is just above normal limits. His actual hearing loss was 65 dB when he was examined the day after stopping work. Of this loss, 10 dB later proved to be a temporary hearing loss, so his permanent hearing loss now appears to be 55 dB. This is not conductive. It is a pure sensorineural hearing loss.

In Chapter 2 we introduced the relatively new term "hearing-threshold level" to take some of the load off hearing loss. Hearing-threshold level is the number of decibels that a person's threshold of hearing lies above the reference zero of the audiometer for that particular frequency (or for that particular speech test). The ASA Standards for Audiometers of 1951 and 1952 required that the intensity dial be labeled "hearing loss," and most audiogram charts were marked the same way; but in the next revision (ANSI S3.6-1969) the term was "hearing threshold level" instead. The sound-pressure levels produced by an audiometer, measured in an appropriate coupler and referred to standard audiometric reference zero level are "hearing levels." The audiometer reading that corresponds to the faintest tone a person can hear is his "hearing-threshold level" for that frequency.

Furthermore, when there is any possibility of ambiguity, we shall call a shift or change of threshold a *threshold shift* and not a hearing loss. The least one can do to avoid confusion when referring to a change of level is to speak of a "loss of hearing" and not a "hearing loss."

In sum, we shall use (1) *hearing level* (HL) to designate the output of an audiometer referred to an audiometric zero level, (2) *hearing-threshold level* to designate the sensitivity of an individual's hearing, and (3) *threshold shift* for any change in his hearing-threshold level; and we shall reserve (4) *hearing loss* for the general condition of impaired hearing or the process that causes it. The implications of "hearing loss" are of a partial handicap or of an abnormality of structure or function. "Hearing-threshold level," however, carries no implication of handicap or even abnormality. It simply states the result of an objective psychophysical measurement. Unless otherwise specified the calibration or reference zero level of the audiometer will always be assumed to be ANSI S3.6-1969, which is the same as the earlier ISO zero levels. (See Chapter 7 for details.) A practical rule to keep the usage of these terms straight is: "If decibels are involved, the proper term isn't 'hearing loss'; it is either 'hearing level' or 'threshold shift.'"

Another rule, to which we shall return in Chapter 9, is: "There is no such thing as percentage of hearing level or even percentage of hearing loss." Occasionally we talk of percentage of handicap, and a lawyer may talk about percentage of disability, but these values are calculated by arbitrary rules and only for particular purposes such as compensation.

Now with our new terms to help us, let us try again that statement made in court by the examining physician. He now says:

This employee suffered a loss of hearing from exposure to noise. The threshold shift was 40 dB. His hearing-threshold level before employment was 25 dB (ANSI), which is just above normal limits. His actual hearing-threshold level the day after he stopped work was 65 dB. Of this, 10 dB proved to be a temporary threshold shift, so his final and presumably permanent hearing-threshold level now appears to be 55 dB. He does not have any conductive hearing loss; his impairment is purely sensorineural.

PERIPHERAL HEARING LOSS

A few moments' study of the anatomy of the ear, described in Chapter 3 and summarized in Figure 4-1, will make clear the distinctions between middle-ear impairment and cochlear impairment. The distinction is important because the prognosis and the treatment, as well as the causes of the two types, differ considerably. It is sometimes very simple to distinguish between the two by tests of hearing, but it is always possible and even probable that any case is really a mixture or combination of the two impairments. Figure 4-1 also shows that the division between the conductive process and the sensorineural processes lies within the cochlea at the hair cells. Conductive hearing loss includes middle-ear impairment but extends beyond it.

Conductive hearing loss may be caused by plugging the external canal, damping the free movement of the drum, or restricting the movements of the ossicles. Any of these will reduce the intensity of the airborne sound that finally reaches the inner ear. Wax impacted in the canal is the commonest form of plug, and wax in contact with the drum or the scars of old healed perforations of the drum may restrict its vibrations. Adhesions of scar tissue on the ossicles or a bony new growth of otosclerosis around the edge of the stapes in the oval window may restrict the normal movements of the ossicles even more severely.

Middle-Ear Hearing Loss

The classical test to distinguish middle-ear from cochlear or sensorineural impairment is the difference between air-conduction hearing levels and bone-conduction hearing levels. With severe impairment of conduction in the middle ear, as from adhesions or otosclerosis, the audiometer may show a hearing-threshold level for airborne sound as high as 60 or possibly 70 dB. The patient may be quite unable to hear a vibrating tuning fork held near his ear. Thus his "air conduction" is said to be "reduced." But if the shaft of the vibrating fork is now applied to his skull, or the bone-conduction vibrator of the audiometer is placed on the mastoid bone just behind his ear, he may be able to hear the sound as well as a normal person does in the same test. There is no reduction in his "bone conduction."

If he can hear normally by bone conduc-

tion, we infer that his inner ear and auditory nerve must be normal and that his difficulty in hearing depends only on some obstacle in the external or middle ear to the conduction of airborne sound. Audiograms showing hearing-threshold levels by air conduction and by bone conduction in sensorineural loss and in middle-ear conductive loss are shown in Chapter 7, where the audiogram is explained in detail. The difference between the hearing-threshold levels by air conduction and by bone conduction is called the "air-bone gap" and, if allowance is made for the "Carhart notch," explained in the next paragraph, it measures the conductive loss in the middle ear.

It is tempting to assume that if *bone* conduction is reduced, there must be a corresponding degree of sensorineural hearing loss. However, there are practical pitfalls. Some skulls and the skin and soft tissues over them do not conduct sound as well as others. As another example, when the footplate of the stapes is firmly fixed in the oval window by otosclerosis, the fluids in the inner ear can no longer move so freely under the influence of bone-conducted acoustic energy. This makes the hearing-threshold level at 2000 Hz for bone conduction 10 to 15 dB poorer than it would otherwise be. At 500, 1000, and 4000 Hz the threshold shift is usually only 5 to 10 dB. The resulting dip in the bone-conduction audiogram is sometimes called the "Carhart notch." Following successful stapes surgery the bone-conduction threshold shifts back toward zero by this amount.

In addition, there are special technical difficulties in obtaining accurate measurements of hearing-threshold levels by bone conduction, such as the presence of too much background noise in the test room. These will also be considered in Chapter 7, but in general the audiologist or otologist hesitates to conclude that he is dealing with sensorineural hearing loss simply on the basis of finding poor hearing by bone conduction without supporting evidence.

Important supporting evidence for middle-ear impairment may be provided by measurements of the acoustic impedance or admittance of the ear. The concepts of impedance and admittance are explained in Chapter 7, together with the methods of measurement that are now available. In simplest terms the measurement of acoustic impedance is a measure of the stiffness of middle ear's conductive system. The stiffness is greatly reduced by interruption of the ossicular chain and is greatly increased by stapedial otosclerosis or by surface adhesions from otitis media. In either case the efficiency of the conductive mechanism is reduced. Normal values for impedance or conductance are strong evidence against middle-ear conductive impairment, but abnormal values do not directly measure the air-bone gap.

Conductive hearing loss is not much of a handicap to hearing in a noisy place. In fact, a man with pure conductive hearing loss of moderate degree can hear conversations just as well as the average person can (and better than a great many) in traffic, in airplanes, and in similar noisy surroundings. Under these conditions he simply does not hear, or hears only faintly, the noise that disturbs his companion with normal hearing and masks the speech at ordinary conversation levels. But in noise all of us automatically talk louder—loud enough so that we can hear ourselves above the noise. The loud speech overrides a moderate conductive hearing loss. The problem for our hard-of-hearing listener is no longer that of *hearing* the speech but only of *distinguishing* it from as much of the noise as also succeeds in reaching his sense organ. Since he does not hear much of the noise and his sense organ is normal, he can distinguish and understand the loud speech as well as anyone. Furthermore, the

training in understanding speech that has been forced on him by his hearing loss is likely to give him an actual advantage over a person with normal hearing. This ability to hear in noisy places as well as, or better than, normal persons has been given the impressive name of *paracusis Willisii* and is characteristic of conductive hearing loss.

Inner-Ear Conductive Hearing Loss

Until recently all inner-ear impairments were automatically classed as sensorineural. It now appears useful to recognize that physical changes can occur in the basilar membrane and the tectorial membrane, or both, and that they may reduce the efficiency with which acoustic energy is delivered to the hair cells. In this chapter we define the sense organ and sensory hearing loss as beginning at the hair cells, as indicated in Figure 4-1. This provides a more logical set of definitions with (1) proper distinctions between anatomical areas and physiological processes; (2) recognition of the tissues of the basilar and tectorial membranes as the potential site of significant physical changes, notably as the result of aging; (3) a more plausible explanation of the results of certain tests of hearing, notably the "recruitment of loudness," which will be discussed below; and (4) a conceptual framework adequate for our rapidly increasing knowledge of the pathology of the inner ear.

Some useful generalizations about conductive hearing loss and its alleviation are as follows:

1. A conductive abnormality always causes more or less attenuation of the acoustic energy that reaches the sense organ. The normal young ear is about as efficient physically as it can possibly be, and can get only worse. Nature does not introduce new amplifiers in the system.

2. The attenuation is usually, though not always, different for different frequencies.

Sometimes the attenuation is greater the lower the frequency. This gives the so-called "rising audiogram" which was once thought to be characteristic of conductive hearing loss or middle-ear impairment. Quite often, however, the audiogram falls toward the high frequencies. This is particularly true of the types of inner- and middle-ear conductive impairment associated with aging.

3. Conductive impairments may occur in different parts of the system simultaneously, and their effects will be additive.

4. Conductive impairments may make the system more nonlinear in its action and thus increase the distortion of the acoustic waveforms that reach the sense organ.

5. The attenuation of conductive impairment can be imitated by electric or acoustic filters and, subject to limitations imposed by nonlinearity, can be offset by amplification, provided also that the frequency characteristics of the amplifier are properly chosen.

6. Any nonlinear distortion associated with the impairment not only will not be corrected, but is likely to become worse when the input signal is increased in order to deliver more acoustic energy to the sense organ. Moreover, the amplifier may introduce additional distortion of its own.

Sensorineural Hearing Loss

Sensorineural impairment is best understood in anatomical and physiological terms. The concept of the sensory unit (see Chapter 3) is helpful. It will be recalled that a sensory unit is an auditory nerve fiber plus the hair cell or cells that excite it. One inner hair excites ten or more nerve fibers, and each fiber innervates only one or two hair cells. Each fiber to the outer hair cells innervates a group of six to ten or more cells. We shall center attention on the nerve fibers rather than on the cells because the nerve is the bottleneck for transmission of auditory information and also because the traffic of impulses

in single fibers has been studied experimentally.

As a simplification, Figure 4-1 shows several groups of fibers running to different segments of the organ of Corti on the basilar membrane. The hair cells of that segment are indicated schematically by a single hair cell and by an intensity scale for each segment. The nerve fibers attach to the scale at different points. This is a graphic representation of the differences in threshold of different sensory units in a given small segment of the organ of Corti. The differences in threshold depend on the sharp tuning of the units, as described in Chapter 3. Even within a frequency range as narrow as a critical band the differences in threshold for a particular frequency may be considerable, although the range of 50 dB, used arbitrarily in Figure 4-1, may prove to be somewhat too large. Note also in Figure 4-1 the scale of frequency along the basilar membrane, which expresses the place principle. Recall also that the threshold of hearing lies at an extremely low energy level, and that in animal experiments most if not all units are actually firing spontaneously at low rates even in the quiet.

In such a system as this we can expect several types of impairment, including: (1) absence of units, (2) abnormal thresholds for some or all units, (3) changes in the sharpness of tuning of units, (4) increase in spontaneous activity, (5) abnormally rapid fatigue, (6) abnormal effects or lack of any effect at all from the efferent nerve supply (not shown in the diagram), and possibly (7) abnormal peripheral interactions among neighboring sensory units. Each of these impairments might affect all units equally, its effect might be graded uniformly in some way, or it might be distributed at random. The different impairments can combine with one another and also with conductive impairment in the middle or inner ear, or both. It is not surprising that there are many auditory signs and symptoms or that a single cause may produce a variety of effects. Nevertheless the concept of sensory units allows us to construct a series of models approximating the major clinical types and etiological groups of impairments. These models are tentative explanations, but they may help us to understand the nature of each impairment and the possibilities for therapy or rehabilitation of the impairment.

Three additional characteristics of the sensory units, in addition to their anatomical distribution and graded thresholds, are important. One is the "all-or-none" character of the nerve impulses they carry. Another is the small dynamic range for each unit between threshold level and saturation level, that is, the level of stimulation at which the sensory unit reaches its maximum number of impulses per second. With a steady stimulus the long-term rate is normally maintained indefinitely, but the long-term rate is considerably below the initial transient maximum output. Still another characteristic of a unit is its sharp tuning near its best frequency (see Figure 3-18). The threshold rises rapidly, although unsymmetrically, both above and below the best or characteristic frequency. The steepness of the boundary helps to explain frequency discrimination. The overlap of response areas explains the wide dynamic (intensity) range over which the total output of impulses from all units increases with increase in the stimulus level. Units that are "tuned" above the stimulating frequency, and also some tuned slightly below it, are progressively activated as the intensity increases.

Particular Sensorineural and Mixed Hearing Impairments

Abrupt high-tone hearing loss The word "abrupt" refers here to the shape of the audiogram, not to any suddenness in time of the onset of the condition. As a matter of fact this type of impairment is very stable and probably has a congenital hereditary basis. It is much more common in males than in females, and it has long been confused with noise-induced hearing loss. The sensitivity of hearing is normal or nearly so for low tones but falls off abruptly at a rate of as much as 80 dB per octave or steeper. Sometimes the loss is total above the abrupt drop. Sometimes the audiogram continues to fall toward the very high frequencies, but less steeply. Very rarely does it rise toward higher frequencies. The loss is usually bilateral and at nearly the same frequency in each ear. The hearing for high tones is so poor that it is usually appropriate to call the condition "abrupt high-tone deafness," meaning deafness for high tones with an abrupt transition.

The handicap in terms of understanding speech depends critically on the frequency at which the drop in sensitivity occurs. If it is at 3000 Hz or above, the practical handicap is very slight. If it is at 1000 Hz or below, the handicap is great. The high-frequency conponents that give character to the plosive and fricative consonants and even to some vowels are lost, and the listener is dependent on recognizing very small differences among the sounds that he is able to hear. His discrimination score for word lists (see Chapter 7) is reduced, although not to zero. He may be able, perhaps with some effort, to understand speech in quiet surroundings, but if much noise is mixed with the speech, he has more difficulty than a person with normal hearing.

The audiogram of one ear of an individual with abrupt high-tone loss is shown in Figure 4-2, together with a "map" of the abnormalities found at postmortem examination of that ear. The sensory units, both the nerve fibers and the hair cells, are missing from the basal (high-frequency) portion of the first

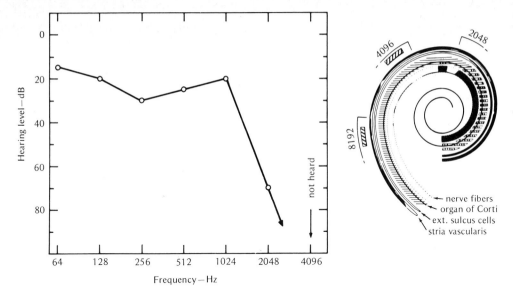

Figure 4-2 Audiogram and chart of postmortem findings in an ear with abrupt high-tone loss. The actual fall in sensitivity of hearing may have been even more abrupt (steeper) than shown because no measurements were made between 1024 and 2048 Hz.

Inner spiral, nerve fibers; black = normal, white = degenerated.

Second spiral, organ of Corti; rectangle with large dots = organ of Corti with normal hair cells, plain line = organ of Corti degenerated.

Third and fourth spirals; black = normal, and white = ab-

normal external sulcus cells and stria vascularis, respectively.

Outside the spiral on the right are indicated the zones required for the normal reception of frequencies 2048, 4096, and 8192 Hz, based on correlation of audiograms and locations of abnormalities of 79 human ears. The shaded rectangles show the most probable locations for 4096 and 8192 Hz. *(Data and chart from Crowe, Guild, and Polvogt, Bull. Hopkins Hosp., 54:315–739; 1934; © The Johns Hopkins University Press; by permission)*

turn. The transition from normal to complete absence of sensory units is very abrupt. This is a clear case of what we may call *subtractive hearing loss,* meaning a loss of sensory units, in contrast to "*conductive hearing loss.*"

Gradual high-tone hearing loss This term also refers to the slope of the audiogram, but as a rule the impairment does develop gradually over a period of months or a few years, as in some forms of otitis media, or over many years, as in chronic suppurative otitis media or in presbycusis. Typically the audiogram is fairly flat up to 1000 Hz but then slopes steadily downward toward the higher frequencies at a rate of 10 to 30 dB per octave. Sometimes the downward slope begins

at 500 or 250 Hz. The bone-conduction audiogram may or may not show a similar, but perhaps less pronounced, slope. These gradually sloping audiograms are frequently associated with conductive impairment of the middle ear and (probably) of the inner ear also, that is, with "mixed" hearing loss.

At postmortem some loss of sensory units, either the nerve fibers or the hair cells or both, has been shown in some cases, particularly in individuals who were 65 years or older at death. The loss of units is usually most severe in the basal turn and progressively greater toward the extreme basal end. But in at least half of the ears examined in the classical study by Crowe, Guild, and Polvogt in 1934 no loss of sensory units could be demonstrated to be sufficient to account for the known hearing loss, particularly when due regard was given to the location in the basal turn of the areas critical for hearing particular frequencies such as 4096 and 8192 Hz (see Figure 4-2). Neither was there in these ears any fixation of the stapes by otosclerosis or any gross adhesion in the middle ear that could account for the hearing loss. In short, no basis in pathology could be found for the hearing impairment.

On the basis of this and other studies we conclude that in gradual high-tone hearing loss without middle-ear disease a loss of sensory units *may* contribute significantly to the impairment in many cases, but loss of units is rarely a complete explanation, and often not even a partial explanation. We must invoke as the primary cause more subtle, and sometimes hypothetical, factors such as elevated thresholds (sensory impairment) or inner-ear conductive changes that cannot be detected under the microscope. Partial loss of units, even if it is most severe in the basal turn, does not explain why the audiogram should slope systematically downward or even why it should be affected at all. In fact in some experimental situations of partial injury of the auditory nerve the loss of units may be considerable even though behavioral thresholds remain normal. This is to be expected from our model. If the loss of units is random, provided some very sensitive units remain and are well distributed along the basilar membrane, the threshold should not be affected. There is no necessary relation between the density of sensory units and the threshold of the most sensitive units.

The gradual, steady slope of the audiogram in typical "gradual high-tone hearing loss" is in sharp contrast to the "4000-Hz notch" that is very characteristic of *noise-induced hearing loss*. In this condition the threshold shift, relative to audiometric zero, is greater for 4000 Hz, and usually for 6000

Hz also, than for 8000 Hz. The origin and certain other characteristics of this type of high-tone sensorineural loss will be described below.

Congenital and toxic impairments   Congenital and toxic impairments will be considered later from the etiologic point of view and with respect to prospects of rehabilitation. They include many very severe hearing losses. In terms of our model we can say that definite abnormalities, such as the complete absence of hair cells, can frequently account for the impairment. In some congenital conditions, however, although the organ of Corti seems to be deformed, the hair cells still are present. Sometimes the tectorial membrane is detached, rolled up in the inner sulcus, and covered with a layer of epithelial cells or perhaps Reissner's membrane is adherent to the organ of Corti, or both. These obvious anatomical defects can logically be classed as "inner-ear conductive impairments." Some may argue that the sense organ as a whole is abnormal even though the hair cells and nerves are present, and that it is therefore a "sensory" impairment. Whichever term is used, however, it is reassuring to know that in some of these conditions many sensory units seem to be present, although it may be difficult to stimulate them.

Loudness recruitment is a symptom that seems to be clearly related to abnormality of the sense organ and cannot be caused by a conductive impairment. The phenomenon, observed by Dr. Edmund P. Fowler in 1928 and named by him in 1939, is an abnormally rapid growth of the sensation of loudness as the intensity of a sound is increased. In terms of the power law, discussed in Chapter 2, the exponent in the power law equation is larger than normal, and therefore the slope of the graph is steeper. In everyday experience we are aware that a fairly intense sound in a normal ear may be masked by background noise and be inaudible until its "masked threshold" is reached. When it emerges from the masking, it quite rapidly becomes louder, and at about 30 dB above the masked threshold it sounds as loud as it does without any noise in the background. This is a perfectly normal form of loudness recruitment. The abnormal form occurs without any masking noise. It can only occur, however, if the threshold is elevated by a sensory impairment. The measurement of loudness recruitment by "loudness balance" is described in Chapter 8.

Loudness recruitment in sensory hearing loss is usually but not necessarily complete at about 90 dB hearing level (ANSI). Sometimes the loudness overshoots (overrecruitment) and a particular tone sounds louder to the abnormal ear than to the normal ear. Sometimes at high hearing levels the growth of loudness becomes less rapid than normal (decruitment), but in the absence of other symptoms the net result of pure recruitment is that the function of the abnormal ear is *less* impaired at high hearing levels than at low levels.

The condition in which pure loudness recruitment is most clearly and regularly seen is a moderate but permanent noise-induced hearing loss or threshold shift. The only clear impairment is elevation of threshold over part or all of the spectrum. The recruitment definitely offsets part of this impairment and can be considered a "benign recruitment."

We emphasize the benign character of pure recruitment because recruitment is often associated with various forms of dysacusis, which will be described below. These may be quite distressing and prevent the understanding of speech. Unfortunately the term recruitment was often used to include all of these other impairments, and it became at one time almost synonymous with what we now call "peripheral dysacusis." This

misuse of the term should be carefully avoided.

As a diagnostic sign, recruitment is very helpful if the patient is able to make the necessary loudness balances reliably. Recruitment is very characteristic of what we call sense-organ impairment, but not of conductive or neural impairment. It is produced by a retrocochlear neural lesion such as an eighth nerve tumor in only about 25 percent of cases. Here partial recruitment is more common, however.

We cannot give a definitive interpretation of loudness recruitment until we resolve the contradictions, set forth in Chapter 3, concerning the sharpness of tuning of auditory units and their thresholds and patterns of innervation. We shall outline two interpretations, although there is a serious objection to each, and there are others.

The most popular theory for many years was based on the obvious anatomical differences between the inner and the outer hair cells. The outer cells were *assumed* to be more sensitive, although their innervation pattern does not seem suitable for any very fine frequency discrimination. The inner hair cells, assumed to have thresholds well above those of the outer hair cells, were thought to provide fine discrimination of frequency and to account for the growth of loudness at high intensities. Recruitment was interpreted as due to a loss of the more sensitive "population," or at least to a temporary or permanent elevation of its threshold. This theory was powerfully supported by the finding in the electrocochleogram of two branches of the input-output curves of the auditory action potentials. Here there are clearly two populations of auditory units, and the one with high threshold and short latency which can generate the larger action potential (due to more nerve fibers) is supposed to be the inner hair cells. Furthermore, the low-intensity branch of the curve is absent from ears with abnormal hearing of the recruitment type. In such ears—for example, those with noise-induced hearing loss—it is the outer hair cells that are most likely to be damaged. All of these points fit together admirably in a consistent pattern. The major objection to this theory is the complete failure of neurophysiologists, with their microelectrodes, ever to find the postulated two populations of auditory units. There should be a large population of high-threshold units and a small population of low-threshold units. Actually they find a *single* population of *low*-threshold units.

The one-population theory attributes the low thresholds that all units show at their characteristic frequencies to an interaction of some sort between the inner and the outer hair cells. The latter are supposed to "sensitize" the former in some way so that the two populations of sensory cells are condensed into a single population of fibers. Thus the response area of each unit consists of a broadly tuned high-threshold portion and a sharply tuned low-threshold portion that provides both sensitivity and selectivity at the characteristic frequency. (See Chapter 3.) Recruitment should occur if the sensitive portion, the "tip," is lost. Powerful support for such a theory is that just such a change in the shape of the response areas (in guinea pigs) of auditory units can be produced by certain ototoxic drugs or by anoxia (see Figure 3-18). The modification by anoxia is reversible. The obvious objection to this theory is that the assumption of an interaction, either excitatory or inhibitory, between inner and outer hair cells is strictly *ad hoc*. Anatomists have sought carefully for neural connections and deny their existence. Other (electrical) mechanisms have been suggested, but none yet seems really plausible.

Peripheral dysacusis The impairments that we have considered so far are quite well grouped together as "hypoacusia," meaning loss of sensitivity of hearing. Elevation of the threshold is the general characteristic.

In conductive hearing loss the equal-loudness contours, described in Chapter 2, are elevated. Their form, like that of the threshold curve, may be changed, but their spacing remains constant. In sensory hearing loss, recruitment usually partially offsets the threshold hypoacusia: the spacing of the equal loudness contours is compressed, usually more at some frequencies than at others. All of this lies in the intensity-loudness domain.

Diplacusis Diplacusis, or "hearing double," is an impairment in the frequency-pitch domain. One symptom is that a given pure tone has different pitches in the two ears. This is *diplacusis binauralis*. Careful comparisons show that most people have a little diplacusis for some parts of the frequency scale most of the time; but unless the condition becomes rather considerable, amounting to differences of a quarter of a tone or more, they are quite unaware of the inequalities. As pointed out in Chapter 2, the brain can average small pitch differences between the ears just as it averages small differences in color vision between the two eyes. There is a limit to this integrative ability, however, and if the tones are heard separately and differently, the symptom may be quite disturbing and distressing, particularly to musicians and music lovers.

Another kind of diplacusis is a loss of the clear musical tonal quality of the sound of a pure tone. The tone becomes "rough," "impure," "noisy," or "buzzing," or may sound like a complex, inharmonious mixture of tones. In extreme cases, two or more distinct tones may be heard simultaneously. In diplacusis binauralis one ear may hear the tone normally while the other hears it as noisy and impure as well as at a different pitch. The hearing of two tones or a tone and noise simultaneously in one ear is called *diplacu-sis monauralis*. It is clearly a form of dysacu-sis, and in its presence the ability to discriminate spoken words is reduced or even lost entirely.

Tinnitus Tinnitus means "head noises" or "ringing in the ears." The subject hears sound or sounds more or less continuously, without any related acoustic stimulus. Most people have some weak high-pitched tinnitus most of the time, although they may not notice it except in very quiet surroundings. The loudness is likely to be matched to that of a tone some 20 dB above threshold. Other people have heard noises that they describe as rushing or roaring, and they may compare them to wind in the trees or to an air blast, or sometimes a low-pitched roar. Such a roar is common in Menière's disease. Sometimes it is related to and therefore "beats" with the pulse. In tense, emotional people tinnitus becomes very annoying and may even interfere with sleep.

There seems to be a close relation between some varieties of tinnitus and the extra noises and "impurities" of diplacusis monauralis. In tinnitus the noise is spontaneous and comes and goes unpredictably. But, as we all know from experience, tinnitus is regularly one of the aftereffects of exposure to a very loud noise, whether a single explosion, a very loud whistle, or the continuing din of a boiler shop. In diplacusis the tinnitus is evoked by speech or other external sounds and is heard at the same time with them. Mild spontaneous tinnitus may be inhibited or masked by speech; strong tinnitus may interfere with speech reception.

In terms of our model with its sensory units, the common, mild tinnitus obviously corresponds to the spontaneous discharge that has been found in most if not all auditory nerve fibers. It should probably be regarded as normal or "physiological." A little

hyperexcitability would drive a unit to a faster rate of discharge, and a more severe "irritation" would cause a still faster discharge and perhaps involve more units. This might be heard subjectively as sound. The discharges of the more sensitive units are accelerated by very small additional mechanical disturbance and could be triggered easily in other ways also, just as burning, tingling, or itching may follow after mechanical bruising of skin. It is not entirely facetious to speak of ringing tinnitus as "an itch in the organ of Corti."

It is often assumed that tinnitus may be associated with the early stages of a progressive degenerative process that will impair hearing. There is no need for concern. A strong tinnitus may continue for years without any change in the audiogram. It is true that irritation within the ear, mechanical as in noise exposure, or biochemical (probably) as in Menière's disease, has an associated tinnitus. Tinnitus *may* be caused by wax impacted against the drum membrane and completely filling the external auditory canal. Perhaps this is only physiological tinnitus that is heard because a conductive impairment keeps out the external sounds that would ordinarily mask it in most environments.

Temporary threshold shift with dysacusis In one set of wartime experiments (1943) normal human ears were exposed to loud, pure tones for many minutes. The chief object of study was the temporary elevation of threshold (threshold shift) that is produced for a restricted range of frequencies above the exposure tone. Frequently continuous tinnitus, tinnitus evoked by speech, and also tonal diplacusis were all produced. Only one ear of each subject was exposed so that the distortion of pitch could be measured by pitch matching. Pitch shifts up to nearly an octave were produced. The shifts were less for loud test tones than for weak ones. Recruitment of loudness was demonstrated by loudness balancing. The threshold was considerably elevated for a restricted range of frequencies a little above the frequency of the exposure tone, producing a partial "tonal gap." (Fortunately the threshold shift, the tinnitus, and the diplacusis were all temporary.) When two tones were heard in response to a single test tone, their pitches usually corresponded to frequencies on each side of the "tonal gap."

Apparently the normal pattern of a continuously graded excitation (the traveling-wave pattern) and correspondingly graded outputs of the sensory units had been temporarily disrupted by the local elevation of thresholds. Some sensory units were depressed, and others, less affected but nevertheless irritated, caused tinnitus. The normal, integrated pattern of neural activity was broken into two (or more) parts, and two (or more) tones or bands of noise were heard. This experiment gives a fairly firm basis for some of our "explanations," and it also points very strongly to an integrating function in the central nervous system that makes a widespread excitation normally sound like a single pure tone. Perhaps this function too can sometimes go wrong and produce a different class of distortions or head noises that do not depend on abnormal or spontaneous patterns of action in or among the sensory units but arise more centrally.

Menière's[1] disease[2] The treatment of Menière's disease is considered in Chapter 6, but its symptoms must be mentioned here as a fine illustration of "peripheral dysacusis." The collection of symptoms known as Menière's disease or Menière's syndrome takes its name from the French physician Prosper Menière, who first described the syndrome in 1861. His descriptions were remarkably complete and accurate. He correctly distinguished a group of cases characterized by sudden onset of vertigo, nausea, vomiting, and loss of hearing from "apoplectiform cerebral congestion," and he also correctly attributed the cause of his syndrome to a disturbance in the labyrinth.

The symptoms occur typically in sudden attacks during which the vertigo is the most distressing and disabling feature. The attacks may persist for hours or days, fluctuating in intensity. In addition to the vertigo there are usually cochlear symptoms consisting of loud, roaring tinnitus, inability to understand speech, elevation of hearing thresholds by as much as 30 to 60 dB, loss of tonal quality, gross distortion of sounds, and often a lowered threshold of discomfort from loud sounds. Recruitment is a very prominent feature, often including overrecruitment. The elevation of hearing thresholds may not appear in the early stages. Some patients have attacks of the cochlear dysacusis without the vertigo. For many others the attacks are purely vertiginous without much impairment of hearing. At first the cochlear symptoms are almost always unilateral. The course of the disease is capricious. The symptoms fluctuate from day to day and subside ultimately, usually leaving a residue of cochlear hearing loss. Also, unfortunately, the symptoms often return at a later date.

---

[1] The spelling of Menière's name has given medical writers some difficulty. Apparently Dr. Menière himself was not consistent. The original form was apparently Méniére, with an acute accent on the first "e," but on his last paper we find it spelled Menière. His son subsequently established the simpler form for the family name, and that spelling is recognized in France. In the fourth edition of this book we continue to follow the French usage instead of the earlier English-American form, Ménière, of our first and second editions. However, under the influence of our typewriters, the name is rapidly becoming Americanized to Meniere.

[2] In this edition we have adopted the term Menière's disease instead of Menière's syndrome because the pathology (endolymphatic hydrops) is now quite firmly established.

One anatomical abnormality has been clearly associated with Menière's disease. The membranous labyrinth is distended like a toy balloon as if the endolymph were under increased pressure. Reissner's membrane may bulge so that the scala media entirely fills the scala vestibuli. This abnormality justifies the name *idiopathic endolymphatic hydrops* as an alternative to Menière's disease. One popular theory relates the attacks to fluctuations of the salt and water balance of the body and a postulated inability of the stria vascularis to cope with it.

Whatever its cause, Menière's disease is an excellent example of sense-organ impairment, and the remissions of the disease show that the impairment is physiological and (except perhaps in the later stages) reversible and not due to destruction of nerve fibers or hair cells. The combination is strongly suggestive of the reversible effect of anoxia on the response areas of single auditory units. In Kiang's terms, the high-threshold "tails" of the response areas remain more or less intact while the sensitive, sharply tuned "tips" are suppressed. In Evans' terms, the "second filter" is out of action. This abnormality would cause elevation of thresholds, recruitment, reduced frequency discrimination, and probably deterioration of tonal quality. Another, but much less common, possibility is a selective (temporary) suppression of low-frequency units as a group, perhaps the entire upper half of the cochlea. This would also cause elevation of thresholds, and reduced frequency discrimination and recruitment for low and middle tones, although hearing should still be quite normal for high frequencies. The low tones would have a rough buzzing quality because they would be heard, through the mechanism of "periodicity pitch," by the relatively normal high-frequency (basal) units. These explanations are all incomplete, however, because we do not know the anatomical and biophysical mechanisms of the sharp but vulnerable tips of the response areas or of Evans' hypothetical "second filter," or the basis of their reversible suppression.

Dysacousia: painful hearing The primary meaning for dysacousia (or its short form, dysacusis) in many medical dictionaries is *painful hearing,* namely pain produced by loud or even by moderate sounds, although we use the term more broadly. Painful hearing may be an isolated symptom, one of the symptoms of Menière's disease, or it may occur in other combinations. The condition may be wrongly attributed to neurosis. There are probably several causes or varieties. For example, if the middle ear is tender from inflammation and the tympanic membrane is tense with pus, the additional mechanical stress of loud sound can be painful. Also, sound can induce mechanical movement reflexly by the contraction of the stapedius or the tensor tympani muscle, or both, and this could be painful in an inflamed ear. Pain is felt even in the toughest normal ear if sound is loud enough, above 140 db SPL, and there are wide individual variations. A sudden sound, whether an explosion, a crash, or a whistle, is more painful than sound at the same level reached in successive small steps. (Incidentally, the thresholds of pain and of discomfort shown in Figure 2-4 were determined by the method of successive small increments of a steady tone. The ears had the advantage that the intra-aural muscles were already contracting reflexly when the last increment of sound pressure level was added.) People complain quite legitimately of uncomfortable loudness at levels well below 120 db SPL, and some may experience true pain at what are ordinarily quite tolerable levels.

A practical aspect of painful hearing is the very sharp limit it may impose at a rather low sound-pressure level on the dynamic range of sound available for communication. If, as is often the case, the threshold is elevated by a sensorineural impairment, and loudness recruitment is present in addition to the painful hearing, the dynamic range between threshold of hearing and threshold of severe discomfort may be no greater than the dynamic range of speech itself. This difficulty is considered again in Chapters 10 and 11 on hearing aids.

Fast auditory fatigue   One more abnormality in the category of abnormal auditory signs and symptoms is *fast auditory fatigue*. This phenomenon is the basis for auditory tests (see Chapter 8) that distinguish quite well between sense organ dysacusis, such as Menière's disease, and neural hearing loss, such as is produced by compression of the auditory nerve by a tumor. This distinction is very important from the neurosurgical point of view because the tumor, if allowed to grow, may become a threat to life. The differential diagnosis is often difficult, partly because the tumor may compress the cochlear artery as well as the nerve and thus cause some cochlear symptoms in addition to the neural injury. The effects of nerve compression on the audiogram and on speech discrimination may be indistinguishable from sensory dysacusis, but as a matter of clinical experience the presence of recruitment points strongly to the sense organ, and fast auditory fatigue points strongly to the auditory nerve.

The fast fatigue appears when a continuous tone is sounded. A normal listener hears the tone loudly at first, then less loudly, due to "per-stimulatory auditory fatigue" or "adaptation" (see Chapter 3), but the tone remains audible and at a fairly steady loudness after the first 15 or 20 seconds. If the nerve is partially compressed by a tumor, however, the loudness continues to fall, and finally the tone becomes inaudible. If its intensity is increased by a few decibels,

it becomes audible again, but it then fades out. On the other hand, a tone that is interrupted (for example, on for half a second then off for half a second) can be heard indefinitely, as it is by a normal ear.

The exact site of the failure of neural transmission in fast auditory fatigue is not known. The nerve fiber seems to be involved, although it is just possible that restricted blood supply to the sense organ is somehow responsible. The failure might be either at the dendritic terminations, at the point of compression, or at the axon terminals, which must all receive essential chemical material from the cell bodies in the spiral ganglion. The phenomenon strongly suggests that there is a metabolic bottleneck somewhere, beyond which only a limited supply of necessary material can be stored during periods of low activity. This supply is exhausted by high or moderate activity. It can be partially restored during a brief rest, but then it can be quickly exhausted again. Continued stimulation, even if there is no evidence of successful transmission, continues to use up the necessary material as fast as it is formed but without ever reaching the threshold necessary to initiate (or conduct) the all-or-none nerve impulses.

Effects very much like this can be produced experimentally in peripheral nerves, and we can consider this hypothetical mechanism to be plausible, although it is unproved. Whatever the details may be, the defect seems to be a failure of sustained transmission of impulses in the neural part of the sensory unit. The defect may be more evident in some groups of sensory units than in others. It is more likely to appear in response to high-frequency tones than to tones of low frequency. The phenomenon is useful diagnostically on a strictly empirical basis, but it may be unnoticed until the test is made because most sounds of interest in everyday life are not long continued but, as in speech, are continually interrupted or else changing in frequency. In the presence of a rapidly growing tumor, however, speech discrimination is usually very bad.

Decruitment   In retrocochlear lesions, and perhaps in some sensory impairments also, a careful loudness-balance test may reveal the opposite of recruitment, namely a failure of the sense of loudness to grow as rapidly as it normally does. This effect is known as "decruitment." It may be confined to one or two audiometric frequencies. It is not likely to cause much practical handicap and is not yet of proved diagnostic significance, but it is of theoretical interest in relation to the model of sensory units.

In the model diagramed in Figure 4-1 the sense of loudness is assumed to depend largely on the *total number* of sensory units that are driven well above their resting rates of discharge. This includes units "tuned" to frequencies above that of the stimulus, even though the tone is heard as single in pitch. Now if there is a reduction in total number of units available, there should be a limit to the maximum loudness that can be heard. The loss might be complete, as in abrupt high-tone loss (compare Figure 4-2), or partial with a random distribution. Such a random or partially random distribution of the blocking of sensory units is just what we might expect in the case of compression of the auditory nerve by a retrocochlear tumor.

Prognosis, Treatment, and Management

The presence of a hearing loss immediately raises a series of practical questions. Will the hearing deteriorate still further? Can progressive deterioration be prevented? Can the hearing be improved by surgery, by medical treatment, or otherwise? Is the hearing loss caused by some infection or tumor that, if untreated, may threaten health in other ways? Is a hearing aid indicated? The answers depend on the medical diagnosis and on the nature and location of the impairment.

In general the conductive impairments of the external and middle ear are easily accessible for treatment, and by their nature most of them are amenable to control: some by drugs, others by surgery, or surgical repair. Nature often assists the surgeon by forming new connective tissue, skin, or mucous membrane as needed. Preventive measures are often quite effective, although we cannot prevent the progressive changes in the tissues associated with advancing age.

The inner ear, on the other hand, is beyond the reach of direct surgical repair. It is almost impossible of access, and its parts are far too small and delicate to repair. Nature does not assist by forming new neurons or hair cells or specialized supporting structures to replace those that may have degenerated or become misshapen. On the other hand, there are several conditions in which diseases affecting the inner ear can be remedied. One set is adjacent tumors of the ear, including cholesteatoma, with associated serous or toxic labyrinthitis. Others are rupture of the round window or chronic otitis media with a fistula, and some cases of sudden deafness. Proper treatment of systemic diseases such as malignant lymphoma, renal disease, or adult hypothyroidism can sometimes improve a sensorineural hearing impairment.

The impairment of neural hearing loss that can be most directly assisted surgically is compression of the auditory nerve by a tumor. The location of the tumor is retrocochlear in the internal auditory meatus or within the cranial cavity. The problem of diagnosis lies in the area of neuro-otology and neurosurgery, and it usually involves signs and symptoms related to the nonauditory vestibular portion of the labyrinth or to other nearby neural structures such as the facial nerve. The chief objective is to find and remove the tumor to protect life. If done in time, however, there may be at least partial improvement of the hearing loss caused by compression block of the nerve fibers.

Use of a hearing aid Conductive impairment offers the best opportunity for the successful use of a hearing aid. Actual success depends on many factors, as we shall see in Chapters 10 and 11, but at least the sense organ is still intact and can respond if stimulated. The prospects for successful use of a hearing aid in sensorineural impairment, as we have defined it, are less favorable. The function of a sensory unit that has degenerated cannot be replaced. In general a dysacusis that involves distortions such as diplacusis or tinnitus cannot be improved by a hearing aid, and the discomfort and confusion are likely to be made worse rather than better. On the other hand, there has been in the past a tendency to dismiss all too easily the possiblity of significant assistance and to say simply, "You have nerve deafness, and a hearing aid won't help. Save your money." We believe that the distinction between conductive and sensory impairment within the cochlea is important. A conductive component in the inner ear, as well as one in the middle ear, can be offset by amplification. Many cases of inner-ear impairment are really cases of *mixed* hearing loss, and should be evaluated as such. A hearing aid may help considerably if the wearer does not expect too much and can adapt to it.

CAUSES OF HEARING LOSS AND DYSACUSIS

In this section we shall review the causes of various types of impairment of hearing. The nature of the medical and surgical problems of prevention and cure will become apparent, but the details of programs of conservation of hearing and of medical and surgical treatment will be reserved for the two following chapters.

Hearing Loss in the External and Middle Ear

Congenital malformations Although cupping the hand behind the ear may amplify speech sounds reaching the eardrum by as much as 10 dB, the pinna or auricle is not very important acoustically. Congenital malformation or absence of the external ear is likely, however, to be associated with malformations in deeper structures, and these may cause a severe loss of hearing. One such malformation is closure, or *atresia,* of the external canal. If normal hearing by bone conduction shows that the inner ear is intact, an operation to relieve atresia of the external canal is occasionally successful. *Malformations of the middle ear* often occur in association with atresia and also in isolation. Many, though not all, of them can be remedied by skillful surgery.

Impacted wax Except for congenital malformations, diseases of the external canal rarely produce permanent hearing loss. The most common cause of hearing loss from within the external canal is wax (cerumen), which may harden in the canal and become *impacted* and thus prevent the sound waves from reaching the drum and the middle ear. Blockage of this type is often first noticed after swimming, washing the hair, or bathing. A droplet of water suddenly closes the last tiny channel that was sufficient for the effective reception of ordinary sounds, and only then does the victim know that something is amiss.

External otitis Occasionally changes occur in the skin of the external canal and thereby permit the growth of bacteria and fungi. Infection of the skin and inflammatory changes involving other structures produce a condition called *external otitis*. This occurs most commonly in hot, wet climates. One type of external otitis is like a pimple or boil in the skin of the external canal, usually near the outer end. It may be produced by scratching the skin of the canal with a fingernail or some instrument such as a hairpin or toothpick. It is usually caused by one of the organisms that are commonly found on human skin and cause no harm unless they invade one or more hair follicles.

External otitis may cause symptoms that suggest middle-ear infection (otitis media) and mastoiditis, but it differs from otitis media in often producing no hearing loss unless the swelling of the skin or the trapped secretions completely close the ear canal. The most prominent symptom is pain on manipulation of the auricle.

Otitis media The middle ear is an air chamber containing the mechanism that conducts sound from the air in the external ear to the fluid in the inner ear. This includes the drum membrane, the ossicles (malleus, incus, and stapes), and their ligaments. Diseases of the middle ear may involve one or more of these structures and produce a conductive hearing loss.

The most common cause of conductive hearing loss is *inflammation in the middle ear.* This inflammation, called *otitis media,* usually develops from a cold in the head. The nasal secretions pass backward and infect the eustachian tube, as shown in Figure 4-3. The infection then travels along the tube

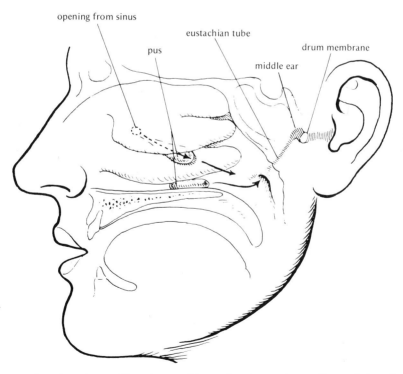

opening from sinus

pus

eustachian tube

middle ear

drum membrane

Figure 4-3 Secretions of pus from the maxillary sinus, and from other sinuses also, easily travel along the floor of the nasal cavity to the mouth of the eustachian tube and can infect the middle ear.

itself or along the lymphatic vessels surrounding it until the middle ear is reached. When the lining of the eustachian tube is inflamed, the tube cannot be opened by swallowing, and the air pressure in the middle ear is no longer equalized. The oxygen in the air of the middle ear is absorbed by the blood that nourishes its mucous lining, and a partial vacuum is produced. The drum membrane is pressed inward and the ossicular chain is forced near to its limit of movement, with all of its ligaments tense. In this situation the conduction of sound is impaired. Furthermore, the reduced air pressure in the middle ear sucks, so to speak, clear tissue fluid from the mucous lining. If much fluid accumulates, sound conduction is impaired further. The condition is called *nonsuppura-*

tive otitis media as long as bacteria do not invade the cavity.

Occasionally otitis media is produced by puncturing the drum membrane from the outside with a dirty instrument, such as a toothpick or a hairpin, and introducing infection in this way. Otitis media frequently starts with a common cold. The cold is due to a virus, but the viral infection weakens the tissues and opens the way to the bacterial infection, with the formation of pus, which is characteristic of otitis media. Furthermore, the middle ear is directly connected in turn with the mastoid air cells, as illustrated in Figure 4-4. Middle-ear and mastoid cells form a single air-filled cavity that is only partly subdivided. Each chamber, large or small, is lined with mucous membrane and

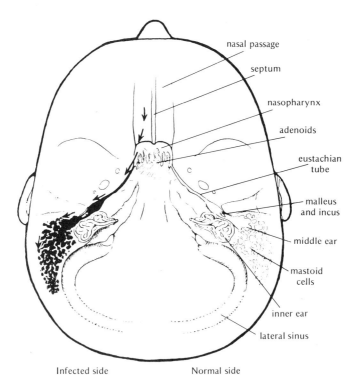

nasal passage

septum

nasopharynx

adenoids

eustachian tube

malleus and incus

middle ear

mastoid cells

inner ear

lateral sinus

Infected side   Normal side

Figure 4-4 In this diagram the head is viewed from above. The dark shading on the left indicates the extent of the air-filled system of middle ear and mastoid cells that is ventilated by the eustachian tube. Notice also how close these cavities, which may become infected, come to the brain cavity and large blood-filled channels, such as the lateral sinus.

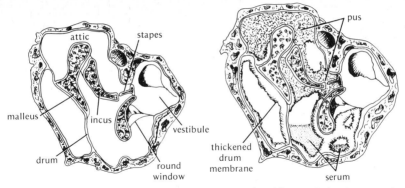

Figure 4-5 *Left:* Englarged drawing of an actual section through a normal middle ear. *Right:* Corresponding section through an infected middle ear. The drumhead is thickened and the middle ear is filled with pus and serum, which restrict the movement of the ossicles. Pus in the middle ear is a more frequent cause of hearing loss than any other, except perhaps senility.

is connected with the others. With every otitis media there is bound to be some inflammation of the lining of the adjoining mastoid air cells.

It will be remembered that in the early stage of a cold the secretion from the nose is watery. In the ear, this stage is properly called *nonsuppurative, or serous, otitis media.* As the disease progresses, the watery secretion thickens into pus. Now, when the material in the middle ear has become infected, the disease is said to be in the acute *suppurative, or purulent,* stage.[3] There is usually excruciating pain until the drumhead breaks or is opened by a surgeon, or until the growth of bacteria is checked by medication. Often there is pain and tenderness behind the ear over the mastoid. (See Figure 4-5.)

When properly treated, the suppuration usually subsides, with or without transient hearing loss, and should then be designated as *healed.* A mild but long-standing otitis media is occasionally called *subacute.* If an ear discharges pus for more than two or three months, and especially if it has a bad odor,

the condition is called *chronic otitis media.*

Aero-otitis media   A fine example of uninfected watery effusion into the middle ear occurs during airplane flight if the eustachian tube is not opened frequently during descent. At the reduced barometric pressure of the higher altitude the middle ear contains less air than at sea level, where the atmospheric pressure is greater and the air is consequently more dense. Normally as the barometric pressure increases during descent, more air enters the middle ear through the eustachian tube, a bubble at each swallow, and equalizes the air pressure between inside and outside. If air does not enter, the differential pressure between the outside air and the middle ear builds up and forces the drum membrane inward. Uncomfortable pressure and finally acute pain is felt, deep in the ear canal. Clear watery fluid gradually collects in the middle ear and partly relieves the difference in pressure. This fluid comes from the tiny blood vessels (capillaries) of the mucous membrane lining of the middle ear. Some actual bleeding usually accompanies the *transudation* or effusion, which is explained below.

There is normally a delicate balance between the mechanical force of the blood pressure, which tends to drive the watery

[3] It is hard for people to think of the word "acute" without considering it as "severe," but severity is not implied in the medical meaning of the word. Nevertheless, a popular misunderstanding persists.

portion of the blood (serum) out into the tissue spaces, and the physicochemical osmotic force, due to the dissolved proteins in the blood, which tends to hold the serum within the capillaries. The mechanical pressure in the tissue, supported by the air pressure in the middle ear, tends also to resist the outward movement of fluid. When the air pressure in the middle ear is reduced, some fluid moves out into the tissue and ultimately into the middle-ear cavity. The action is literally a suction of serum into the cavity from the blood. The resulting condition is called *aero-otitis media*, or otitis media due to *barotrauma* (injury from change in barometric pressure). Similar nonsuppurative otitis often occurs among caisson workers and submarine crews. Diving, especially high diving and skin diving, may also produce effusions of fluid.

Serous and mucous otitis A subacute form of nonsuppurative otitis media has recently become very prevalent throughout the world. Why it was previously so rare no one knows. When the fluid in the middle ear is thin and watery, the disease is called *serous otitis* or middle-ear effusion or (formerly) catarrhal otitis media. When the effusion is thick, the condition is called *mucoid* or *mucous otitis*, or even "glue ear." Some otologists deny that there is any inflammation involved. They therefore object to the suffix "-itis" and prefer to speak of "otic transudates." However, the cellular and chemical content of the fluids of the middle ear in such cases both indicate that there is inflammation and closure of the eustachian tube, so we shall class this condition as a nonsuppurative otitis.

The cause or causes of serous and mucous otitis are not clear. One possible cause is the treatment of suppurative otitis with antibiotics or other biochemicals but without adequate drainage. The bacteria are destroyed or held inactive, but the fluid in the middle ear remains. Another cause is allergy. Some cases are certainly allergic in origin, but it is impossible to explain all cases on this basis. Still another cause is obstruction of the eustachian tube.

The fluid that collects in the middle ear causes a hearing loss. The loss may vary all the way from a mild gradual high-tone loss to a very considerable loss for all tones. When thick mucus is present, the hearing loss is most severe and may resemble that seen with otosclerosis. The treatment is to remove the effusion from the middle ear by puncture or incision of the drumhead, usually with the insertion of a plastic ventilation tube. The consequent relief of hearing loss is one of the most dramatic affairs in otology.

Since the use of antibiotics for treatment of acute otitis media has become so popular, many physicians not in the specialty of otology have felt complacent when the pain and other symptoms of otitis media disappear following the use of antibiotics. They may have neglected to inspect the ear carefully or may have failed to incise the drumhead in spite of the possibility that some fluid remained in the middle ear. The only remaining symptom is a hearing loss, which may be noticed by the parent or detected by routine testing of hearing in schools. The diagnosis is not always easy, but characteristically the drumhead is opaque in color with loss of the light reflex and a shortened, retracted chalky-white malleus. Occasionally fluid can be seen through the membrane, either as bubbles or as a meniscus. The drumhead does not move when positive and negative pressures are applied through a pneumatic otoscope.

In these cases incisions should be made in the drumhead because it is sometimes peculiarly difficult to evacuate the thick gluelike material from the middle ear. If this mucoid material is not removed by the surgeon, it will remain, since it is obviously impossible for it to drain spontaneously through the eustachian tube. The conductive hearing loss will persist, and the condition may in time lead to the formation of adhesions in the middle ear that firmly fix the ossicular chain with bands of fibrous tissue. Also, one of the most important sequelae is the condition known as tympanosclerosis, which can invade the ossicles and promontory and fixate the stapes.

Cholesteatoma Another important cause of hearing loss, and one of the main pathologies in chronic otitis media accompanied by chronic mastoiditis, is cholesteatoma. This is simply a cyst that is lined internally with skin. This cyst grows from the upper part of the drumhead as a pouch within the middle ear (see Figure 4-6). It seems to originate either from a congenital remainder of embryonic tissue or from chronic wetting of the deep parts of the external canal or from inflammation of the middle ear. In any case, a pouch forms, and then the lining desqua-

mates into the pouch. It will be remembered that the outer layers of the human skin come off in thin, tiny sheets. As these cornified layers of skin come off in the pouch, the cyst becomes larger and larger. Eventually such a soft-tissue cyst may erode away the ossicles or other bony structures and cause symptoms. It consitutes a foreign body in the middle ear and favors suppuration.

There are several clinical varieties of cholesteatoma, but all of them represent keratinizing skin in the wrong place, with or without a clearly defined cyst. Usually the patient complains of an intermittent discharge from the ear that has a peculiarly foul odor. The hearing level may be quite good, either within normal limits or perhaps 25 or 30 dB HL. Examination of the ear usually shows a small perforation at the margin of the drumhead, usually at the flaccid upper part.

Allergy Hypersensitivity of the tissues of the middle ear, the eustachian tube, and the inner ear to various foreign proteins in the

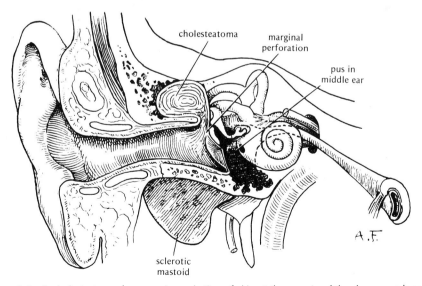

Figure 4-6 A cholesteatoma forms an impocketing of skin at the margin of the drum membrane.

air or bloodstream has been described. One variety is the sensitivity to bacteria called "bacterial allergy." Occasionally, a patient has tinnitus or a hearing loss whenever he or she eats particular foods, such as wheat, milk, eggs, chocolate, nuts, or citrus fruits. Certainly, severe pollen allergies contribute to blockage of the tubes and may make an individual more susceptible to the various types of otitis media.

Other abnormalities of the middle ear It is not necessary for us to include in this general discussion of medical problems the numerous other conditions that may involve either the external, the middle, or the inner ear. Tumors, syphilis, tuberculosis, bullet wounds, fractures of the skull, and a variety of other medical and surgical conditions may involve the ear as well as other parts of the body. The audiologist can assist in the medical diagnosis of these conditions, but detailed descriptions of them are not necessary here. By far the most important causes of conductive hearing loss in order of numerical occurrence are (1) inadequate attention to normal function of the eustachian tube and inadequate treatment of infections of the middle ear and (2) the special disease of the middle and inner ear known as *otosclerosis*.

Otosclerosis Otosclerosis is a unique bone disease that affects the bony capsule surrounding the inner ear. This bone, normally the hardest in the body, becomes invaded by a different kind of softer bone, which grows intermittently and then becomes hard again —that is, "sclerotic." The most common site for the growth of this new bone is in the region just in front of and below the oval window. The most common effect of the new bony growth, if it does anything at all, is to fix the footplate of the stapes firmly in the oval window so that the stapes no longer moves freely. The effect is much like that of

some forms of arthritis which limit the movements of fingers, the knee, or the spine; in fact the two diseases have many points in common. When the stapes becomes fixed, the vibrations carried to it from the drumhead through the malleus and the incus are not effectively transmitted to the fluid of the inner ear. Fortunately, *otosclerosis causes fixation of the stapes and hearing loss in only about 10 percent of the cases in which it occurs.*

Otosclerosis is a hereditary disease. It is frequent among the Caucasoids (whites and East Indians) but extremely rare among the Mongoloids (Japanese, Chinese, Indonesians, American Indians) and among Negroids. The distribution suggests that the disease very likely arose as a single genetic mutation. Its rare appearance in Mongoloids and its presence in American, but not African, blacks are well explained as the result of restricted interbreeding. In the incidence there is a slight but definite unexplained predominance of the female sex. These statements are based on a 1967 survey, entitled "The Incidence of Otosclerosis as Related to Race and Sex" by Altmann, Glasgold, and MacDuff. The authors point out that "the data on the racial distribution of otosclerosis are amazingly scarce for all races, even for Negroes living in the U.S.A. The above statements must therefore be regarded as still subject to future modification."

Part of the data on the incidence of otosclerosis expresses the relation between the number of cases of otosclerosis confirmed at operation and the size of the entire population of the hospital clinics. Another large part of the data comes from examination of temporal bones for evidence of fixation of the stapes in the oval window. Here we must make a distinction between *clinical otosclerosis*, in which fixation of the stapes actually occurs, and *histological otosclerosis*, in which the presence of the otosclerotic process is demonstrated postmortem some-where in the otic capsule. From the point of view of heredity, all persons with histological otosclerosis are carriers of the trait. Those with clinical otosclerosis are simply the less fortunate members of the much larger group of carriers. It is thus easy to understand why, although the disease is hereditary, the hearing loss very frequently skips one or more generations.

More precisely the survey of Altmann, Glasgold, and MacDuff gives the incidence of histological otosclerosis among whites as 8.3 percent and for stapedial fixation as 0.99 percent. The female predominance in both classes is about seven to six. Histological otosclerosis among blacks in the United States (chiefly in New York) is about one-seventh as common as among whites.

Otosclerosis begins in youth. There have been cases presenting the clinical picture of otosclerosis in young children from 4 to 6 years of age, and fixation of the stapes has been observed at operation as early as the seventh year; but these fixations are probably congenital, not otosclerotic. The hearing loss of otosclerosis is *usually* first noticed at adolescence or in the early twenties. Nearly always the hearing loss is evident before the thirtieth year, although in a few cases it makes its appearance when the patient is still older. Otosclerosis may become worse during pregnancy, but since the disease is often progressive during early adulthood in any case, until the hearing loss reaches the 50 or 60 dB level, and since pregnancy by no means always accelerates the process, *otosclerosis should not be considered a deterrent to the bearing of children.*

The fixation of the stapes occurs only gradually over a period of years. As the hearing loss comes on, more and more powerful sound is required to overcome the increasing resistance to movement. However, with the help of a good hearing aid, speech may be understood almost perfectly. Ultimately, however, in most cases of otosclerosis in which the hearing loss is severe, there is, in addition to the conductive hearing loss, some sensorineural loss as well. The combination may cause a very severe loss of hearing.

The otosclerotic process may invade the niche of the round window as well as the area near the oval window. In very rare cases the round window may be closed by the bony overgrowth while the stapes remains mobile. Hearing is impaired because fixation of the round-window membrane deprives the cochlea of its "elastic release." The immobilization of the fluids reduces hearing for bone conduction as well as for air conduction.

Erosion of the hard bony wall of the cochlea by the abnormal, spongy vascular tissue can be demonstrated by X ray, using the technique known as "tomography" or "polytomography." This method blurs the details of the X-ray shadow of structures that are nearer to or farther away than the desired depth of focus. By reducing the confusing overlay it reveals changes in the bony structures that do remain in focus. The decalcification caused by otosclerosis can be detected readily in a tomogram taken at the proper depth and angle. "Tomography" or "planigraphy" is also the best method for identifying small acoustic neuromas in the internal auditory meatus.

Otosclerotic invasion of the cochlea itself is more common than was formerly supposed, and opinion differs concerning the extent which hearing may be impaired by it. The stapes is usually involved as well. The audiogram of "cochlear otosclerosis" is said to be flat or U-shaped. It is assumed that some unspecified chemical or "toxic" effect is responsible for the sensorineural component. It is worth remembering that certain forms of congenital impairment, including maternal rubella, also frequently show U-shaped audiograms. Simple fixation of the stapes does not. Stapes surgery can restore normal hearing if only the stapes is affected; it cannot relieve a cochlear sensorineural component.

In the *early stages of otosclerosis* the hearing loss is *purely conductive.* The bone conduction is normal, or nearly so, but air conduction is impaired. At first the tones in the middle range, 1000 to 2000 Hz, are often less affected than the lower tones. As a rule, the highest tones, 4000 Hz and above, are still less affected at first. However, as the disease progresses—and in a few cases it progresses very rapidly—there is a greater and greater hearing loss for the higher tones by air conduction, and the loss of sensitivity by bone conduction centering at 2000 Hz begins to appear. When these hearing losses for the higher tones appear, tinnitus may become troublesome. Its high-pitched, musical character is evidence of a localized irritation in the sense organ.

We have also mentioned the symptom of *paracusis Willisii,* which is characteristic of conductive hearing loss in general. The patient with otosclerosis seems to hear better in a noisy place, for example in an airplane, in an automobile, or in a factory. The reason is that people with normal hearing naturally raise their voices to overcome the surrounding noise. The man who has only a partial conductive hearing loss can discriminate the voice from the noise as well as anyone else, if only the voice is loud enough to reach his inner ear. He also hears fairly well over the telephone. But as the otosclerosis progresses, and perhaps if sensorineural difficulties are added to the mechanical obstruction at the stapes, the patient can no longer distinguish conversation so easily, and he is much handicapped at a party where more than one person is speaking. The more he tries to hear, the less he hears. When he becomes fatigued or nervous, his hearing becomes appreciably worse.

Diagnosis of otosclerosis The chief points on which a diagnosis of otosclerosis is made are (1) a progressive but moderate loss of hearing, particularly in a young person; (2) a history of hearing loss in the family; (3) no previous infections or other diseases of the ear that might account for the hearing loss; and (4) normal eardrums. The drum membrane may perhaps show a pink glow (Schwartz's sign) during the active period, but nothing more. Impedance measurements, described in Chapter 9, give very valuable supporting evidence.

The hearing threshold levels by air conduction are about equal for all frequencies, or, in the early stages, a little worse for the low frequencies. Hearing by bone conduction is substantially normal or a little depressed from 1000 to 4000 Hz. Otosclerosis may, of course, be combined with other types of conductive hearing loss, such as those due to chronic infection of the middle ear. In such cases it may be very difficult to decide how much of the hearing loss may be due to the otosclerosis and how much to the chronic otitis media. Otosclerosis may also be combined in later years with some degree of presbycusis, in which case the audiometric tests show worse hearing for the high frequencies.

The course of otosclerosis Otosclerosis rarely progresses to very severe hearing loss. To call otosclerosis "progressive deafness," as it was once known, is therefore misleading. Many patients believe that this diagnosis means that they will soon be totally deaf. For this reason the term should never be used. Usually there is very little, if any, further loss after the hearing has reached a level of 50 to 60 dB (ANSI). The hearing may stay the same for 20 years or more, with a gradual additional loss when the high-tone neural hearing loss of old age adds itself to the conductive hearing loss of otosclerosis.

For many years it was believed that inflation of the eustachian tubes and pneumatic massage of the drum would loosen the bony fixation of the stapes and improve the hearing in otosclerosis. This has been proved false. The improvement reported by some patients was apparently purely illusory or psychic in origin.

Since the hearing loss of otosclerosis in its early stages is a conductive loss, the patient can anticipate good results with a hearing aid. If the inner ear is reasonably intact, as shown by bone conduction, the patient, with advice from his otologist, should consider overcoming the mechanical barrier by means of stapes surgery, which is described in Chapter 6.

Inner-Ear Impairments

Presbycusis (presbyacusis, presbyacousis)   By far the most common cause of inner-ear hearing loss, and probably of all hearing loss, is advancing age. Actually aging also affects the middle ear, and it affects the inner ear in several ways. We shall here consider presbycusis as a whole.

The possibility that aging may cause *conductive impairment in the middle ear* has been generally overlooked for many years. Of course the older a person grows, the more opportunity he has for episodes of otitis media, either acute or as recurrence of a chronic condition. If there is a history of chronic otitis media with discharge from the ear and other symptoms, this point of view is reasonable. It is also true that the older a person becomes, the amount of accumulated exposure to noise, with its effects on hearing, increases. It now seems, however, that even without severe noise exposure or recurrent otitis media elderly people, particularly those beyond 80 years of age, do develop a middle-ear conductive hearing loss. The impairment is greater for high than for low frequencies. Also it is greater for air conduction than for bone conduction. The presence of an "air-bone gap" in the audiogram clearly establishes *this part* of the hearing impairment to be due to changes in the middle ear.

The nature of the changes in the middle ear with age have not been clearly established, but it is well know that connective tissue loses much of its elasticity in elderly people. Their skin becomes flabby and wrinkled. If such changes occur in the ligaments of the joints between the ossicles so that the bones are not held snugly together, or if the drum membrane loses its stiffness and becomes flabby, there should be just such conductive impairments.

The characteristic audiogram in elderly people is a gradual high-tone loss, as described in the previous section. The slope is very gradual below 1000 Hz, although the sensitivity may be depressed at all frequencies. The slope is steepest above 2000 Hz. There may be an air-bone gap in more advanced age or if the presbycusis is added to a previous middle-ear impairment, but the cochlea is clearly the area chiefly involved. There is little or no recruitment of loudness in this condition unless there is a noise-induced component.

Actually changes in the sensitivity of hearing begin in adolescence. Children not only have a wider frequency range than adults, but throughout the entire range their thresholds tend to be lower. This fact was not clearly appreciated until the results of a systematic survey of the hearing of children in certain public schools in Pittsburgh were published in 1963. In this study it was necessary at the very start to modify the audiometers to provide test tones 20 dB below the usual lower limit of clinical audiometers of that date (about 0 dB ANSI). Of course additional precautions to provide sufficiently quiet test booths were also needed.

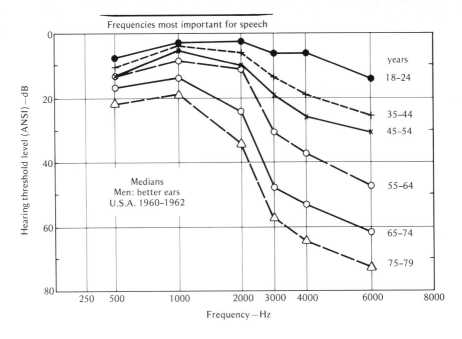

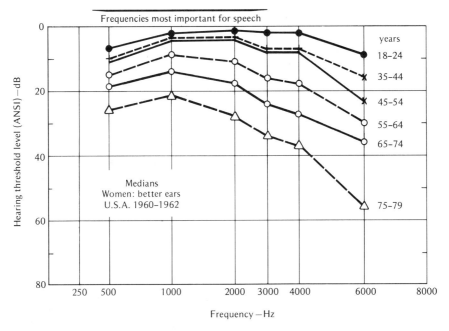

Figure 4-7 Composite audiograms for the better ear in men and women, by age groups. The values plotted are the medians or 50-percentile values. Some of these data are shown in another form in Figure 9-3; there the 25- and 75-percentile values are also shown. (Data of the National Health Survey from Hearing Levels of Adults by Age and Sex, United States, 1960–1962. Public Health Service Publication, No. 1000, Series 11, No. 11; data recalculated to the ANSI zero reference level)

A few years later a survey of adult hearing was carried out by the U.S. Public Health Service, also using modern audiometric instruments, methods, and test booths. More details concerning this survey of 1960–1962 will be found in Chapters 7 and 9, but the trends of the relations of hearing threshold to age and to frequency are shown in Figure 4-7. The hearing of men for high frequencies falls off faster than that of women, but the general trends are the same: from the age of 18 years onward the median sensitivity of hearing falls. The fall is slight at and below 1000 Hz. The fall is greater, the higher the frequency and the older the person.

In Figure 4-8 a series of curves are drawn showing the *change* in hearing thresholds with age, as deduced by Drs. Spoor and van Laar from a study of several surveys made in several countries. Here the curves have been smoothed and are drawn according to the mathematical equation that yielded the best fit for the median values. The trends suggest that the fall in sensitivity actually begins at birth, not at 18 years of age. The U.S. Public Health Service data were not available for inclusion in this study, but the agreement between the two sets of data of Figures 4-7 and 4-8 is noteworthy.

The association of hearing loss with advancing age is proverbial. Actually this association accounts for much of the resistance to the use of hearing aids by young and middle-aged persons who could use them to good advantage.

Most clinical studies of presbycusis during the past 60 years were directed toward describing the impairment due to age alone and finding the specific pathological changes associated with age that would account for the hearing loss. In order to isolate the effects of the aging process it was customary to exclude from the studies all patients who had any significant conductive impairment as revealed by an air-bone gap.

This arbitrary exclusion delayed the recognition of significant changes in the middle ear due to age. Also, it was often tacitly assumed that there is a single "disease process" or pathological change responsible for presbycusis. When one such change, namely loss of sensory units in the basilar turn was found, this change was accepted as an adequate general explanation. This attitude was reflected in early editions of this book, in which we dismissed presbycusis in a single cursory paragraph. In it we wrote:

The structural change that is responsible is perfectly well known. The sensory cells in the part of the organ of Corti toward the base of the cochlea simply degenerate and vanish as do the nerve fibers that connect with them. . . . We can only wonder why the part of the organ sensitive to high tones is almost invariably first involved.

Our present view is that at least five different aging processes contribute to the overall pattern of presbycusis. One is a conductive middle-ear impairment that develops late in life, in the eighth decade and beyond. The second is the conductive cochlear component discussed in a previous section. Its nature is hypothetical, but loss of elasticity and increase of internal friction in the basilar membrane, that is, a more "leathery" character, would give the characteristic pattern of gradual high-tone loss. Other tissues show just such changes as part of the aging process. The third component is the loss of sensory units, which occurs chiefly in the basal turn. The decrease in the number of sensory units is not significant, however, in more than half of the ears with high-tone, sensorineural impairment that have been studied. A fourth category should perhaps be reserved for possible chemical or metabolic abnormalities that may follow changes in blood vessels or in the stria vascularis. Finally, we must emphasize the loss of neurons in the

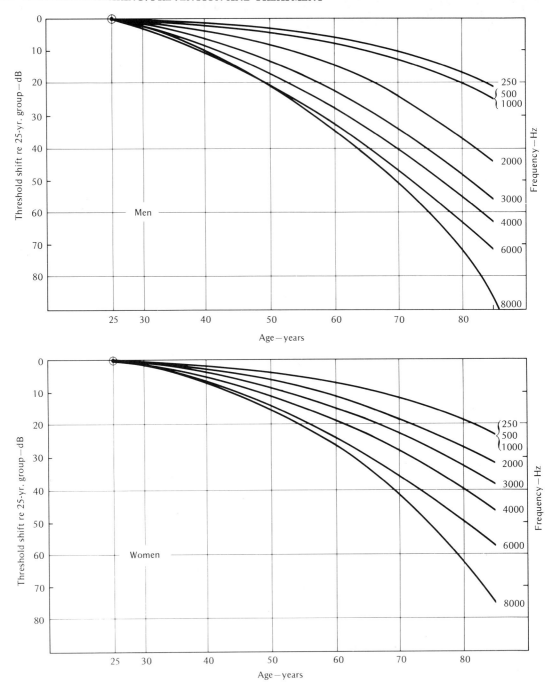

Figure 4-8 The change in sensitivity of hearing with age for men and women. The parameter is frequency in Hz. Data for men and women from eight different publications from four different countries were combined, taking as reference in each study the hearing level of the age group centering at 25 years. In these studies individuals with histories of otological disease or severe noise exposure had been eliminated. A mathematical equation was found that describes the combined data well, with different values of its parameters for men and for women. The curves are smooth curves derived from the equation. (*Adapted from Spoor and van Laar*, International Audiology, *July 1967*)

central nervous system that occurs with aging, particularly if there is severe arteriosclerosis. In a later section we shall describe "phonemic regression" and other well-known symptoms of old age that contribute very importantly to the overall clinical picture of presbycusis.

Drugs, poisons, and allergens There has been much speculation in the past as to possible injury to hearing from excessive use of certain drugs, notably quinine and the salicylates (aspirin). It seems probable that both of these drugs *may* have caused some sensorineural hearing loss in particularly hypersensitive or allergic individuals. Permanent injury will almost certainly be avoided, however, if the use of the drug is stopped as soon as tinnitus occurs.

More recently a group of antibiotic drugs, notably dihydrostreptomycin, kanamycin, neomycin, and gentamicin, have been found to be definitely ototoxic. Apparently these drugs become concentrated in the endolymph, and they injure or kill hair cells. The process is slow, and the hearing loss may not appear for as long as two or three months after the medication is given. This is why for several years dihydrostreptomycin was not suspected as a cause of hearing loss. It was routinely used at one time, in mixtures with other antibiotics such as penicillin, for so-called prophylactic therapy. Now it is used only when there is a specific and compelling indication for it, as a matter of life or death, and then only as a calculated risk.

Many other chemicals and drugs have been incriminated from time to time as ototoxic agents. The following list, which is fairly inclusive, is taken from a recent (1973) review of diseases of the inner ear. (See Paparella and Shumrick in Suggested Readings and References at end of chapter.)

Chemicals

carbon monoxide
mercury
oil of chenopodium
tobacco
gold
lead
arsenic
aniline dyes
alcohol

Drugs

Antibiotics
  streptomycin
  neomycin
  gentamicin
  viomycin
  chloramphenicol
  dihydrostreptomycin
  kanamycin
  vancomycin
  ristocetin
  polymixin B
Diuretics
  ethacrynic acid
  furosemide
Miscellaneous
  salicylates
  polybrene
  quinine
  nitrogen mustard

Circulatory disturbances? This group of causes is largely hypothetical, invoked as the most probable cause of the sudden attacks of Menière's disease and of sudden loss of hearing without other symptoms. Vascular spasm is often mentioned without proof and, as we shall see in Chapter 5, therapy is guided accordingly. "Sludging of the blood," a condition in which the red blood corpuscles adhere to one another to an abnormal degree, has also been implicated. There are suggestions of a strong psychogenic factor in Menière's disease, as in peptic ulcer, and this might operate by way of the blood supply.

Very puzzling indeed are the rare but well-documented cases of sudden loss of hearing, usually unilateral, without apparent adequate cause. There may or may not have been a precipitating event, such as exposure to cold. A vascular spasm, embolism, or other "accident" is as good a guess as any and better than most. The important point is to know that such sudden losses *can* happen.

Noise

Temporary hearing loss Whoever has worked in a really noisy factory, driven a tractor on a farm, or indulged in much pistol or skeet shooting can recall how his ears rang for hours afterward, and voices sounded muffled and indistinct. Loud sounds could be heard as well as ever, but he was temporarily hard of hearing. After a few hours, or by the following day at least, his hearing had recovered. Recovery from this hearing loss is usually so complete that the hearing loss may properly be considered a fatigue rather than an injury. We call this a *temporary threshold shift*.

It is a curious fact that the temporary threshold shift produced by exposure to a loud tone or noise is confined almost entirely to frequencies *higher* than the frequency of the offending tone or noise. *The greatest shift is for tones about half an octave above the exposure tone,* but all of the higher frequencies may be more or less affected.

Hearing for lower tones, on the other hand, remains almost as good as ever. Furthermore, the high tones, in addition to being more annoying (although not more painful), also cause a more rapid shift of threshold. The greater susceptibility of the ear to fatigue by high tones offsets the greater intensity of the low components in most loud noises, both natural and man-made. For most noises, therefore, the temporary effect is usually a partial high-tone loss, *most severe for high frequencies above the range essential for speech*. Ears vary so much in their susceptibility, and noises vary so much in

their spectra, that isolated numerical statements are not very meaningful, but an example may be given from some wartime experiments. Exposure to a 1000-Hz tone at 120 dB SPL (about at the threshold of discomfort) for half an hour usually caused a temporary threshold shift of about 35 dB over the upper half of the speech range. Hearing was usually normal the next day, but the last part of auditory sensitivity to recover completely was almost always the band *between 3000 and 5000 Hz*. This band seems to represent a vulnerable spot in the sense organ of hearing that recovers more slowly, regardless of what tone or noise produces the threshold shift.

Permanent injury from noise Temporary threshold shift may be called "fatigue," but somewhere injury begins. We know that the muzzle blast of a big gun or the explosion of a nearby shell may rupture the drum membrane or cause permanent sensorineural hearing loss. (Curiously enough, if the membrane *does* rupture, there is likely to be less permanent sensorineural loss of hearing than if it does not. Blast deafness is rarely total in any case.) In animal experiments it has been found that blasts may disorganize the organ of Corti or shake great pieces of it loose into the surrounding fluid. The injured part of the organ does not regenerate but instead is replaced by a layer of simple cells. The same sort of permanent injury is produced by a sufficiently intense noise or pure tone. The intensity required to cause such breaking of the organ of Corti depends in part on how long the noise lasts.

Acoustic trauma Injury to the ear by a single brief exposure to sound, particularly to an explosion or gun blast, is called "acoustic trauma." This term has been, and in European countries still is, used to include loss of hearing from prolonged and repeated exposure to noise. It is useful to distinguish the two conditions, however, particularly for medicolegal reasons. In acoustic trauma, as we shall use the words, it is easy to identify the actual incident and the time that it happened, and usually the responsibility for it. From the audiological point of view the loss of hearing may be very severe at first, but much recovery can be expected, and improvement usually continues for several months. This degree of recovery is in sharp contrast to the chronic noise-induced hearing loss among industrial workers in very noisy trades. Their improvement in hearing after the first 48 hours off the job is very slight indeed.

Another form of acute injury to hearing is a loss resulting from a blow to the head. A blow on the external ear, the old-fashioned "boxing the ears" of children as a form of punishment, can cause not only severe pain in the middle ear and possible injury to the drum membrane or fracture or dislocation of the ossicles but even permanent injury to the inner ear. The injury is caused by a violent wave of air-conducted "sound." Similar damage to the inner ear may even be caused by a very sharp blow on the skull, such as one that may occur in an automobile accident. Here the injury is best described as acoustic trauma by bone conduction.

Noise-induced hearing loss is the preferred term for what was once called "boilermakers' deafness" or "industrial hearing loss." It is a loss of hearing that develops gradually over months and years. With most industrial noises the loss *almost always begins at 4000 or 6000 Hz,* where the recovery from temporary threshold shift is slowest, but this depends significantly on the spectrum of the noise.

Noise exposure The ear can tolerate for a few seconds a painfully loud noise that would disrupt the organ of Corti or at least cause degeneration of some of its sensory cells if continued for minutes. In other words, the duration as well as the intensity of the exposure is important. Injury from noise exposure depends on decibels, on frequency, and also on duration measured in seconds, hours, months, or years. The sound levels necessary to produce rapid injury, say 150 dB or more, rarely occur as sustained sound except near the exhaust of some jet engines and rockets. Those who work in such situations must take special precautions, and certain areas may be forbidden entirely as too hazardous for hearing. But for the more ordinary, less severe noise exposures, the usual practical question about injury is: "Will the temporary hearing loss produced day after day and week after week ultimately become permanent?" The answer is "yes" *if* the noise is loud enough and if a long exposure is repeated often enough; but we do not know how loud and how often is "enough." Some ears are more susceptible to temporary threshold shift than are others, and there are probably similar differences in resistance to permanent injury. In the practical situations of the drop forge worker or the skeet shooter who has suffered a permanent hearing loss, we rarely know how loud the sound was that finally caused the permanent injury. Rules, criteria, and methods for the prevention of noise-induced hearing loss are considered in the next chapter. It is comforting to know that the sound levels of sonic booms caused by supersonic aircraft are far below the pressure levels that can cause a permanent hearing loss, even with repeated exposures.

CONGENITAL AND CHILDHOOD DEAFNESS

Congenital means strictly "existing at birth," but according to common usage we extend it to include those conditions that are caused by or associated with the birth process, such as birth trauma, or that develop in the first few days of life, such as icterus

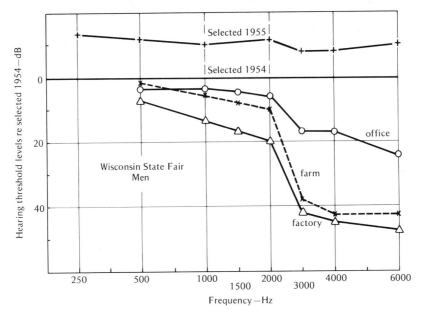

Figure 4-9   Hearing threshold levels. The two "selected" groups were young adults visiting the Wisconsin State Fair in 1954 and 1955 who were judged to be otologically normal and with no history of noise exposure or otic pathology. The three other groups were self-selected from among visitors to the Wisconsin State Fair in 1954 only. The self-selection probably introduced some bias toward impaired hearing. Factory and farm workers showed more high-tone hearing loss than did office workers. The median hearing-threshold levels, relative to the selected 1954 group, for office workers, for farm workers, and for factory workers are shown separately. The divergences from the selected group express the combined effects of age, noise exposure, previous diseases of the ear, and the biases of self-selection. The difference between the "selected" levels of 1954 and 1955 is discussed in Chapter 7. The "Selected 1955" levels were included in the calculation of the ANSI reference zero level.

neonatorum. A condition that is congenital may or may not be hereditary.

In children and young people the most common "cause" of sensorineural hearing loss, if we are to accept medical statistics at their face value, is "congenital," but the meaning of the term as it appears in medical records is not entirely clear. It is a sort of wastebasket classification in which are placed all cases of impaired hearing in children for which no likely cause can be found. The term "congenital" may be wrongly applied to cases in which the impairment is actually due to scarlet fever, meningitis, or some other disease of childhood that destroyed hearing before the child learned to talk. There is no doubt, however, that babies may sometimes be born deaf and also that

there is a hereditary tendency, fortunately rare, for the sense organ of hearing and the auditory nerve to degenerate at an early age without apparent cause.

Bacterial Infection

The inner ear may be the site of a bacterial pus-forming infection somewhat similar to infection in the middle ear. This is not a congenital condition, but it may occur during the first year or two and lead to very severe or total loss of hearing and its attendant handicap in the failure to develop speech. (Such infection may also occur later in life after speech has developed.) The infection usually reaches the inner ear through the perilymphatic connection between the inner

ear and the cranial cavity. Infection and inflammation of the coverings of the brain and
spinal cord, the "meninges," is known as
meningitis. The agent is most frequently the
meningococcus which has a special predi-
lection for the meninges. Sometimes it is a
pneumococcus, a staphylococcus, the tuber-
cle bacillus, Hemophilus influenzae, or some
other variety. If the infection reaches the inner ear, it may destroy the auditory nerve,
the organ of Corti, and most or all of the
other delicate auditory structures. This is illustrated in Figure 4-10.

In the 1920s and 1930s meningitis was the
most common single, clearly identified
cause of acquired total deafness in childhood. Since that time preventive innocula-
tions have greatly reduced the prevalence of
the disease, and antitoxins and antibiotics
have saved the lives of a larger proportion of
patients. But the life may be saved only after
destruction of the inner ear, and bacterial infection still appears on our lists of causes of
childhood deafness.

Typhoid fever and *diphtheria* are two
bacterial diseases that probably affect the ear
remotely by the *toxins* formed by the bacteria in the gastrointestinal tract or the respiratory tract, respectively. The result is more or
less complete degeneration of the organ of
Corti and associated structures. These diseases were formerly a relatively common
cause of acquired deafness, but thanks to the
widespread practice of immunization they
are now quite rare in the United States.

There is obviously no hope of regeneration
or repair of a missing organ of Corti, and no
type of treatment, medication, or stimulation
will improve the hearing of anyone whose
deafness is due to meningitis or any similar
bacterial infection. This proposition applies
also to toxic degeneration and to viral infections such as mumps and measles, which
also cause severe and permanent anatomical
changes.

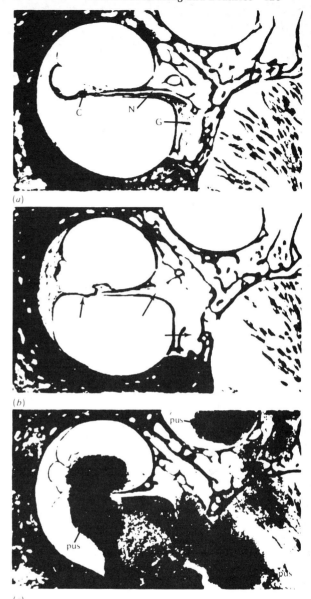

Figure 4-10 Two types of sensorineural impairment. *4-10a:* Normal cochlea. The location of this section in relation to the inner ear as a whole is shown by the rectangle
in Figure 3-8. C, organ of Corti; N, fibers of the auditory
nerve; G, ganglion cells. *4-10b:* The lower turn of a cochlea
of a person with high-tone loss. The arrows indicate where
the organ of Corti, nerve fibers, and ganglion (nerve) cells
are absent. This is typical of abrupt high-tone loss. Compare
Figure 4-2. *4-10c:* Destruction of the organ of Corti, basilar
membrane, and nerve by pus, as in meningitis.

A less severe form of labyrinthitis, which may cause only temporary threshold shift, is *serous* labyrinthitis. This may occur as an irritative reaction to middle-ear pathology or cholesteatoma.

Viral Infections

Almost any of the common infectious diseases of childhood, which in general are viral rather than bacterial, may in severe cases affect the inner ear. Frequently, as is usual with mumps, only one ear is damaged, but all too often both ears suffer. A virus is submicroscopic in size, much smaller than a bacterium, and it usually reaches the ear directly from the bloodstream instead of from the cerebrospinal fluid of the cranial cavity. As mentioned above, a virus does not stimulate the formation of pus, but it may severely injure delicate specialized structures such as the organ of Corti and the tectorial membrane. One type of end result is an intact basilar membrane with a formless mass of cells covering it, usually heaped up near the limbus. Many of the cells are endothelial cells that have replaced other dead cells. Sometimes remains of the tectorial membrane, all curled up and covered with endothelium, can be identified. Sometimes a few hair cells and nerve fibers remain, particularly at the extreme apical or the extreme basal end of the basilar membrane. If the sensory units do survive and function, there is a remnant of hearing which may be reached with a hearing aid. The hearing loss may be very severe, but it tends to be very stable.

In 1928 an extensive study was made, under the leadership of Dr. G. E. Shambaugh, Sr., of the causes of deafness and severe hearing loss in children enrolled in a number of public schools for the deaf. In more than half of the pupils, most of them studied in retrospect on the basis of their medical and family histories, no cause could be assigned, but "infectious diseases of childhood" including typhoid fever, diphtheria, and "high fever" (not otherwise identified) accounted for deafness in about 15 percent of the pupils. Some of these diseases, notably typhoid fever, diphtheria, and scarlet fever, have now been brought under control and cause few impairments, but other diseases are still very significant as causes. No precise recent statistics are available, however.

Maternal rubella One particular viral disease, however, has now emerged as a major cause of congenital deafness. It is *rubella* or "German measles." Particular strains of this virus that are unusually virulent have appeared, and the disease has twice assumed epidemic proportions. The first recognized outbreak occurred in Australia about 1942. It was following this epidemic that it was recognized that rubella in the mother during early pregnancy could cause a congenital deafness. The largest recent epidemic was in 1963, 1964, and 1965. The northeastern seaboard of the United States suffered most severely, but the disease was quite widespread throughout the midwestern and Pacific Coast states. By good fortune a continuing cooperative long-term study of a large group of expectant mothers was in progress in Baltimore and other medical centers when the epidemic appeared. This study was sponsored by the United States National Institutes of Health. In it several important features of rubella and its effects on the developing embryo or fetus were discovered.

For the mother the disease is usually a mild infection. Actually about half of the Baltimore mothers who gave birth to infants in whom the virus or antibodies were detected by laboratory tests had had no clinical symptoms of rubella themselves. It is the developing embryo, not the mother, that suffers. In the Baltimore study there were 165 children with confirmed prenatal rubella. Of these, 73 failed to pass their hearing test. But congenital deafness is only one of the many developmental defects that may occur. Vision may be impaired, the heart may be defective, and the nervous system may be abnormal in a variety of ways, ranging from minor defects to complete idiocy.

The chances of developmental defects, including severe hearing loss, proved to be greatest when the maternal illness occurred during the first three months of pregnancy. Previously it was believed that the embryo was vulnerable *only* during the first trimester, but it is now clear that the virus may persist and injure an embryo that is conceived weeks or even a few months after the infection, and injury to a fetus can occur at least as late as the seventh month of pregnancy. Nineteen mothers in the Baltimore study contracted rubella during the second trimester of pregnancy. Two fetuses were stillborn, with positive viral cultures. Six viable infants showed abnormalities compatible with prenatal rubella. Only five of the infants failed to give laboratory evidence of rubella at birth.

It had been generally assumed that the mechanism of the injury was an interference with the control of development. Heart, nervous system, eyes, and ears go through important and complex stages of development in the first trimester. But the length of time that the child carries the virus is also significant. The children who carry it for long periods after birth tend to suffer more severely than those from whom it disappears after birth. Here inhibition of normal growth appears to be involved.

The anatomical appearance of the inner ears of infants with congenital rubella deafness that have been studied is rather like that seen following postnatal viral infection. There is severe but incomplete injury to the organ of Corti and what looks like a "heal-ing" regrowth of epithelium. It is quite possible that the virus, as well as toxins, can pass through the placenta and that the embryo or fetus is damaged in utero. Very likely the protective mechanisms of the fetus are less effective than those of the mother. The ear and other developing organs may be directly infected, and some of their cells destroyed by the virus.

The rubella virus was isolated in the middle 1960s, and by 1968 a successful vaccine against it was announced. Programs for systematic inoculation are now active in many places in the United States. One such program, in Massachusetts, administered the vaccine to children in the first two grades of school, and later extended it to adolescent and postadolescent females. A primary concern was the possible prevention of another major epidemic, which without a program of extensive inoculation was expected in the early 1970s. Actually no such epidemic occurred.

Rubella is not the only viral infection that can cause congenital deafness or dysacusis. Almost any severe infection can do so, particularly during the first trimester when the embryo seems to be more vulnerable than later during fetal life. Influenza and mumps seem to be the most dangerous, after rubella, but at the other extreme the common cold creates no such hazard.

Rubella rarely causes total deafness. The children with this type of congenital impairment may be severely hard of hearing and educationally deaf in the sense that they do not hear speech sounds well enough to learn speech and language spontaneously. They need hearing aids. Very frequently they retain fairly good hearing for the very high frequencies (4000 Hz and above) or for low frequencies (250 and 125 Hz), or both. They respond to many environmental sounds, including the human voice, and it may be several years before it is realized that they actually have a serious hearing handicap. The consequences of such delay in diagnosis can be very unfortunate, as we shall point out in the discussion of central dysacusis. These children with serious but incomplete hearing losses have frequently been misdiagnosed as aphasic, mentally retarded, or "brain damaged."

Encephalitis   Encephalitis or infection of the brain is a final member of our list of infections. It can cause a great variety of symptoms of "brain injury," including central dysacusis. The impairments are usually neurological, not audiological, but sometimes there is peripheral cochlear impairment, just as in so many viral infections, and the hearing loss or deafness may be the greatest handicap.

Rh and Other Incompatibilities

Another cause of congenital dysacusis, either peripheral or central, is the incompatibility of certain blood proteins of the parents. More specifically, the rhesus or "Rh" factor may be present or absent. Other factors are "A," "B" and "O." The incompatibilities all operate according to the same pattern and cause their injury to the ears or to the nervous system during the first few days of life, either directly or by the condition known as "jaundice of the newborn," *icterus neonatorum*, or *kernicterus*. The jaundice of kernicterus is caused by abnormal destruction of red blood cells when or before independent life begins at birth. One of the degradation products of the red blood pigment, hemoglobin, is bilirubin, one of the bile pigments. Its yellow color causes the jaundice, and its selective accumulation in certain areas or "nuclei" in the brain causes brain injury. The auditory system is one of the systems that is likely to be injured.

The dangerous parental combination is father Rh-positive and mother Rh-negative, or the corresponding ABO combination. The common feature is that the father's tissues contain a protein that the mother's lack. To her body it is a foreign protein. If this hereditary characteristic is transmitted by the father to the embryo, the mother's system may react against the embryo (or later the fetus) by the same mechanism that develops immunity against any foreign proteins, such as those of pathogenic bacteria. A critical condition is that enough of the "foreign" Rh (or A) factor cross the placental barrier. Then the mother's system forms "antibodies" against it. These antibodies in turn may cause a miscarriage or toxemia or, if they in turn cross the placental barrier, either injure the fetus immediately or through a postnatal kernicterus. Fortunately this biological accident is less likely in a first pregnancy, but it seems as if a first pregnancy may sensitize the mother's system and make difficulties more probable in any later pregnancies in which the heredity is Rh-positive. It may be possible in the future to protect an Rh-negative mother with an anti-Rh antibody that inactivates any Rh-positive fetal blood cells that may pass into her circulation.

The treatment for icterus neonatorum is massive blood transfusions for the infant. It must be done promptly and thoroughly, amounting to complete blood replacement. Too little or too late may still save the life, but only after permanent injury has been done by the bilirubin. Infants who have had even a mild "bilirubinemia" (20 mg or more of bilirubin per cubic centimeter of blood) for any reason should be considered "at risk" with respect to their hearing.

Birth Injury, Anoxia, and Other Nonhereditary Causes of Dysacusis

For completeness and convenience we mention here a few other causes of congenital dysacusis, even though their usual area of injury is central rather than peripheral. Almost all of these relate to various complications of labor, such as prematurity (best defined as a birth weight of 1500 grams or less), either prolonged or precipitate labor, or difficult delivery involving the use of obstetrical forceps with traction on the neck, or birth injury from any cause. Such injuries are usually complicated by hemorrhage in or around the brain. Premature babies are particularly liable to intracranial hemorrhage. Toxemia of pregnancy from any cause, quite apart from Rh incompatibility, carries a risk of injury to hearing.

At birth a very common cause of injury is apnea or failure to breathe, particularly if it goes to the stage of cyanosis (blueness). Certain midbrain auditory centers are among those most susceptible to injury from such asphyxia.

A rather rare accident, one that deserves passing mention, is the use for a premature infant of an incubator that is too noisy.

Injuries may occur at any age. We must remember that not only skull fractures that might crack the temporal bone but blows to the ears ("boxing the ears") and even blows to the skull can sometimes cause acoustic trauma.

Metabolic and Endocrine Disorders

A completely different type of difficulty arises from certain metabolic or endocrine disorders in childhood. The clearest association of dysacusis is with hypothyroidism (cretinism). Impairment of hearing, very likely of a mechanical conductive sort, may accompany the slow skeletal and muscular development, the low metabolic rate, the sluggishness of movement, the mental retardation, the pudgy thickening of the skin, and other abnormalities.

Hereditary Deafness

One of the first questions one asks about childhood deafness, particularly if it is congenital, is whether it is hereditary. The maternal history may include a viral infection or streptomycin intoxication, or the child may have suffered birth injury or an illness such as meningitis. But the family history often reveals relatives with hearing difficulties. These data may strongly suggest a familial or hereditary deafness. In addition, sporadic cases without a family history are frequent, and often no certain diagnosis can be made. As we have noted elsewhere, a large proportion of sporadic cases of deafness are probably due to genetic causes.

There are many types of hereditary deafness. Some hereditary deafness occurs as part of a syndrome—that is, in association with other abnormal traits. Other types have deafness as their only characteristic. The latter, however, may differ according to the age of onset, the severity of hearing loss, and the part of the ear or nervous system affected. In addition, as we shall see below, the genetic bases of hereditary deafness may vary.

Genes are the units of heredity, and are carried on the chromosomes in each cell of the body. There are many thousands of genes in humans, and they are distributed among 23 pairs of chromosomes. Because chromosomes come in pairs, each type of gene is represented by a *gene pair* in every individual. One of each pair of chromosomes comes from the mother, the other from the father. The individual in turn will contribute only one set of chromosomes to his or her children by way of eggs or sperm. Some of these chromosomes will be derived from the individual's mother, and some from his or her father. The distribution of genes in different types of matings is illustrated in Table 4-1.

Genetic abnormalities are due to abnormal or *mutant* genes. If only one member of a gene pair is mutant and yet is expressed as an abnormal characteristic such as deafness, we say the mutant gene is *dominant*. A person having one normal and one dominant

TABLE 4-1
GENETIC CONSEQUENCES OF DIFFERENT MATINGS

		Parents	Gametes	Children
1. Gene pairs pure in each parent (homozygote × homozygote)	(a)	EE × EE	E E	all EE
	(b)	EE × ee	E e	all Ee
	(c)	ee × ee	e e	all ee
2. Mixed gene pair in one parent (homozygote × heterozygote)	(a)	EE × Ee	E ½ E, ½ e	½ EE, ½ Ee
	(b)	Ee × ee	½ E, ½ e e	½ Ee, ½ ee
3. Mixed gene pair in both parents (heterozygote × heterozygote)		Ee × Ee	½ E, ½ e ½ E, ½ e	¼ EE, ½ Ee, ¼ EE

A *homozygote* is an individual in whom the two members of a particular gene pair are the same, either both normal or both mutant. In a *heterozygote* the members of the gene pair are different. A *gamete* is one member of a parental gene pair, after separation, in the ovum or spermatozoon. Each one is either normal or mutant. The fractions ½ or ¼ represent probabilities, not exact ratios.

mutant member of a given gene pair will transmit the normal one to about one-half of his or her children, and the mutant member of the gene pair to the other half of the children. Because the mutation is dominant, the latter children will show the abnormality even if they receive normal genes from their other parent. Children who receive the mutant gene can transmit it in turn to half their children. Thus, where in a family history an abnormality occurs in each generation, and where marriages of affected with unaffected people yield about 50 percent of affected children, a dominant gene is indicated.

A *recessive* mutation is one that cannot be expressed unless *both* members of a gene pair are mutant. (Here, the normal form of the gene is dominant to the mutant form.) A person who is deaf because both members of a gene pair are mutant must have received a mutation from both of his or her parents. Such a person will transmit one mutation to all offspring.

Let us consider in more detail the relation between the abnormality and the mutation. Even though an affected person transmits a recessive mutation to his or her children, the children will be normal if their other parent contributes a normal member of the gene pair. The children who have both a mutant and a normal member of the gene pair, are *carriers*; that is, they can transmit a mutant gene to their offspring. If a carrier of a recessive mutation marries another carrier of the same mutation, about one-quarter of their children will suffer the abnormality. A summary of the types of matings involving dominant and recessive mutations is shown in Table 4-2.

The patterns of dominant and recessive

genetic disease described above are relatively simple, but certain complications and different patterns are often encountered. The first complication is the variation in the severity of the effect of a mutant gene or gene pair. Obviously many thousands of genes interact in the development of the individual, and no two organisms (except identical twins) will have the same genes. Moreover, no two organisms (even identical twins) will

TABLE 4-2
CONSEQUENCES OF MATINGS INVOLVING MUTATIONS FOR DEAFNESS

			Parents				Children
1. Matings involving a rare dominant mutation, A'	(a)	AA $\times$ AA'	(normal) (deaf)		$\frac{1}{2}\,AA$ $\frac{1}{2}\,AA'$	(normal) (deaf)	
	(b)	AA' $\times$ AA'	(deaf) (deaf)		$\frac{1}{4}\,AA$ $\frac{1}{2}\,AA'$ $\frac{1}{4}\,A'A'$	(normal) (deaf) (deaf, or lethal)	
2. Matings involving a recessive mutation, a	(a)	AA $\times$ Aa	(normal) (normal, carrier)		$\frac{1}{2}\,AA$ $\frac{1}{2}\,Aa$	(normal) (normal, carrier)	
	(b)	AA $\times$ aa	(normal) (deaf)		all Aa	(normal, carrier)	
	(c)	Aa $\times$ Aa	(normal, carrier) (normal, carrier)		$\frac{1}{4}\,AA$ $\frac{1}{2}\,Aa$ $\frac{1}{4}\,aa$	(normal) (normal, carrier) (deaf)	
	(d)	Aa $\times$ aa	(normal, carrier) (deaf)		$\frac{1}{2}\,Aa$ $\frac{1}{2}\,aa$	(normal, carrier) (deaf)	
	(e)	aa $\times$ aa	(deaf) (deaf)		all aa	(deaf)	
3. A mating of deaf people bearing different recessive mutations, a or b		$AAbb$ $\times$ $aaBb$	(deaf) (deaf)		all $AaBb$	(normal, carrier of two mutations)	

In this table "deaf" means a more or less severe impairment of hearing, depending on the nature of the mutation and its penetrance. Sometimes the combination of two dominant mutations ($A'A'$) is lethal, meaning that the embryo dies.

develop in identical environments in utero or thereafter. For these reasons, people having exactly the same dominant mutation or the same recessive mutant gene pair may differ greatly in the severity of their deafness or other abnormality. In the extreme, some individuals may give little or no evidence at all of having the mutation(s). When this happens, the mutant gene is said to have *incomplete penetrance*. If partial deafness is due to an incompletely penetrant dominant gene, the gene is often not recognized as dominant, or even the deafness as genetic. This is especially true if both parents of an affected child have normal or nearly normal hearing.

A second aspect of gene action is that a single mutant gene may affect several characteristics of the person bearing it. While some forms of deafness are limited to this trait, deafness also occurs as a part of "syndromes" in which the skeletal system (Treacher-Collins disease), nervous system, visual system, integumentary system (Waardenburg's disease), renal system (Alport's disease), or endocrines are also abnormal. Such associations indicate that the gene in question participates in the formation or function of several body structures.

A third complication, well known to geneticists, is that two different recessive mutant genes may both affect the same trait. A large number of genes contribute to hearing, and any one of them can cause hearing loss if it is mutant. *A child receiving a recessive mutation from each parent will not be deaf if the mutations belong to different gene pairs.* If this is the case, each parent will have contributed a normal gene to mask the mutation contributed by the other parent (Table 4-2). Diagrammatically, consider two parents *AAbb* and *aaBB*, where *a* and *b* are recessive mutations of different genes. The gametes of these parents, having one of each type of gene, will be *Ab* for the first parent and *aB* for the second. Their children will be of the type *AaBb*, where the normal genes *A* and *B* are dominant to the recessive mutations, *a* and *b*. A well-documented case of this phenomenon, from a study in Northern Ireland, is shown in Figure 4-11. Because deaf people often marry one another, a number of such instances are known.

A fourth complication of hereditary deafness is the "sporadic" case of deafness. Where deaf children arise in family lines with no history of deafness, a disproportion-

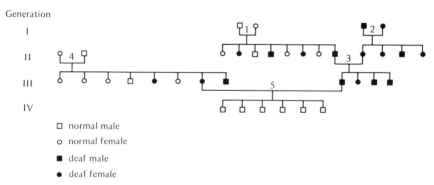

Figure 4-11 Pedigree of deafness in four generations involving two family lines. Mating 5 between two deaf parents produced all normal children. The mating is thus probably of type 3 of Table 4-2 *(AAbb × aaBB)*. Matings 1 and 4 are of type 2c *(Aa × Aa or Bb × Bb)*. The excess of deaf children over the one-quarter expected is not significant statistically in such a small sample. Matings 2 and 3 are of type 2e *(aa × aa)*. Progeny are given in order of birth. *(After A. C. Stevenson and E. A. Cheesman, "Hereditary Deafmutism with Particular Reference to Northern Ireland," Ann. Hum. Genet., 20;177; 1956)*

TABLE 4-3
CONSEQUENCES OF CONSANGUINITY: A COUSIN MARRIAGE INVOLVING A RECESSIVE GENE

Generation	Mating		Description
I		$Aa \times AA$	Original mating
II	$AA \times Aa$	$Aa \times AA$	Two Aa children marry unrelated people, both AA
III		$Aa \times Aa$	Two grandchildren (cousins) marry one another
IV		aa (deaf)	Certain great-grandchildren may receive two copies of the original mutation

ate amount of *consanguinity,* or marriage among relatives, is almost always seen. Most of the deleterious recessive genes in a population are relatively rare and exist mainly in carrier individuals. Therefore, by chance alone carriers will almost always marry people who have two normal members of the gene pair in question. Such unions cannot yield affected offspring (see Table 4-3). However, marriage of first cousins bears the risk that they will both be carriers of the same recessive mutant gene, derived from their common ancestor. In such families recessive genetic diseases frequently gain expression for the first time in a family line. One question to be asked of a couple who have a congenitally deaf infant, therefore, is whether they do in fact have a common ancestor. The pedigree in Table 4-3 illustrates this phenomenon.

Finally, sex linkage must be noted as a characteristically different mode of inheritance. In humans and many other animals, one pair of chromosomes is unusual in that females have two X chromosomes, while males have one X and one Y chromosome. The X chromosomes are similar to other chromosomes, whereas the Y chromosomes carry a particular set of genes that make the individual a male. Of importance here is the

fact that females have two of every X-borne gene, whereas males can have only one. Thus a female may have two, one, or no mutant member of a gene pair. If she has one recessive mutant gene, she is a carrier. A male, by contrast, either has one mutant gene or one normal gene. If he has a mutant gene, he will express it, even if it is recessive. This is because there is no normal counterpart of the mutant gene on the Y chromosome. The pattern of inheritance of sex-linked genes differs from the usual (Table 4-4). Males always pass their Y chromosome to their sons and their X chromosome to their daughters. This means that a father cannot transmit an X-linked genetic disease to a son. Sons always get their X chromosome from their mothers. If the mother is a carrier for an X-linked genetic disease, half her sons will display the disease, regardless of who the father of these sons is. The characteristics of a sex-linked disease, then, are that it appears much more frequently in males; it is not transmitted from father to son; and unaffected carrier mothers transmit the disease to half their sons. Hemophilia (the bleeding disease) and certain forms of color blindness are probably the best known cases of sex-linked disorders. In pedigrees, a sex-linked recessive mutation can frequently be traced

TABLE 4-4
GENETIC CONSEQUENCES OF A MATING INVOLVING A SEX-LINKED MUTATION (a)

(1)	$X^A X^a$ (normal, carrier female) × $X^A Y$ (normal male)	$\frac{1}{4}$ $X^A X^A$ (normal female) $\frac{1}{4}$ $X^A X^a$ (normal, carrier female) $\frac{1}{4}$ $X^A Y$ (normal male) $\frac{1}{4}$ $X^a Y$ (deaf male)
(2)	$X^A X^A$ (normal female) × $X^a Y$ (deaf male)	$\frac{1}{2}$ $X^A X^a$ (normal, carrier female) $\frac{1}{2}$ $X^A Y$ (normal male)

The gene pair that includes a sex-linked mutation (a) is shown borne on the X chromosome. "Normal" means normal hearing.

from an affected man through an unaffected daughter, to her affected son. A small proportion of hereditary deafness follows this pattern.

Among the hereditary forms of deafness, a great variety exists, and a useful, complete, and well-illustrated compilation of over 60 of them has been made by Konigsmark. The hereditary forms may be distinguished on the basis of their associated traits, the anatomical basis of hearing loss, the frequency ranges affected, the age of onset, and, of course, the pattern of inheritance (dominant, recessive, sex-linked; completely or incompletely penetrant). We summarize very briefly by noting that the other abnormalities associated with impaired hearing include bizarre skeletal deformities, abnormal pigmentation, and defects of eyes and central nervous system. Each syndrome is known by the name of the doctor who first described it in the literature and they are well described in medical monographs. Examples are the *Waardenburg* syndrome, the *Klippel-Feil* syndrome, and the *Treacher-Collins* syndrome; and there are others.

We also name certain types of abnormality of the labyrinth or of the middle or the external ear which may occur in isolation. One of these, *Scheibe's* type (sacculocochlear type),

is worth mentioning because Drs. Whetnall and Fry (1964) state in their monograph that it occurs in about 70 percent of cases of hereditary deafness. The abnormalities are confined to the cochlear duct and saccule. The organ of Corti shows the greatest change in the apical turn, where it may consist of only "a mound of undifferentiated cells." The stria vascularis is degenerate. The tectorial membrane is flattened over the organ of Corti, or rolled up in the internal sulcus, or attached to Reissner's membrane. The cochlear duct may be dilated, but more often it is collapsed. Reissner's membrane may be adherent directly to the organ of Corti. This description is strangely similar to our description in an earlier paragraph of the effects of viral infection.

Another type to recall, mentioned earlier, is the delayed degeneration of the organ of Corti that occurs during childhood. The immediate reason for and mechanism of the degeneration is not known, but the same kind of thing happens in waltzing guinea pigs, in albinotic cats, and probably in other kinds of hereditary deafness in animals.

An interesting suggestion, made by Dr. E. Wedenberg of Stockholm, is that the carriers of the gene for at least some form(s) of hereditary deafness may be identified by careful audiometry. They show dips in the high-frequency range of the audiogram that are not reasonably explained by noise exposure, and their stapedius reflex is weak or absent. Wedenberg believes that these are incomplete expressions (associated with the low penetrance) of the gene in question. This is very interesting theoretically, but it does not point as yet to any practical application unless it be to alert parents to the possibility of sporadic deafness so that it will be detected early and managed appropriately.

With the recognition of the low penetrance of some genes that produce deafness *it becomes reasonable to suppose that the majority of cases of unexplained severe congenital hearing loss and deafness are actually sporadic hereditary deafness.*

Konigsmark and Gorlin estimate that over one-half of profound congenital deafness is hereditary, and that four-fifths of these cases are due to recessive gene pairs. From intermarriages of the deaf in Northern Ireland and the eastern United States, investigators have concluded that there are about five or six different recessive genes that may be responsible for these cases. It is of interest that there is almost complete penetrance of this type of genetic defect. By contrast, the dominant genes responsible for 10 percent or so of congenital deafness are not completely penetrant, may vary in severity, and in some cases may affect one ear much more severely than the other.

Several forms of hereditary deafness without associated traits are either late in onset and incomplete, or progressive, or both. A good example of these characteristics is otosclerosis, one of the major causes of hearing loss. In one study in Sweden cited by Konigsmark, a familial pattern of otosclerosis was seen in 80 percent of the cases. The disease, which appears in the teens or twenties, is ascribed to one or more types of dominant mutations having penetrance of 25 to 40 percent.

Little can be done to reverse the primary symptoms of hereditary deafness. No measures can eliminate the many rare mutant genes from the human population. However, two points should be made. First, the detection and the management of hereditary deafness is the same as for nongenetic deafness. This is particularly true of profound or early-onset deafness, where speech and language impairments can be minimized by appropriate early training. If the deafness is progressive during childhood, hearing aids can extend the period in which speech can develop normally.

The second point is that there is a role for genetic counseling. Familial patterns of hearing loss, combined with accurate diagnosis, can help decide the risk of hearing loss in the descendants of affected parents. When deaf people marry one another, diagnosis and counseling may in some instances predict with good accuracy and confidence that they will or will not have deaf children. In many other cases, unfortunately, because of the incomplete family histories or the uncertain diagnosis of other nongenetic causes of parental deafness, the estimated risk of having affected children is very uncertain. These children must always be considered "at risk" for congenital deafness and be tested carefully, as described in Chapter 8. Of course, effective counseling recognizes the requirement of mature sensitivity to the ethical, moral, and psychological factors involved in the delicate process of advising people about family planning.[4]

CENTRAL DYSACUSIS

Organic Impairments

In general, the more peripherally a lesion is located in the nervous system, the more

[4] For major assistance in rewriting this section the author is indebted to Prof. Rowland H. Davis of the University of California, Irvine.

clear-cut are the signs and symptoms and the easier it is to make a diagnosis and to locate the lesion anatomically. Lesions of the auditory system within the brain can rarely be localized, or even clearly identified, by their symptoms, except perhaps to say that the lesion is more probably on the right side or on the left. More often the questions asked will be whether there is *any* pathological condition that would be visible postmortem and, if so, whether it has any clear localization, like a tumor, or is completely generalized, like arteriosclerosis.

Among the numerous causes of central impairment are generalized infections such as encephalitis and meningitis, specific infections such as syphilis, degenerative diseases such as multiple sclerosis, the progressive death of individual neurons due to old age, "cerebral vascular accidents" of various sorts such as cerebral hemorrhage or the blocking of blood vessels by local clotting (thrombosis) or by a clot originally formed elsewhere (embolism), and clearly local injuries such as gunshot wounds, skull fractures, birth injuries, and the scars and adhesions resulting from these. Congenital abnormalities, either specific malformations or generalized conditions such as Down's syndrome, should be mentioned also. A subtle general or partially localized injury may follow prolonged asphyxia, either at birth or from drowning (with delayed resuscitation) or carbon monoxide poisoning. Some areas of the sensory systems in the brain stem seem to be particularly susceptible to such asphyxial injury. Finally, and very important, there are brain tumors, cysts, and abscesses.

Acoustic neurinoma In a previous section we considered the type of impairment that is most commonly associated with a tumor of the eighth nerve—the so-called acoustic neurinoma or neuroma. From the audiological point of view it is logical to class the impairment as *neural*, although from the anatomical and surgical point of view these tumors are *central* lesions.

Acoustic tumors are not malignant, and they may grow very slowly over the years, but the earlier they are recognized and removed, the better the chance of preserving the facial nerve and possibly the eighth (auditory) nerve also. The symptoms of pressure on the eighth nerve are hearing loss, mild tinnitus, and vertigo, and sometimes there are also symptoms due to pressure on other cranial nerves or the brain stem. The position of these tumors at the base of the brain makes their removal a serious operation. Audiological tests, described in Chapter 8, and tests of vestibular functions may be very helpful in establishing the diagnosis firmly.

The overlap between otology and neurology is well illustrated by the problems of diagnosis and surgical removal of acoustic neurinomas. The overlap includes also the lesions, disorders, and malfunctions of the central auditory system. The auditory dysacuses may be accompanied by equally or more important impairments of other systems, as in cerebral palsy. But, regardless of which specialist first recognizes the case or which one makes the final diagnosis or who handles the treatment, the audiologist can assist by performing the tests that are described in later chapters and by evaluating the results for the benefit of his medical and surgical colleagues. The audiologist does not make diagnoses, but his tests often indicate a strong probability of one diagnosis or anatomical localization as opposed to another. And it makes little difference whether the joint specialty that the audiologist serves is known as "neuro-otology" or "otoneurology."

The foregoing list of cerebral diseases, injuries, and impairments is not exhaustive, but it illustrates the variety of conditions that must be considered by the neurologist in making a diagnosis, and it also illustrates the specific localization of some lesions and the diffuseness of others. And even if a lesion like a tumor is perfectly definite and discrete, the symptoms that it causes may be very vague indeed, particularly if it is located in one of the "association areas" of the cerebral cortex. But sometimes the audiologist, by appropriate tests that involve the understanding of speech under difficult listening conditions, or presented at high speed, or requiring the fusion of information delivered to the two ears, may assist the neurologist to a diagnosis or a localization. The basis of such tests will be considered in Chapter 8. An impairment of hearing associated with any of the foregoing diseases or conditions is said to be an "organic" dysacusis.

Functional Dysacusis

There is another major class of central auditory impairments that do not have any apparent organic basis but relate instead to distortions of attention, motivation, and understanding, that is, to psychological factors. These are known as *nonorganic* or *functional dysacuses.*

We call attention here to what may be, for some, an extension of the concept of dysacusis to include psychological factors such as inattention, hysterical deafness, deliberate feigning, and so on. It seems useful to include them all, however, in the blanket term because it is often very difficult to distinguish one from another and from organic dysacuses. Some of the psychological factors will be considered specifically below.

It is particularly important to recognize that the functional impairments may be combined with, and to some extent arise from, organic impairments, particularly from peripheral hearing loss. We then speak of a *functional overlay.* It is often very difficult to determine the extent of the overlay, or

even to distinguish between the organic and the functional components. Here three major questions must be considered.

1. What is the degree of motivation and cooperation of the subject? Is a child incompetent because of mental retardation or the psychiatric condition known as *autism* or *childhood schizophrenia*? Is an adult deliberately exaggerating a hearing loss, that is, feigning or simulating for reasons of his own? More technically, is it a case of *pseudohypoacusis*? Or does he fail to understand what he is expected to do? Is his *span of attention* too short? Obviously, a test of peripheral hearing that does not require active cooperation by the subject can be of great help in answering such questions (see Chapter 8).

2. What is the extent of any peripheral hearing loss, that is, true hypoacusis? A severe or even a moderate hearing loss, such as might be caused by a congenital defect, an infection, or acoustic trauma, may establish certain patterns of attention and behavior that become firmly established but may nevertheless be reversible with proper management and training. In other words, how great is the functional overlay?

3. At what age did the impairment appear? If a child has had sufficient hearing in his first two or three years of life to learn speech and develop language spontaneously, his overall prospect for rehabilitation will be very much better than that of the child who has never developed speech. On the other hand, the "plasticity" of the nervous system of the young child mentioned in Chapter 3 may make learning or relearning easier if he suffers a partial organic impairment early, rather than later in life. As we shall point out below, we simply do not yet know how much the development of the nervous system is influenced by early sensory deprivation, either partial or total. Here the distinction between organic and functional

ceases to be very meaningful. We shall return to this question in Chapter 17.

Audiometric Tests in Central Dysacusis

Central dysacusis does not cause elevation of the threshold of hearing, except for what may be attributed to failure of attention and cooperation, nor does it impair hearing for particular frequencies as in abrupt, high-tone hearing loss. The characteristic difficulty is *difficulty in understanding speech* or even the failure to recognize the meaning of simple acoustic signals. The term *central auditory imperception* is sometimes used to describe the difficulty. One of the best diagnostic clues to central dysacusis is a discrepancy between the ability to understand speech and the prediction based on pure-tone audiometry. A patient may say "I hear you, but I can't understand the words." Or he may just seem bewildered. Another major characteristic, particularly of certain functional impairments, is a variability of thresholds from one test to another.

Pure-tone audiometry may be very important for the recognition and assessment of a peripheral organic component, but it is practically useless for the description of a functional overlay. Central dysacusis is not measured in hertz or in decibels. Better dimensions are to be found in speed of perception, in synthesis, and in understanding. This point is illustrated in the following descriptions of several particular forms of central dysacusis.

Phonemic Regression in Old Age

The term "phonemic regression" was coined by Dr. John H. Gaeth to describe a condition that he noticed fairly often in elderly people who came to the hearing clinic at Northwestern University. They complained of difficulty in understanding what other people said. By pure-tone audiometry these elderly people showed nearly normal hearing-threshold levels, at least up to 2000 Hz, if the tests were carried out carefully, deliberately, and sympathetically, and with adequate rest periods. But with speech audiometry, particularly with recorded speech tests, as described in Chapter 8, these people had great difficulty. They understood only a few words correctly and soon became discouraged.

It is easy to recognize in this the pattern of old age. The attention span becomes short, and the person will not and cannot be hurried. Given time, he may answer correctly, but seldom quickly. He has much more difficulty with the complicated acoustic patterns of speech than with simple pure tones. That is why Dr. Gaeth called it *phonemic* regression. These people usually have the high-tone sensorineural hearing loss of presbycusis, but their failure to understand words is far greater than can be explained by this loss alone.

The cause of phonemic regression lies in the brain, not in the ear. Generalized cerebral arteriosclerosis is probably the most common cause. Many individual cells have died throughout the brain, and there may be many bits and patches where the loss is more than just a thinning of the cell population. The brain still remembers old experiences and habits, but it learns or remembers little that is new. Attention is short. Naps become frequent. And even familiar performances, like recognizing the meaning of words or sentences, although often still possible, may require special motivation and plenty of time. These elderly people have particular difficulty understanding speech in a background of noise. For those with phonemic regression a hearing aid is of little help, nor does it help to shout at them. It is more important to speak *clearly*, *simply*, and, above all, *slowly*.

Verbal Dysacusis (Sensory Aphasia)

Verbal dysacusis means specifically the failure to understand the meanings of words even though the sounds are presumed to be heard quite perfectly and correctly. "Word deafness" is a reasonable popular translation, but the term aphasia has been used more and more widely. Strictly, aphasia refers to the inability to say, or perhaps to find, the word one wants to express an idea. But understanding incoming words and finding the proper word to say are closely related to one another, and both functions are likely to be impaired by the same organic lesion, and it is reasonable to use the same term for both. We may, however, wish to distinguish *motor* or *expressive aphasia* from *sensory aphasia* in some circumstances.

Verbal dysacusis may be caused in adults by an injury, as in an automobile accident or a "cerebral vascular accident," to the parietal-temporal area of the hemisphere (usually the left) that is dominant for speech. This speech area and also another more anterior area (Broca's area) and a third supplementary speech area are shown in Figure 4-12, but we shall not go into the details of the anatomy of the areas. The management and rehabilitation of such patients and current issues and theories are considered in a later chapter.

The relearning of speech, both motor and sensory, may be slow and tedious, but it is usually possible. Our understanding of the neurological and physiological basis of the aphasias, the "agnosias," and the related conditions of cerebral injury, epilepsy, and the like is advancing rapidly, but we must always approach the practical problems of the clinic on the basis of direct observation and experience and not rely on neurological or physiological theory.

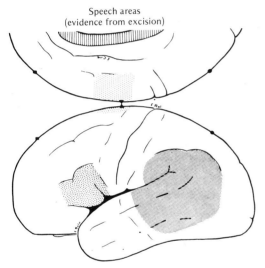

Figure 4-12 The three speech areas, shown in this diagram by Penfield and Roberts, are believed to be of different values. The posterior, or parietotemporal, area is the most important. The anterior, or Broca's, area is the next most important but is dispensable—in some patients at least. The superior, or supplementary motor, area is dispensable but probably is very important after damage to one of the other speech areas. This diagram is based on postoperative study of patients from whom known areas of the cortex had been removed to relieve them of epileptic seizures. Very similar speech areas can be deduced from the interference with speech that has been produced at operation by electrical stimulation of the exposed brain. Note that the speech areas are located only in the hemisphere that is dominant for speech, usually the left. *(From W. Penfield and L. Roberts, Speech and Brain Mechanisms. Princeton, N.J.: Princeton University Press, 1959; London: Oxford University Press; by permission)*

Congenital Aphasia Based on Birth Injury

Some children who do not learn to talk spontaneously resemble in many ways the aphasic adult. Their hearing is good to the extent that their attention can be attracted by sounds, including voice sounds, but the sounds seem to convey little or no meaning. They may imitate speech sounds and intonations, but they do not learn words. With patience, and by reducing speech to its elemental parts and gradually building up a series of associations with sounds and written symbols, they can be taught to understand

and to speak, but an outstanding characteristic is a *difficulty in learning*, particularly in learning language. This condition has been given the name *congenital aphasia* or "childhood aphasia." (Aphasia here does not mean the loss of a function [speech] that was once learned but instead a *failure to develop* speech in the first place.) In addition there are some children who, after learning speech, do become truly aphasic following a severe illness such as encephalitis. This is an *acquired aphasia*. Then there is the final combination in which an injury occurs early in life and apparently prevents the normal learning of speech.

Following the analogy of aphasia in adults, the failure to develop speech has usually been attributed to a congenital defect or birth injury or to a brain injury in early childhood before speech was learned that has affected certain critical areas of the brain. Actually in only one such case, a boy with multiple congenital defects, has a postmortem examination been reported. This brain did indeed show extensive malformation and degeneration in both temporal lobes and in the medial geniculate bodies of the thalamus. In spite of the anatomical absence of the primary auditory projection areas of the cortex, this boy had been taught with fair success at an oral school for deaf children and at the time of his death (at 10 years of age) had a vocabulary of several hundred words. His use of language was best in structured lessons, but spontaneous speech was effective. He comprehended oral language best when it was spoken slowly. He understood only the most familiar expressions when they were spoken at a normal rate. His pure-tone audiogram was within normal limits. This case meets the criteria for congenital aphasia.

It now appears, however, that this type of case, with no significant hearing loss, is rare.

Certainly the organic defect that must be assumed to account for congenital aphasia, namely an extensive injury limited to both cortical auditory areas (like that in the case described above), is very improbable. This improbability has led many to question whether the implicit diagnosis of "brain injury," particularly when it is not supported by other neurological signs or symptoms, is a reasonable explanation for failure to learn speech. At least one alternative explanation is available for many cases.

Congenital Aphasia Based on a Partial Hearing Loss

Careful audiometric study of one group of so-called "aphasic children" showed that nearly all of the children had a very significant loss of hearing for frequencies in the middle range, that is, for the frequencies important for the understanding of speech (Dr. L. L. Elliott at Central Institute for the Deaf). Often, however, they had fairly good hearing for either the very high or the very low frequencies, or both. This pattern of hearing loss is actually rather common among children whose mothers have suffered from rubella early in their pregnancies. It was rather characteristic in the history of these children that the hearing loss was not recognized until the fourth or fifth years. They had often been wrongly diagnosed as mentally retarded, and they frequently had developed serious problems of behavior. This situation and its management will be considered more fully in Chapter 17.

The alternative hypothesis invoked to explain the difficulty in learning is essentially developmental. It is postulated that the auditory system requires sensory input during the early years—particularly during the second year, when the normal infant begins to learn speech—in order to complete its development, and that if this normal organization does not occur, it is more difficult to bring it about later, even though sounds are then made audible by amplification. The failure to recognize the partial hearing loss leads to false expectations and inappropriate management. The child develops what may be called a "habitual disregard" for sound as a means of communication. It makes no difference whether the hearing loss is hereditary, congenital, or acquired, but it is important that the loss is present during the years when children normally learn to talk.

This interpretation is still a hypothesis, but it is supported by experiments on the visual system in kittens that are deprived of eyesight by suturing their eyelids closed for the first weeks or months of life. These kittens develop long-lasting visual defects that persist after their eyes are opened. Anatomical abnormalities of organization and even degenerative changes have been demonstrated by the work of Wiesel and Hubel. It is not appropriate here to describe these experiments in detail, but the analogy is very suggestive. Much more important, however, is the clinical experience that young children in whom the partial hearing loss is detected early and who are given the benefit of early and habitual exposure to loud speech, with a hearing aid as soon as they are old enough, do develop speech and effective use of their residual hearing much better than children with similar audiograms who have not had the advantage of early auditory exposure and training.

The practical implication of this hypothesis is, of course, to recognize early the auditory defect and to initiate the proper management, as described in Chapter 17. In any case the diverse usages of the term "congenital aphasia" and the connotations that have become attached to it have made it very confusing and almost useless. We recommend

that it be used only when the diagnosis is unquestionable. Most of the children in our experience to whom it has been applied are now known to be hypoacusic, many of them quite severely so; but their really important impairment is their failure to have learned speech and a *difficulty in learning* in general. Above all, we as audiologists or speech therapists must not postulate a brain injury without a clear history of trauma or illness or supporting neurological signs or, preferably, both.

Dyslogomathia: A New Term

Dysmathia is a more appropriate term than aphasia. Dysmathia is an old Greek word that means exactly what we want to say, namely, *difficulty or slowness in learning.* If we wish to be more specific and say *difficulty in learning speech and language,* we can form a new word, *dyslogomathia.*[5] The familiar root "logos" carries the connotation of both speech and language.

In summary, true congenital aphasia based on an anatomical defect or birth injury does occur, but it is rare. Dyslogomathia, based on partial sensory deprivation, is a more probable explanation in a majority of the cases in which children show some reactions to fairly loud sounds but do not spontaneously develop speech, and often have great difficulty learning speech later. Further study should clarify the situation and allow us to accept, reject, or modify this working hypothesis.

---

[5] The writer is indebted to Prof. W. M. Sale of the Department of Classics at Washington University for suggestions and advice concerning the new word "dyslogomathia." Plato used *dysmathia* for "difficulty in learning." The root *math* survives in English in *mathematics. Logo-* is a familiar Greek combining form meaning *word, speech* or *discourse,* or *reason.*

Psychogenic Dysacusis versus Feigning (Pseudohypoacusis)

An extreme form of functional or nonorganic dysacusis is so-called *psychogenic dysacusis*. This condition is caused by psychological changes in the personality. By definition there is either partial or total inability to hear, either as an isolated condition or as a psychogenic overlay in addition to an organic dysacusis. Nerve impulses initiated in the ear by sound waves reach the brain, but *they are not consciously heard*.

Psychogenic deafness or a psychogenic overlay merges imperceptibly into *feigning*, or *pseudohypoacusis*. The difference is that the person who feigns *knows* that he can hear, whereas the patient with psychogenic deafness does not know that his peripheral hearing is as good as it actually is. This is a very difficult distinction for the audiologist to make, and as a matter of fact the diagnosis can logically be made with confidence only in retrospect when either the patient has been cured by appropriate psychiatric treatment or has confessed to deliberate deception. As we shall see in Chapter 8, the detection of malingering is easy, with the help of special audiometric tests, but the measurement of actual threshold levels and the proof of motive usually depend on a battle of wits between the audiologist and the subject. The assessment of motivation becomes very important. In general the *diagnosis of psychogenic deafness or overlay is made as a last resort and when it is in keeping with an overall pattern of behavior and medical history* that suggests a particular pattern of *emotional stress and conflict*.

In civilian life in the United States at the present time, psychogenic deafness should be regarded as a rare condition. No case reports have appeared in the literature during the past 25 years. Nevertheless it was apparently fairly common among military personnel in World War II and also in certain other cultures. There are few descriptions of the condition, and for this reason we retain from the first edition of this book the following account, written in 1945.

Laymen in general have been unaware of the existence of psychogenic dysacusis, or functional deafness, and the medical profession has tended to underestimate its importance, in spite of occasional obvious cases of "miraculous" cures at shrines, by faith healers, or for no evident or reasonable cause. The experience of World War II showed, however, that psychological factors may be among the common causes of deafness and hearing loss in military service. Of course, hearing loss is not necessarily *either* organic *or* psychogenic. Very often it is both, in uncertain proportions. The best estimate we can find is based on a careful study of the last 500 cases admitted to the Hoff General Hospital (United States Army) at the end of World War II for auditory rehabilitation. Fifteen percent of these men were found to have indications of a psychogenic factor in their hearing loss. For some of them the history of the hearing loss did not coincide with the usual clinical history or with the results of the otological examination. For others the audiogram varied widely from day to day, or the hearing loss for speech was much more or much less than the audiogram suggested it should be. Perhaps a hearing aid gave no improvement at all or else a startlingly great improvement. These 15 percent, a total of 75 men, were treated by appropriate methods (which we shall not attempt to describe) for psychogenic dysacusis. The accuracy of the original estimate was substantiated by the fact that 60 of the 75, or "12 percent of all patients admitted, had either a complete return of hearing to normal or a substantial improvement" at the time of separation from the Army.

This figure, high enough to make some

otologists incredulous, does not mean that 12 to 15 percent of the cases of hearing loss were *purely* psychogenic, but it does mean that psychological factors accounted for at least a significant part of the hearing loss in approximately one in eight men whose hearing became inadequate in military service. The special stresses of combat service obviously increased the proportion of cases of psychogenic dysacusis. Psychogenic hearing loss was a prominent factor in the army cases studied, and in all probability it is more prevalent and important in civilian life than has previously been suspected, but the importance and prevalence in civilian life of psychogenic deafness, as distinct from a mild psychogenic overlay and from malingering, is still an open question.

Hysterical deafness The most common type of psychogenic deafness is called *hysterical deafness*. In this type, deep emotional conflicts within the personality structure involve the sense of hearing and manifest themselves in a total loss of hearing. Conflicts of which the individual is unconscious, rather than an impairment of the auditory mechanism, are the real cause. The disturbing emotional problem is converted into an impairment of hearing. Such substitution for the emotional problem is called *conversion*, and the resulting deafness is termed a *conversion hysteria*. Hysteria may involve senses other than hearing. A man may suffer from hysterical blindness or from anesthesia or paralysis of any part of the body without any physical impairment of the eye, or nerves, or muscles. But in any case of hysterical loss, the individual is unaware of the conflict that has found a substitute solution, or at least he does not understand its true nature.

It is impossible in this chapter to describe the different types of emotional disturbance that find their solution in hysterical symp-

toms. In every personality there are some emotional conflicts that do not present any problem in the ordinary course of living. In general, however, the more severe the emotional conflict the less able is the individual to withstand strain of any kind. Actually, 38 percent of the cases of "blast deafness" (acoustic trauma) admitted to Hoff General Hospital were diagnosed either as purely psychogenic or else as organic hearing loss with a large functional overlay. For example, a soldier exposed at close range to the burst of a large shell or a land mind escaped with his life, but was temporarily deafened by the noise. Later his ears recovered, but his unconscious emotional forces prevented his regained "hearing" from becoming conscious. What was probably a true physiological deafness at first was continued as a psychogenic dysacusis. Some men who regained most of their hearing spontaneously after a temporary blast deafness have reported that their recovery of hearing was quite sudden, or that for a time their hearing fluctuated with their mood or condition. They heard poorly when tired or nervously tense and better than usual when relaxed by a convivial dose of alcohol. These stories clearly suggest a *temporary psychogenic dysacusis* that passed off without recognition or special treatment.

A particular kind of emotional conflict may be the basis of hysterical deafness in time of war. Since hearing serves to create, through language, a structure for the moral code, and since war liberates the basic aggression in human nature, conflict is inevitable. From childhood on, we have been taught not to kill. War reverses that moral prohibition as well as many others. It is not surprising, therefore, that the conflict present in accepting this reversal should, in some persons, result in the rejection of hearing. To liberate his basic aggression, such a man must say, "I will not hear the voice of conscience." The hearing apparatus through which the moral code was formulated then becomes involved in a basic emotional conflict that is sometimes solved by a complete or partial rejection of the apparatus itself—with consequent deafness. This rejection is, of course, not conscious but takes place at the unconscious level. The soldier is utterly unaware that his deafness is *psychogenic* and was not caused by physical injury to his ears.

When a civilian becomes hysterically deaf (which apparently happens only rarely), we can infer that his inner conflict is correspondingly more severe, since the loss of hearing is precipitated by a milder stress. We must also infer that hearing has an unusual importance for such a person. There are, of course, great individual differences in the relative importance of the sense of hearing. In most of us one type of imagery plays a stronger part than do the others; vision, hearing, or the sense of motion may predominate in our relation to the world. When asked to recall the melody of a song, one person may *picture* the printed score, another may *hear* the melody, while a third may *feel the finger positions* required to play it.

In addition to these individual differences, however, auditory images generally affect most of us powerfully in the emotional field. This is particularly true in emotionalized memory. In terrifying situations, it is often the sounds involved in the experience, rather the sight of it, that convey the horror. If one has witnessed an accident in which a man was hurt, his cries may persist in memory long after the visual image of the experience has faded.

This tendency of auditory imagery to persist in memory is strengthened in the man whose perceptive interests and imaginative capacities are integrated around hearing. If the experience which he is trying to forget is charged with emotional material, as it always is in war, it is possible for repression to blot out hearing and to make him deaf.

As for the civilian who becomes hysterically deaf, previous experience must contain incidents or situations that threaten him as deeply as combat does the soldier. An understanding of these incidents or situations can be gathered only through a careful case study of his development.

Therapy of psychogenic dysacusis The prevention and the therapy for all other forms of dysacusis, deafness, and hearing loss will be found in the next chapter. It is appropriate, however, to consider the therapy of psychogenic dysacusis here because it illustrates very vividly the nature of the disorder. In fact, the diagnosis of psychogenic dysacusis usually rests almost entirely on the success, at least temporary, of some attempt at therapy.

The most effective treatment of hysterical deafness is based on the *positive suggestion* that the hearing loss is only temporary. To make the patient accept positive suggestion is difficult because in many of the hysterically deaf we see what Charcot, the great French psychiatrist, has called *la belle indifférence* to their conversion symptoms. Since they have achieved even a false resolution of their emotional conflict, they appear placid and quite undisturbed by the fact that they have given up their hearing. When they describe their deafness, they rarely emphasize their own feelings about the loss, but instead point out the objective or practical inconvenience of not being able to hear a car start, for example, or to hear directions. Even these practical difficulties are usually brushed aside by such a remark as "But that is not important."

It is better to teach the patient how to *listen* than to teach him speechreading, for speechreading may only help to confirm the symptom of deafness and make it less accessible to treatment. By suggestive therapeutic methods the hysterically deaf may be encouraged to regain their hearing. But unless some relief from the basic emotional conflict is achieved by the therapeutic process, the cause for the conflict remains, and the conversion symptom may merely shift over into another sensory field or take the form of a partial paralysis. A "cure" of psychogenic dysacusis may be only temporary, but this at least demonstrates that part or all of the deafness or hearing loss is functional. It does not mean that the cure is necessarily permanent or that the fundamental problem may not again appear in some other incapacitating symptom. If the hearing losses of the soldiers at Hoff General Hospital were purely the result of combat pressure, release from army service might have been sufficient to make their cure permanent. It is probable that a civilian who becomes functionally deaf from the pressures of living cannot be cured without psychiatric therapy deep enough to change the patient's personal concept of himself and his relationships with others.

Depression Deafness

Hysterical deafness does not include all the cases of deafness or dysacusis that should be classified as psychogenic. Dr. D. A. Ramsdell (see Chapter 19) has differentiated a type, which he terms "depression deafness," in a schizophrenic personality structure. Personality tests, case histories, and the presence of recognized schizophrenic symptoms indicate that this type of dysacusis is not due to conversion, as had been previously supposed. (Schizophrenia is a type of mental disorder characterized by a progressive isolation of the individual from reality. Feeling unable to meet the practical demands of his environment, the patient escapes into an unreal world of fantasy.)

An intensive study of depression dysacusis reveals that there is a particular pattern in the case histories of such patients. The patients emphasize the subjective effects of their hearing loss and show definite hypochondriacal symptoms. They speak not of the objective inconvenience of their impairment, as does the hysteric, but of the change in their own feeling state. They are perplexed and frightened, and find the world about them incomprehensible and overwhelming. Failure of the sense of hearing to operate normally in such a patient is not due to conversion as a means of solving a basic conflict. The simulation of hearing loss or deafness acts as a protective defense against the precipitation of a schizophrenic episode. Hearing, more frequently than any of the other senses, becomes involved in the schizophrenic's escape from reality.

It is a well-known fact that hearing may be accentuated in early schizophrenia to the point where the patient hears imaginary voices or has "auditory hallucinations." The reverse may also be true, and the patient may become deaf as part of the schizophrenic process. Such a patient is basically suicidal, but since he stops short of an actual biological death, the case may more properly be described as one of partial suicide. By giving up hearing, the patient succeeds in arriving at the state that one individual has described as "being buried alive." The patient restricts himself to a world that lacks the movement and flow so characteristic of the complete world of reality. He severs the auditory coupling, which is the chief link in maintaining an experience of aliveness and of identification with a moving world. In schizophrenic depression, the reward for the deafness, which corresponds to *la belle indifférence* in the hysteric, is the maintenance of only a visual orientation to the world around him.

In any case of psychogenic deafness or hearing loss, careful diagnosis should always be made before therapy is undertaken. Superficially the two types of psychogenic dysacusis appear much alike, but the treatment appropriate for depression deafness is quite different from that indicated in hysteria. For cases of depression deafness, therapy should be as painstaking and as careful as if one were dealing with threatened suicide because the wrong type of therapy may precipitate a psychotic episode.

It would be unwise to attempt here a detailed explanation of the therapy for either type of psychogenic dysacusis. If medical examination and tests of hearing indicate that the hearing loss is not due to impairment of the hearing apparatus, professional psychiatric aid should be obtained.

The variety of types of central dysacusis is illustrated by the experience of one particular clinic. Here 8 percent of the children referred for communication disorders were eventually diagnosed by psychiatrists as having autism or infantile schizophrenia, another 7 percent had severe emotional disturbances, 14 percent were mentally retarded, 15 percent had auditory agnosia or verbal dysacusis, and 19 percent had one or another type of central dysacusis as well as deafness or a hearing loss.

SUGGESTED READINGS AND REFERENCES

Nearly all of the readings cited below are primary publications in the scientific literature that give evidence on which statements in the text are based. The titles are good guides to their subject matter.

Altmann, F., A. Glasgold, and J. P. MacDuff. "The Incidence of Otosclerosis as Related to Race and Sex," *Ann. Otol.*, 76:377–392 (1967).
This supersedes the 1944 study by S. R. Guild.
Bordley, J. E., P. E. Brookhouse, J. Hardy, and W. G. Hardy. "Prenatal Rubella," *Acta Otolaryng. (Stockholm)*, 66:1–9 (1968).
Chung, C. S., and K. S. Brown. "Family Studies of Early Childhood Deafness Ascertained through the Clarke School for the Deaf." *Amer. J. Hum. Genet.*, 22:630–644 (1970).
Special consideration is given to penetrance of dominant genes, the number of recessive genes involved, and genetic risks.
Clarke, C. A. "The Prevention of 'Rhesus' Babies," *Sci. Amer.*, 219:46–52 (1968).
Committee on Hearing and Equilibrium: Otologic Homograft Transplantation Program. *Trans. Amer. Acad. Ophthal. Otolaryng.*, 80:ORL30–ORL72 (1975).
A series of papers on various aspects of homografts.
Davis, H., "A Functional Classification of Auditory Defects," *Ann. Otol.*, 71:693–704 (1962).
———, C. T. Morgan, J. E. Hawkins, Jr., R. Galambos, and F. W. Smith. "Temporary Deafness Following Exposure to Loud Tones and Noise," *Acta Otolaryng. (Stockholm)*, Supplement 88 (1950).
An experimental study of temporary threshold shift and peripheral dysacusis in man, carried out in 1941–1942.
Elliott, L. L. "Descriptive Analysis of Audiometric and Psychometric Scores of Students at a School for the Deaf," *J. Speech Hearing Res.*, 10:21–40 (1967).

————, and V. Armbruster. "Some Possible Effects of the Delay of Early Treatment of Deafness," *J. Speech Hearing Res.*, 10:209–224 (1967).

Fraser, G. *The Causes of Profound Deafness in Childhood.* Baltimore: Johns Hopkins University Press, 1976.

> *This volume on hereditary deafness presents detailed findings from three surveys conducted by the author of more than 3500 deaf individuals. The subjects are classified by recognizable hereditary deafness syndromes or indirectly through analysis of pedigree data.*

Gallaudet College Public Service Programs. *What Every Person Should Know About Heredity and Deafness.* Washington, D.C.: Gallaudet College, 1975.

> *This is the second booklet in a series developed by Public Service Programs for deaf high school students and deaf adults.*

Glorig, A., and H. Davis. "Age, Noise and Hearing Loss," *Ann. Otol.*, 70:556 (1961).

————, and K. S. Gerwin (eds.). *Otitis Media.* Springfield, Ill.: Charles C Thomas, 1972.

Huizing, E. H., A. H. Van Bolhuis, and D. W. Odenthal. "Studies on Progressive Hereditary Perceptive Deafness in a Family of 335 Members, I. Genetical and General Audiological Results. II. Characteristic Pattern of Hearing Deterioration," *Acta Otolaryng. (Stockholm)*, 61:35–41; 161–167 (1966).

Knapp, P. H. "Emotional Aspects of Hearing Loss," *Psychosom. Med.*, 10:203–222 (1948).

> *A good discussion of psychogenic overlay.*

Konigsmark, B. W., and R. J. Gorlin. *Genetic and Metabolic Deafness.* Philadelphia: W. B. Saunders, 1976.

> *A scholarly comprehensive compilation. Includes genetic hearing loss as it occurs with no associated abnormalities, and with other abnormalities such as of the external ear and diseases of the eye, and of the musculoskeletal, integumentary, renal, and nervous systems.*

Landau, W. M., R. Goldstein, and F. R. Kleffner. "Congenital Aphasia," *Neurology*, 10:915–921 (1960).

> *A case of true "congenital aphasia" with autopsy report.*

Lindenov, H. *The Etiology of Deaf-Mutism with Special Reference to Heredity.* Copenhagen: Einar Munksgaard, 1945. (Translated from the Danish by A. Anderson.)

> *A fine historical summary and a source book of results. Interpretation is in Mendelian terms without the concept of penetrance.*

Martin, N. A. "Psychogenic Deafness," *Ann. Otol.*, 55:81–89 (1946).

> *One of the rare clinical papers on this topic.*

Paparella, M. M., and D. A. Shumrick. *Otolaryngology.* Philadelphia: W. B. Saunders, 1973.

> *In Basic Sciences and Related Disciplines (Volume 1) the health sciences as they relate to otolaryngology are outlined in traditional manner, obviating the need, in most instances, for the reader to search for additional information in a basic science textbook. Following this, fundamental principles of surgery and of medicine are discussed. Ear (Volume 2) is concerned with*

the medical and surgical aspects of otology.

Penfield, W., and T. Rasmussen. *The Cerebral Cortex of Man.* New York: The Macmillan Company, 1950.

Based on studies of conscious patients during brain surgery.

————, and L. Roberts. Speech and Brain-Mechanisms. Princeton, N.J.: Princeton University Press, 1959.

An important book for speech pathologists.

Schmidt, P. H. "Presbycusis: The Present Status," *Int. Audiol.,* Supplement 1 (1967).

In our opinion this is the best summary of presbycusis to date.

Ventry, I. M., and J. B. Chaiklin (eds.). "Multidiscipline Study of Functional Hearing Loss," *J. Aud. Res.,* 5:179–262 (1965).

Extensive studies carried out under the auspices of the Veterans Administration.

Whetnall, E., and D. B. Fry. *The Deaf Child.* London: William Heinemann Ltd., 1964.

This monograph contains some excellent descriptions of various syndromes of congenital deafness, and much more concerning assessment and management of deaf children.

Wiesel, T. N., and D. H. Hubel. "Extent of Recovery from the Effects of Visual Deprivation in Kittens," *J. Neurophysiol.,* 28:1060–1072 (1965).

A very important animal experiment.

Williams, H. L. *Ménière's Disease.* Springfield, Ill: Charles C Thomas, 1952.

An authoritative monograph by an eminent otologist.

Hallowell Davis, M.D.

5

Conservation of Hearing or Prevention of Hearing Loss

The term *conservation of hearing* was introduced about 1920 when a group of local organizations for the hard-of-hearing united to form what later became the American Hearing Society. Its program included the phrase "to stimulate scientific efforts in the prevention of deafness and the conservation of hearing." Its first meeting, in Boston in 1921, was held in conjunction with a meeting of the Otological Section of the American Medical Association. About 1924 its first Committee on Hard-of-Hearing Children appealed to the Bell Telephone Laboratories for an instrument that could test the hearing of large numbers of children. The response to this appeal was the Western Electric 4C audiometer, which is described in Chapter 7.

A few years later the Committee on Conservation of Hearing of the American Academy of Ophthalmology and Otolaryngology was established, and with the American Hearing Society it successfully promoted the widespread establishment of screening audiometry in many school systems throughout the country.

For a long time the conservation of hearing movement was directed chiefly toward the medical and surgical treatment of otitis media. Gradually, with the development of vaccines and of chemotherapy and antibiotic drugs, the scope of prevention has broadened greatly, and it has finally come to include adults as well as children and environmental threats to hearing as well as disease. The great environmental hazard is excessive noise. Here the most serious and obvious risks are in heavy industry and in military activities, but the noises of jet aircraft, trucks, subways, farm tractors, and "rock" music now constitute significant noise exposures of a large fraction of the population. In this chapter we shall consider briefly the prevalence and the seriousness of the various threats to hearing and the form and the effectiveness of various preventive measures. We shall follow roughly the sequence of age, beginning with possible prevention of deafness in infants by prenatal measures, then the problem of otitis media, which is predominantly a disease of childhood, and then the hazards of noise, particularly in the industrial context. Details of aural hygiene and the remedial measures of medicine and surgery will follow in the next chapter.

PREVENTION OR CURE OF DISEASE

The ideal form of prevention to eliminate a disease entirely has now been very nearly accomplished for smallpox. Another form is to protect individuals, as by immunization, illustrated by poliomyelitis. Another is effective treatment of diseases that cannot be prevented, as with otitis media. Still another is the control at the source of environmental hazards such as noise. And finally there is the detection and protection of individuals who begin to suffer impairment.

Many forms of prevention of hearing loss require systematic and accurate measurements of hearing of many individuals. This is a task for audiology, as in screening tests of hearing of schoolchildren and monitoring audiometry in heavy industry.

Much conservation of hearing has been achieved indirectly by public health measures that have limited the infectious diseases of childhood that were formerly common causes of acquired deafness. Widespread immunization has greatly reduced

the incidence of diphtheria, scarlet fever, measles, mumps, and to a lesser degree influenza, and has reduced their severity for those who may still contract them. One form of meningitis (meningococcal) is now relatively rare, and effective treatment for another form (Hemophilus influenzae) is advancing rapidly.

Two viral diseases that are prenatal threats to hearing have become targets for immunization largely because they are rather specific threats to hearing. One of them is *cytomegaly virus* disease. This one is not very common, but it has recently been recognized as a disease entity and a threat, and protection by immunization should become available in due time. The other, very well known and far more prevalent, is *rubella*. Here also the particular danger is to the developing fetus if a pregnant woman contracts the disease, particularly in the first trimester of pregnancy. The virus may enter the fetus and cause very serious damage, not only to the developing ear but to eyes, heart, or central nervous system or any combination of them, as described in Chapter 4. From time to time a particularly virulent strain of rubella has spread as an epidemic in various parts of the world. Australia in 1942 and the United States and other countries in 1963–1965 suffered severely, and in every case there was a dramatic increase in the number of congenitally deaf infants. Efforts to develop an immune serum were undertaken promptly and were successful. The serum was licensed for general distribution in the United States in 1969 and has been more and more widely used, particularly to immunize adolescent girls. There is mute testimony to the effectiveness of the protection. Another U.S. epidemic of rubella had been predicted to occur about 1972. Actually there was no increase in the incidence of the disease, and epidemiologists give the credit to the immunization program. Sporadic cases of rubella deafness continue to appear, but epidemics can now be prevented.

In short, for childhood deafness caused by viral or bacterial disease, protection is possible in principle and this protection is continually being spread more widely in practice.

Hereditary Conditions

A preventable form of congenital deafness is caused by the development of *neonatal kernicterus* or jaundice of the newborn. The pigments, especially bilirubin, that cause the injury to the ear and particularly to parts of the midbrain are formed by destruction of blood cells in the newborn infant. This is part of a complicated sequence of immune reactions that originate in an incompatibility between certain blood proteins of the mother and the father, as explained in Chapter 4. The so-called "Rh factor" is the best known, but there are others. What is important for conservation of hearing is that the mechanism is quite well understood, that the incompatibility can be detected in advance, and that effective treatment is possible, either by means of immune globulin or by massive blood transfusion of the infant during the first days of life. A mild "bilirubinemia" of 20 mg per ml of blood in the infant is an accepted indication that its hearing is "at risk," and that treatment should be initiated.

A quite different variety of congenital deafness is strictly *hereditary*. Hereditary deafness is now well understood as a genetic problem, but *in a practical sense the prevention of hereditary deafness is not possible. This is true both for sensorineural defects and for otosclerosis.* The only available tool is genetic counseling, and unless the defect is clearly present in both families, any general advice such as to avoid consanguinous marriage is rarely, if ever, effective. The basic difficulty in regard to hereditary deafness (other than otosclerosis) is that there are many different genes that may cause such a defect if the child receives the same abnormal gene from both parents. As explained at some length in Chapter 4, these genes are almost always recessive, they are relatively rare, and they are rather widespread in the general population, particularly in a mobile population such as that of the United States. The net result is that the defect appears as "sporadic deafness," unpredictably here and there. These cases are usually listed as "cause unknown," but probably most of them are actually hereditary deafness, even though they may not conform to the better known patterns such as the Waardenburg, the Treacher-Collins, or the Klippel-Feil syndromes.

Otitis Media and Screening Audiometry

The major original target for prevention of hearing loss was otitis media. The various forms of the disease are described in some detail in Chapters 4 and 6.

It is often difficult to identify an ear with chronic otitis media unless the ear is actually discharging pus. A fully trained otologist may not always be available to look at the eardrum membrane with his otoscope. Another method for picking out children who may need attention is to test their hearing. Tests of hearing, including pure-tone audiometry, are described in Chapter 7, but it is obvious immediately that it would be both time-consuming and wasteful to test every ear at all frequencies when most ears are perfectly normal. The answer has been "screening audiometry." All of the children in a school are tested briefly and quickly to identify or screen out, as by a sieve, those whose sensitivity of hearing is below some arbitrary hearing level. Those who are thus screened out are then given a full, careful, audiometric test and otologic examination. Of course, a good many of them turn out on the full test to be normal or very nearly so. The screening test is planned to screen out the borderline cases so as not to let any really abnormal cases go undetected.

It must not be assumed that screening audiometry in schools will detect every child who has a mild or incipient otitis media or enlarged adenoids or even frank cholesteatoma. Children have such sensitive hearing that audiometers with extended dynamic range and correspondingly good quiet audiometric booths are required to determine their hearing thresholds. It is often difficult to provide quiet enough locations to carry out the screening test at a level low enough to detect all of those who should be screened out for further study.

Actually, a recent survey of the hearing of children in certain selected schools in Pittsburgh, continued over several years, showed a very disappointing correlation between the results of the hearing tests and direct otological examination of the ears of all of these same children. The tests were actual determinations of the hearing threshold levels, not merely screening tests. The children whose ears were judged abnormal otoscopically in one way or another did indeed average some 10 dB less sensitive by audiometry, but there was a large overlap between the groups. In the conclusions of the survey, published in 1963, we read the following:

It has been assumed in the past that conventional audiometric screening will reveal not only those children with "hearing loss," but also those with ear conditions needing medical care. The Pittsburgh data indicate that audiometric testing, however complete it may be, cannot identify all children with physical abnormalities which may have predictive value, or who may need medical treatment. In addition to failing an audiometric screening procedure, some other means is needed to identify children needing special otological and audiological attention. A history of earaches and ear discharge, especially when accompanied by otoscopic evidence of past or present infection, indicates a child who needs special otological and audiological services. The frequency of occurrence of these conditions appears to be a measure of the urgency of this need.

The inadequacy of screening audiometry as a sole method of identification of otitis media was noted also at the National Conference on Otitis Media in 1970. We quote from the summary chapter on prevention:

The prevention of otitis media and associated hearing, language, and speech impairments must begin well before the age that routine public or preschool audiometry might indicate that such problems exist. The screening of infants and very young children for otitis media must, therefore, be carried out by medical doctors or paramedical individuals especially trained in the detection of middle ear disease. Should such disease be detected, appropriate referrals will be made to those individuals qualified to provide definitive diagnosis, treatment, and follow-up care, including audiologists and speech pathologists.

The summary chapter on diagnosis contains the two following paragraphs:

The diagnosis of otitis media depends on visual inspection of the ear drum through a clean ear canal, preferably with magnification and a pneumatic otoscope.[1] A good history, examination of the nose and throat, and a test of hearing are required to evaluate the individual case. A radiological examination and other laboratory tests may also be necessary.

We strongly recommend that medical students, interns, and paramedical personnel receive more training in the proper examination of the ear.

In spite of all, however, screening audiometry does detect the children with moderate or severe impairment of hearing

---

[1] The pneumatic otoscope is described in Chapter 9 in connection with diagnostic audiologic tests.

even if it will not detect those with mild impairments who nevertheless suffer from otitis media. It remains a primary method for the conservation of hearing in children. Tympanometry (impedance measurements), described in Chapter 9, has now been simplified enough to make it a practical addition to or substitute for screening audiometry. In principle, it should assist materially in detecting mild otitis media.

Otitis Media and Socioeconomic Factors

In the *Proceedings of the National Conference on Otitis Media* (1970) is an excellent review of the literature on the epidemiology of otitis media by D. McEldowney and D. M. Kessner, as well as a full discussion of its etiology, pathology, prevention, diagnosis, treatment and rehabilitation. The epidemiology shows a higher incidence in children than in adults, and particularly high rates among Alaskan Eskimos and North American Indians. Some special racial susceptibility, based perhaps on anatomical differences, had been suspected, but a much more definite correlation with poor socioeconomic conditions, notably crowded housing and limited health services, is now revealed.

In the aforementioned review of the literature we read why otitis media was selected as a "tracer" or "indicator" for a study of contrasts in health status.

In response to the current national concern for the development of effective, efficient and equitable health services, the Board on Medicine of the National Academy of Sciences has recently initiated a program entitled, "Contrasts in Health Status: A Comparative Inquiry into the Health Needs, Barriers, and Resources of Selected Population Groups." A major part of this program involves a searching examination of the organization, delivery, and financing of ambulatory health care. Its design centers about the use of *tracer* morbidity conditions as indicators of broad health system functions. In addition to the collection of social, economic and medical care utilization information, a clinical-epidemiologic study of the tracer disease and a survey of medical providers who deliver care to the populations at risk will be undertaken. We have selected middle ear disease and associated hearing loss in a pediatric population as the first tracer condition for this study of contrasting forms of health care delivery.

The strengths of middle ear disease and associated hearing loss an an *indicator* of broad health system functions can be summarized as follows: the etiology of the condition appears to be related to social factors; the disease has a high prevalence rate and can be diagnosed with relative ease; the major medical complication, hearing loss, can be measured with a high degree of accuracy; primary ambulatory medical care and sophisticated restorative surgery can effectively alter the course of this condition; and the social services system can play a major role in rehabilitation both at the biologic level (hearing aids) and at the social level (job placement).

This succinct summary tells why otitis media should remain as a major target in our efforts to prevent hearing loss.

Ototoxic Drugs

It is clear from the foregoing discussion of otitis media that it is not always easy to separate the hazards to hearing into disease versus environmental. The same may be said for ototoxic drugs, which are a significant cause of deafness. Ototoxic drugs are a threat to hearing when they must be employed as life-saving measures. In a sense it is a probem of preventive medicine to identify such drugs and alert physcians to their danger. In Chapter 4 we have noted *dihydrostreptomycin*, *kanamycin*, and *gentamicin* as such ototoxic drugs. Sometimes they must be used, as a calculated risk. It is not feasible to control the dosage by monitoring the patient's hearing; first, because the patients are usually too ill for accurate audiometry, and second, because the loss of hearing may be delayed for days or even a month after the course of treatment. The chief safeguards for prevention are an alert medical profession and avoidance of these particular antibiotic drugs in any routine or prophylactic medication.

A list of other drugs and poisons that have been suspected of ototoxic action is given in Chapter 4 and need not be repeated here, except to mention two diuretics, *ethacrynic acid* and *furosemide,* whose ototoxic properties are quite well documented.

One helpful note is that tinnitus generally occurs in association with developing deafness and usually precedes it. It may be a helpful warning sign.

NOISE

Noise is the major environmental threat to hearing, and major efforts have and are being directed to the control of noise at the source, to protecting people from excessive noise exposure in industrial and military situations, to assessing the exact degree of risk from particular noise exposures, and to identifying and protecting individuals who begin to suffer from noise-induced hearing loss.

Possible General Effects of Noise

We need not fear any mysterious general effects, such as fatigue, headache, neurosis, or sudden death, from any special sounds or combination of sounds. On careful investigation the persistent rumors about such effects have proved to be unfounded. The ears are much more sensitive to noise than is any other part of the body, and they are always injured first. To be injurious, sounds must be powerful, and usually long-lasting or repeated as well. *There is no magic in any strange disharmony or in any high-frequency "ultrasonic death ray" at any practical intensity.* Noise is unpleasant, but in a wartime experiment designed to imitate piloting an airplane a steady loud noise did not measurably impair the performance of men in any of a large variety of tests of coordination, steadiness, memory, puzzle solving, and the like. Those who *must* work in noise soon learn to disregard it. We may guess that those who dislike their work and are irritable tend to blame noise for their ills more than it really deserves.

With the increase in the noise from traffic and from airplanes there has been increased popular protest against the noise, and concern is frequently expressed that the "nervous strain" of the noise of our industrial civilization may impair mental health. This problem goes beyond the limits set for this book. The literature on the subject is very extensive. Several summaries of the effects of noise on people have been prepared for the Environmental Protection Agency and other governmental agencies and are listed at the end of this chapter.

A more limited concern, however, is the proposition that the habitual noise exposure of Western civilization causes a significant impairment of hearing, not only in industrial workers but in all urban dwellers. The poorer hearing of high frequencies in men as compared with women, mentioned in Chapter 4, is interpreted by many as due to more frequent, more prolonged, and more severe noise exposure of men. Actually the noise exposure of the average U. S. male is well below accepted industrial warning levels, particularly if he is an office worker. Some, however, have had dangerous temporary exposures in military training, in driving a tractor, in skeet shooting, and so on. It is possible, however, that lesser but more habitual exposures in subways, dance halls, airports, and so on may have a similar effect on men and women alike. In this connection the case of the Mabaans, studied by Dr. Samuel Rosen and his associates, is often cited.

The Mabaans are a primitive African tribe who live in a remote area near the border between Sudan and Ethiopia. Their agrarian culture is that of the Stone Age, and they live particularly quiet, peaceful, well-ordered lives, go nearly naked, and eat a simple vegetarian diet. They do not engage in warfare, beat drums, or even sing loudly. They apparently live to a considerable age, although they keep no records of births or deaths. It was actually much easier for Dr. Rosen to measure their hearing than to determine exact ages, but they do not seem to suffer from presbycusis. The point is that the hearing of these primitive people, who live their entire lives in these quiet surroundings, is very sensitive, *even in old age and for high frequencies.*

Does this mean that *our* presbycusis is due to noise? Not necessarily. The Mabaans differ from us in more ways than one. They are notably free not only of social stress and turmoil but also of arteriosclerosis and cardiac disease. On the other hand, if a Mabaan moves to an Egyptian city such as Cairo and joins our world and eats our food, he does develop some presbycusis, and he becomes liable to cardiac and circulatory troubles, peptic ulcers, and so on. His life is no longer serene. It is troubled and it is noisy—and the Mabaan does not hear so well.

Other studies of other well-defined groups in different climates with different dietary habits and cultures—for example, in Finland, Yugoslavia, and Germany—have confirmed the association of the retention of good high-frequency hearing with freedom from arteriosclerosis and coronary disease.

Such studies should throw more light on the causal relations here and help us to evaluate the relative contributions of heredity, way of life, diet, and noise.

Hazardous Noise Exposure in Industry

In Chapter 4 we described the effects on hearing, both temporary and permanent, of exposure to loud noise. Noise hazards for hearing have for many years been associated with certain industries, notably boilermaking, drop forging, and weaving. The growth of heavy industry has increased the noise levels and also the number of workers exposed to them. The aircraft industry, particularly since the development of jet engines, has added new problems. Moreover, quite recently it has become clear that gunfire, including skeet shooting as well as artillery, machine guns, and small arms, and even the tractor on the farm are significant hazards to hearing. But noise-induced hearing loss develops slowly. Noises that are not painful or even really uncomfortable after the first week or two may gradually impair hearing if exposure to them is habitual.

For many years a sort of tacit conspiracy of silence kept the problem of noise-induced hearing loss from public view. Workers in very noisy places were pleased with their relatively high wages, and industry feared litigation, insurance problems, and compensation payments. (The problem of handicap and compensation is discussed in Chapter 9.) Now, however, "noise control" has become practical and popular, thanks to technical advances in acoustical engineering, to community concern about aircraft noise, and to a variety of military problems, including communication in noise. Court decisions in New York and Wisconsin first recognized noise-induced hearing loss as compensable under workmen's compensation laws, and similar recognition is being given in a rapidly increasing number of other states. It is now possible to state with considerable confidence just what is a hazardous noise exposure to some, but not all, industrial noises, as we shall see in a later section.

Now that it is common knowledge that hazardous noise exposures actually do exist, a major objective in the conservation of hearing of adults is to do something about the hazard. There are several approaches to the problem: to reduce the noise, either at the source or in transmission; to remove all personnel from noise areas; to use protective devices such as earplugs or earmuffs; to identify noise-susceptible persons and remove them from noisy situations; and to institute "monitoring audiometry" to identify the persons who are actually beginning to develop a noise-induced hearing loss before they develop enough permanent threshold shift to constitute any practical handicap.

Monitoring audiometry was first formally defined and named in a symposium on "Problems in Military Audiometry," sponsored by what was then the Armed Forces–National Research Council Committee on Hearing and Bio-Acoustics. The concept is very much the same as that of screening audiometry for children. We watch or "monitor" the hearing of all those who have a hazard of noise exposure and find which ones require special attention. That attention may involve the use of earmuffs, or it may involve removal from the noise. Monitoring audiometry is regarded as part of a routine periodic health examination or physical checkup. The audiometry required is more elaborate than for screening schoolchildren, less elaborate than for diagnostic purposes.

Conservation of Hearing in Noise

The literature on the effects of noise on hearing is voluminous. Several summaries are listed at the end of this chapter. One such statement concerning hazardous exposure to noise and the application of a "damage-risk criterion" is a report prepared in 1968 by a working group of the National Academy of Sciences–National Research Council Committee on Hearing, Bioacoustics and Biomechanics ("CHABA") at the request of the U. S. Army.

The simpler but very useful "Guide for Conservation of Hearing in Noise," prepared for the benefit of industry, was issued in a revised edition in 1973 by The Committee on Hearing and Equilibrium of the American Academy of Ophthalmology and Otolaryngology, and is available on request. It is oriented to the criteria for industrial noise set by the Occupational Safety and Health Act (OSHA) of 1970. This act, which is considered further in Chapter 16, makes a hearing conservation program *mandatory* whenever there is habitual exposure to steady noise levels above 90 dBA. The guide gives appropriate criteria and methods of measurement and assessment of noise exposure in detail and also contains a very helpful section on practical aspects of industrial audiometry.

A report compiled by J. C. Guignard at the Aerospace Medical Research Laboratory for the Environmental Protection Agency (EPA) was cleared for open publication in 1973. It is entitled "A Basis for Limiting Noise Exposure for Hearing Conservation." The approach of the EPA is quite different from that of OSHA. Its congressional mandate, under the Noise Control Act of 1972, requires a statement of "recommended levels of environmental noise requisite to protect the public health and welfare with an adequate margin of safety." This major document does not take economics and technology into account. The following is either quoted or paraphrased from some of the conclusions of the AMRL document prepared for the ERA:

Sufficient basic data now exist to enable the

risk to hearing from specified noise exposures to be predicted on a statistical basis. There is however a need to reevaluate the question of what constitutes a real or "significant" noise-induced hearing loss. Hitherto, in the case of continuous, spectrally distributed noise (the commonest variety in urban and industrial settings), this question has been considered only in the context of occupationally related hearing loss. Now it has to be considered in the wider social context of possible damage to the hearing from environmental noise to which the general population may be exposed, either voluntarily or unwittingly, in the course of day-to-day living.

Such an extension of the preventive concepts worked out over many years of industrial hearing conservation raises new administrative questions concerning the social and ethical criteria by which hearing conservation standards should be set. These standards recommend noise-exposure limits in various living and working contexts in order to protect certain portions of the population against a specified amount of Noise-Induced Permanent Threshold Shift (NIPTS). It must be recognized that decisions of this kind necessarily become even more arbitrary than they have been hitherto in the area of hearing conservation at the "speech frequencies" when the hearing is threatened daily by regular occupational exposure to noise. It is, for instance, inherently more difficult to define acceptable margins of safety governing the selection of exposure limits to protect general populations against nonoccupational exposure; for such populations differ much more widely than, say, a relatively homogeneous group of industrial workers (presumed all to be adults below the age of retirement) in regard to their health, range of susceptibility to noise-induced permanent threshold shift, life-style (determining circumstances of noise exposure) and the personal and social significance of any hearing loss that may be sustained.

Such difficulties notwithstanding, however, the present report provides basic information from which predictions of hazard to the hearing from a variety of noise (both occupational and nonoccupational) can be made.

Continuous noise exposure. The present consensus is that, in the case of daily exposure to a continuous noise without strong tonal components, a level of 75 dBA sustained for 8 hours (or 70 dBA for 24 hours) per day is the threshold for detectable noise-induced permanent threshold shift; exceeding that threshold may cause a shift exceeding 5 dB in up to 10 percent of the people after a cumulative noise exposure of 10 years. This hearing change is predicted for the most sensitive audiometric frequency, namely 4000 Hz. For the conventional speech frequencies (0.5, 1, and 2 kHz), the threshold may be 10 dB higher, that is, 85 dBA for a daily exposure of 8 hours.

Intermittent noise exposure. In the case of daily exposure for cumulative durations other than 8 or 24 hours, an equivalent continuous sound level (that is, an effective level normalized to an 8-hour exposure) may be calculated in order to evaluate the risk.

Impulsive noise. Detectable injurious effects on hearing may occur in some people (< 10 percent) who are exposed to impulses exceeding a peak sound-pressure level as low as 125 dB (grazing incidence at the ear) for more than 3 milliseconds; and a level of 150 dB SPL exceeded for more than 3 milliseconds may be taken to be the threshold of hazard for many purposes, depending on the duration, number, rate and pattern of repetition, character, and spectrum of the impulses. With certain provisos, isolated exposures up to 165 dB peak SPL may be permissible in some circumstances when the impulse duration is very brief (less than 1 millisecond). *Note:* Impulsive noises must be identified and measured using an oscillographic analytical technique in order to evaluate the hazard properly; an ordinary sound-level meter is not suitable to the purpose.

Education and protection of the public. There is a real need to raise public awareness (and indeed that of many physicians, engineers, and administrators) regarding the hazard of environmental noise to the hearing mechanism. Programs designed to educate the public about noise hazards can be envisaged. There is much to be said for encouraging the public to regard a periodic hearing test as a desirable and routine part of health care throughout life. Graphic posters and warning notices can be used to reinforce public awareness in specific situations (for example, at work or in certain recreational settings such as shooting ranges) where the noise is hazardous to the hearing.

Uncertainties and Differences of Opinion about Noise

At this writing (1977) there are still many simplifications and arbitrary decisions involved in setting criteria for hazardous noise exposures. Fortunately, there has been a convergence of opinion on one point: the use of dBA as a single number for the intensity of the noise in question. We quote from the AAOO Guide mentioned in the previous section:

The sound level meter A-filter network and scale were devised originally to assist in predicting the overall loudness of relatively faint noises. The filter attenuates or excludes both high and low frequencies which may be physically present but to which the ear is relatively or completely insensitive. By coincidence, the "weighting" it gives to the different parts of the spectrum corresponds closely to the tendency of each part to produce a significant impairment of hearing. (By "significant" we mean an impairment of hearing in the range of frequencies important for the understanding of speech.) This correspondence is now widely recognized. The A scale has been incorporated in the method of assessing noise-exposure.

Concerning intermittent noise there is strong difference of opinion between supporters of the "5-dB rule" and of the "3-dB rule." Again we quote from the Guide:

The Department of Labor Occupational Noise Standards now applicable to practically all industries in the United States stipulate that "90 dBA is the limit for eight hours per day habitual noise-exposure and a permissible increase of 5 dB in intensity for each halving of exposure time up to a maximum of 115 dBA."

The next simplification relates to changes of the intensity of the noise during a typical workday. If a steady noise is continuous at a given intensity over the entire workday, we can predict with considerable confidence what the workers' average hearing levels will be after a given number of years of such noise-exposure. Often, however, the noise is not continuous. It may change in intensity or perhaps cease entirely at certain phases of the operation, or the worker may not remain continuously in one place. The second simplification made is to *calculate from the measured durations and intensities of noise-exposure the equivalent sound level A, or "l_{eq}," which carries the same risk of impairment of hearing as the actual exposure.* Such a single number is needed for the next step in the calculations.

The calculation of equivalent sound level A makes use of the "trading relation" that has been established between intensity (dBA) and exposure-time in minutes and hours. Laboratory studies of temporary threshold shift have contributed greatly to establishing this relationship. The simplest rule assumes that the risk of injury depends on the total sound energy of the noise-exposure, regardless of how the energy is distributed in time. *Thus for every halving of the duration of exposure, doubling the energy (i.e., an increase of 3 dBA) is permissible without increasing the risk.* This is the rule recommended by ISO/TC43/SC-1 (International Standards Organization, Technical Committee 43/Subcommittee 1) in 1969.

Some other organizations believe that the equal energy rule is too conservative when short noise-exposures are concerned. Also, it may not allow adequately for the ability of the human ear to recover partially, during intervals of low noise levels, from the effects of brief intense noise-exposures. For these reasons they recommend a 5 dB rule instead of the 3 dB rule, namely, *for every halving of the duration of a partial exposure the intensity of the exposure can be increased by 5 dBA without increasing the risk.* The 5 dB rule has been adopted by the Department of Labor in implementing the Occupational Safety and Health Act of 1970. The American National Standards Institute has not yet made its choice.

The definition of risk from long-term noise exposure is based on studies of hearing of industrial populations habitually exposed to noise. The increase in percentage risk of developing a hearing handicap due to noise exposure, as opposed to presbycusis alone, is given in Table 5-1, with exposure level in dBA and years of habitual exposure to the

TABLE 5-1
PERCENTAGE RISK OF DEVELOPING A HEARING HANDICAP

Age		20	25	30	35	40	45	50	55	60	65	Years
Exposure		0	5	10	15	20	25	30	35	40	45	
80	Total	0.7	1.0	1.3	2.0	3.1	4.9	7.7	13.5	24.0	40.0	
	Due to Noise	no increase in risk at this level of exposure										
85	Total	0.7	2.0	3.9	6.0	8.1	11.0	14.2	21.5	32.0	46.5	
	Due to Noise	0.0	1.0	2.6	4.0	5.0	6.1	6.5	8.0	8.0	6.5	
90	Total	0.7	4.0	7.9	12.0	15.0	18.3	23.3	31.0	42.0	54.5	
	Due to Noise	0.0	3.0	6.6	10.0	11.9	13.4	15.6	17.5	18.0	14.5	
95	Total	0.7	6.7	13.6	20.2	24.5	29.0	34.4	41.8	52.0	64.0	
	Due to Noise	0.0	5.7	12.3	18.2	21.4	24.1	26.7	28.3	28.0	24.0	
100	Total	0.7	10.0	22.0	32.0	39.0	43.0	48.5	55.0	64.0	75.0	
	Due to Noise	0.0	9.0	20.7	30.0	35.9	38.1	40.8	41.5	40.0	35.0	
105	Total	0.7	14.2	33.0	46.0	53.0	59.0	65.5	71.0	78.0	84.5	
	Due to Noise	0.0	13.2	31.7	44.0	49.9	54.1	57.8	57.5	54.0	44.5	
110	Total	0.7	20.0	47.5	63.0	71.5	78.0	81.5	85.0	88.0	91.5	
	Due to Noise	0.0	19.0	46.2	61.0	68.4	73.1	73.8	71.5	64.0	51.5	
115	Total	0.7	27.0	62.5	81.0	87.0	91.0	92.0	93.0	94.0	95.0	
	Due to Noise	0.0	26.0	61.2	79.0	83.9	86.1	84.3	89.5	70.0	55.0	

Exposure level in dBA (left axis); Percentages of exposed population (right axis).

The criterion for hearing handicap is an average hearing level at 500, 1000, and 2000 Hz of 26 dB (ISO) or more.
Noise exposure is assumed to be habitual from 20 years of age onward.
The percentage risk due to noise is the total percentage at each age and exposure level minus the corresponding percentage risk at 80 dBA or less (first line), which is due to causes other than noise.

noise as parameters. The user of the table must decide what percentage of risk is to be considered acceptable. We reproduce the table here even though it is likely to be modified in the future by inclusion of British as well as American data in an International Organization for Standardization (ISO) document.

The percentage risk also depends on the hearing levels and the frequencies chosen to define a "significant" hearing handicap. This question is discussed in Chapter 9, but the choices confirmed by an Intersociety Committee in 1970 are open to future revision. (The Intersociety Committee consisted of representatives of the American Academy of Occupational Medicine; American Academy of Ophthalmology and Otolaryngology; American Conference of Governmental Industrial Hygienists; Industrial Hygiene Association; and Industrial Medical Association.) The choices of the Intersociety Committee to define hearing handicap were "25 dB for the average hearing levels at 500, 1000, and 2000 Hz." Opinions differ as to whether a higher frequency should be included and, if so, whether it should be 3000 or 4000 Hz.

It is worth noting that with this definition of handicap and on the basis of data from the Research Center of the Committee on Conservation of Hearing, 40 percent of the population who have not had habitual exposure to noise above 80 dBA nevertheless surpass the threshold of beginning handicap by the age of 65 years. It is obvious that even the most complete noise control program will not protect individuals from developing hearing impairments from causes other than noise.

NONINDUSTRIAL NOISE HAZARDS

Aggravation of Hearing Loss by Noise

It is a legitimate question whether exposure to noise that is not loud enough to damage a normal ear might nevertheless injure a hard-of-hearing ear. The question is most often raised with respect to the use of a hearing aid, which may deliver speech sounds at very high levels, as described in Chapter 11. Some people have been advised against the use of a hearing aid on this account by physicians who have made a diagnosis of sensorineural hearing loss, for fear that the noise would accelerate the process of degeneration that was thought to be the cause of the hearing loss. In many cases this advice amounted to conservative cruelty. There are, indeed, certain types of hearing impairment in which such caution is proper, but they are few.

In the first place it should be obvious that if the impairment is conductive in nature there is no danger. The handicap of a hearing loss is not great enough to require an aid until hearing thresholds are 30 dB or higher. This is about the equivalent of a good earplug, and the conductive impairment gives protection against the noise, like an earplug. It may do much better! Remember that all middle-ear impairment and also much inner-ear impairment is conductive (see Chapter 4).

The conservative view with respect to hearing aids was undoubtedly based in large part on the interpretation of presbycusis as a progressive degeneration of sensory units. We pointed out in Chapter 4 that this is only a part—and probably the smaller part—of the story of presbycusis. Nearly all presbycusis probably has considerable built-in protection provided by its conductive components.

Noise will not accelerate the progressive conductive changes of presbycusis or otosclerosis, and neither will it delay them. If the user of a hearing aid finds that his hearing has continued to fail, this is no evidence that the hearing aid is responsible.

Caution concerning noise is legitimate in all cases of sensorineural impairment that show signs of irritation, such as diplacusis and loud tinnitus. Often these conditions carry their own warning sign in the form of painful hearing. This type of pain or serious discomfort should be carefully respected.

An unfortunate condition without warning signs is a hereditary form of progressive degeneration of hearing in childhood. It is doubtful that noise influences this condition, and it is probably wiser to use a hearing aid to help the child learn as much language as possible before his hearing fails entirely than to withdraw the aid and make the child educationally deaf immediately.

Another problem lies in the application of hearing aids to congenitally deaf infants. To solve it we need to know, first, how reliably and accurately the diagnosis of impairment of hearing has been made and, second, at what age an infant with near-normal hearing will give reliable indication of auditory pain or discomfort from a hearing aid. Opinions on these points differ, but obviously some caution and common sense are in order here.

The problem will be considered again in Chapters 9 and 12.

Incubators for Infants

Premature infants may be exposed to hazardous noise in incubators or oxygen tents. The fans employed have not always been chosen with this risk in mind, and it is not known whether the safe level for the infant is as high as the 75 dBA recommended by the EPA for adults.

Loud Music and Auditory Analgesia

In the presence of very loud noise or music most subjects become less sensitive or insensitive to certain kinds of pain. Dental pain and obstetrical pain may be controlled in this way sufficiently to allow tooth extractions or childbirth without local or general anesthesia. Either music or white noise is given by earphones, and the patient has the volume under his own control, turning it up as necessary. Not all pain can be controlled in this way: for example, auditory pain in the ears at very high sound levels still persists. This form of analgesia has been given limited clinical trial, but concern about possible injury to hearing has discouraged its widespread use. Minimum standards to protect against this hazard were issued in 1961 by the American Dental Association.

The physiological and psychological mechanisms of auditory analgesia are not at all clear. We may think of a "saturation of the sensorium" and the principle of counter-irritation, but these are little more than descriptions of the phenomenon. High sound levels of the order of 120 dB SPL are required. The experience is unusual and psychologically impressive, and it may explain in part the fascination of the very high noise levels in some modern dance halls. Playing in such orchestras night after night should be recognized as a hazardous noise exposure.

OTHER CONSERVATION CONSIDERATIONS

Infants

Neonatal screening of infants in maternity hospitals to identify those who are deaf and require special management has been tried repeatedly, but the methods so far have not been sufficiently reliable to justify the expense. When confined to infants who are known to be "at risk" for deafness, however, such screening becomes feasible. It and the "high-risk register" are considered in Chapter 8.

Elderly People

For elderly people the problem of hazardous noise exposure becomes less and less important, and the maintenance of reasonable hygiene of the ear becomes more and more routine. There are fewer and fewer risks, as people grow older, from dirt and water or even from the common cold. The characteristic hearing loss of old age (presbycusis) is chiefly an inner-ear impairment, but we have no idea about how to protect against it. Neither can we protect against cerebral arteriosclerosis and the other conditions that we lump together as "senile changes." They are in the province of the new branch of medicine known as *geriatrics*.

Something can be done, however, to *protect communication by speech*. As hearing begins to deteriorate in elderly persons, they can begin to wear hearing aids and learn how to use them to their advantage. They can also take lessons in speechreading, and, as their hearing losses become severe, they can even learn how to keep their own voices pleasant and intelligible. These suggestions sound very simple and obvious, but the people who could benefit from them find them difficult to carry out, even if they can be persuaded to try. The problem is to *start soon enough* while the elderly man or woman is still adaptable, able to learn, and willing to make the necessary effort. As will be explained in other chapters, the person who becomes hard of hearing, particularly the elderly person, often does not recognize or admit his incapacity. He may blame others for not speaking up or for mumbling. By the time his hearing loss has become an obvious handicap it may be too late to "teach the old dog new tricks" and to alter his habits of a lifetime. To overcome such individual inertia and to create a healthy, constructive social point of view toward these and other problems of aging are the objectives of conservation of speech communication in elderly people.

SUGGESTED READINGS AND REFERENCES

Burns, W. *Noise and Man*, 2d ed. Philadelphia: J. B. Lippincott, 1973.
An excellent survey of all aspects of the noise problem.
———, and D. W. Robinson. *Hearing and Noise in Industry*. London: Her Majesty's Stationery Office, 1970.
Coles, R. R. A., G. R. Garinther, D. C. Hodge, and C. G. Rice. "Hazardous Exposure to Impulse Noise," *J. Acoust. Soc. Amer.*, 43:336–343 (1968).
Committee on Hearing and Equilibrium of the American Academy of Ophthalmology and Otolaryngology. "Guide for Conservation of Hearing in Noise." (Rev. 1973). Supplement to *Trans. Amer. Acad. Ophth. Otolaryngol.*
This guide is oriented to the Occupational Safety and Health Act of 1970 (OSHA 70).
Council on Dental Therapeutics. " 'Audio Analgesia': Supplementary Report." *J. Amer. Dent. Ass.* 66:420–434, 1963.
This report contains the revised minimum requirements for apparatus for "audio analgesia." Safety for hearing is the dominant objective.
Davis, H., G. Hoople, and H. O. Parrack. "The Medical Principles of Monitoring Audiometry," *AMA Arch. Industr. Health*, 17:1–20 (1958).
Eagles, E. L., S. M. Wishik, L. G. Doerfler, W. Melinick, and H. S. Levine. "Hearing Sensitivity and Related Factors in Children." Special monograph issue of *Laryngoscope*, 1963.
This is the "Pittsburgh Study" on schoolchildren, discussed near the beginning of this chapter.
Glorig, A., and K. S. Gerwin (eds.). *Otitis Media*. Springfield, Ill.: Charles C Thomas, 1972.
An important symposium volume.
Guignard, J. C. *A Basis for Limiting Noise Exposure for Hearing Conservation*. (Joint EPA/USAF Study), 1973. AMRL-TR-73-90 and EPA-550/9-73-001-A.
Copies are available from National Technical Information Service, 5285 Port Royal Road, Springfield, Va. 22151.
Harris, C. M. (ed.). *Handbook of Noise Control*. New York: McGraw-Hill Book Company, 1957.
Chapters 4 and 7 are particularly pertinent.

Henderson, D., R. L. Hamernik, D. S. Dosanjh, and J. H. Mills (eds.). *Effects of Noise on Hearing*. New York: Raven Press, 1976.
  A symposium dealing with basic problems of noise-induced hearing loss and criteria related to it.
Kryter, K. D., W. D. Ward, J. D. Miller, and D. H. Eldredge. "Hazardous Exposure to Intermittent and Steady-State Noise," *J. Acoust. Soc. Amer.*, 39:451–464 (1968).
  Prepared by NAS-NRC CHABA Working Group 46 to specify damage-risk criteria for exposure to sound.
Miller, J. D. "Effects of Noise on People." *J. Acoust. Soc. Amer.*, 56:729–764 (1974).
Rosen, S., M. Bergman, D. Plester, A. El-Mofty, and M. H. Satti. "Presbycusis Study of a Relatively Noise-free Population in the Sudan," *Ann. Otol.*, 71:727–743 (1962).
  This is the study of the Mabaan tribe.

Michael M. Paparella, M.D.
Hallowell Davis, M.D.

6

Medical and Surgical Treatment of Hearing Loss

OTOLOGY AND AUDIOLOGY

In Chapter 1 we reviewed briefly the relations between otology and audiology. Otology is the medical and surgical specialty that deals with the organs of hearing and balance from the point of view of their diseases and the prevention or treatment of these diseases, as well as safeguarding the life of the patient. Otology is a part of the field of otorhinolaryngology, the medical specialty that deals with disease of the ear, nose, and throat. Its point of view is primarily biological. Audiology is a specialty that is concerned with the function of hearing, with strong emphasis on its educational and social aspects and on providing assistance, where appropriate, in the form of hearing aids.

The two specialties, though separate, obviously interact strongly and provide much mutual support. These interactions will be a major concern of this chapter and several subsequent chapters. The otologist can do much to relieve conductive hearing impairment due to abnormalities or pathology of the external or middle ear and can give relief medically to some disorders of the middle and inner ear. The audiologist in turn can provide the otologist with very useful information from several audiological tests, particularly those designed to locate the anatomical site of a lesion. Sometimes when a differential diagnosis, such as that between an auditory neurinoma and Menière's disease, is vital, it may be greatly assisted by tests performed by the medical audiologist. Such tests will be considered specifically in Chapters 7 and 8.

A final principle, already noted in Chapter 1, is that although both fields share responsibility for the management of the individual patient, decisions on otological management should always precede decisions on audiological management. Biological safety must be insured, and function should be restored as fully as possible. On the other hand, surgical or medical intervention to improve or restore auditory function must be evaluated in terms of the auditory potentialities that remain as well as many local and general clinical considerations.

OTOLOGIC TREATMENT OF HEARING LOSS

Congenital Malformations

Congenital malformations of the external and middle ear are well-recognized developmental defects that may or may not be hereditary. They range in severity from just noticeable deviations from normal to complete absence of the external ear (anotia), complete closure of the external canal (atresia), absence or fixation of ossicles, and failure of development of the inner ear.

Abnormalities of the pinna alone cause very little practical impairment of hearing. They present a cosmetic problem but not an auditory one, and the surgical building of a cosmetically acceptable pinna is a task for a plastic surgeon as much as for an otologist. Sometimes a complete artificial pinna, molded from plastic, is the best solution. However, functional considerations take precedence over cosmetic ones. The way the ear works is more important than how it looks.

A child with bilateral atresia will benefit from surgical intervention in one ear by an experienced otologist before age 5 or when the child starts school. The mastoid should be adequately developed and pneumatized (air spaces) to permit surgery with safety. Unilateral atresias may be repaired later in life, for example, during the teens.

A meatus (opening) and canal can be surgically created (canalplasty), a new tympanic membrane can be provided by grafting techniques, and the middle ear can be reconstructed (tympanoplasty). Inner-ear defects are not treatable, but fortunately they rarely occur with atresia since the middle ear and the inner ear have different embryological origins.

Special X-ray studies such as polytomography, along with other studies, can help reveal defects in advance, and other essential information and audiological tests may indicate whether enough cochlear function is present to warrant attempts at reconstructive surgery.

Aural Hygiene

Certain rules of aural hygiene are worth a brief review. Blockage of the external canal by wax is rather frequent, particularly in later adult life. Complete final blockage may occur very abruptly, when perhaps a droplet of water closes the last tiny air passage, and the patient suffers an abrupt although partial loss of hearing. If the patient visits an audiologist before he sees a physician, the audiologist should habitually inspect the ear canal to assess the probability of blockage; but the removal of the wax is a procedure for a physician, who can remove it without injury to the canal or the drumhead. Normally the wax will work its way out unnoticed, bit by bit; but there are some people whose wax simply does not come out of the canal in this way, and once or twice a year they should have the wax removed by a doctor before it "macerates" or otherwise injures the skin of the canal. Hydrogen peroxide or cerumenolytic agents (such as Cerumenex) are sometimes used to soften the wax, which may then be washed out by irrigation with warm water. If this is done, the canal should be thoroughly dried afterward. Actually, if the ears are kept clean, the average person does not develop impacted wax. The constant insertion of the earmold of a hearing aid, or of matchsticks or hairpins, often pushes the wax so deep into the canal that it must be removed by a doctor. Impacted wax sometimes causes, by reflex, an annoying dry cough.

External Otitis

The skin of the external canal is in some areas very closely attached to the underlying cartilage and bone, so any infection of it is very painful. It is unwise, as a rule, to open a limited external otitis with a knife, as is often done with similar abscesses elsewhere in the body, to let out the pus. Incision, and other types of manipulation as well, will often spread the infection and may produce a diffuse external otitis.

The physician can treat external otitis quite effectively with a variety of local applications. The old-fashioned eardrops of alcohol and boric acid are sometimes effective, but often painful. For the patient, the important thing is to keep water out of the canal and to avoid self-inflicted trauma (as with cotton swabs, paper clips, or the like), which worsens the infection. Water softens the skin and spreads the infection more widely. If the canal has been wet, either from essential washing away of dead skin or wax, or inadvertently from ill-advised use of any watery medication, such as hydrogen peroxide, the canal should be dried out with 90 percent ethyl alcohol. The alcohol will sting for a few minutes, but the ultimate benefits justify the temporary discomfort.

Another variety of external otitis (the "eczematoid" type) is a chronic scaling of the skin that is very difficult to treat success-

fully. Fortunately, this type rarely causes deafness unless the canal is neglected and allowed to fill with wax and the cast-off scales of skin.

Aerotitis (Barotrauma)

Aerotitis media depends entirely on failure to ventilate the middle ear through the eustachian tube while descending from a high to a low altitude, leading rapidly to a collection of serum and blood in the middle ear. The best way to avoid aerotitis[1] is not to fly while suffering from a cold. Colds inflame the tissue at the mouth of the eustachian tube and prevent its proper function. If the tubes are partially blocked, continual swallowing on descent will help to equalize the pressure. This is helped by chewing gum, which produces enough saliva to allow for sufficient swallowing to open the tubes and equalize the pressure while the subject is making a normal descent. It is helpful to tilt the head back while swallowing. Airline pilots are instructed to descend or to depressurize a cabin at a rate of not more than 300 feet a minute. Occasional swallowing during such a slow descent will suffice for most people. Passengers who are asleep should be awakened before descent, and children and others who constantly have trouble with their eustachian tubes during flight should be given water to drink. Inhalants such as benzedrine that tend to shrink swollen mucous membranes may also be very helpful. A systemic decongestant or antihistamine may also be helpful.

Professional pilots and commercial travelers who must do a great deal of flying and who have recurrent aerotitis should have their eustachian tubes treated medically if they wish to continue flying without developing some permanent loss of hearing. In a similar category are submarine crews, deep-

[1] Aero-otitis is an alternative form.

sea divers, skin divers, and caisson workers. If the eustachian tubes do not open with swallowing, yawning, or moving the jaws about, an attempt should be made to open the tubes by strong blowing of the nose. If this does not work, a doctor may employ a drug like ephedrine to shrink the mucous lining of the nose temporarily, or he may have to inflate the tube with various blowing or swallowing maneuvers (Valsalva or Politzer), or with a catheter passed through the nose (Figure 6-1). In rare instances of severe aerotitis, incision of the drum may be necessary to remove the fluid.

Allergy A condition akin to aerotitis media but less abrupt in its onset may occur as the result of blockage of the eustachian tube by swelling of lymphoid tissue as part of an allergic reaction. This results in the retraction of the tympanic membrane and secretion of fluid, but the fluid is sterile and does not form pus unless infection enters secondarily. In time the fluid may become sufficiently thick and mucoid that drainage through the eustachian tube is impossible, even if the allergic reaction subsides. Surgical intervention to remove the secretion may be necessary. Other treatment is obviously to identify the cause of the allergy and deal with it appropriately.

Blowing Out the Ear

Inflation, whether performed by an instrument fitted to the nostril or by a silver catheter passed through the nose to the pharyngeal orifice of the tube, will improve the hearing, temporarily at least, if there is a plug of mucus blocking the tube. Often inflation is the only effective relief for temporary middle-ear hearing loss, but the method can be abused, and it is useless in cases of otosclerosis or of neural hearing loss. An old

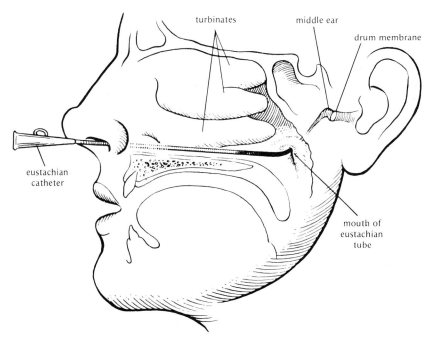

Figure 6-1 A catheter can be introduced through the nostril and inserted into the opening of the eustachian tube.

theory has been proved false: that wiggling the ossicles back and forth by blowing air up the eustachian tubes will loosen them and improve the hearing. Inflation through a catheter is now reserved for diagnostic purposes and for patients who have a temporary blocking of the tubes by excessively thick secretions. Many people can clear their own tubes by yawning or blowing the nose. The self-inflation maneuver of Valsalva is familiar, that is, blowing while holding the nose. If this does not work, the Politzer maneuver may succeed. The otologist places the olive-shaped tip of an air-filled "Politzer bag" in the patient's nostril and squeezes the bag as the patient swallows. Too much strong inflation may produce a loose, floppy drumhead, however, and there is always the danger, too, of forcing infected material up the tube from the back of the nose.

Otitis Media (Infection)

The various forms of otitis media have been described in sufficient detail in Chapter 4. Here we shall emphasize the prevention, the early treatment, and finally the surgical intervention that often is necessary in this condition.

Infection is the basis of most forms of otitis media, and by far the commonest pathway for the entry of infection is through the eustachian tube. The spread of infection up the eustachian tube is frequently increased by the improper forcible blowing of the nose that is so commonly practiced. Children in particular should be instructed to blow the nose gently with both nostrils open so that the pressure does not force infected material from the nose up the eustachian tube to the middle ear.

Periodic opening of the eustachian tube, associated with swallowing, is necessary not only for equalizing the air pressure between the middle and the external ear but also to al-low the normal drainage of secretions in the middle ear to the nasopharynx. This periodic slow movement of material is a powerful barrier to the spread of infection into the middle ear. Both blockage of the eustachian tube and infection in the nasopharynx favor the entry of infection into the middle ear.

One cause of partial or complete blockage of the eustachian tube and also a source of potential infection is enlarged lymphoid tissue of the nasopharynx (adenoids). In addition, tonsillitis, sinusitis, and the common cold can lead to otitis media. Enlarged tonsils and adenoids can easily be removed surgically, and this materially reduces the risk of otitis media in properly selected patients. The operation of tonsillectomy and adenoidectomy is probably the one most frequently performed by otorhinolaryngologists, though much less frequently than a generation ago. Some children are prone to otitis media, and immunological factors may play a role. Genetic predisposition also seems significant in certain patients.

Unfortunately the surgical removal of the adenoids does not always enable the eustachian tubes to open readily, particularly if chronic nasal or sinus infection is present. At one time radium treatments or X rays were used to shrink the lymphoid tissue that makes up the adenoid since this tissue is extremely sensitive to radiation. This form of treatment has been generally abandoned, however, because of the possibility of injury to other nearby tissues, notably the pituitary gland and midbrain structures.

Detailed discussion of the many methods of medical treatment of chronic nasal infection would extend beyond the scope of this book.

Acute Otitis Media *Drainage* For acute otitis media, and sometimes also for the chronic condition, the surgeon easily provides drainage by incising the lower back portion of the drum, where the incision has been found to cause no loss of hearing. If the drum is not opened, it will usually rupture spontaneously sooner or later. It has been found that more hearing loss and more mastoiditis requiring surgical attention occur after spontaneous rupture of the drum than after surgical incision. *Prompt attention to infection of the middle ear will do much to prevent the loss of hearing that frequently accompanies perforation of the drumhead and chronic diseases of the middle ear.*

Drug Therapy The bacteria that usually cause acute infection of the middle ear can be killed by various antibiotics, notably penicillin. Some physicians treat all otitis media with these drugs without surgery. This is not good practice, however, because subacute or chronic otitis media is likely to recur in certain cases if drainage is not provided in addition to drug therapy. *Acute otitis media should not be treated by patients themselves or by druggists.* The tendency is to stop the drug as soon as the pain of the discharge subsides, and this is too soon. On the other hand, prolonged use of the drugs without medical supervision is dangerous. Inadequate dosage only extends the disease and makes the bacteria less susceptible to the drug being used. It is the recurrent, subacute, or chronic types of otitis media that cause hearing loss, and it is in these conditions, as a rule, that complications develop.

A very mild inflammation or an infection treated by antibiotics may not develop into purulent or suppurative otitis media but may become instead a *chronic mucous otitis media*. The chief problem concerning mucous otitis media, particularly in children, is to recognize the condition. The treatment is to open the ear, remove the thick viscous fluid and to insert a ventilation tube through the tympanic membrane. During the past two decades, these ventilation tubes, properly utilized, have been of immense importance in treating and preventing otitis media with middle-ear fluid formation. They assist the eustachian tube in its primary functions of ventilation and drainage. They are left in place and may remain as long as one or two years, after which they extrude spontaneously. In certain patients, replacement is necessary. It is preferable to open the ear earlier when the inflammatory process is a little more acute and the secretions still thin and watery (*serous otitis media*).

Chronic otitis media Chronic otitis media, particularly if it is recurrent or frequently reactivated, forms adhesions that impede the transmission of sound and may destroy the eardrum membrane, the ossicles, and other structures. It is a common and important cause of hearing loss. Of course, the first concern of an otologist confronted with a case of otitis media is with the general health and safety of the patient. If some loss of hearing must be risked or even deliberately produced by removal of the ossicles together with the pus and diseased tissue in order to be sure to check the infection, the otologist does not hesitate to remove them. Where possible, of course, he spares or improves the hearing, but his first concerns are life and health. Treatment of otitis media by drugs may help restore or save hearing, but unless the infection is very mild, it is best to provide drainage for it. Drainage is nature's most effective way of getting rid of infection and the products of infection. When refractory pathological tissues, such as cholesteatoma or granulation tissue, are located within the middle ear and mastoid, surgical removal is necessary to achieve a safe, dry ear.

Mastoidectomy The mastoidectomy operation for chronic otitis media may have been considered a terrible and dangerous procedure by laymen, especially before the days of antibiotics. It can be, however, a lifesaving operation, and in the hands of a competent otologic surgeon it is not dangerous.

There are several kinds of mastoidectomy from a historical point of view. The "simple" mastoidectomy, performed for acute mastoiditis, aims to remove the diseased tissue in the mastoid bone and to establish free drainage of pus from the mastoid and the middle ear. "Radical" mastoidectomy is performed in chronic cases when the disease is not only in the air cells of the mastoid bone but in the middle ear as well. Its object is to remove all diseased tissues from both cavities and to create a single cavity that will eventually become lined with skin and cause no further trouble. "Radical" mastoidectomy can also be used to remove tumors. "Simple" mastoidectomy, performed for acute infection of the mastoid air cells, causes no appreciable hearing loss if there are no other complications. The hearing may be expected to stay within normal limits. "Radical" mastoidectomy, on the other hand, performed most frequently for chronic running ears, usually leaves a hearing level for speech of about 45 dB because the middle-ear contents are removed in the operation, even if they have not already been destroyed by the infection.

In about one-third of all cases the final level actually represents an improvement of hearing over the condition of conductive loss that existed before operation while the middle ear was plugged with pus and other disease products. For another one-third there is no significant overall change in hearing, and for the remaining third the hearing is worse after the operation than it was before. Of course, if, as is frequently the case, there is also some sensorineural hearing loss, the impairment due to it will remain and will be added to some 40 dB of conductive impairment produced by the operation. It should be clearly understood that radical mastoidectomy is a lifesaving operation or is performed to prevent further deterioration of the inner ear and not for the sake of any possible improvement of hearing.

At the present time, most mastoid operations are modifications of the above "classical" procedures and are done in combination with tympanoplasty, which will be described later. The objective of these mastoid procedures is to remove pathological tissues to make the ear safe and dry and thereby enhance the opportunity for improving hearing through reconstruction of the middle ear.

SURGICAL ALLEVIATION OF CONDUCTIVE HEARING LOSS

The two major diseases of the middle ear, otitis media and otosclerosis, have been discussed in some detail in previous chapters. The surgical treatment of acute otitis media is an important procedure, but there are now other surgical operations that aim not only to combat the disease process but also to improve the conduction of sound to the inner ear. One of these is *myringoplasty*, or repair of a persistent perforation of the drum membrane. Closely allied to this operation is the use of a "prosthesis," which is a mechanical substitute of some sort for a missing ossicle. The commonest use of a prosthesis is in the operation of stapedectomy to restore acoustic transmission after fixation of the stapes in otosclerosis.

Myringoplasty and Tympanoplasty

There are many cases of chronic otitis media in which the disease is not sufficiently severe to warrant a radical mastoidectomy. However, the hearing in such cases is decreased because of the scarlike adhesions and perhaps because of other anatomical changes that have taken place in the middle ear, and perhaps also because of perforation of the tympanic membrane. For many years plastic operations have been performed in such cases either to re-form the middle ear or perhaps only to close the hole in the drum membrane. The more extensive operation was formerly known as "modified radical mastoidectomy," but it has recently been improved and popularized under the name *tympanoplasty*. Here we should remember that "tympano-" refers to the entire middle ear, and not merely to the drum membrane. For the simpler operation, directed to closure of a hole in the membrane and nothing more, we use the term *myringoplasty*.

The Committee on Conservation of Hearing of the American Academy of Ophthalmology and Otolaryngology approved, in 1964, the following statement and recommended set of definitions:

Until recently the modified radical and the radical mastoidectomy were the common operative procedures performed for chronic ear infection. These operations were designed primarily to eradicate this infection. More recently, the concept of surgery in chronic ear infection has changed to include both eradication of disease and reconstruction of the destroyed hearing mechanism. These more complex surgical procedures are being described by a multiplicity of terms. This multiplicity of terms to describe similar surgical procedures has caused considerable confusion. The common operations performed in surgery for chronic ear infection are listed below. It is felt that, with rare exceptions, any operation for chronic ear disease could be classified as one of the following procedures. Technical surgical variations peculiar to one or another surgeon do not alter the fundamental classification:

1. Radical or Modified Radical Mastoidectomy
2. Mastoid Obliteration Operation
   An operation performed to eradicate infection when present, and to obliterate a mastoid or fenestration cavity.
3. Myringoplasty
   An operation in which the reconstructive procedure is limited to repair of a tympanic membrane perforation.

4. Tympanoplasty without Mastoidectomy
   An operation performed to eradicate disease in the middle ear and to reconstruct the hearing mechanism, without mastoid surgery, with or without tympanic membrane grafting.
5. Tympanoplasty with Mastoidectomy
   An operation performed to eradicate disease in the middle ear and mastoid, and to reconstruct the hearing mechanism, with or without tympanic membrane grafting.

Myringoplasty   In many cases the tympanic membrane has been perforated as the result of an old healed otitis media. The ear is perfectly dry. There is no discharge, but the patient's hearing is depressed because of the hole in the drumhead. Such holes can sometimes be closed by cauterizing, cutting, or scraping the edge of the perforation, and then providing some sort of scaffolding, such as cigarette paper or cotton, to assist the epithelium to grow across and thus heal the perforation. Some surgeons have had considerable success with these procedures, but others have not. A recent approach to the closure of perforations is to separate the epithelium from the fibrous portion of the drum membrane for a distance of about 2 or 3 mm from the edge of the perforation. A graft is prepared, usually from subcutaneous tissue (fascia) that covers the temporalis muscle, and is placed over the raw surface that has been exposed. It receives its blood supply from the raw surface. Such operations may improve the hearing for speech from levels between 20 and 30 dB to a level of 15 dB or better, that is, within normal limits.

Tympanoplasty   When disease is still present in the upper part of the middle ear (the attic), a more extensive operation is required. The objectives are to remove all diseased tissue from the middle ear, the attic, and the mastoid, and then to re-form a middle ear and ossicular chain. Defects in the drum membrane, or indeed a total loss of the membrane, can be repaired by the use of fascia from the temporalis muscle, skin, or a tympanic membrane transplant. When, as is most commonly the case, the incus is diseased, and its long process (that part which is joined to the stapes) is missing, the remains of the incus (the body and short process) can be removed and a hollow drilled in the body. This hollow will then be placed on the head of the stapes and the short process under the handle of the malleus so that the vibration from the drum membrane and malleus are conveyed to the movable stapes (called *incus transposition*). There are, in addition, many other techniques of ossicular reconstruction depending on the defects observed at the time of surgery. In the event that the crura of the stapes are destroyed by disease, the graft that forms a new drum membrane is invaginated into the oval window (so-called Type IV tympanoplasty). Later, if air reaches the round window through the eustachian tube (allowing for phase differential), and the hearing is still not satisfactory, the normal ratio of areas may be restored through appropriate ossicular reconstruction.

A variety of grafts are useful in tympanoplasty. As mentioned, fascia grafts are the most popular. Skin grafts were originally used in tympanoplasty and are still essential for certain cases. Other grafts such as vein grafts have been used. Tissue banks are a new and useful development for the otologist who performs tympanoplasty. These banks contain *homografts*, a term that refers to tympanic membranes or ossicles, removed from donors, that can be successfully used in tympanoplasty.

Fenestration

The concept of forcibly breaking loose a fixed stapes and thus restoring its function is as old as it is simple. It was tried many times during the last quarter of the nineteenth century and in the early nineteen hundreds, but without much lasting success, and the operation was finally abandoned. The two major difficulties were infection and the formation of new bone to close the oval window. However, in the 1930s the advent of new and more powerful drugs gradually reduced the danger of infection, and a new approach was developed, based on making an entirely new opening (a *fenestra*, or window) into the horizontal semicircular canal and covering this opening with a skin flap. This operation temporarily restored hearing to about the 30-dB hearing level, but windows as wide as a millimeter still closed all too frequently within a few weeks. Finally, in the 1950s, Julius Lempert and his disciples solved the problem of how to prevent the bone from healing over. The principle was merely to grind the edges of the fenestra thin and smooth and then press a skin graft from the wall of the ear canal firmly over the fenestra, in contact with the membranous labyrinth, within the horizontal semicircular canal. The membranous labyrinth, the endosteum, and the skin flap heal together, thus preventing the growth of new bone from endosteum and periosteum from closing the fenestra. Only about 1 percent of the fenestras close, and those that do close do so within the first six months.

The principle of the fenestration operation is illustrated in Figures 6-2 and 6-3. In Figure 6-2, which is a diagram of the anatomical relations described in Chapter 3, the normal path of sound across the middle ear and into the inner by way of the stapes and oval window is indicated by arrows. Figure 6-3 is intended to show: (1) the fixation of the stapes by otosclerosis; (2) the degeneration of some of the sensory cells of the cochlea, which so frequently occurs in the later stages of otosclerosis; (3) the opening of a fenestra through the bony wall of the middle ear into the horizontal semicircular canal; (4) the

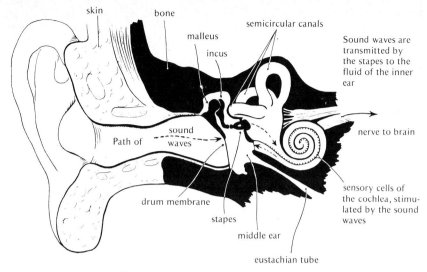

Figure 6-2 Normal path of sound waves.

skin flap from the ear canal covering the fenestra; and (5) the displacement of the eardrum and removal of the incus and most of the malleus. The new path of the sound waves is indicated, for simplicity, as entering the inner ear through the fenestra. Of

course, both windows must be mobile, and both are affected by the sound pressure outside. The movement inside occurs because of the *difference* in pressure on the two windows at each instant. The pressure is probably greater on the average on the new fe-

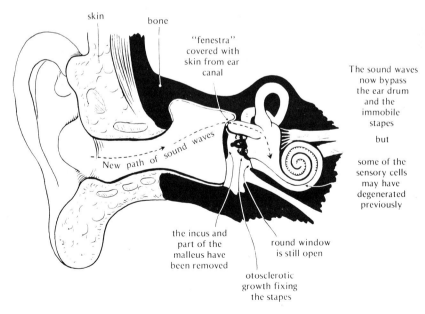

Figure 6-3 New path of sound waves after fenestration.

nestra than on the round window, which lies behind what is left of the drum membrane. The pressure wave at the round window may also be a little earlier or a little later than at the fenestra ("out of phase," as we say), and this phase difference may increase the difference in instantaneous pressure. It does not matter much which way the fluid in the cochlea moves during the compression phase of a sound wave in the canal. What is important is *how much* it moves. It has been found through experience that the drum membrane over the round-window niche is an important factor in getting a good differential between the two windows.

In the previous editions of this book a detailed historical account and description of the operation were included. They are omitted from the present edition because, although the fenestration operation is still performed in rare cases, it has been almost entirely superseded by the operation of stapedectomy, which is described below. The major reason is that fenestration cannot restore normal sensitivity of hearing. The tympanic membrane and the ossicles are removed and bypassed, and the acoustic gain that they normally provide is lost. This loss is approximately 30 dB. The resulting unavoidable hearing impairment is a great improvement over preoperative levels of 50 to 70 dB, but even with a good surgical result and a normal cochlea the patient still suffers a mild but real hearing handicap. The operation of stapedectomy has now been made equally reliable, and because the ossicular mechanism is retained (with an artificial stapes) hearing is usually restored to about the 10 dB hearing level or even better. Also the fenestration operation entails considerable postoperative discomfort from dizziness and usually requires hospitalization for a few days. Furthermore, even after complete healing, the cavity must be cleaned periodically, and swimming must be forbidden.

Stapedectomy

About 1955 Dr. Samuel Rosen of New York revived the simple stapes mobilization. Although the immediate results were moderately successful, a rather high percentage of successfully mobilized stapes became immobile once more. In 1958, Dr. John Shea of Memphis suggested removal of all or part of the stapes. He used a piece of vein to close the oval window. He attached a small piece of plastic tubing to the incus, and the end of this tube rested on the vein. The sound vibrations were now carried from the ossicles to the fluids of the inner ear by this tubing. The hearing by this method was restored almost to normal in many cases. As time went on, other materials were tried for closure of the oval window and for the attachment to the incus. Gelfoam, fat, and vein were used, and also stainless steel wire. Teflon took the place of the plastic tube.

In stapes surgery the middle ear is approached by way of the external canal. The incision is made in the skin of the canal, and the skin is lifted off the bone and reflected forward, carrying the tympanic membrane with it. The head of the stapes is not readily visible from the ear canal, but by careful curetting with fine instruments under a powerful microscope enough bone is removed to obtain a good view. With very fine knives, hooks, probes, and chisels, all specially made for this purpose, the stapes is dissected out, usually piecemeal.

The head of the stapes is separated from the incus. The crura of the stapes are removed; the footplate is cracked across and removed in pieces. The oval window is now open. A prosthesis of connective tissue and wire (premade) is placed over it to close it and prevent the escape of perilymph. The wire is attached to the incus and connects to the middle of the graft closing the oval window. If the otosclerosis of the oval window is so extensive as to be obliterative, a micro-drill can be safely used to create a smaller opening (at least 1 mm). In this case, a piston prosthesis made of Teflon and wire is inserted to prevent reclosure of bone and to permit good hearing to persist. When anatomical conditions permit, and when the otosclerotic focus is localized to only the anterior margin of the oval window, a conservative stapedectomy (partial stapedectomy) or anterior crurotomy is preferable. In this case the anterior crus and footplate only are dissected out, and the oval window is grafted, thus preserving the incudostapedial joint, the posterior crus, and the functional attachment of the stapedial muscle. This may be important to a patient who must work in a noisy environment. The drum membrane and the skin of the canal wall are then replaced and are held in position with a pack.

The advantages of stapes surgery are: (1) it is, for the patient, a relatively minor operation requiring only a brief stay in the hospital, usually two nights and one day; (2) it is performed prudently, under local anesthesia; (3) it leaves a normal ear canal and drum membrane when healing is completed; (4) when successful, the hearing level for speech is well within normal limits, often better than 10 dB, depending of course on the patient's cochlear reserve.

Postoperatively there is very little discomfort. There is a slight earache, which usually can be controlled by aspirin. There may be a very slight dizziness, but much less than that following the fenestration operation. Sometimes the sense of taste on the side of the tongue corresponding to the side of the operation may be modified so that food tastes unnatural and somewhat metallic. This effect, undoubtedly due to manipulation of the chorda tympani in the middle ear, is usually only temporary.

For the majority of patients who achieve a good hearing result, the result will be a lasting one. Occasionally a conductive loss may subsequently reappear due to regrowth of the otosclerotic bone or due to failure of the ossicular chain to conduct sound because of fixation of the malleus or mechanical failure of the stapes prostheses. A judicious stapedectomy revision may correct the problem. In certain cases a sensorineural hearing loss can result, either related to the surgery (not more than a 2 percent likelihood in the hands of an experienced otologist) or, more commonly, to a progressive longterm sensorineural hearing loss caused by the effects of otosclerosis on the cochlear membranous labyrinth.

MENIÈRE'S DISEASE

As it was described in Chapter 4, Menière's disease is characterized by a triad of symptoms: sensorineural hearing loss, episodic vertigo, and tinnitus. In certain cases, Menière's disease appears in a cochlear form (hearing loss only) or the vestibular form (vertigo only). A very thorough medical diagnostic workup, including studies during hospitalization, is indicated in some patients.

Most patients with Menière's disease can be managed medically. There is an important psychological component in Menière's disease, but this does not mean that it is a psychosomatic disease; rather, the vertigo causes an anxiety reaction. Recent studies have shown that diazepam (Valium) is helpful, apparently because it exerts some selective sedative effect on the vestibular nuclei. The physician can also prescribe antivertiginous drugs. Other agents used include vasodilative agents, betahistine hydrocholoride (Serc), low salt diet, diuretics, and bioflavonoids. Since Menière's disease is probably a chemical disorder of the relation between blood and endolymph, a useful drug might one day be forthcoming.

The patient should be treated conservatively and reassured that he does not have a more serious disease. The more the patient understands the self-limiting, waxing and waning characteristics of Menière's disease, the better he can cope with it. If the patient has incapacitating or disturbing vertigo in spite of strenuous and extended medical management, several procedures may be considered. Surgical procedures may be either conservative, designed to decompress the endolymphatic hydrops and allow the endolymph to escape, or else destructive (labyrinthectomy), in which the entire inner contents are removed or destroyed. The vestibular labyrinth only can be selectively destroyed by ultrasonic techniques.

Drainage of the Endolymphatic Sac

Drainage of the endolymphatic sac was introduced by Portmann many years ago, and House has repopularized it in recent years. A simple mastoidectomy is done, and the endolymphatic sac in the dura over the posterior cranial fossa is exposed between the lateral sinus and the posteroinferior semicircular canal. One method consists of incising the sac and inserting a T tube made of silicone elastomer (Silastic) sheeting to drain endolymph into the mastoid cavity, over which tissue or gel foam is then placed. Thus, drainage of endolymph occurs in a location remote from the cochlea. Another method is to establish a shunt between the sac and the subarachnoid space.

Most patients have virtually no or little difficulty with episodic vertigo thereafter. The operation may improve hearing in some patients and seems to prevent further development of sensorineural deafness. Sometimes tinnitus is reduced. There is approximately a 5 percent chance of sensorineural deafness resulting from this procedure, however, and this must be compared to the natural progression of sensorineural hearing loss that invariably develops in the long-term patient with Menière's disease.

If hearing is poor (for example a speech reception threshold of 50 dB HL and only 50 percent discrimination of words) and a conservative procedure is not feasible for anatomic or other reasons, labyrinthectomy (total desctruction of the inner ear) can eliminate the vertigo. Disequilibrium requires a few weeks or months for compensation. A certain few patients have a lasting sensation of positional dizziness. The procedure is relatively simple. The surgeon enters both windows of the inner ear by a transcanal approach and mechanically removes the inner ear contents, using an operating microscope.

Another development in recent years is the successful repopularization of the method of selective vestibular nerve section. This method was previously tried unsuccessfully many years ago by a very famous neurosurgeon.

If incapacitating vertigo persists after the conservative therapy in patients with bilateral Menière's disease, ablation of both vestibular labyrinths through parenteral administration of streptomycin can be considered. The patient is hospitalized and carefully monitored with caloric and audiometric tests. Streptomycin sulfate, 1 gram twice daily, is given until vestibular function, as measured by maximum caloric tests (using 30 to 50 ml of ice water) ceases. This process requires one to several weeks.

OTHER FORMS OF SENSORINEURAL HEARING LOSS

It is not within the purview of this chapter to attempt a comprehensive discussion of medical and surgical treatment. The emphasis, for proper reasons, has been to discuss treatment of conductive losses since these represent the bulk of hearing losses, which in the main are amenable to medical therapy. There are examples of sensorineural hearing loss that, after proper diagnosis, can be managed. The hope for the future is that, through research, more patients with sensorineural hearing loss will receive specific medical diagnoses which may lead to improved methods of treatment.

Prevention

The most effective form of treatment is prevention. Early medical diagnosis and treatment will help, not only in the management of an immediate problem, but also to prevent a progressive sensorineural hearing loss. Examples here include cochlear otosclerosis, acute otitis media, serous otitis media, mucoid otitis media, noise-induced hearing loss, ototoxicity, genetic hearing losses and X-ray treatments. G. E. Shambaugh, Jr., has fairly well demonstrated that in some patients sodium fluoride with a calcium supplement will help arrest a progressive sensorineural hearing loss due to otosclerosis by converting the spongy vascular bone (*otospongiosis*) into a safe, hard sclerotic bone (*otosclerosis*). It has also been shown by Paparella through audiological and temporal bone studies that patients with otitis media, especially chronic otitis media, frequently develop a progressive hearing loss for the high frequencies with evidence of pathology localized to the round window and the basal turn of the cochlea. Products of infection can spread from the middle ear through the round-window membrane in these patients. Early medical and surgical treatment of middle-ear effusions in children can prevent a serious sensorineural hearing loss from chronic otitis media in adulthood. As noted in Chapter 5, the best way to prevent noise-induced hearing loss is to avoid noise when possible or to wear protective

devices when necessary to attenuate sound energy to a safer, more tolerable level.

Many powerful drugs are introduced each year for treatment of serious generalized diseases. Many presently available drugs are known to be ototoxic, and others yet to be identified may be ototoxic. Examples of ototoxic drugs include aspirin, quinine, diuretics such as ethacrynic acid, streptomycin, kanamycin, and neomycin. It is important for the physician to save the patient's life first, even if it requires causing a hearing loss, but in most cases, through early audiometric monitoring and recognition, a dangerous ototoxic agent can be safely replaced with a nonototoxic one. Finally, again we mention X-ray treatment of the temporal bone. It is known that high doses of irradiation therapy to the temporal bone can cause sensorineural hearing loss. Thus, when managing patients with tumors in this region, the physician should take this possibility into consideration.

Surgical Management

Surgery can improve a sensorineural hearing loss occasionally in patients with acoustic neuromas (tumors), cholesteatoma with a fistula complication, middle-ear tumors, and sudden deafness. If the loss is due to pressure on the auditory nerve or the cochlear artery from a tumor of the auditory nerve, removal of the tumor may restore some or all of the lost hearing. Improvement is more likely if the hearing loss came on rather rapidly and if the operation is performed promptly than it would be if the tumor grew slowly. In this case, the nerve cells and hair cells are likely to be injured or starved beyond hope of recovery. The operation for removal of the tumor is not undertaken to restore hearing, however. It is undertaken to protect life, because further growth may cause pressure on vital centers in the lower brain stem. Another example where surgery can improve sensorineural hearing loss is in certain patients who have a cholesteatoma that has destroyed the bony labyrinth, such as in the region of the horizontal semicircular canal, causing a complication called a *fistula*. The patient may have serous labyrinthitis, causing a temporary threshold shift and impending suppurative labyrinthitis, which would result in permanent deafness. After proper and preferably early removal of the cholesteatoma through mastoidectomy, the sensorineural hearing loss may be improved dramatically in certain cases. This same phenomenon may be seen when tumors of the middle ear and mastoid are removed. A final example of sensorineural hearing loss improved through surgery is in certain cases of so-called sudden deafness. Goodhill has described, and others have confirmed the presence of, a rupture of the round-window membrane in certain patients with sudden deafness. When this is identified early, and treated with application of a graft to the round window through an exploratory tympanotomy, hearing may be restored.

Medical Management

There are examples in which medical treatment can result in improvement of cochlear function. In addition to Menière's disease described above, these include fluctuant hearing losses due to allergy or vascular phenomena, as well as kidney-cochlear disease, syphilis, and hypothyroidism. In some patients the identification and avoidance of an allergen will help restore hearing. Vascular problems causing fluctuant sensorineural hearing losses have been described by many. Treatment is empirical at present because of a lack of scientific substantiation. This is an area where future research holds great promise for identification and treatment of many of these disorders, but at the present time, treatment must necessarily re-

main empirical. Kidney transplants have become a standard procedure in many medical centers. This has led to an ever-increasing incidence of cochlear losses in patients on dialysis or those who have received transplanted kidneys. Some of this hearing loss is probably due to ototoxic drugs, but there are many other patients for whom this explanation does not suffice. A relationship, such as an immunological one, is assumed to exist between the glomerulus of the kidney and the stria vascularis of the cochlea. It is possible that such hearing loss may be prevented or treated with immunosuppressive drugs. Hypothyroidism has clearly been associated with cochlear dysfunction as seen in both animal studies and in man. The sensorineural hearing loss is fortunately not usually of severe magnitude and is readily improved with proper restoration of thyroid function through medical treatment. Syphilis is still a significant cause of sensorineural hearing loss today. It was thought that syphilis would disappear with the introduction of penicillin in the early 1940s, but such is not the case. Indeed, there seems to be an increasing problem in this regard. Both congenital and acquired syphilis can cause sensorineural hearing loss. Endolymphatic hydrops and vertigo can also result in certain patients. Treatment consists of steroid medication and high doses of penicillin provided over an appropriate period of time. With this treatment in hospitalized patients a dramatic improvement of sensorineural function occasionally can be observed and documented in the audiograms.

THE COCHLEAR IMPLANT FOR TOTAL DEAFNESS

The basic idea of the cochlear implant is very simple. Its objective is to restore hearing in a deaf ear by electrical stimulation of the auditory nerve. The idea must be as old as the discovery of the electrophonic effect, which is described in Chapter 3. Although there are many ways in which an electric current passed through a normal ear can give rise to mechanical movement of the basilar membrane and thus stimulate the auditory nerve through the usual sensory channel, the current can also excite the nerve fibers directly. The sensation so elicited is not a pure tone but a noise. This effect has been produced also in ears with impairment of the organ of Corti. Speech has not been made intelligible by this method, although its temporal and stress patterns can be appreciated. The missing item is the mechanical frequency analysis performed by the basilar membrane. Exploratory studies of direct stimulation of the nerve were first carried out in favorable cases during aural surgery. The second stage of development has been to implant one or more electrodes permanently in cochleas of deaf ears.

The objectives of the implant are, first, to provide a permanent indwelling prosthesis that can deliver electrical stimuli to whatever auditory nerve fibers remain in a deaf ear; and, second, to provide selective stimulation, related to acoustic frequency, for different nerve fibers through several electrodes. For the second objective, electroacoustic filters carry out a frequency analysis instead of the basilar membrane so that each group of nerve fibers is stimulated in response to selected incoming acoustic frequencies. There is good reason to hope that subdivision of the acoustic spectrum into as few as four or five bands will result in intelligible speech if the outputs can be matched anatomically to nerve fibers (sensory units) with approximately the corresponding characteristic frequencies.

We can say, in summary, that the first objective has been achieved to a limited but useful extent. There are at the present writing (1976) about a dozen individuals in the United States who are wearing and using implants that have been in place for more than one year and in one case for as long as five years. The second objective, however, has not been successfully achieved. Although multiple electrodes have been tried, the technical difficulties are still formidable, and the present implants in the United States all employ only a single intracochlear electrode. These implants restore hearing in a limited sense, but they do not render speech intelligible. There are, however, some real benefits from only a single channel, and efforts to improve the system will probably continue.

The cochlear implant is in an intermediate stage of development. We shall therefore not attempt to describe details but rather to assess its demonstrated performance and its apparent potentialities. Likewise we do not attempt a detailed history of its development but will only mention in passing the names of several otologists and associates who have pioneered in the development and assessment. Prominent among these are Drs. William F. House, F. Blair Simmons, R. P. Michelson and M. M. Merzenich in California, and Drs. C. H. Chouard and P. MacLeod in Paris. Among the electrical engineers associated with Dr. House are P. Doyle and J. Urban. The early efforts have been very controversial and have been severely criticized, but enough positive results have been achieved to raise high hopes as well.

The most favored approach has been to introduce one or more fine-wire electrodes through the round window or holes drilled into the scala tympani. Sometimes the stimulation has been monopolar, with the second electrode outside the cochlea; sometimes it has been bipolar, with two electrodes closely spaced within it. The electrode wires have sometimes been connected to a plug, surgically implanted in the mastoid bone and extending externally through an opening in the skin. Sometimes the coupling to the external electrical stimulating circuit has been inductive, with one coil implanted under the skin and another outside, held in contact with the skin like a bone vibrator. Sometimes the stimuli have been alternating currents with waveforms corresponding to sound waves. Sometimes they have been brief pulses in the temporal pattern of sound waves, and sometimes a high-frequency (such as 16-kHz) carrier wave has been amplitude-modulated in the pattern of speech or other acoustic signals. As yet the choice has been that of each experimenting team, with no consensus or standardization. As a practical proposition, however, the direct connection by means of an exposed "hard-wired" plug has not endured satisfactorily. Ultimately the connecting electrode wires have broken, or the plug has been rejected biologically and failed mechanically. The subcutaneous coil with inductive transdermal coupling has fared better, but it requires accurate positioning of the external coil.

As noted above, the efforts to introduce multiple electrodes (in the form of a miniature cable extending as far as possible up into the cochlea) have not proved successful, and an alternative approach employed by the French team, to make multiple fenestrations of the cochlea, requires much bolder surgical procedures. Each American effort has resulted in a single effective electrode, without selectivity of frequency. The French effort seems to have been suspended, at least temporarily, because of technical engineering difficulties. Perhaps in the near future multiple electrodes will function in the cochlea and be maintained successfully for more than a few months, and also wearable electronic equipment for selective stimulation by different bands of acoustic frequency will be provided. These seem to be the prerequisites for a really successful cochlear implant.

So far the American efforts, all in California, have yielded fewer than 20 cases of successful implants, the majority placed by Dr. William House. (The title of Dr. House's recent monograph is given in the list of references at the end of this chapter.) From a follow-up study by Dr. R. C. Bilger of about a dozen available cases several important generalizations emerge. Without going into detail we summarize them in paraphrase as follows:

1. The cases considered suitable candidates for the implant are young or middle-aged adults who have learned speech and language but have later been deafened totally or profoundly. Two congenitally deaf adults have been implanted, but the prelingually deaf, and particularly children, should *not* be considered suitable candidates for the implant.

2. The implanted subjects experience a true sensation of hearing. This restoration of hearing for those who have not benefited from hearing aids is a great psychological boon to them, for reasons explained in Chapter 19. To them the world is no longer "dead." They feel a part of it once more.

3. Many familiar environmental sounds can be recognized as "signals," partly by their contexts and temporal patterns. The subject's own speech is rendered more intelligible, unless it is already either very good or very poor without using the implant.

4. The subjects are delighted with the restoration of hearing by only one channel, but later they become frustrated by their inability to learn to understand speech.

5. Incoming speech is *not* intelligible to any subject, except in the special case of a very restricted vocabulary in which temporal cues, such as the number of syllables, are significant. Remember that the implants under consideration here all have only a single channel. (The preliminary results of the French team with multiple channels show that four or five may be sufficient, but at least

one or two electrodes must be located in the apical half of the cochlea. With such placements and a month or two of relearning, good speech recognition scores were obtained.)

6. Intensity discrimination is excellent. The problem of compressing the wide dynamic range of everyday sounds into a very restricted dynamic range of effective but tolerable electrical stimulation seems to be fairly well solved.

7. Frequency discrimination is poor. It corresponds quite well to what is predicted theoretically on the basis of "periodicity pitch," explained in Chapters 2 and 3. Frequency discrimination is not effective at all above about 1000 Hz, with a single channel.

8. Ambient noise is very troublesome for these subjects.

One very general comment is that the greatest benefits to date from the cochlear implant are psychological. Another is that limited frequency discrimination is exactly what is expected theoretically with only one channel, and so is the failure to understand speech. A third is that the procedure is still very much in the experimental stage, and awaits considerable improvement with respect to the placement of multiple electrodes and the availability of effective and wearable electronic equipment. Preoperative electrical tests should allow the surgeon to be sure that a sufficient number (and distribution) of auditory nerve fibers remain to take advantage of multiple-electrode stimulation. Finally, the method at present offers no real hope for those who are prelingually deaf.

SUGGESTED READINGS AND REFERENCES

Bilger, R. C., and others. "Evaluation of Subjects Recently Fitted with Implanted Auditory Prostheses," *Ann. Otol. Rhinol. Laryngol.*, Suppl. 38 (1977).
Evaluation of fifteen subjects presently fitted with implanted auditory prostheses.

Davis, H., and T. E. Walsh. "The Limits of Improvement of Hearing Following the Fenestration Operation," *Laryngoscope*, 60:273–295 (1950).

Glorig, A., and K. S. Gerwin. *Otitis Media*. Springfield, Ill.: Charles C Thomas. 1972.
An important symposium volume.

Hawkins, J. E. "Drug Ototoxicity," *Handbook of Sensory Physiology*, vol. 5 (The Auditory System, part 3), 707–748. Berlin, Heidelberg, New York: Springer-Verlag, 1976.
An extensive, up-to-date and authoritative review.

House, W. F. "Cochlear Implants," *Ann. Otol. Rhinol. Laryngol.*, 85:1–93, Suppl. 27 (1976).
A full historical account written by one of the most active proponents of the method.

Paparella, M. M., and D. A. Shumrick (eds.). *Otolaryngology*. Philadelphia: W. B. Saunders, 1973.
In Volume 1 (Basic Sciences and Related Disciplines) the health sciences as they relate to otolaryngology are outlined in traditional manner, obviating

the need, in most instances, for the reader to search for additional information in a basic science textbook. Following this, fundamental principles of surgery and of medicine are discussed. Volume 2 (Ear), is concerned with the medical and surgical aspects of otology.

Schuknecht, H. (ed.). *Otosclerosis.* Boston: Little, Brown & Company, 1962.

This symposium volume surveys authoritatively and exhaustively the subject of otosclerosis and its surgical treatment.

Williams, H. L. *Ménière's Disease.* Springfield, Ill.: Charles C Thomas, 1952.

An authoritative monograph by an eminent otologist.

Part III
AUDITORY TESTS

Hallowell Davis, M.D.

7

Audiometry: Pure-Tone and Simple Speech Tests

Audiometry means the measuring of hearing. There are many tests of hearing: some old and many new; some crude and some very refined and elaborate; some intended for screening and others designed for medical diagnosis. We shall make a rapid survey of these tests and name and classify or characterize most of those that are in current use in hearing clinics. We shall, however, be content to point out the principles that are involved and the kind of information that each test yields. We shall not discuss the details of technique and precautions. This is not a "cookbook of audiometry." Neither do we go far into controversial questions of theory or the "last word" from experimental psychophysics. Other authors and the current journals provide adequate treatment of these various topics. We are writing only a guide for the beginning student or the interested worker in a related field.

OBJECTIVES OF AUDIOMETRY

There have always been two quite different reasons for measuring hearing. It is well to recognize these immediately because the choice of what aspect of hearing to test, the instruments and test materials or signals to be employed, and the whole conduct of the test depend on the objectives that are sought. A test or an instrument that is good for one purpose may be quite useless for another. Failure to understand the differences in objectives has led to considerable confusion and misunderstanding in the past.

One clear purpose of audiometry is to *assist in medical diagnosis*. The question to be answered is, *"What is wrong with the auditory system and where is the problem?"* The early simple tests, notably those that employed tuning forks, were clearly oriented to this purpose, and the first American Standard for electric audiometers was specifically entitled "Audiometers for General Diagnostic Purposes."

Another purpose is *overall assessment of hearing* to determine the fitness of the individual for certain tasks or duties, his need for special education or other assistance, his claim for compensation or insurance, and so on. The need for a hearing aid and the assessment of the benefit provided by a hearing aid fall in this general category. The central question usually is, *"How well can this person hear and understand everyday speech?"*

A third purpose is to identify quickly in a large population those with an impairment of hearing sufficient to require special attention. The final objective may be to cure or check the progress of the impairment or to provide special assistance to override it. This type of audiometry is called *screening audiometry*. The question is, *"Who is in trouble but may not know it?"*

The fourth purpose is to detect any changes in hearing that may occur as a result of some recognized hazard to hearing. The typical hazard is habitual exposure to loud noise, usually in a military or industrial situation. This is called *monitoring audiometry*. Hearing is tested regularly, just as weight and blood pressure may be monitored by annual physical examinations. A record of the status of hearing, year by year, is kept. The question is, *"Has anyone's hearing changed enough that his hazardous exposure should be reduced?"*

We shall consider below how audiometers, particularly electric audiometers, have been developed and how tests with them have been specialized for each of these purposes. In general, diagnostic audiometry requires the greatest range of frequencies and the greatest dynamic range without sacrifice of accuracy. The assessment of hearing puts much more emphasis on speech audiometry, and screening and monitoring audiometry deal with large numbers of people; speed and simplicity of test are important.

Organization of Chapters 7, 8, and 9

The following description of tests of hearing and their interpretation is divided broadly according to the main purposes of the tests as outlined above, but in part the organization is determined by the nature of the tests and the instruments employed.

In this chapter, after a brief historical survey of simple tests of hearing, we give special attention to the electric audiometer as defined in the American National Standard Specifications for Audiometers, ANSI S3.6-1969 (R1973). We explain in some detail the standardization of audiometers and the audiogram, that is, pure-tone threshold audiometry as used for general diagnostic purposes. We include here the use of pure-tone threshold audiometry for monitoring and screening purposes. In the second part of the chapter we describe speech audiometry and the determination of the speech-reception threshold and discrimination scores. The discussion is organized around the standardized instrument and familiar materials.

In Chapter 8 we describe tests of hearing other than the determination of thresholds of hearing and simple articulation curves. The use of audiometry to assist in the selection of a hearing aid is included here. We consider many (but not all) of the audiometric tests that have been proposed for diagnostic purposes, particularly those oriented toward sensorineural and central impairment. Here we also describe certain physiological tests of the ear, notably evoked-response audiometry and the measurement of acoustic impedance.

Chapter 9 is oriented to the problem of auditory handicap and to military and other standards of hearing. Special attention is given to the relation between audiometric measurements and workmen's compensation. The question of "normal hearing" in medicolegal contexts is also considered.

NONELECTRICAL TESTS OF HEARING

In Chapter 2, "Acoustics and Psychoacoustics," it was pointed out that there are several different aspects of hearing. We may be interested in testing any or all of them, and different types of test are appropriate for each one. First and most obvious is *sensitivity*. How weak a sound can be heard? Then there is the *recognition of pitch*. Do pure tones sound pure and musical, and is the ear "in tune," so to speak? There is also auditory *discrimination*. How small a difference in pitch or in loudness can a person detect? Can he recognize difficult words? Can he pick out speech from a background of noise or of many voices as well as he should? And finally there is *tolerance*. At what intensity does a sound become uncomfortable or painful?

Originally the interest in audiometry lay almost entirely in sensitivity. From the medical point of view the object was to determine whether the fault lay in the sound-conducting mechanism of the middle ear or in the neural mechanism of the inner ear. More recently, however, the importance of tolerance, of correct recognition of pitch, and of auditory discrimination has been recognized, and tests for these other aspects of hearing have been developed. The otologist now wants to distinguish impairments of the sense organ from those of the auditory nerve or brain stem, and both such conditions from what we now call central dysacusis.

Crude Tests of Sensitivity

To bring the study of hearing out of the realm of guesswork and to guide the medical treatment of its problems, we need tests and, above all, *measurements* of hearing. When someone is totally deaf in both ears, there is usually no doubt about it. However, to devise a simple and reliable test to determine whether a man's hearing is good enough for him to enter military service or bad enough to entitle him to compensation for injury is a very different matter. It is not easy to measure the sensitivity of hearing accurately, partly because it requires complicated apparatus to deliver sounds of known intensity to the ear and partly because physical sound has two major dimensions—frequency and intensity—and the loss of hearing for some frequencies may be much greater than for others. The difficulties are overcome by the electric audiometer; but the instrument is expensive, and the quiet surroundings required for accurate measurements of hearing may be expensive and difficult to provide. For rapid and approximate testing, therefore, the crude but time-honored methods—the *conversational voice*, the *whisper*, the *coin click*, and the *watch tick*—will still be used.

These four simple tests solve in different ways the problem of which frequencies to test. The voice and the whisper represent two kinds of sound that are most important for a man to hear, and if he can hear (and understand) the human voice, we do not much care whether or not he can hear the cricket's chirp. The frequencies most important for good understanding of speech extend from about 400 to 3000 Hz, and the voice test therefore gives some idea of the usefulness of hearing over this range. The watch tick and the click of coins, on the other hand, are high-frequency sounds, mostly above the range that is really needed to understand speech. They are useful because loss of hearing often begins with a loss of sensitivity for high frequencies, and the defect can be detected much earlier by the coin or the watch than by the voice or the whisper. In a very general way the hearing for speech is impaired most by conductive hearing losses, which affect all frequencies. Sensorineural loss is most often a high-tone hearing loss, most severe above 2000 Hz. The spoken voice and the watch tick or coin click supplement one another in just this way, and to the extent that they can be standardized they are useful tools for rough-and-ready testing.

Two major difficulties with all simple tests, in addition to the necessity of providing a quiet room for testing with walls that do not reflect the test sounds, are standardizing the sounds and measuring their intensity. We have to assume that one man's voice is as easy to understand as another's, that watch ticks are alike, and that any two coins struck together in various ways will give off the same sound. Of course, many efforts to standardize these tests have been made. For example, certain key words, usually numbers such as "66" and "99," are regularly used in the voice test. Those who do much testing of this sort try to speak always with the same loudness and distinctness, and they do produce reasonably reproducible signals, but it is more difficult to match one voice with another.

The whisper test has the advantage over the conversational voice in that it is relatively easy to standardize the loudness of a whisper by whispering only at the end of an expiration. Incidentally, the whisper represents at fairly even intensity the range of frequencies needed for good understanding of speech. In an ordinary conversational voice the low frequencies are much more powerful than most of the high frequencies.

The intensity with which the sound of the voice, watch, or coin reaches the ear is varied by the tester coming closer and closer to the subject. This is theoretically a reasonable method because the intensity of sound varies inversely as the square of the distance it travels. (Twice as far away, one-fourth the intensity at the ear; three times as far, one-ninth; and so on.) In practice this rule almost always breaks down badly because of echoes from the walls of the room. Only in special sound-absorbent rooms does the rule mean much for distances of more than 6 feet or so.

When we test the sensitivity of the ear, we do not merely want to know that someone can hear our voice at 20 feet and our watch at 5, or that he can detect a tone of 1000 Hz at one ten-thousandth of a dyne per square centimeter. We want to know how the sensitivity of his ear compares with that of his fellowmen. We therefore establish the performance of a number of "otologically normal" men and women and express the performance of the man with poor hearing as a ratio with respect to the average expectation. "Otologically normal" means free of any obvious otological defect or impairment such as wax in the canal, a perforated drum membrane, or a history of earaches, discharge from the ear, or obvious difficulty in hearing. On the average, an "otologically normal" person just understands the standard whispered voice at 20 feet. If we must come closer to a man with poor hearing, say within 5 feet, before he can understand our whisper, we say that his hearing is 5/20 ("five over twenty" or simply "five-twenty"). Many standards of performance or hearing requirements, discussed in Chapter 9, are expressed in such ratios. The analogy to the Snellen chart test for visual acuity is obvious.

Early tests of frequency range. Among the first instruments employed for quantitative measurements of hearing were musical instruments (a small organ), the Galton whistle, and the Struycken monochord. The Galton whistle emits very high frequencies, like present-day ultrasonic dog whistles, but the frequency is adjustable by a calibrated micrometer screw. The monochord is a taut, metal wire activated by a bow like a violin or struck by a hammer like a piano. The intensity of neither instrument is closely controlled, but the threshold of hearing rises so sharply at the upper frequency limit that intensity is not very critical (see Figures 2-4 and 2-5).

The determination of the lower frequency limit of hearing was never satisfactory, but the broad distinction between high-frequency loss, as in presbycusis, and flat or low-frequency loss, as in otosclerosis, could be made. The whistle and the monochord are no longer used to any great extent.

Tuning forks. The most satisfactory and versatile simple instrument for testing hearing, one that is still a very important part of an otologist's equipment, is a set of tuning forks. The octave frequencies of 64, 128, 256, 512, . . . Hz became established early as the standard frequencies. The forks emit a quite pure tone. Moreover, their damping is small and thus the intensity decays slowly but regularly. With practice the fork can be activated by striking it a standard blow. One quantitative measure is then the length of time that the patient can hear the tone when the vibrating tine is held close to his ear canal. More often however, the otologist uses his own ear as a standard of reference. When the patient ceases to hear the tone, he quickly brings the fork to his own ear and hears for himself the loudness of a tone just below the patient's threshold. In this way a quick survey of the patient's sensitivity of hearing, octave by octave, can be obtained— at least by an otologist who himself has at least average hearing.

Tuning forks are particularly useful to the otologist because with them he can test hearing by bone conduction as well as by air conduction. If the rounded tip of the hilt (han-

dle) of a vibrating tuning fork is pressed gently against a person's skull, either at the mastoid process, the forehead, the top of the head, or on a tooth, its sound is heard by bone conduction at pretty much the same loudness, for the average listener, as by air conduction. The following common diagnostic tests are based on this property.

The *Schwabach test* is a test of bone conduction. Instead of holding the vibrating fork close beside the entrance to the ear canal, the otologist places the tip of its hilt gently but firmly against the mastoid process of the skull behind and below the patient's ear. He then notes by how many seconds the hearing of the fork is shortened or prolonged relative to a normal ear, usually his own, in the same environment. "Schwabach-shortened" or "bone-conduction–decreased" means that the patient's bone conduction is not as good as the average. This will be the situation if the patient has a sensorineural hearing loss. If bone conduction is "lengthened" or "increased," a conductive hearing loss is suggested. The patient's hearing by bone conduction may actually be better than the examiner's because a conductive loss protects the bone-conducted tone against masking by air-conducted background noise, and it also prevents the radiation of acoustic energy out from the ear canal after it has reached the inner ear by bone conduction.

The *Rinne test* compares the patient's hearing by bone conduction with the patient's own hearing by air conduction. Like the Schwabach test, it is really a test of how much the ambient noise masks air-conducted as opposed to bone-conducted sound. The hilt of the tuning fork is applied to the mastoid as in the Schwabach test; however, when the patient no longer hears the sound, the fork is held close to the patient's ear instead of near the otologist's ear. If the patient again hears the tone he is said to have a "positive Rinne." It is normal to hear about twice as long by air- as by bone-conduction with the usual initial standard blow. If the patient does not hear the tone again by air, it is a "negative Rinne." The presumption in this case is a middle-ear conductive hearing loss in that ear.

The *Weber test* compares the hearing by bone conduction in the patient's two ears. This test also depends largely on differences in masking by the ambient room noise. The hilt of the vibrating fork is applied to the center of the patient's forehead and he is asked where he hears the tone. If both ears are normal, they will be equally stimulated and equally masked, and the sound will be heard as if it is in the center of the head. If there is conductive loss on one side, the sound is heard better by that ear (by bone conduction, of course). Thus the sound is heard in the abnormal ear, which is less masked. The Weber is said to be "lateralized" to the right or the left, as the case may be. If, however, one ear is normal and the other has a *neural* loss, the Weber is lateralized to the normal side. If the two ears are both abnormal but symmetrically so, the Weber will not be consistently lateralized to either side.

Still another tuning-fork test, directed to detecting the middle-ear conductive impairment, is the *Bing* or occlusion test. It depends on the increase in the loudness of bone-conducted sounds that occurs in the normal ear when the external auditory meatus is occluded. It will be recalled that one of the several pathways and mechanisms of bone conduction is a compression of the middle ear, with consequent movement of the tympanic membrane and ossicles, including the footplate of the stapes. This compression becomes much more effective when the meatus is closed. (Actually the placement of an air-conduction earphone with a flat cushion over the ear produces a significant occlusion effect.) Sounds below 2000 Hz are particularly enhanced. The effect

does *not* depend simply on the exclusion of ambient masking noise from the occluded ear, although this may sometimes contribute to the effect.

The tuning fork, usually 512 Hz, is applied to the mastoid as usual. While the sound is still comfortably loud, the otologist applies the palm of his hand over the auricle, or presses the tragus enough to close the meatus, or inserts the tip of his finger or perhaps an earplug into the meatus. The patient simply reports whether the sound remains the same (Bing-negative) or becomes louder (Bing-positive). (One precaution is to avoid trapping air under the finger or earplug, thereby increasing the air pressure in the meatus and reducing the mobility of the tympanic membrane.)

In Europe many otologists routinely determine bone-conduction thresholds (with the electric audiometer) with the meatus open ("relative" bone-conduction threshold) and also with it occluded ("absolute" bone-conduction threshold). The comparison of absolute with relative bone-conduction thresholds is the equivalent of the Bing test.

Another old (1881) tuning-fork test is the *Gellé test*. This test is intended to detect fixation of the stapes, and depends on changing the air pressure in the external auditory meatus by means of an accessory nozzle, a tube, and a bulb. The sound from the hilt of the tuning fork is delivered through the nozzle or by bone conduction. Changes in pressure diminish the hearing, more for air conduction than for bone conduction and more for negative than for positive pressure in the meatus. Such changes constitute a "positive" result. If the stapes is fixed, there is no change in threshold with change in pressure: the test is "negative." With obstruction of the eustachian tube, negative meatal pressure may *improve* hearing, particularly by air conduction. There is some disagreement whether hearing for low tones is more affected by changes of pressure than medium tones, and it is troublesome to standardize the equipment and procedure precisely, but when properly performed the test is valid and useful.

Many other tuning-fork tests have been suggested, but most of them are variations on the same themes. All of them, including those described, have their pitfalls and difficulties, but their value for initial orientation and for final confirmation, combined with their speed and simplicity, should not be overlooked by the electronically oriented audiologist. It should be noted also that all of these tuning-fork tests can be carried out with an electric audiometer. The advantage of the tuning fork lies in its speed and simplicity.

THE ELECTRIC AUDIOMETER

Definitions

There are several types and classes of electric audiometer. The following definitions and classification are inspired by the draft of a proposed revision of the American National Standard Specifications for Audiometers. As of 1976 the new draft is under consideration by the American National Standards Institute (ANSI), and agreement has been reached on all major points. It probably will be approved by the time this book is in print.

Audiometric measurements can be made with pure tones or with spoken words or sentences. We therefore recognize two major classes of audiometer, namely the *pure-tone audiometer* and the *speech audiometer*. A single instrument may be designed to serve as both types.

Another distinction is *manual* versus *automatic*. This refers to the way in which the test tones or spoken material are selected

and the results recorded. Still another distinction is according to their complexity or the range of auditory functions that they test.

More explicitly a *pure-tone audiometer* provides pure tones at discrete frequencies and controlled output levels. In an *automatic* pure-tone recording audiometer the signal presentations, the frequencies, the levels and the recording of the subject's responses are implemented automatically. Automatic recording audiometers may be either the diagnostic, type I or type II, or the simpler monitoring type. A *speech audiometer* provides means of presenting speech at controlled sound-pressure levels, either through earphones or loudspeakers.

A general classification of audiometers can be based on the number of features, including the range of frequencies and intensities, that a given instrument provides. In the ANSI specifications of 1969 the terms *wide-range*, *limited-range*, and *narrow-range* are employed. These will probably be replaced by terms that refer to the uses to which the instruments are adapted; namely, *diagnostic*, *monitoring*, and *screening* (see Figures 7-1 and 7-2). The special features and primary uses of each class will be considered in detail below, and they are conveniently summarized in Table 7-1.

One class of audiometer defined in the ANSI 1969 specifications but omitted from Table 7-1 is the *group audiometer*. A group audiometer presents either pure tones or spoken words to a group of persons simultaneously. The original speech audiometer (Western Electric 4C) was such an instrument but no other group instrument has ever proved popular.

Three acoustic definitions are important for audiometry. The *sound-pressure level* is understood to refer to the root-mean-square (rms) sound-pressure level developed in a National Bureau of Standards 9-A coupler, which is defined in ANSI S3.6-1969 (R1973).

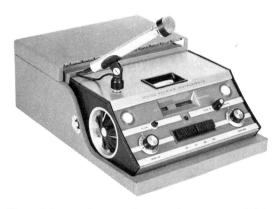

Figure 7-1 A wide-range electric audiometer intended for general diagnostic purposes has air-conduction receivers and also a bone-conduction vibrator (not shown). Masking noise is provided. *(Maico Electronics, Inc.)*

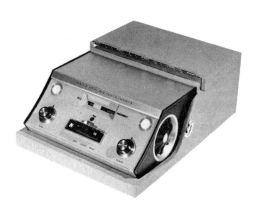

Figure 7-2 A limited-range audiometer, suitable for monitoring or screening, does not have a bone-conduction vibrator; nor does it provide masking noise. Its range of intensities may be restricted and often the frequency range may be, also. *(Maico Electronics, Inc.)*

Other couplers may be used only if suitable comparison data are available. The levels are expressed in decibels relative to 20 μPa. (See Chapter 1.) The *hearing level* is the sound-pressure level relative to a standard audiometric reference level, also given in ANSI specifications. The *hearing-threshold level* of an ear is the number of decibels by which its threshold of audibility exceeds the standard audiometric reference level for the frequency in question.

Common Features of Pure-Tone Audiometers

In a pure-tone audiometer an alternating current of the desired frequency is generated by an electronic oscillator circuit. Standard models provide a series of fixed frequencies in octaves based on 1000 Hz, except for the patient-controlled automatic recording type, which may provide a continuously varying frequency. Intermediate steps in frequency above 500 Hz are provided in most models. The number and choice of frequencies is one basis of defining the classes of audiometers in Table 7-1.

The intensity of sound output is regulated by means of a dial graduated in steps of 5 dB or less. The electric current produces sound in a receiver or in an earphone that is held by a spring headband snugly against the subject's ear. Usually two receivers, carefully matched to one another, are provided, with a switch on the instrument so that the sound can be delivered to either ear at the choice of the operator. Sometimes one of the earphones is a dummy, provided simply to exclude distracting sounds from the ear not under test. The receiver is provided with a rather firm sponge-rubber cushion that makes a good, comfortable acoustic seal against the side of the subject's head. Future diagnostic audiometers will probably provide a range of intensities of 120 dB at the middle frequencies. An additional 10 dB of intensity is provided in some special instruments in use in schools for the deaf, but it is questionable whether the sense of hearing or the sense of feeling is being tested at these very high intensities. A remnant of hearing at such a high level is not very useful even with modern hearing aids. For ordinary testing the range of 120 dB is quite sufficient. Additional

TABLE 7-1
CAPABILITIES OF VARIOUS TYPES OF AUDIOMETER

Features	Advanced Diagnostic[a]	Diagnostic		Monitoring	Screening	Test Objectives
		I	II			
Pure tone: air	125 to	125 to	250 to	500 to	500 to	Determine hearing
Frequency range	8000 Hz	8000 Hz	8000 Hz	6000 Hz	4000 Hz	threshold levels
Intensity range[b]	−10 to	−10 to	−10 to	0 to	0 to	
(500 to 6000 Hz)	110 dB	110 dB	110 dB	70 dB	45 dB	
Pure tone: bone	X	X	X	O		Differentiate
Frequency range	250–4000	250–4000	250–4000			conductive from
Intensity	−10 to 70	−10 to 70	−10 to 70			sensorineural
(1000 to 3000 Hz)						
Masking	X	X	X			Differentiate between ears
Speech test	0 to 90 dB					Establish level of
Air conduction	X	X	O			speech communication
Sound field	X	X	O			Hearing aid evaluation
Intercom. system	X	O				Communicate with subject
Special tests						
Pulsed tone	X	O	O	O	O	
Automatic (Békésy)	X	O	O	O		
ABLB	X	X				Alternate binural loudness balance
SISI	O	O				Short increment sensitivity index

X = required; O = optional.

[a] The Advanced Diagnostic type is not listed as such in the ANSI specifications. It is a diagnostic type 1 instrument with all or nearly all of the optional features.

[b] Intensities given are hearing levels. Lower maximum values are allowed at 125, 250, and 8000 Hz. See Table 7-2.

steps toward either very high or very low levels introduce considerable engineering difficulties.

The reference zero levels constitute a point of special interest and importance and will be discussed in some detail below.

The test tone is turned on and off by the operator. A special switching circuit is pro-vided to cause the current to fade in and out gradually enough to avoid any audible click that might be produced by a sudden start or stop. On the other hand, the rise time is not more than one-tenth (formerly one-half) of a second, so it is quite practical for the opera-tor to use very brief pulses of tone as test sig-nals if he wishes. In the earliest models the test tone faded in and out very gradually and was normally on unless the operator interrupted it by means of the switch. Most modern audiometers can be operated with the tone either normally on or off. The thresholds obtained with the earlier models are practically identical with those obtained with more rapid interruption or pulses, but the subject can usually make up his mind more rapidly and with less effort with the briefer signals. The net result of using rather brief pulses is a saving of time and fatigue on the overall test.

Sometimes a signal circuit is provided whereby the subject holds down a push button as long as he hears the tone and releases it when he ceases to hear. Most audiometrists, however, now prefer to have the subject raise his finger when he hears the tone rather than press a button. The speed and promptness with which the finger is raised give an observant operator much additional information as to the certainty with which the subject feels he hears the tone.

The heart of the audiometer, from the engineer's point of view, is not the generator that determines frequency or the "attenuator" that varies the intensity, since these are now routine in the electronic art; it is the receiver, which converts the electric energy into acoustic energy. It is not easy to design and construct an earphone that is reasonably efficient for all the frequencies we wish to test and will maintain its original efficiency year after year. And the operator is at the mercy of the earphone. If the earphone is put out of adjustment by accidentally falling on the floor, its loss of efficiency in generating the sound will be interpreted as a lack of efficiency of the ear in detecting the sound. The scale on the instrument does not actually measure the sound but only the electric current that generates it. The careful operator therefore periodically tests his own ear, and

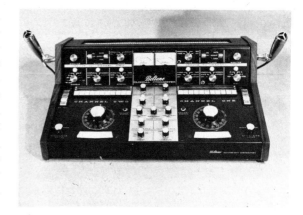

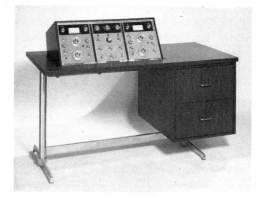

Figure 7-3 For certain tests, such as loudness balance, an audiometer requires two channels. *Above:* In this audiometer, each channel contains a microphone and a VU meter with which to monitor speech. Various other features may include automatic pulsing of the test tone and a "warble" (frequency modulation) of adjustable degree. *(Beltone Hearing Aid Company) Below:* In this two-channel audiometer, the console is mounted as part of a desk-like unit.

if the instrument says that his ear is losing its sensitivity, he tests other presumably normal ears. If most of them show the loss of sensitivity, it is fairly certain that the "calibration" of the audiometer is no longer correct.

An important item for an audiometer intended for diagnostic purposes is a *bone vibrator*, which delivers vibrations to the mastoid process of the temporal bone instead of generating sound waves in an earphone. The same electric circuits are employed with no change except in the scale on which the hearing level is read.

Still another accessory is a circuit that generates a *masking noise* to be delivered to the ear opposite to the one being tested. This may be necessary if the ear being tested is quite hard of hearing and the opposite ear hears well by bone conduction, and it is always required in tests of bone conduction.

The types of masking sound recommended in ANSI S3.6-1969 (R1973) are a narrow band of noise near the frequency of the test tone or a wide band of noise covering at least the range from 250 to 4000 Hz. The latter alternative was usually chosen by manufacturers, but in the proposed revision of the ANSI standard an additional option of weighted random noise will be provided. There will be closer specifications for the spectra of the masking noises and for *effective masking*. ("An audiometer is calibrated in effective masking when, for any frequency, dial markings on the masking-level control indicate the hearing level to which a pure-tone test signal is elevated in the presence of the masking signal in the same ear.") The use of narrow-band masking noise facilitates the calibration in effective masking, and should be a very useful improvement. Narrow-band masking is not appropriate for speech audiometers, for which other alternatives will be specified.

Standardization of Audiometers

The American Standards Association, renamed in 1966 as the United States of America Standards Institute (USASI), and renamed once more in October 1969 as the American National Standards Institute (ANSI) is a voluntary association of manufacturers and consumers, which has written standards for many branches of U.S. industry. These standards are a convenience for all concerned and are regularly made the basis of specifications or procurement both by government and by industry. In the field of acoustics, for example, there are ANSI standards not only on acoustical terminology, but on such items as sound-level meters, octave-band filters, microphones, meters, and methods of sound measurement. These standards are revised from time to time to keep pace with technical progress and the state of the art.

The National Bureau of Standards also cooperated in the development of the American National Standard Specifications for Audiometers, and it preserves the instruments on which the definition of the zero levels for audiometry rests. It serves as the final arbiter in any questions that may arise concerning the accuracy of calibration of new instruments in this country.

In addition to the various national standards organizations, like the American National Standards Institute and the British Standards Institution, there is an International Organization for Standardization (Organization Internationale de Normalisation). The name of this organization is abbreviated "ISO." It is composed of ISO "member bodies" in the various countries, and it develops and issues ISO recommendations for standards in various fields, including acoustics. Actually there is also another very similar affiliated organization, the International Electrotechnical Commission (Commission Électrotechnique Internationale), abbreviated IEC, which develops and issues recommendations for electrical instruments and equipment. Due to this division of interests at the international level one organization, ISO, deals with the reference zero levels for audiometers, because they are related to the sensitivity of human hearing, and its affiliate, IEC, deals with the audiometer as an electroacoustic instrument. The collaboration between ISO and IEC is so close that we may think of them as virtually a single organization.

Neither ISO nor IEC has any authority to enforce its recommendations. Like the American National Standards Institute, they are voluntary associations. They issue recommendations on the basis of a consensus that must represent close, if not complete, unanimity among the national member bodies, but for each country the only valid standard is the national standard of that country. In general, however, the ISO and IEC recommendations serve as models and are usually incorporated almost completely into the corresponding national standards. In some countries the member bodies are government bureaus, and their national standards have the force of government regulations. This is not the case in the United States.

As noted above, the American National Standard Specifications for Audiometers of 1969 are now (1976) in process of revision by a working group, sponsored by the Acoustical Society of America. This group consists of representatives of the American Otological Society, the American Academy of Ophthalmology and Otolaryngology, American Speech and Hearing Association, National Bureau of Standards, audiometric manufacturers, and other interested individuals.

The revised audiometer standard covers in detail such things as the standard reference levels for pure tones and speech signals, test frequencies, accuracy, distortion, masking sounds, and safety requirements. The specified standard reference threshold levels values for the various earphones on a 9A coupler are in agreement with those of the International Organization for Standardization as published in ISO 389-1975. The new standard provides additional requirements for more complex audiometers and provides specifications for the measurement of per-formance. The basic requirements for performance, accuracy, and safety are the same for all instruments.

In the past few years some progress has been made in determining the reference threshold levels for bone conduction. American National Standard Artificial Head-Bone for the Calibration of Audiometer Bone Vibrators, ANSI S3.13-1972, contains values for headbone impedance and also contains specifications for bone vibrators.

Considerable attention has also been given to the safety of audiometers to assure consistency with the pending American National Standard on Safety of Medical and Dental Equipment. Because of the influence of Underwriters Laboratories on medical facilities, efforts have been coordinated to be consistent with their requirements. One of the problems encountered is that the earphones specified in the audiometer standard (ANSI S3.6-1969) all have exposed metal that may come in contact with the patient. These earphones cannot meet Underwriters Laboratories Specifications UL 544 for Medical and Dental Equipment. Earphones with a plastic case have now been developed, and the new threshold values for these earphones will soon be determined, as explained below.

In doing audiometric testing, the result will be dependent upon the test method and the acoustic environment in which the test is being conducted. To minimize the intertest differences due to test methods, a new ANSI standard, "Method for Manual Pure-Tone Threshold Audiometry," is being prepared. This standard will outline the sequence for frequency and intensity presentation and define the method of determining the threshold of hearing of the patient.

The Reference Zero Level for Audiometers: The Audiogram

When the famous Western Electric Company 2A audiometer was designed in the

Bell Telephone Laboratories in the early 1920s, a basic decision was made concerning the reference zero level. An obvious choice from the engineering point of view would have been the dyne per square centimeter, the same for all frequencies. Then the sensitivity curve for hearing would have been plotted like the threshold curves in Figures 2-3, 2-4, and 2-5. This form of plotting facilitates comparison of human hearing with other sounds, as in Figure 2-3, or specifically

with the average intensity of speech, as in Figure 7-4. However the otological consultant to the project, Dr. Edmund P. Fowler, saw the new instrument as a *diagnostic tool* for the otologist, and wished to emphasize the *deviation from normal* of each subject. He believed, probably quite correctly, that this form of presentation of the results would promote the acceptance and general use of the electric audiometer by otologists. Dr. Fowler's counsel prevailed, and the inten-

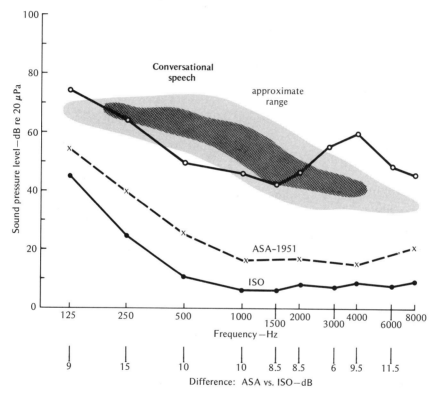

Figure 7-4   The two lower curves show the ISO recommended reference zero levels (solid line and dots) and the ASA-1951 levels (dashed line and crosses). The numerical differences in decibels are given beneath the frequency scale. These *differences* are the same regardless of the type of earphone or coupler employed. The actual sound pressures plotted are for the WE 705-A earphone and NBS 9A coupler, and are the same as the data points shown by crosses (+) in Figure 2-5.

The upper curve (solid with open circles) is the hypothetical threshold curve of a man with impaired hearing, discussed in the text. The shaded area (dark and light) shows

the approximate range of the intensities and frequencies of the sounds of conversational speech at 1 meter. It is not strictly accurate to plot such *field* measurements of acoustic pressure on a graph of *coupler* pressures, for reasons explained in Chapter 2, but the orders of magnitude are correct, nevertheless, and the comparison is valid for something as poorly defined as the area of conversational speech. The intensities measured from moment to moment would fall most often in the darkly shaded area, less frequently in the lighter area, and only rarely either above or below the light area.

sity dial of the audiometer was labeled "hearing loss," meaning "decibels less sensitive than normal." The format of the audiogram (Figure 7-5) was devised with the reference zero level represented by a straight horizontal line near the top of the sheet and hearing loss (poorer hearing) plotted downward.

The next step was to determine experimentally for each frequency the voltage to be applied to the earphones that would produce a sound at the threshold of normal hearing. The particular earphone employed was the WE 705A, which was specially designed for stability of performance. Dr. Fowler selected a group of 85 young adults who worked in the offices or laboratories of the Bell Telephone Laboratories, people whom he found to have no signs or symptoms of disease of the ear. Such persons we now call "otologically normal subjects" (defined in the ISO Standard 389-1975 as "a person in a normal state of health who is free from all signs or symptoms of ear disease and from wax in the ear canal, and has no history of undue exposure to noise"). The engineers at the Bell Telephone Laboratories then measured the thresholds of the 85 subjects with the laboratory model of the new audiometer. The actual readings were the voltages that had to be applied to produce a barely audible tone at each frequency. Each instrument was adjusted or "calibrated" so that when the intensity dial (later labeled "hearing loss") was set at zero decibels, the appropriate voltage was delivered to the earphone.

In the actual manufacture of audiometers, production control of earphones is maintained by measuring the acoustic pressure produced by each earphone in a small cavity known as a coupler or "artificial ear." The cavity is about the same size, 6 cm³, as the human external canal and middle ear plus the space under the diaphragm of an earphone, but the walls are metal and the shape

is simple. The pressures produced in this "coupler" are not quite the same as the pressures produced in the ear by the same earphone. The coupler pressures are, however, *reproducible* and serve to show that one earphone of a particular model is like another. A coupler was standardized by the National Bureau of Standards, and the present ANSI standard for the zero hearing level is "stored" in the form of sets of acoustic pressures produced by certain models of earphone in an "NBS-9A coupler."

The actual set of threshold pressures, measured in the NBS-9A coupler, have turned out to be very close to later laboratory studies at the Bell Telephone Laboratories and elsewhere and also to the values finally recommended in 1964 by the International Organization for Standardization. The latter values are plotted as the lower curve in Figure 7-4. The pressures differ slightly from one another for different frequencies from 500 Hz upward, and are significantly greater at 250 and 125 Hz than for higher frequencies.

In Figure 7-4 the upper solid curve shows an abnormal threshold curve such as might be obtained from a patient with a moderate conductive hearing loss. The approximate range of frequency and intensity of the sounds of conversational speech are also shown on the same diagram, and it is evident that he will not hear the higher speech frequencies, which are relatively weak, although the lower speech sounds lie mostly above his threshold. As pointed out in Chapter 2, this comparison of sound in an open acoustic field with sound pressures measured in a coupler is not exact, but as explained in Chapter 2 the error is only a very few decibels, and the diagram illustrates a principle.

In Figure 7-5 the same threshold curve is plotted on an audiogram. The horizontal zero line represents the ISO curve of Figure

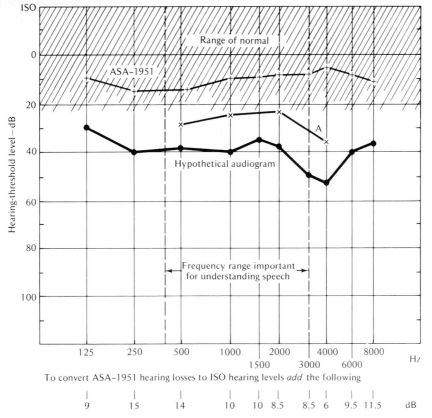

To convert ASA-1951 hearing losses to ISO hearing levels *add* the following

9	15	14		10	10 8.5	8.5 6	9.5 11.5	dB

Figure 7-5   On this ISO audiogram blank are shown (1) the reference zero level (horizontal at 0 dB), (2) the "range of normal," extending from the faintest tone provided by an audiometer to a transition zone between 15 and 22 dB hearing level, (3) the ASA-1951 reference zero level for pure-tone audiometers, (4) the U.S. Army "profile A," from AR 40–501 (see Chapter 9), (5) a hypothetical "flat" audiogram with a slight "4000 Hz notch," and (6) the range of frequencies important for understanding speech. The audiogram points do not fall exactly on the horizontal guide lines because the thresholds are supposed to have been measured on an audiometer calibrated to the ASA-1951 standard. The "hearing losses" were converted to ISO hearing threshold levels by adding, at each frequency, the number of decibels given below the frequency scale. For a discussion of the range of normal, see Chapter 9. For otologically normal young adults the 95th percentile lies at about 12 dB HL (see Figure 2-5), but for older people it is lower, particularly at high frequencies.

In this figure the hearing threshold curve of 7-4 is plotted in the conventional format of the audiogram. The ISO reference levels are now the horizontal zero line. The positions of the ASA-1951 zeros relative to ISO are also plotted.

The range of normal hearing is not precisely defined (see Chapter 9) but extends to 15 dB (ISO) and shades off gradually over the next 10 dB or thereabouts. This form of shading on an audiogram chart is a useful reminder.

7-4. The hearing-threshold levels are the differences between the ISO points and the actual threshold levels, plotted with increasing hearing-threshold levels (poorer hearing) downward. (These values are read directly from the dial of the audiometer.) In this diagram the emphasis is on the difference in sensitivity of the patient from "otologically normal subjects" of the 18- to 30-year group, and not on how well the patient hears ordinary speech.

In this way the reference zero hearing levels of the audiometer came to be associated with "normal hearing." We will consider in

Chapter 9 the unfortunate and unforeseen difficulties that have arisen because of the various interpretations and connotations of the word "normal." Suffice it to say here that the word normal should be used only to refer to the subjects, not the hearing-threshold levels. We should say that *the reference zero hearing levels of the audiometer are the average (or mean or median) of the thresholds of otologically normal persons between 18 and 30 years of age.*

In the 1930s each manufacturer determined experimentally his own set of reference zero levels, just as the Bell Telephone Laboratories had done for the Western Electric Company, and inevitably differences appeared among them. When the Council on Physical Therapy of the AMA prepared its first set of Minimal Requirements for Audiometers it adopted for the reference zero levels the values that had been determined in a field health survey that had been conducted by the United States Public Health Service (USPHS) in 1935–1936. The audiometric equipment, including the soundproof booths, was excellent. The survey was planned to obtain a cross section of the population of the United States, both rural and urban. Questionnaires and physical examinations made it possible to select from the data the threshold values for otologically normal subjects between 18 and 30 years of age. The modal values for each frequency were chosen, and later (1951) became the American Standard reference levels. These values, as coupler pressures, are plotted in Figure 7-4.

Those responsible for this choice were aware, of course, that the new reference levels were higher than the original Western Electric 2A values, but the difference was ascribed to the more representative selection of subjects in the USPHS survey, and they were accepted without question by otologists in the United States. The values seemed "realistic" in clinical practice.

Soon after World War II, however, when electric audiometers began to be used extensively in Europe and when various countries considered establishing national standards for audiometers, widespread dissatisfaction with the American Standard reference values appeared. Studies in England of the threshold of hearing, mentioned in Chapter 2, were carried out, and a British Standard, B.S. 2497 (1954), quite different from the American Standard, was based on them. Also independent studies were made in France, Germany, the U.S.S.R., and by several investigators in the United States.

The problem of the "normal" threshold of hearing was taken up by the ISO in 1955, and a recommendation (R389) entitled "Standard Reference Zero for the Calibration of Pure-Tone Audiometers" was issued in 1964. The values were based on 15 published studies (nearly half of them carried out in the United States) that seemed comparable in technique, precautions, and the selection of subjects. It is important to note that the subjects were not specially trained or experienced listeners, and the only "selection" was to reject those who were not "otologically normal."

The results of these 15 studies were in very good agreement. It was necessary to determine experimentally the relations between the coupler pressures produced by the different earphones in the different couplers used in France, Germany, the United Kingdom, the United States, and the U.S.S.R. In the ISO recommendation, values are given for five different combinations, but each one represents the same loudness produced in the human ear. Now these ISO values have been incorporated in the 1969 standard and they have been almost universally adopted by all European countries.

After the publication of the ISO values, the results of another U.S. Public Health Service survey became available. The data were collected in 1960–1962. The population samples were chosen with great care, and the hearing levels have been analyzed with respect to age, sex, race, region, and area of residence. The data that most closely correspond to the previous USPHS survey are those for the hearing in the better ear of men and women in the 18- to 24-year age group. These data are shown in Figure 4-7. From 1000 to 4000 Hz the average value is 3 dB (ISO). If the worse ears are included, the average hearing-threshold level is about 4 dB. (At 500 and 6000 Hz the divergences are greater, and no measurements were made in the survey at 125, 250, or 8000 Hz.)

The differences between the ASA-1951 levels and ISO average about 8 dB from 1000 through 4000 Hz. Thus the USPHS survey data fall between the ASA and the ISO reference levels but somewhat closer to ISO than to ASA-1951.

The reasons for the difference between ASA-1951 and ISO have been debated at length, and the answers are not very clear. Evidently less than half of the difference can be attributed to the use of restricted populations (ISO) as opposed to a national survey with proper demographic sampling. Perhaps the audiometric technique and the time taken to determine each end point or perhaps the motivations of the subjects are the important differences. No one is sure (see also Chapter 9).

(This rather lengthy section dealing with the reference levels for audiometers has been retained from the third edition for historical reasons. The ISO-recommended values are now firmly established in ANSI and most national standards. It is important, however, that anyone dealing with American audiometric data collected before 1969 be fully aware of the difference between the present reference levels and those of ASA-1951. For example, the tabulations of hearing levels by the U.S. National Health Survey dated as late as 1970 are all based on ASA-1951.)

Calibration for Bone Conduction

The bone vibrator is more difficult to standardize than the air-conduction receiver, and bone-conduction tests are more difficult to carry out properly. Skulls and skin differ to an annoying degree in their ability to conduct sound, and the force with which the bone-conduction receiver is applied to the mastoid is important. Some audiologists prefer to apply it to the forehead instead. The ear not under test must be masked by noise delivered through an air-conduction receiver. The ear under test must be open to the room. This makes it more vulnerable to masking by room noise than an ear that is snugly covered by an air-conduction receiver.

The new ANSI specifications for audiometers will contain details concerning the bone vibrator. The reference levels for its calibration are already available in ANSI S3.13-1972 (Artificial Head-Bone for the Calibration of Audiometer Bone Vibrators). In the meantime the calibration has been left to each manufacturer. The standard practice has usually been to label the scale for bone-conduction hearing levels in such a way that there will be no air-bone gap when air conduction and bone conduction are determined on subjects with no conductive (middle-ear) impairment. The ears may be normal or may have pure sensorineural impairment.

Like the air-conduction part of the equipment, the bone-vibrator portion should be tested periodically on presumably normal subjects. Calibrations are never permanent, and one of the great weaknesses of audiometry in the United States has been neglect of recalibration. *Annual recalibration by the*

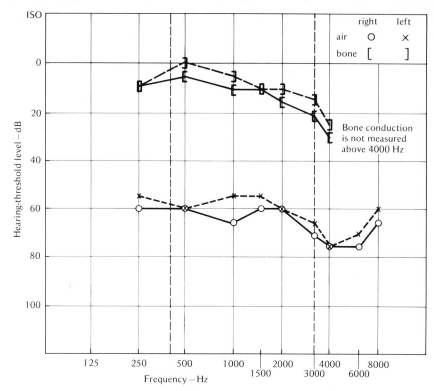

Figure 7-6 These air-conduction and bone-conduction audiograms show the hearing-threshold levels in a hypothetical case of symmetrical middle-ear hearing loss with a slight additional inner-ear loss at the higher frequencies. Most of the bone-conduction thresholds are within normal limits. Note that each audiogram blank should carry the notation ISO (or ANSI) and also the code of symbols to be employed. The latter are not standardized. Often arrow heads (< and >) are used instead of brackets for bone conduction and often the convention for right and left is reversed. It is helpful to use color with red = right. This is a universal convention. Note also that it is difficult to make an audiometric chamber quiet enough to measure zero hearing-threshold levels by bone conduction at 250 Hz and particularly at 125 Hz.

manufacturer is strongly advised, particularly if audiometric data are to be used in relation to insurance or other compensation.

Automatic Audiometry

Probably the first automatic audiometer was the instrument developed by Békésy in 1947. This instrument introduced the novel feature of control of intensity by the subject, combined with graphic recording of his adjustments. The frequency of the test tone is automatically increased, slowly and steadily, as the audiogram chart advances under the recording pen. The patient presses a button when he hears the tone. The tone may be steady or else interrupted two or three times a second (see Chapter 8). The intensity of the signal is gradually reduced as long as the button is held down. When the subject no longer hears the tone, he releases the button. Now the signal becomes stronger and stronger until the subject presses the button again. Thus the pen zigzags up and down across the chart, reversing its direction each time the button is pressed or released. Usually there is an interval of 5 to 10 dB between the pressing (hears) and release (does not hear) of the button, as in Figure 7-7, but this range becomes very narrow in an ear that shows loudness recruitment.

The Békésy audiometer has been put to use in many research laboratories and hearing centers. It has yielded a vast amount of new experimental information on such topics as masking and auditory fatigue. Its accuracy is comparable with or better than clinical pure-tone audiometry. The proposed ANSI specifications for audiometers include a section on the automatic recording audiometer, with detailed specifications concerning the rate of frequency change, hearing level control, and the pulsing of the tone.

The field of automatic audiometry at the present time (1977) is practically reduced to two representatives of the subject-controlled type, at present known as the Békésy and the Rudmose, respectively. (In the next ANSI specifications the names Békésy and Rudmose will probably not appear.) The Békésy audiometer (Figure 7-8) provides either a continuously changing frequency ("sweep frequency") or a single selected frequency, and it yields a graph of the adjustments of intensity made by the subject. The Rudmose instrument (Figure 7-9) tests each ear at six predetermined frequencies and records the thresholds on a card. With each type the operator only needs to start the machine.

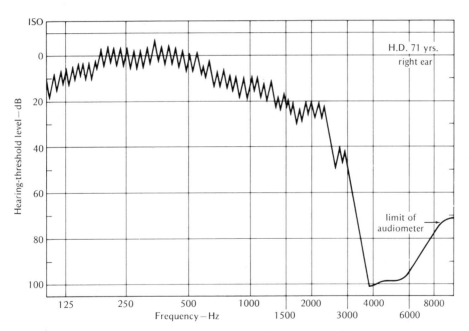

Figure 7-7 Audiogram produced by an automatic patient-controlled (Békésy type) audiometer *(Grason-Stadler Co., Type E-800).* The chart moved steadily to the left as the frequency of the test tone changed continuously at the rate of 1 octave per min. The pen moved up or down at a rate of 2.5 dB per second. The direction of movement of the pen was upward (less intense) as long as the patient held his switch closed ("I hear the tone") but was downward (more intense) when the switch was open ("Don't hear the tone").

The subject for this test has an abrupt high-frequency sensorineural hearing loss beginning just below 3000 Hz. He hears nothing above 3600 Hz in this ear. Part of the loss from 500 to 2300 Hz is due to presbycusis (71 years). The results of a monaural loudness balance test of this ear, 3000 vs. 2000 Hz, are shown in Figure 8-8 (seven years earlier). This ear does not show the narrowing of the trace that is very often associated with recruitment.

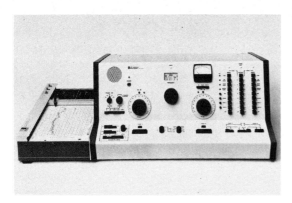

Figure 7-8 This complete diagnostic two-channel audiometer incorporates the recording patient-control principle as one of its options. The latter may be used either at a fixed frequency to study changes of threshold with time or with steadily changing frequency to trace an audiogram like that shown in Figure 7-7. An audiometer with this feature is usually known as a Békésy audiometer. *(Grason-Stadler instrument, courtesy of GenRad)*

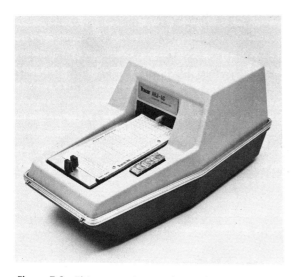

Figure 7-9 This automatic recording audiometer uses the patient-control principle to test hearing at six frequencies in each ear. It does not require an operator except to start the machine. It is usually known as a Rudmose audiometer. *(Tracor, Inc.)*

The Békésy instrument is versatile and well suited to diagnostic and research use, and the Rudmose instrument is particularly adapted to monitoring audiometry.

Monitoring Audiometry and Identification Audiometry

The CHABA Council published, as part of the report of the meeting of 1955, a summary of the purposes and objectives of audiometry in the armed forces. The problems are the same as for audiometry in industry. In this summary "monitoring audiometry" was first formally defined. A later report (1967) of CHABA Working Group 43, concerned with intraservice standardization of audiometric tests, employs also the term "identification audiometry." The distinction between these two terms is stated in the following note:

Identification audiometry, or reference audiometry, deals with the initial preinduction tests that establish [a man's] reference hearing level. Recommendations for identification audiometry also hold for monitoring audiometry which deals with periodic check-ups.

The 1967 report strongly recommends individual automatic audiometry of a type that makes unnecessary any intensity adjustment by the tester.

We quote from the report of 1955.

PURPOSES AND OBJECTIVES OF AUDIOMETRY

The purposes and objectives of audiometry in the Armed Forces, including their civilian employees, fall into five major categories:

1. to select or reject men as a part of the regular initial physical examination;
2. to provide information for the otologist concerning the extent and nature, the probable cause, and the progress of individual hearing losses in relation to the disease and to the effectiveness of treatment and preventive measures;
3. to establish the amount of hearing loss for compensation purposes, including the determination of the original state of hearing before any service-connected or employment-connected hearing loss has developed;

4. to enable personnel officers to determine whether certain individuals are qualified for certain military specialties that involve special kinds of hearing ability;
5. to obtain new information as to (a) the causes and the prevention of hearing loss; (b) criteria for hazards to hearing; and (c) the effectiveness of particular tests and instruments for accomplishing the above objectives.

A clear distinction must be made between: (1) the kind of hearing test; (2) the way in which the test is administered; and (3) the particular instrument or technical means that embodies both the chosen test and the chosen method of administration. Not all types of hearing test will suit all of these purposes equally well. There is at the present time no single "best" test of hearing, and much less is there any single "best" instrument for administering hearing tests in all situations. The kind of test best suited for each purpose will depend upon the kind of information that must be obtained from the test.

For example, the most generally useful kind of hearing test is pure-tone threshold audiometry by air conduction. This was developed originally for diagnostic medical purposes and is also well suited for screening at induction centers, for monitoring hearing conservation programs, for estimating disablement and appropriate compensation, and for many types of medical research. Another kind of hearing test is speech audiometry, including tests of ability to hear speech in noise. These special tests are appropriate for determining special hearing abilities needed in particular military specialties.

It is assumed that a pure-tone test of hearing is desired. There are a number of ways in which pure-tone tests can be administered, each with its advantages and disadvantages. Furthermore, the different choices are not all mutually exclusive, but can be combined in many ways, just as an aircraft can be designed for combat, transport or reconnaissance, may be large or small, may be piloted or a robot drone, and may be powered by reciprocating, jet or turbo-prop engines.

Among methods and types of pure-tone audiometry there are major choices that must be made between: (1) screening audiometry vs. monitoring audiometry vs. diagnostic audiometry, which implies a choice between a pass-fail test, a limited audiogram, or medically oriented audiometry including complete audiograms; (2) individual audiometry vs. group audiometry; and (3) manual vs. semiautomatic or fully automatic audiometry.

As to the means of embodying the chosen type and method in an actual instrument there are several choices at the engineering level, such as between electronic oscillators vs. tests recorded on discs or magnetic tape. The various choices listed above are more or less independent but, just as in the cases of aircraft, certain useful combinations are already well established. Audiometry was developed as a medical tool to assist in diagnosis and for this purpose the complete audiogram individually administered is universally employed. Furthermore, nearly all audiometers for diagnostic audiometry are manually operated and contain electronic oscillators. Semiautomatic recording audiometers for diagnostic purposes are under development, however, and may soon prove to be a useful supplementary tool in certain situations. The medical interest in diagnostic audiometry seem to lie in the development of new audiometric tests, rather than in new ways to facilitate the administration of pure-tone threshold audiometry.

For audiometry, as for aircraft, the choice of purpose is primary and the way of accomplishing the purpose depends on a balance of many factors, which include expense, personnel, and the availability of a particular instrument of established merit. The development of a means or instrument may make feasible a method that was previously not possible or practical. Such development is often an essential step, but a careful review of both old methods and new developments is mandatory before commitment is made on a large scale. There have been important recent developments in pure-tone audiometry for survey, monitoring, compensation and particularly for screening purposes. Such large-scale audiometry as is obviously required by the Armed Forces should be greatly facilitated by such new methods and instruments for group and individual pure-tone audiometry, both automatic and semiautomatic.

New methods and instruments alone will not insure good audiometry. Three other requirements are absolutely essential for *all* forms of audiometry. They are: (1) adequate acoustic environment, which means specially sound proofed, properly located booths and/or rooms to house the instruments and subjects; (2) trained personnel to administer the tests or to service any automatic devices that may replace the trained audiometrist; and (3) provision, both instrumentally and administratively, for periodic verification of the accuracy of audiometers in the field.

The uncertainties as to what are the best methods of audiometry for the Armed Forces appear to arise from the interplay of several factors. The most important factor is the recent laudable trend toward pure-tone audiometry as a required test of hearing to replace the outmoded voice and coin-click tests. The trend establishes a demand for audiometry on a large scale, but for audiometry that is quite different from the elaborate diagnostic audiometry that has for some time been employed as an adjunct to a medical specialty. Yet the concepts and the instruments for audiometry were developed for just these medical diagnostic purposes.

More recently screening audiometry, and group audiometry as a way of performing such screening, has been developed. Screening audiometry arose as a part of preventive medicine with particular orientation to the conservation of hearing in school children. The objective here was to identify rapidly those children who require closer examination and perhaps medical treatment. Such audiometry is roughly equivalent to the old voice tests and it has been rather taken for granted that it is the most appropriate type of audiometry for induction centers where a quick pass-or-fail test of hearing adequacy is the primary requirement. Screening audiometry, like diagnostic audiometry, is now a familiar and well-established concept.

An intermediate type of audiometry that we here term "monitoring audiometry" has more recently been developed in connection with conservation of hearing programs in industry. Its objectives are twofold. One is to establish the state of hearing of a relatively large number of individuals and to provide reference audiograms from which subsequent changes in their hearing are measured. The reference audiograms, particularly if they are pre-employment or so-called pre-placement audiograms, may be used to determine subsequent liability for later changes in hearing in connection with workmen's compensation. Its other objective is to detect changes in the hearing of individuals, relative to their reference audiograms, before the hearing losses become a practical handicap. Monitoring audiometry thus gives warning in time for instituting effective protective measures, such as the reduction of the noise itself, the reduction of the noise exposure of the individual or the use of individual protective measures.

Monitoring audiometry is more restricted than diagnostic audiometry. Only air-conduction tests are required for monitoring audiometry and a more restricted range of frequencies and intensities [is] sufficient. It differs from screening audiometry, however, in that it must measure auditory acuity and not merely give a pass-or-fail result. Usually, within the range that it covers, it must yield an audiogram comparable in accuracy with a diagnostic audiogram. The restricted range of a monitoring audiometer favors the development of group and of automatic or semi-automatic methods of administration. On the other hand, the necessity for accuracy and for an audiogram that is complete within the chosen range imposes serious difficulties both in the design of automatic instruments (particularly automatic group instruments) and in insuring their continued accuracy.

It seems clear that at present it is feasible to design and develop screening audiometers and monitoring audiometers that will expedite and make practical the screening and/or the monitoring of large numbers of individuals within reasonable limits of time, expense, space and trained personnel. It is not clear, however, that the same instrument should be expected to perform both functions. It is also possible that all monitoring audiometry need not be done in just the same way. In some situations an automatic individual audiometer, in other situations a manually operated group audiometer may have clear and overriding practical advantages. The general concepts of screening, monitoring, and diagnostic audiometry are well established, but there are several audiometric tests that fall in each class. There are various means or instruments for administering a given test and these differ in respect to expense, space, time and personnel required.

Reduced Screening

Reduced screening employs 4000 Hz as a single monitor frequency to detect the beginning of hearing loss in situations that involve hazardous noise exposure. It is at this frequency that the first permanent threshold shift is noticed in exposure to most industrial or military noises. This shift produces the well-known "4000-Hz notch." *Single-frequency screening* at 4000 Hz may greatly simplify and expedite routine monitoring audiometry. It is very quick, and it has the great advantage of not requiring an acoustic environment any quieter than that of the average office. Some audiologists prefer to employ a second frequency, usually 2000 Hz, to back up the single-frequency test at 4000 Hz. Of course, all soldiers or workers whose hearing levels are found to lie above the screening limit, whatever limit may be chosen, must then be tested at all the regular monitor frequencies, and, if the loss is confirmed, should be given a full otological examination and diagnostic audiometry.

At the present writing opinion is still divided as to whether *reduced screening* at two or perhaps three frequencies is sufficiently reliable to be used to expedite conservation of hearing programs for schoolchildren as well as for adults.

The Pittsburgh survey of hearing in children, mentioned earlier in this chapter, showed that even complete pure-tone audiograms were not as effective as had been hoped in identifying the ears with otological abnormalities that might be helped by proper treatment or preventive measures.

Frequencies for Audiometers

When audiometry was new emphasis was placed on the measurement of hearing for very low tones, such as 64 Hz, and very high tones, such as 16,000 Hz. The trend over the years has been to concentrate attention on the range from 500 to 6000 Hz (see Figure 7-10). It gradually became clear that measurements at the extreme frequencies are unreliable. At the high frequencies there are technical difficulties due to resonances in ears and earphones, and at the low frequencies it is expensive to provide adequate exclusion of sound from audiometric booths at 250 Hz and below. Furthermore, the hearing levels for the whole lower half of the frequency range, from 1000 Hz down, can be very well predicted from the hearing level at either 500 or 1000 Hz. 4000 Hz is important as the most sensitive indicator of high-tone loss. The otologist may desire measurements at 250 Hz and perhaps at 8000 Hz, but for screening, monitoring, and identification these frequencies are quite unnecessary. More important are the intermediate frequencies of 1500 Hz (see Figure 7-10) and particularly of 3000 and 6000 Hz.

The frequencies for audiometers required

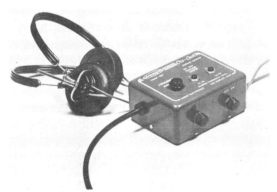

Figure 7-10   A simple, two-tone (2000 and 4000 Hz) narrow-range audiometer with only two levels of output can be made very compact indeed. *(Ambco Electronics)*

in the proposed ANSI standard on audiometers and those generally used for certain particular purposes are given in Table 7-2.

Noise Levels in Audiometric Booths

In all audiometric work it is assumed that the tests are carried out in a room that is quiet enough that the background noise does not interfere with the test. This is not a very difficult condition to meet if the patients are all very hard of hearing, as they are in a school for the deaf. If, however, we wish to measure normal or nearly normal hearing, special sound treatment for both the exclusion and the absorption of unwanted background noise is necessary. Prefabricated audiometric booths (see Figure 7-11) are available commercially, and, in general, have proved more satisfactory than reconstruction of a room in an existing building.

In a new building, however, acoustical engineers can design satisfactorily quiet rooms for audiometry at reasonable cost if they are consulted early enough in the planning. Sometimes the problem is very difficult for the acoustical engineer, as when the audiometric rooms must be located near washrooms, elevators, ventilating fans, or other machinery. The low frequencies are the most difficult and the most expensive to exclude.

The expense of a satisfactory booth will also depend critically on just what kind of audiometry is to be done in it. Are we content with measuring thresholds down to (but not below) 10 dB (ISO), that is, the old ASA-1951 zero? Such measurements are quite sufficient for monitoring audiometry in either military or industrial situations. Will an earphone always be over the ear under test or will we want to measure bone-conduction thresholds with an open ear canal? Do we

TABLE 7-2
REQUIRED FREQUENCIES (Hz) AND MAXIMUM HEARING LEVELS (dB HL) OF AUDIOMETERS

Class and Purpose											
Audiometers											
Diagnostic I	125	250	500	750	1000	1500	2000	3000	4000	6000	8000 Hz
	75	90	←————— 110 —————→								90 dB
Diagnostic II		250	500	750	1000	1500	2000	3000	4000	6000	8000 Hz
		90	←————— 110 —————→								90 dB
Monitoring			500		1000		2000	3000	4000	6000	
			←————— 70 —————→								
Screening			500		1000		2000		4000		
			←————— 45 —————→								
Military physical standards (U.S. Army)			500		1000		2000		4000		
Calculation of hearing handicap (AAOO rule)			500		1000		2000				

Intensity levels are ANSI (1969) hearing levels (dB HL). Data on audiometers are taken from proposed ANSI specifications as of 1976.

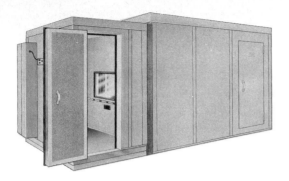

Figure 7-11 Prefabricated sound-treated booths provide the quiet that is needed for accurate determination of auditory thresholds. The subject sits in a separate compartment from the tester. Both compartments are ventilated, but without raising the ambient noise level sufficiently to affect the desired threshold measurements. Specifications for such levels are given by the American National Standards Institute. *(Industrial Acoustics Company, Inc.)*

A recent development that may assist materially in carrying out audiometric tests when the ambient noise is still a little above the desired standard levels is an earphone that provides *a circumaural noise-excluding shield in addition to the standard flat MX41/AR cushion that is applied against the auricle.* This device is known as an Otocup (Figure 7-12). The circumaural seal is made by means of a fluid-filled doughnut-shaped sac attached to the plastic shield. The advantage of the Otocup is that the earphone can be calibrated on the NBS 9A coupler. An alternative uses only the circumaural seal. The volume of air enclosed is more than the standard 6 cc, and coupler calibration is difficult above 2000 Hz. This form is excellent for communication in noisy situations but is not suited to precise audiometry.

want to measure thresholds at 125 and 250 Hz for diagnostic purposes, or will we be content to start at 500 Hz, as in monitoring audiometry?

Of course, the amount of sound treatment needed depends on the sound levels expected outside as well as on the permissible levels inside. The outside levels depend on local conditions, but for the guidance of acoustical engineers American National Standard Criteria for Background Noise in Audiometer Rooms, ANSI S3.1-1960 (R 1971), tells what octave-band sound levels are permissible if we wish to measure hearing levels down to 10 dB (ISO). At present (1976) this standard is undergoing another revision to provide for two or three alternatives for different minimum hearing levels, such as 0 dB and even -10 dB (ISO). The latter specification is difficult to meet unless the booth is located in a quiet area, but it is necessary if the threshold of hearing is to be measured in children. On the other hand, the requirements for screening audiometry at perhaps 20 dB are relatively easy to meet.

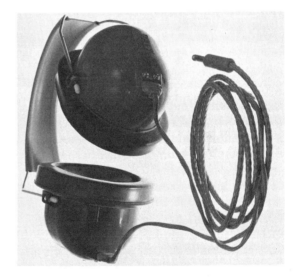

Figure 7-12 The Rudmose RA-125 Otocups are earphone enclosures which allow the standard MX-41/AR audiometric cushions to rest against the pinna in normal fashion but provide noise attenuation by an outer plastic case with a conforming seal that fits around the edge of the case and makes circumaural contact with the side of the subject's head. Such devices supplement sound-treated booths in reducing background noise for audiometric tests. *(Tracor, Inc.)*

Tests of Tolerance

A simple audiometric test that is very important in the selection of a hearing aid is the test of tolerance for loud sounds. It is usually performed with pure tones at 500, 1000, and 2000 Hz. One of the most important choices in the selection of a hearing aid relates to its maximum acoustic output, and this is determined by the subject's tolerance for loud sound (see Chapter 11). There are definite advantages in using a hearing aid that comes close to but never quite reaches the threshold of real discomfort.

The sensations of discomfort, of tickling in the ear, and of pain that are produced by very loud sounds have already been mentioned in Chapter 2 in the description of the auditory area. Here again, individuals differ as to the intensities of sound that merely cause discomfort, tickle, and pain. There seem to be tough ears and tender ears, or, rather, tough men and tender men. (Women, by the way, seem to be just as tough as men in this respect.) The man with one tough ear usually has another tough ear on the other side of his head. This toughness can be increased by simply listening to loud sounds for a while, even if the sounds are never made so loud as to tickle or become definitely uncomfortable. The increase in tolerance is likely to be greatest if the ear is unusually tender to begin with.

A test for tolerance is very simple in principle. It is like an audiometer or a speech test except that very loud sounds are used. Special apparatus may be required to make the sounds loud enough without distortion. The intensity is increased gradually until the listener indicates that he has had enough. Any such test, however, must be conducted with care, particularly on anyone with impaired hearing who has not yet become once more accustomed to hearing loud sounds. He may be startled, antagonized, or even frightened if the sound is made too loud too rapidly.

It was surprising to learn through a series of experiments conducted about 1944 at the Central Institute for the Deaf that the tolerance thresholds of the hard-of-hearing are on the average the same as those of normal ears. The hard-of-hearing may scatter a little more widely above and below the average, with some ears more tender and some tougher than the usual run of normal ears, but the differences are much smaller than had been expected.

Speech Audiometry

Speech audiometry supplements pure-tone audiometry, although, as we shall see, it tests more than the ear. Its chief diagnostic use, as we shall see in Chapter 8, relates to impairments of the central nervous system. But if a *test of the overall performance* of a subject in hearing, understanding, and responding to speech is desired, the directness and high face validity of speech audiometry appeal to audiologists and to subjects alike. They all *like* speech tests. Also the tests for threshold, usually called the *speech-reception threshold* (SRT), have proved to be very reliable, and they have the advantage of giving the result as a single number.

Speech audiometry is particularly suitable for the general *assessment* of hearing and the estimation of the degree of practical handicap. The speech-reception threshold has an advantage for *screening* audiometry also because a single pass-fail criterion can be established. Actually the screening by speech audiometry of the hearing of schoolchildren in 1927, using the Western Electric 4C audiometer, was the first use of speech audiometry and also of group audiometry. The success of this instrument and its method did much to promote the general acceptance of electric audiometers.

The principle of a *speech audiometer* is

very simple. The test material is speech. Words or sentences may be spoken into a microphone ("live-voice testing") or, better, they may be recorded in advance in standard form and at known levels on either magnetic tape or a phonograph disc (Figure 7-13). In either case the speech signal becomes an alternating electric current. Its strength is varied by a calibrated attenuator. The listener may wear earphones, or sometimes listen with both ears to a loudspeaker. The listener determines, not when he can just hear the voice sounds, but when he can *identify* the words. He may repeat the test words aloud; check them on a multiple-choice list; or write them down; or perhaps, if the speech material is a set of questions, he may answer the questions. Usually we take the "50 percent correct" level as the threshold. Or the subject may simply listen to the reading of some simple text and himself set the volume control so that he can just get the gist of what is being said. Of course, each form of test and each sample of speech material must be calibrated separately; that is, we must find the median (or modal) threshold for a reasonably large group of otologically normal listeners.

There are several *difficulties with speech audiometry*, some of which are quite apparent, although others are not. An obvious one

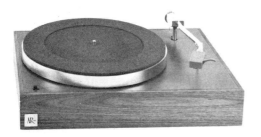

Figure 7-13 A turntable is needed for recorded speech tests. *(Acoustic Research, Inc.)*

is the problem of physical measurement of the intensity of the speech signal; others concern the choice of words or sentences; others, the voice of the talker; and others, the purpose of the test.

The problem of *physical measurement* has been adequately solved, even though measurement of speech is never as precise as measurement of pure tones because the intensity of the sound-pattern of speech is continually changing. The usual convention is to take a sort of running average of the largest of the excursions of the meter as it swings in response to the syllables of the words. A particular kind of meter, the VU ("vee-you") meter, or "volume indicator," is used for this purpose. (See sections 3.2 to 3.5 of American National Standard Volume Measurements of Electrical Speech and Program Waves, ANSI C16.5-1954 [R1961].) The term "volume" in electrical engineering is used to mean exactly this kind of measurement of electrical speech signals, and the dial on a radio or a hearing aid that controls the intensity (loudness) of the output is therefore known as the "volume control." If the talker has the meter in sight himself, he can adjust, or *monitor*, his speech to a chosen standard level. A practiced talker can hold such a general level of conversation, or repeat a given word, within a couple of decibels, which is quite sufficient for our purpose.

More disturbing is the realization that all words, spoken naturally and in sequence, do not have the same physical power. Here we adopt the convention that all the words are to be spoken with the same *effort*, and the monitoring is done only on the strongest syllables. If single words are used, they are introduced by the same carrier phrase or word, such as, "Say the word ———" or "Would you write ——— now." The talker monitors on the carrier and lets the test word come naturally without any extra emphasis. The carrier also serves to warn the listener that the test word is coming so that he is at attention.

But now the *choice of material* becomes important because all words are not equally intelligible even when carefully monitored. Some can be understood even when barely audible, whereas others must be at a much higher level before even a practiced listener can identify them correctly. Familiar words are more intelligible than the unfamiliar; words of many syllables are easier than monosyllables; and words with weak vowels and high-pitched consonants, such as "thin" and "sift," are particularly difficult.

Still other factors affect the *intelligibility of speech*. Everyone knows that it is much easier to recognize a word in context in a sentence than when it is heard alone. Everyone knows also that it is easier to identify familiar words or names than those that are not familiar, and also that words are easiest to identify if they are spoken in a familiar dialect. It is obvious that nonsense syllables, which are used in research on the intelligibility of speech, are so difficult that they are not suitable for clinical use. What is not so generally recognized is the principle that *the size of the vocabulary that is used is important*. It is much easier to identify a digit— "one," "three," "eight," and so on—if we know that the test words are all numbers than if the word may be any word in the English language. Context reduces greatly the number of probable alternatives among which the listener must choose. Certain combinations of words or phrases are probable; others are not.

The development of speech audiometry The development of speech audiometry in the United States originated in the studies at the Bell Telephone Laboratories of the acoustic characteristics of speech, the psychoacoustics of human hearing, and the use there of samples of human speech to test the effec-

tiveness of an electrical communication system, the telephone. We have already referred to the important part played by these laboratories in the early development of the pure-tone audiometer (the Western Electric 2A) and of the first screening speech audiometer (the Western Electric 4C). Another innovation was their use of speech material, ranging from nonsense syllables through single words to complete sentences, to test the effectiveness of a communication system.

This idea was exploited during World War II at the Psycho-Acoustic Laboratory at Harvard University. There the communication systems under test were at first military radio systems, used in the presence of loud noise or in other difficult acoustic conditions. Attention was later turned to hearing aids and the question of their best design. In each of these problems the intelligibility of standard lists of words or of sentences was the best, if not the only, basis on which to compare one radio system or one of its components with another or one hearing aid with another.

In the tests of radio systems the listeners were average young men with average hearing. In the tests of hearing aids the listeners were hard-of-hearing men and women with different kinds and severity of hearing loss. It seemed a very simple and direct extension of speech testing to compare the hearing of people with impaired hearing (without hearing aids) with that of people with average hearing, using the same speech material and method of scoring that had been used to compare the radio systems or the hearing aids with one another. Those who took this step did not realize that two important hidden assumptions were involved. Unfortunately the assumptions were not justified, and speech audiometry has been overvalued for 30 years as a result!

This statement must be qualified immediately by recognizing that one type of measurement, a measurement of *sensitivity,* can indeed be made very successfully by speech audiometry. The speech-reception threshold, measured with suitable material such as digits, two-syllable (spondaic) words, simple sentences, or connected discourse, is as precise and reproducible as the pure-tone hearing-threshold levels of the audiometric frequencies of 500, 1000, 2000, or 3000 Hz. In fact the correlation between these two measures of sensitivity, using easy speech material and pure tones, respectively, is so good that the measure of the speech-reception threshold is redundant and therefore unnecessary in most cases. The more serious overvaluing has related to the measurement of the "speech-discrimination score" or the "discrimination loss."

The two major types of test for sensitivity and for discrimination, respectively, must be carefully distinguished. Very different types of material are (or should be) used, the administration of the tests is different, and the kind of information derived is very different also. The two types of speech test will be considered separately.

Speech-reception threshold tests   The speech-reception threshold is measured in decibels, like the hearing-threshold level for pure tones. The subject listens to simple, easy speech material. The level is sought at which the material is either "just intelligible" or perhaps "50 percent correct." His performance is compared with the average performance of a large number of otologically normal individuals of similar age, education, and linguistic background.

The important requirements for the test material are *familiarity of the test words* and *uniformity of presentation.* The vocabulary must be suited to the level of education of the subject, and the subject must be thoroughly familiar with the language (and dialect) in which the test is given. If it is a word test, such as Auditory Tests W-1 and W-2 (see Appendix), *the subject should be allowed to read a list, alphabetically arranged, of the words that he may hear.* This step in the procedure is very often neglected, but it is assumed if the standard calibration is to apply. Another general principle for threshold tests of speech is that *the listener must understand all of the items correctly at some high intensity.* If he does not, the test material is not suitable for him, or else a threshold test is not the proper kind of test to apply for the disorder that he has. Most listeners hear correctly if the intensity is high enough, but as the intensity is reduced, mistakes begin. The level at which half of the items are correctly understood is usually taken as the end point, or *threshold.* A rapid, but reasonably accurate, method is to adjust the volume of continuous speech, such as a simple text read from a book, until the listener can just easily follow the sense of what is being read. Such a continuous, even sample of simple, unemotional text is known in some laboratories as "cold running speech."

Probably the most popular recorded threshold tests for speech are the word tests known as W-1 and W-2, prepared by the Central Institute for the Deaf. They are direct developments from Auditory Test No. 9, standardized by the Psycho-Acoustic Laboratory of Harvard University for wartime use at the Army and Navy Aural Rehabilitation Centers. The words are all familiar words of two syllables with equal stress on each syllable (spondees) such as "railroad" (see Appendix). The very similar earlier list, used by the Western Electric Company in its 4C group audiometer, is a series of two-digit numbers, as, for example, "six four," "two three." Both sets of lists have been recorded on phonograph discs, with the words in groups, and each group weaker by a known number of decibels than the preceding group. Both sets have been carefully standardized, and the performance of listeners with otologically normal ears for each of them is known. With either list properly administered, the *hearing level for speech* may be measured with at least the same precision and reliability that we attain with the puretone test of a clinical audiometer. This accuracy is possible because, as their volume is reduced, the words pass quite abruptly from intelligible words to a mere trace of speech sound. The words were selected for uniform intelligibility by a laborious series of experiments. The use of several words in each group minimizes any errors introduced by a lucky guess or momentary inattention.

Slightly less, but still satisfactory, accuracy can be obtained by a trained talker reading the words into a microphone. Of course, he has his monitoring meter before him, and he adjusts the attenuator until the listener repeats half of the words correctly. Each talker must "calibrate" his own voice as well as the earphones (or loudspeaker and test room) by measuring the threshold of many otologically normal listeners of appropriate educational level. The calibration cancels out the effects of the talker's particular voice and tricks of pronunciation.

The Western Electric Company 4C group audiometer is now of only historic interest. A few of these instruments may still be in use for screening tests of schoolchildren, but they are no longer manufactured. The instruments had a magnetic pickup, no amplifier, and 20 or 40 pairs of earphones.

The ANSI 1969 specifications for audiometers give important technical requirements concerning the amplifier, the earphones or loudspeaker, and the recording and playback characteristics for phonograph discs and magnetic tapes. Additional details will be specified in the next revision. An important specification is a calibration tone of 1000 Hz, which is recorded with the test material at the level determined as the running average of the largest excursions of the VU meter. According to the proposed (1976) new ANSI standard, the amplification is to be adjusted so that the coupler pressure produced by the earphone is 12.5 dB above the reference level for the 1000 Hz tone. This is to be the *standard reference zero level for speech audiometry.* For a TDH-49 earphone on a NBS 9A coupler this becomes 20 dB re 20 μPa. It is a slight readjustment from the original ASA-1953 value of 22 dB.

The above standard reference zero level is based on extensive studies of the speech-reception threshold, particularly at Northwestern University, using the W-1 and W-2 recordings prepared at Central Institute for the Deaf. However the speech-reception threshold is very nearly the same for these recordings, for simple sentences or for simple continuous discourse.

Uses of the speech-reception threshold The standard reference zero level for speech of 20 dB is, of course, higher than the ISO thresholds for the speech frequencies. The difference corresponds, obviously, to the difference between the threshold of *audibility* and the threshold of *intelligibility* of speech. Actually, as we have already noted, the speech-reception threshold level can be predicted very well from the average hearing-threshold level for 500, 1000, and 2000 Hz (or from the average of the two best of these three hearing-threshold levels). The greatest practical use of the speech reception threshold in a hearing clinic is as a confirmation of the results of pure-tone audiometry. If the two hearing-threshold levels, for pure tones and for speech, do *not* agree, it strongly suggests either a sense-organ disorder, such as Menière's syndrome, or a psychological or motivational situation, such as simulated hearing loss (pseudohypoacusis), or an error of technique or failure of cooperation of the patient in one or both of the tests.

The improvement in hearing that can be achieved by the use of a hearing aid (Chapter 11), or perhaps by surgery or other treatment (Chapter 6), can be very well described by the change in the speech-reception threshold.

Speech discrimination tests and "articulation scores"   The second type of speech test aims to measure how well the listener hears words in general—all words. The test material is intended to be a sample of English speech as a whole, or at least that portion of English that is appropriate to the age, education, and linguistic background of the listener. It is not a question of the level at which easy words become intelligible, but of (1) how rapidly words become intelligible as speech becomes louder, (2) the maximum percentage of words (or nonsense syllables or sentences) that are intelligible at the most favorable intensity, and (3) how great that intensity is. Telephone and other communication systems, including hearing aids, are compared with one another on the basis of such information.

All the words in the English language are usually heard correctly by the average listener in ordinary face-to-face conversation; otherwise, the words would not have crept into the language in the first place. But some speech sounds, and therefore the words in which they are used, have a much wider margin of safety than others; that is, some of them can be understood at a much lower volume than others. (It will be recalled that by *volume* is meant the running average of the intensity of the strongest syllables in speech, and it is assumed that the weaker words and syllables are spoken with the same effort that is used in producing the stronger ones.) If we take a generous sample of familiar English words and speak them one at a time in a "carrier phrase" that offers no context to help the listener to identify the word, we

find that some words, which we may call the "difficult" words, require a volume of 25 dB or more above the volume at which the first "easy" words are understood. By contrast, the lists of spondee words, matched experimentally to be equally intelligible, go from "first word intelligible" to "all words intelligible" in a range of about 6 dB (see Figure 7-14).

It is not always realized that the intelligibility of various word lists is a matter of the way the talker utters the words quite as much as it is of the "phonemic composition" of the words. Of course, some sounds—the weak fricatives, such as "th," "f," and "s," for example—depend for recognition on high frequencies in speech, and in speech the high frequencies generally carry less energy than do the low frequencies (see Figure 7-4). Actually the voice and enunciation (or "articulation") of the talker are just as important. To be sure, an ear with severe high-tone hearing loss will not hear the high frequencies in speech; but the careless talker may fail to put them in in the first place.

Actually, in ordinary conversation we probably fail to hear correctly and completely many of the difficult words, but we do not realize that we have missed them because we hear part of the word, and the context gives us the rest. The context guides us in our choice among several possible words, any one of which we might have heard, just as it tells us which of several meanings of the same word, such as "run," "turn," "meat (meet)," or "so (sew)," is intended. Only when we come to unfamiliar proper names or something out of context do we realize that the speech to which we are listening is something less than 100 percent intelligible.

We can describe someone's ability to hear speech *or* how well speech is transmitted by a communication system by means of an *articulation curve*. This tells us what percentage of a specified list of words the listener

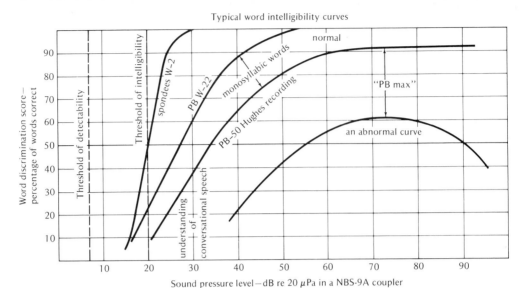

Typical word intelligibility curves

Word discrimination score — percentage of words correct

Sound pressure level — dB re 20 μPa in a NBS-9A coupler

Figure 7-14 The sound-pressure level for speech tests is defined relative to 20 μPa for the calibration tone (1000 Hz) that is usually recorded on each disc. This meter reading for the calibration tone should match approximately the peaks reached by the VU meter during the carrier phase.

The articulation curve for spondees rises more steeply than for monosyllables and is fairly constant from one talker or recording to another. The threshold of intelligibility for simple sentences and for connected discourse is practically the same as for spondees. This threshold is often called the speech-reception threshold. For monosyllables, however, the steepness and position of the curve vary from one talker or list of words to another. For some talkers, even normal listeners do not show perfect discrimination scores. For some abnormal ears the articulation curve goes through a maximum and falls again at high speech levels. The plateau or maximum is called the "PB max" (maximum for phonetically balanced word lists).

can identify as the words are spoken to him louder and louder. Of course, we should keep the talker constant from test to test, and the best way to do this practically is to use recorded word lists. The basic idea of describing speech reception by means of a curve instead of by a single index is no more complicated or subtle for the articulation curve than it is for the audiogram, although the quantities that are related to one another (that is, the percentage of words correctly understood and their intensity) are different from the intensity and frequency that enter into the audiogram. The articulation curve obtained for a group of listeners for one communication system is compared with the curve obtained for the same listeners with a standard comparison system. Or, in the context of a listening test, we can compare a man's articulation curve with an average or normal articulation curve for that particular recorded sample of speech.

The term "articulation" has been used to designate tests in which the listener tells what syllable, word, or sentence he has heard. This use of the term was introduced by communication engineers who were primarily interested in telephone or radio transmission between a talker and a listener. In a later chapter the term "articulation" will be used in its original sense (as it is employed in phonetics) to indicate how well a talker forms his words. In forming the consonants and fricatives, the tongue, lips, teeth, and other parts of our vocal apparatus fit together, or "articulate," with one another like the bones in our joints. The meaning has become extended, however, because the engineers speak of the "good articulation" of a telephone circuit when they mean that it effectively transmits to the listener the articulation of the talker. The tests by which engineers measured the articulation of telephones were called "articulation tests," and now, when the same kinds of tests are used to study the defects of someone's hearing, they are still called "articulation tests." The usage makes sense if we think of the word as meaning *the listener's ability to benefit by someone else's articulation* of the words to which he is listening.

Many *lists of sentences* as well as lists of words have been compiled for auditory tests of this sort. The earliest were the lists of the Bell Telephone Laboratories. They are framed as questions or as directions to tell or explain something, and the listener either answers the question or repeats the sense of it. Sample sentences include the following:

What are some of the personal characteristics of the people of Japan?

Is the Hudson River salt or fresh water?

What punishment is inflicted upon a murderer in this state?

Explain how Jersey milk is obtained in Ohio.

More of the Bell Telephone Laboratories' sentences as well as sentences and words of the other tests that will be mentioned are given in the Appendix. Long lists are necessary because the same sentence cannot be used twice with one listener. His memory makes it much easier for him to recognize a sentence again even from a single key word. Sentence tests are therefore not so suitable for phonographic recording, but they have the advantage of being more interesting to the listener, and they have high face validity as samples of English speech.

The Bell Telephone Laboratories' sentences are too difficult in vocabulary and also require too much local knowledge of New York City to be satisfactory for general use elsewhere; and other lists based on more limited vocabularies and special interests— the military, for example—have been used to good advantage. Some sentences from a simplified Psycho-Acoustic Laboratory list (see the Appendix), designed as questions to be answered by a single word, are

Which is larger, a man or a mouse?

Can you burn your mouth with ice cream?

Does a cow have kittens or horns?

What month comes after February?

In an effort to obtain more accurate scoring, still another list was developed in which each sentence contains five key words. The subject repeats the entire sentence, but only errors in the key words are counted. This is a special sort of "word in context" intelligibility, useful for research work. A few samples, with key words italicized, are

Clams are *small, round, soft* and *tasty.*

Sport is *fun,* but *we need money.*

The *boat tipped,* and the *fat lady screamed.*

It is a *shameful act* to *wipe* your *mouth* on a sleeve.

Plug the *leaky pipe* with a *wad* of *gum.*

Another set of sentences was developed at Central Institute for the Deaf to provide a sample of "everyday speech." Special attention was given to the vocabulary, the length and form of sentences, and to idiom. The talkers, both male and female, were chosen as average with respect to "articulation." These sentences were intended for tests to determine the threshold of handicap (see Chapter 9), but they could also be used for easy material in an articulation test.

The best-known *lists of words used for articulation tests* are probably the *PB-50 Word Lists.* These lists, 50 words each and of reasonably familiar monosyllables, were developed at the Psycho-Acoustic Laboratory at Harvard for wartime research on equipment for communication. Several complete lists are given in the Appendix. The abbreviation "PB" stands for "phonetically balanced." This means that nearly all the phonemes of the English language are represented in every list of 50 words. If only the initital consonants and the vowels are considered, the frequency of occurrence of the various sounds is fairly representative of English speech as a whole.

A rather similar set of 50-word lists, using a somewhat smaller and more familiar vocabulary, was prepared at Central Institute for the Deaf. Two recordings of the CID lists have been made with different talkers. It so happened that one talker (Ira Hirsh) is highly intelligible, so intelligible in fact that the test has many of the properties of the spondee lists and does not reveal the limitations of hearing that we wish to measure. The other talker (Rush Hughes) clips his words so badly that some sounds are entirely missing by physical analysis, and even the best listener makes a perfect score only with the help of some fortunate guesswork. This recording is too "difficult" to constitute a good standard.

A list of words suitable for children was developed at the Clarke School for the Deaf, and other tests based on multiple choice rather than on simple repetition or writing down of the test word have been tried. Some of the most useful of these are given in the Appendix.

American National Standard Method for Measurement of Monosyllabic Word Intelligibility, ANSI S3.2-1960 (R1971), specifies how word lists should be used to compare one communication system with another. The word lists contained in it are not quite identical with the PB lists used at the Psycho-Acoustic Laboratory or by the Central Institute for the Deaf, and represent an improvement with respect to familiarity of vo-

cabulary. Still another set of lists, prepared by Peterson and Lehiste, is cited in the Appendix.

We are still without a proper standard articulation test for which normal values have been established. The administration of PB word lists by "live voice" is not satisfactory because talkers are not interchangeable. And even with the same talker the percentage of words correctly repeated by a given subject at a given intensity level may vary 5 or 10 percent from trial to trial even if the full 50-word lists are employed.

Nevertheless, certain generalizations can be made that are useful, assuming an "average talker." If a PB list (or any other list) is read too faintly, none of the words can be understood. As the voice becomes louder, more and more of the words are recognized, but even a normal listener does not make a score of 99 or 100 percent on a PB list until the intensity is at least 25 dB above the intensity at which he just recognizes one or two words. If lists are read at several different intensities, say 10 dB apart, the scores can be plotted, and an *articulation curve*, such as the one in Figure 7-14, can be drawn through the points. We know from thousands of experiments that the articulation curve is in general a smooth curve that is steepest at or a little below its middle, and that at the upper end it levels off rather gradually to a plateau.

In Figure 7-14 it is evident that the articulation curve for the spondee words of tests W-1 and W-2 is much steeper than that for the PB-50 lists, and it lies farther to the left at lower sound-pressure levels. The steepness of the curve is due to the "homogeneity" of the list. The words were chosen and the level of each adjusted in the process of recording to bring about just this matching of intelligibility. As a result, the sound level corresponding to 50 percent correct can be determined very precisely. The less steep slope of the articulation curve for the PB words expresses the much greater spread in the "difficulty" of these words. The threshold for the PB words as recorded in test W-22 lies at a sound-pressure level about 7 dB higher than the threshold for the spondee words. This is chiefly because the monosyllabic PB words are more difficult as a group.

Another factor is the *larger vocabulary* employed. For the spondees the vocabulary is 36 words, and the subject reads the list before the test. For the PB test the vocabulary is very large. There are more than a thousand reasonably familiar monosyllables in the English language from which the listener makes his choice. If, however, a list of only 25 monosyllables is used and the listener has read the list (alphabetically arranged) before the test, the monosyllabic threshold will lie appreciably closer to the spondaic threshold. Practically speaking, the effect of size of vocabulary becomes small for sets of more than 100 items.

If a few of the words are *unfamiliar*, it will have very little effect on the *threshold* (50 percent correct) *but will significantly reduce the level of the plateau, or "PB max."*

In Figure 7-14 the difference between a "good" talker (W-22) and a "difficult" talker (Hughes) is well illustrated. The articulation curve for Hughes lies some 7 dB higher than for the W-22 recording, and its PB max is well below 100 percent.

For normal ears under good listening conditions, the plateau of the articulation curve is at 100 percent of words correctly understood; but if the words are heard through a communication system that does not transmit all the speech frequencies (or otherwise distorts the sounds) or if the words are spoken against a background of noise, the curve may level off at some lower value such as 70 or 80 percent. This means that with an infer-

ior communication system some words are never correctly understood, no matter how loud the speaker talks or how much amplification is introduced in the system. Just so, *a man with severe high-tone sensorineural loss will always fail to hear certain sounds and will never make a perfect articulation score.* On the other hand, the same man may hear some words, the easy low-frequency words, as well as anyone else does. He may even have a normal speech-reception *threshold*.

It is a very convenient, though accidental, property of the PB and similar lists of familiar monosyllables that the volume at which 50 percent of the words are correctly understood when they are well spoken is about the level at which we can easily understand ordinary connected speech. It may seem remarkable that speech is readily understood when only about 50 percent of isolated monosyllables can be identified separately; but that is the experimental result both for normal and for hard-of-hearing listeners. In fact, if the connected speech is simple and deals with familiar material, it may be intelligible if the listener really pays attention at a level at which only about 25 percent of monosyllabic words can be correctly understood.

Practically, an important thing to know about someone's hearing is whether or not he can follow ordinary conversation. Is his hearing *socially adequate*? If not, the position of the 50 percent point on his PB articulation curve tells us how loud speech must be made (by a hearing aid) in order to make him socially adequate. Or we can measure his speech-reception threshold and add 8 or 10 dB to estimate the level for 100 percent correct on easy sentences or everyday speech.

We have described the articulation curve in general and the PB lists in particular because they show us the fundamental relations between the *intensity* of speech and its *intelligibility*. The position of an articulation curve on the intensity scale is primarily a measure of *auditory sensitivity* (a threshold) and secondarily of the difficulty of the material for that listener. The height of the plateau that can be reached is a measure of *auditory discrimination*, that is, of how well difficult words are heard. For some abnormal ears the articulation curve not only reaches a plateau but actually goes through a maximum. Very loud speech is *less* intelligible than speech 10 or 15 dB less intense.

The important concept here is that there are two independent properties of speech and hearing. One is intensity. Usually this dominates the situation, and the intensity determines completely (for a given recorded test and a given listener) what the score will be, and if we know the threshold for speech we can predict the rest. But this is not always true. Ears with the same threshold for speech may differ in the maximum percentage of test words they can hear correctly. To test this maximum, the words are given well above threshold. It is the maximum or the height of the plateau that is determined. This is the PB max referred to earlier. A common cause for a PB max less than 95 percent is high-tone hearing loss. Another is poor enunciation by the talker. Another is distortion of the speech signal by a poor hearing aid.

General Remarks on Speech Audiometry

When speech audiometry was first introduced, the idea of the articulation curve as a measure of hearing was received with considerable enthusiasm by most audiologists and many otologists. It now appears that both the administration of the test and the interpretation of the results are more difficult than was then appreciated. We have pointed out in this chapter some of the sources of variability and uncertainty. For example, there is no accepted standard word list of monosyllables. Too much importance has been attached to phonetic balance of the word lists and not enough to the diction of the talkers, the familiarity of the words, the size of the vocabulary employed, and the test-retest variability of patients. The latter point is particularly troublesome because it obscures what we had hoped would be very useful information relating to the choice of hearing aids for particular patients. (We shall return to this question in Chapter 11.)

One reason for the present writer's early optimism in regard to the value of PB articulation scores and their possible use in diagnosis and assessment was an oversimplified concept of the phoneme as a unit of speech. He assumed that the difficulty in correctly hearing certain words depends primarily on the lack of intensity of certain elementary speech sounds (phonemes), notably the weak fricatives. These particular phonemes are rich in high frequencies, and therefore an ear with a high-frequency loss should be unable to hear them, and a poor ("low-fi") communication system would not transmit them adequately. The spectral composition of a phoneme was thought to be constant and to be a necessary and sufficient condition for its correct recognition. Words were thought of as mosaics of acoustically constant phonemes that are perceived and recognized independently. This is one reason why the phonetically balanced word lists were valued very highly.

The writer is now told by his colleagues that a given phoneme does not always have the same sound spectrum, that the transitions from vowel to consonant and consonant to vowel are as characteristic and as important as the steady state (if any) of either the vowel or the consonant, and that the duration of a speech sound or the presence of a silent period may determine what it "sounds like" in a word. In short, speech is much more complicated than he once supposed.

Of course, the complexity of speech and the lability of the phoneme do not mean that the assumptions on which speech audiometry were founded are entirely wrong. It means that the assumptions were oversimplified. If high frequencies are not heard, as in the hypothetical case illustrated in Figure 7-4, the listener will certainly suffer some handicap in understanding speech. The extent of the handicap is hard to predict, however, because it will depend largely on how well the listener can employ other cues of timing, the modification of adjacent phonemes, emphasis, context, and so on, to offset his inability to hear the high-frequency components of some phonemes.

On the other hand, when large numbers of listeners and many trials are involved, articulation scores become quite stable and predictable. A very elaborate method of calculation of what is called the "articulation index" makes it possible to calculate from the spectrum and intensity level of a noise what the articulation scores (for monosyllabic word lists) will be for people listening in that noise, and a "speech-interference level" for that noise can be predicted. The method and concepts serve as useful guides in architectural planning and in noise-abatement programs.

We shall consider in Chapter 9 the "Social Adequacy Index of Hearing" that was proposed in 1948 for assessment of an individual's hearing. The difficulty in practice seemed to lie in the variability of the "PB max" scores of an individual and also in the dynamic aspects of speech. One clearly important factor that has not been explicitly standardized is the speed of talking—both the length of time devoted to each word and phoneme and also the rate at which words or test items follow one another.

In summary, speech tests have several possible clinical uses, and different forms of test are required for each. One use is to measure the speech-reception threshold. For this the spondee word lists are very satisfactory, and easy sentences and connected discourse are acceptable. Speech-threshold audiometry has been standardized. Another use is in medical diagnosis. The basic articulation curve gives only limited diagnostic information, such as a grossly reduced maximum score, but special speech tests appropriate to central auditory impairments have been developed. Some of these will be noted in the following chapter. Another use is overall assessment of hearing. The monosyllabic (PB) curves are descriptive and quantitative: but they test much more than the ear, and they are still inadequately standardized. A final use, the evaluation of hearing aids, would seem to be theoretically possible, but here articulation scores work poorly in practice. They are the right kind of a tool, but the tool is not sharp enough. Uncontrolled factors of various sorts make the test-retest reliability too low to assess the importance of actual differences among instruments except in extreme cases. In research, speech tests such as those involving articulation scores are a very useful tool in such areas as hearing in noise and ascertaining the advantages of binaural hearing, as well as in the study of the relation of the physical characteristics of speech to speech perception and to linguistics. Here many special tests have been devised for special purposes.

SUGGESTED READINGS AND REFERENCES

American National Standards Institute, Inc., 1430 Broadway, New York, N. Y. 10018:

ANSI C16.5-1954 (R1961). *Volume Measurements of Electrical Speech and Program Waves.*

ANSI S1.1-1960 (1971). *Acoustical Terminology.*

ANSI S3.1-1960 (1971). *Criteria for Background Noise in Audiometer Rooms.*

ANSI S3.6-1969 (R1973). *Specifications for Audiometers.* (Work is in progress on a forthcoming revision of this standard.)

ANSI S3-13-1972. *Artificial Head-Bone for the Calibration of Audiometer Bone Vibrators.*

ANSI S3.21-197-. *Methods for Manual Pure-Tone Threshold Audiometry.* (Forthcoming.)

Bunch, C. C. *Clinical Audiometry.* St. Louis: The C. V. Mosby Company, 1943.
A monograph devoted to the early development and use of the pure tone audiometer. Now chiefly of historical interest.

Davis, H., G. D. Hoople, and H. O. Parrack. "The Medical Principles of Monitoring Audiometry," *AMA Arch. Industr. Health,* 17:1–20 (1958).
This paper is based on the report of a CHABA working group to the Air Force.

————, and F. W. Kranz. "The International Standard Reference Zero for Pure-Tone Audiometers and Its Relation to the Evaluation of Impairment of Hearing," *J. Speech Hearing Res.,* 7:7–16 (1964); also, *Trans. Amer. Acad. Ophthal. Otolaryng.,* 68:484–492 (1964).

Eagles, E. L., S. M. Wishik, L. G. Doerfler, W. Melinick, and H. S. Levine. "Hearing Sensitivity and Related Factors in Children." Special monograph issue of *Laryngoscope,* 1963.
This is the "Pittsburgh Study," also cited in Chapter 5.

Egan, J. R. "Articulation Testing Methods," *Laryngoscope,* 58:955–991 (1948).
This is a condensation of the reports of the same title prepared at the Psycho-Acoustic Laboratory for the Office of Scientific Research and Development (OSRD Report No. 3802). It contains a full description of the original phonetically balanced (PB-50) word lists.

Fletcher, H. and J. E. Steinberg. "Articulation Testing Methods," *Bell System Tech. J.,* 8:806–854 (1929).
A classic article from the Bell Telephone Laboratories. It contains the complete list of BTL sentences.

Hirsh, I. J. *The Measurement of Hearing.* New York: McGraw-Hill Book Company, 1952.
An authoritative monograph that deals with psychoacoustic methods and principles.

————, H. Davis, S. R. Silverman, E. G. Reynolds, E. Eldert, and R. W. Benson.

"Development of Materials for Speech Audiometry," *J. Speech Hearing Dis.* 17:321–337 (1952).
This gives the background of the CID auditory tests.

International Electrotechnical Commission. *Pure-Tone Audiometers for General Diagnostic Purposes,* IEC Publication 177. Geneva: Bureau Central de la Commission Electrotechnique Internationale, 1965.
Also available from the American National Standards Institute.

ISO Standard 389-1975. *Acoustics—Standard Reference Zero for the Calibration of Pure-Tone audiometers.* Geneva: International Organization for Standardization, 1975.
Also available from the American National Standards Institute.

Jerger, J. F., R. Carhart, T. W. Tillman, and J. L. Peterson. "Some Relations between Normal Hearing for Pure Tones and Speech," *J. Speech Hearing Dis.,* 2:126–140 (1959).

Katz, J. (ed.). *Handbook of Clinical Audiology.* Baltimore: Williams & Wilkins Company, 1972.
Good for practical details of audiometric tests.

Kranz, F. W. "Audiometer: Principles and History," *Sound,* 2:20–32 (1963).
Excellent historical review, including discussion of the reference level and the ISO standard.

Rose, D. E. (ed.). *Audiological Assessment.* Englewood Cliffs, N.J.: Prentice-Hall, Inc., 1971.

Silverman, S. R., and I. J. Hirsh. "Problems Related to the Use of Speech in Clinical Audiometry," *Ann. Otol.* 64:1234–1245 (1955).

The citations in the literature for several additional word or sentence lists are given in the Appendix.

Hallowell Davis, M.D.

8

Audiometry:
Other Auditory Tests

In the previous chapter we described the electric audiometer and also its use in determining pure-tone thresholds, the speech-reception threshold, the PB word-articulation curve, and the "PB max." This survey included most of the tests that are useful in the selection of hearing aids. We also described a number of simple diagnostic tests that can be performed with tuning forks or with a single-channel, pure-tone audiometer with a bone-conduction vibrator.

In the present chapter we consider a basic diagnostic strategy using simple tests and then describe several other diagnostic auditory tests that are suitable for cooperative adults and older children. Second, we consider the various tests for feigned impairment of hearing or pseudohypoacusis. In a third section we consider the auditory tests that are appropriate for young children, from neonates to the age of full understanding and cooperation. This includes reflex audiometry and electric response audiometry: tests which are sometimes grouped together as *objective audiometry*. We include these tests of young children here, although their purpose is more often assessment than diagnosis, because implicit in such testing is a search for conditions that can be treated medically or surgically. The final section of the chapter considers some of the tests used in otoneurology (or neuro-otology) to assess overall auditory function and to assist in neurological diagnosis of disorders of the central nervous system.

We shall not describe the practical details of the various auditory tests. As in Chapter 7, we shall be concerned with the principles involved and with the logical relations among the tests. Full details of the instruments and tests, their historical development and their use, together with references to the publications in which they were originally described, are given in the books and review articles cited at the end of Chapters 7 and 8.

DIAGNOSTIC TESTS FOR ADULTS AND OLDER CHILDREN

A primary reason for testing hearing is to assist in making a medical diagnosis. On the diagnosis rests the decision for treatment and also the forecast of the improvement or deterioration of hearing. Advice concerning use of a hearing aid, surgery for improvement of hearing, and so on, also depends in large part on a correct medical diagnosis. Furthermore, tests of hearing may be of real assistance to the neurologist and neurosurgeon in the diagnosis of disorders of the central nervous system, whether the basic trouble is auditory or not.

The otologist is always interested in the cause of the condition he finds. In order to treat it intelligently he should know not only *where* it is, but also *what* it is and, whenever possible, *what causes* it. Of course, the anatomical and physiological distinctions establish certain classes of possible causes. Rarely, however, even for so simple a diagnosis as conductive hearing loss, does a physician base his opinion and course of action on a single symptom, a single sign, or the result of a single test. He always seeks confirmatory evidence, and he bases his final diagnosis on the balance of evidence in a total picture. Only the fully trained physician is competent to do this, although it is very tempting for an audiological specialist to be-

gin to make diagnoses on the basis of the results of his hearing tests alone. An audiologist may be correct more often than not, but the experienced physician who considers audiometric findings as only one part of the total examination is in a better position to make a correct diagnosis. Above all, the physician will usually avoid the tragic mistakes that can so easily follow from oversimplification or from dependence on a single kind of information. For him the improbable but serious alternative, such as a brain tumor or a metabolic disturbance, is a very real alternative. He is better able to recognize these conditions that actually threaten life and to realize that the auditory symptoms that result from them are of only secondary importance for the welfare of the patient.

Diagnostic Strategy

The diagnostic strategy of audiology is directed primarily toward identifying the anatomical location of impairments of hearing, whether in the middle ear, the inner ear, the auditory nerve, the central nervous system, or in some combination of two or more areas. This objective is desirable because it directs the otologist or neurosurgeon to the appropriate area and suggests the probable nature of the impairment. It is possible because the nature of the impairments that affect these areas cause characteristically different disturbances of function.

From the description of the anatomy and function of the different parts of the system given in Chapters 2, 3, and 4, it is evident that, broadly speaking, the impairments of the external and middle ear cause a conductive hearing loss, measurable in decibels, and that impairments of the central nervous system cause a quite different type of disorder, in general not describable in terms of hertz or decibels. The disorders of the inner ear cause impairments that may be partly conductive in nature, but usually show other characteristic disturbances that may be identified with some degree of confidence by appropriate auditory tests. The major difficulties occur when two or more types of impairment occur in combination.

The interview: informal spoken-voice testing
An important first step toward a diagnosis can be made very simply in adults and older children on the basis of a direct interview, with only the voice of the examiner as the test instrument. If the patient has difficulty in understanding the spoken voice at a conversational level but can hear and understand a loud voice, it is a strong indication that the difficulty is conductive and probably chiefly in the middle ear. In terms of audiometry, the thresholds for pure tones and for speech are elevated, but the articulation score at high intensity levels is high. Some otologists say, in this situation, that the patient's "cochlear reserve" is good. The prospects are good for alleviation of the impairment by aural surgery or for circumventing it by means of a hearing aid. Actually, if high-intensity speech is well understood, both the cochlear reserve and the central functions of perception and understanding are good.

On the other hand, if the hearing and understanding of speech at high level are poor, or if the patient says that he hears but cannot understand the words, or complains of poor quality of musical tones or of interfering "head noises," or if he requires a very slow and deliberate presentation of words in order to repeat them correctly, then he probably has a more complicated disorder of inner ear, nerve, or central nervous system.

Bone-conduction tests for middle-ear (conductive) impairment Let us suppose that by the simple spoken-voice test the patient's cochlear reserve appears good. The logical next step is to seek for evidence of middle-ear impairment. Most of the appropriate audiological tests relate to bone conduction and the presence or absence of an air-bone gap (see Chapters 3 and 4). Air conduction is impaired by middle-ear disease, but bone conduction is affected little or not at all. The simple tuning-fork tests described in Chapter 7 give a quick approximate assessment of bone conduction. The Rinne test compares air and bone conduction, the Schwabach test compares the patient's bone conduction with that of a normal listener, and the Weber test compares the bone conduction of the patient's own two ears. The Bing test and the Gellé test are essentially quick tests for mobility of the stapes. These tests are not quantitative, however, and as performed in an otologist's office they may sometimes be confused by ambient noise.

The equivalent of the tuning fork tests can, of course, be performed with an electric audiometer if desired. The usual first step with this instrument, however, is the pure-tone audiogram, and then, unless the pure-tone audiogram is well within normal limits, a bone-conduction audiogram. As a first approximation the bone-conduction audiogram measures the inner-ear impairment, and the air-bone gap measures the middle-ear (conductive) impairment, including what may be due to fixation of the stapes. We repeat, however, that (1) the calibration of the bone-conduction vibrator is more difficult than that of the earphone, and the reference zero values are less clearly defined; (2) masking of the ear not under test is always necessary and may be disconcerting to the patient; and (3) very quiet surroundings are needed to avoid unwanted masking of the ear actually under test. Finally there are many anatomical pathways for bone conduction, some of which include the ossicles, and there is acoustic interaction between the inner and the middle ears. It is beyond the scope of this book to discuss the pitfalls and the limitations of bone-conduction tests. They are complex, particularly those related to masking a relatively good ear while testing the opposite (poorer) ear. In order to avoid some of the difficulties a modified bone-conduction test was proposed by Rainville in 1955.

Rainville and sensorineural acuity level (SAL) tests of bone conduction The new principle introduced by Rainville was to measure the masking effect on *air-conducted tones* produced by *bone-conducted noise*. The most familiar application (Jerger and Tillman, 1960) of the Rainville is the so-called sensorineural acuity level or SAL test, but there are other modifications. The masking noise is applied to the mastoid (Rainville) or the forehead (SAL). A normal ear and an ear with only middle-ear impairment both have normal sensitivity for the bone-conducted masking noise. The difference in air-conducted sound level required to be heard, in the presence of this bone-conducted masker, between a normal listener and the patient under test measures the conductive loss (attenuation) of energy in the patient's middle ear. Of course the system must be calibrated on a group of otologically normal individuals, but it is not necessary to have the surroundings completely quiet, either for the calibration or for the actual test.

The SAL test is carried out by measuring two air-conduction thresholds: the threshold in quiet and the threshold in the presence of a fixed high-level bone-conducted noise. The difference in decibels between these two thresholds is then subtracted from the shift produced by the same noise in normal ears. The resulting number is the sensorineural hearing level in decibels. This level is not quite the same as the conventional hearing level by bone conduction because it is determined with the ear partially occluded by the air-conduction receiver, although in the conventional method the ear is not occluded. The estimates of the air-bone gap, however, seem to be perfectly valid. The masking procedure is simpler than for the conventional bone-conduction measurements, but there still remains (1976) a technical difficulty in providing reliably a noise level by bone conduction as high as is desired for severe impairments.

Acoustic impedance-admittance measurements Much information as to the nature of middle-ear impairments can be obtained from purely physical measurements of certain acoustic properties of the ear. These measurements do not require active participation by the subject, and it is more accurate to call them *acoustic measurements* than audiometric tests. We shall consider them here, however, because they can strongly support bone-conduction tests. Within the past decade very effective commercial electroacoustic instruments have been developed, and the method has come into widespread use. It has the advantage that it can be conducted on very young children, with little or no sedation. It is simple and rapid enough to be a candidate for use in auditory screening of children.

The transformer function of the middle ear in matching the acoustic impedance of air to that of the fluid-filled inner ear is described in Chapter 3. The impedance of a system is the opposition it offers to the flow of energy through it. The acoustic impedance of air is low, whereas the impedance of water or bone is high. The efficiency of the impedance-matching function of the middle ear may be assessed by measuring the proportion of the acoustic energy that is reflected back when a probe tone is presented to the ear.

In more detail, the acoustic impedance depends on the acoustic resistance, the stiffness, and the mass of the system. The resistive or "real" component is due to friction, and represents a loss of acoustic energy. In the ear this component is small, and in one popular method of measurement it is neglected entirely. As in a spring, energy is stored during compression in one phase of a sound wave and is released in another phase. The spring may be stiff (high impedance) or it may be loose and compliant (low impedance). The other component of the "reactive" impedance is the mass or inertia of the moving parts. This also stores energy and returns it, but a quarter of a cycle out of phase with the stiffness. The relative importance of stiffness and mass depends on the frequency. The mass component is least at low frequencies and greatest at high frequencies. Stiffness dominates at low frequencies. The system is "resonant" at the frequency for which the two reactive components are equal (but different in phase). Measurements of the impedence of the ear are usually made with a relatively low-frequency tone, such as 220 Hz, for which stiffness is the dominant component.

For certain calculations and types of measurement it is more convenient to consider the reciprocal of impedance, that is, the acoustic *admittance* of the ear. This means the ease with which the acoustic energy flows into or through the system. One of the popular instruments, the Grason-Stadler 1722 (Figure 8-1), is actually an *otoadmittance* meter. Other commercial instruments, such as the Madsen Z070 or ZS76-I (see Figure 8-2), yield their values in terms of *impedance* (acoustic ohms). The unit of admittance is the acoustic mho (ohm spelled backward). It is somewhat confusing to have these two different, though closely related, sets of units, but the important point is not the absolute value of the impedance or the admittance but its relation to the normal range of values, and each class of instrument

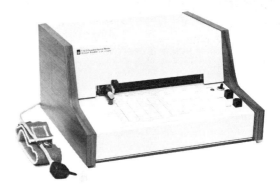

Figure 8-1 The Grason-Stadler 1722 Otoadmittance Meter is fully automatic in its operation and is suitable for rapid semi-screening procedures. *(GenRad)*

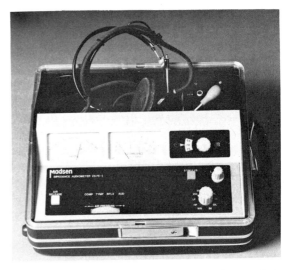

Figure 8-2 This portable "impedance audiometer" is combined with a pure-tone audiometer. It allows measurement of compliance, absolute impedance, tympanic mobility, reflex threshold, and reflex decay. An x-y writeout (not shown) can produce tympanograms like those shown in Figure 8-5. *(Madsen Electronics)*

is appropriately calibrated. With either system the contrast is clear between the normal range of values and the high impedance (low admittance) of a stiff otosclerotic ear or the low impedance (high admittance) of a loose and compliant ear with disarticulation of the ossicular chain.

We shall not go into the history of the development of clinical acoustic impedance bridges (Metz, 1946; Zwislocki, 1963) or the subsequent electroacoustic developments. Figure 8-3 shows the basic principle of an early Zwislocki bridge. This bridge and many later models yield measurements in terms of the equivalent volume (in milliliters) of air that is required to bring the bridge to a balance. These values can be translated to acoustic ohms or mhos, but the situation is confusing. We hope that standardization of units will soon be achieved. A step in this direction has been the introduction of a scale of *compliance* as a substitute for equivalent volume of air. Compliance is measured in acoustic ohms and refers to the reactive component, neglecting resistance. The less stiff a system is, the more compliant it is. We shall not discuss further the physics, terminology, or mathematics of acoustic impedance and admittance or the theoretical and practical advantages of each approach. Excellent and authoritative treatments of these topics by

Dr. Alan S. Feldman and by Dr. James Jerger are available (see References), and simplified versions are provided in the handbooks provided with the commerical instruments.

Important additions to impedance-admittance measurements have been two "dynamic" measures that relate impedance-admittance to some other parameter. The first parameter is the air pressure in the ear canal. The second is the activation of the acoustic (stapedius) reflex by sound delivered to the contralateral ear. This dynamic measure is the most important contribution of the method. It will be considered in a later section.

In order to relate the impedance-admittance measures to air pressure, the ear canal must not only be tightly sealed with a well-fitting plug, just as for a static measurement, but a tube and air-pump must regulate the pressure within. Thus there are three tubes that pass through the plug: one for the probe tone, one for the measurement of the incident plus the reflected sound, and one for

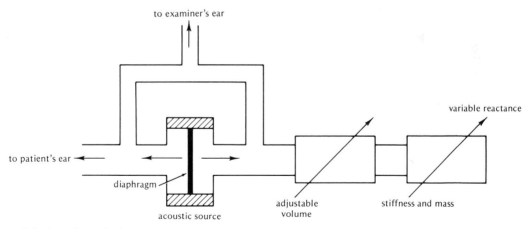

Figure 8-3 Impedance bridge: schematic diagram; after Zwislocki (1961). The acoustic source is a symmetrical earphone, which produces equal intensities of sound in the tubes that lead to the opposite faces of its diaphragm. The sound waves generated in the two tubes are in opposite phase and will cancel one another at the examiner's ear provided the sound reflected from the patient's ear at the left matches the sound reflected from the variable reactance at

the right. An adjustable volume in series with the variable reactance is first set to match the volume of the patient's ear canal. Then the variable "reactance," which corresponds to a combination of stiffness and mass components, is varied until the bridge is balanced and the examiner hears no sound. (Annals of Otology, Rhinology and Laryngology, 70:604; 1961; by permission) regulation of air pressure. Figure 8-4 is a simplified schematic diagram of such an electroacoustic impedance bridge. (The otoadmittance meter is slightly more complex electrically.) In most normal ears the air pressures in the external and middle ears are equal and the tympanic membrane is in its most mobile position. At zero pressure, as indicated on the manometer, the impedance will therefore be minimum (admittance maximum). Increasing the air pressure to $+200$ mm of water stretches the tympanic membrane and stiffens it, and practically eliminates acoustic transmission across the ossicular chain. The difference between this reference level of impedance-admittance and the minimum (or maximum) found as the

pressure is systematically reduced to -200 mm of water is one of the most significant measurements. A second significant measurement is the air pressure at which minimum impedance (maximum admittance) is reached. The curve relating impedance or admittance to air pressure is called a *tympanogram* (Figure 8-5). The relations of deviations of the tympanogram to various pathological conditions in the middle ear, notably otosclerosis, otitis media, and eustachian tube functions, are being developed so rapidly at the present writing that we shall not attempt to summarize them. Instead we paraphrase from an editorial by Dr. J. Jerger (in *Archives of Otolaryngology (Chicago)*, October 1975) that summarizes his very extensive experience:

1. The threshold of the acoustic reflex, both crossed and uncrossed, is the most important contribution of impedance measurements.

2. The shape of the tympanogram is an extremely useful diagnostic tool. It does not make much difference how it is measured as long as the probe tone is kept below 500 Hz and resistance (or conductance) is avoided. Whether it relates air pressure to the impedance vector or to reactance, susceptance, or admittance is largely irrelevant to the clinical application of tympanometry.

3. No absolute impedance measure has much clinical value, on whatever scale it is measured. They are all of equally questionable value. The clinical value of impedance measurements lies in the unique interactions among the audiogram, the tympanogram, and the acoustic reflex threshold. The clinical value of the last two is largely independent of the exact vehicle of measurement.

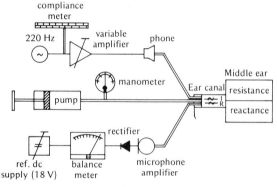

Figure 8-4 Electroacoustic bridge: schematic diagram. This bridge measures the amplitude differential between incident (I) and resultant (R) signals in the ear canal. The resultant is rectified to a dc voltage and compared to a reference voltage (lower left) by the balance meter. Adjustment of a potentiometer (upper left) brings the meter to balance, usually at a specified sound pressure level in the ear canal of about 85 dB. The compliance meter readout (upper left) may be calibrated in milliliters of air or in acoustic ohms or both.

The air pressures are adjusted by the pump and measured on the manometer. Points may be plotted manually one by one as a graph, but in recent models of impedance or admittance meters the air pressure is automatically reduced slowly from its maximum to its minimum value. The movement of an x-y plotter on its x scale is controlled by the pressure, while the y value shows the compliance or admittance. The resulting graph is a tympanogram, recorded automatically. *(From L. J. Bradford, ed., Physiological Measures of the Audio-Vestibular System,* Academic Press, *1975; by permission)*

We also quote in full Dr. A. S. Feldman's concluding paragraph of his chapter on acoustic impedance-admittance measurements (Bradford, 1975):

While the isolated measurements within this battery of tests may sometimes fail to provide the examiner with definitive diagnostic information about the middle-ear or sensorineural status, the

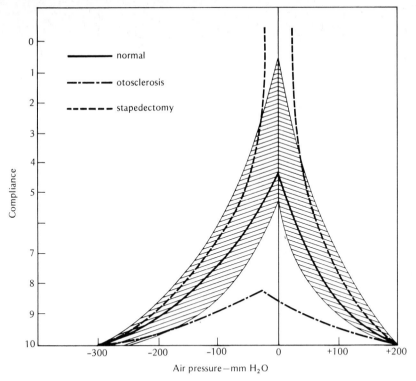

Figure 8-5 Tympanograms, as made with a Madsen Z070 electroacoustic bridge. Normal range of compliance is shaded. Typical tympanograms for ears with normal impedance, high impedance (otosclerosis), and low impedance (stapedectomy) are also shown. The units of air pressure are millimeters of water. The scale of compliance-impedance is arbitrary. *(From L. J. Bradford, ed.,* Physiological Measures of the Audio-Vestibular System, *Academic Press, 1975; by permission)*

combined battery of static and dynamic acoustic impedance measurements constitute the fastest and most effective means at our disposal for this determination. The short battery of tests completely eliminates the need for bone conduction audiometry in cases of pure sensorineural losses, and lends objective support to the examination of the auditory system medial to the middle ear. Although it does not supplant much of the traditional audiological battery, it may reasonably substitute for some procedures and provide a substantial reinforcement for other clinically obtained data.

Simple speech audiometry in the diagnostic sequence Following the determination of pure-tone thresholds by air and by bone conduction the usual next step is to measure the speech-reception threshold and the maxi-

mum word-articulation score. These measures confirm and make quantitative the impressions gained in the initial interview. A numerical value can be assigned to the "cochlear reserve," namely, the percentage of monosyllables correctly repeated when heard at a comfortably loud level, at least 25 dB above the speech-reception threshold. At this level we sample the plateau of the articulation curve, that is, the PB max.

The speech-reception threshold itself usually gives little new information because it correlates so well with the average pure-tone hearing-threshold levels at 500, 1000, and 2000 Hz. A discrepancy is important, however. It immediately points to something more than a conductive impairment. Of course a close agreement of speech and pure-tone hearing-threshold levels can be expected only if the patient has in the past had sufficient hearing to have learned speech and language in his mother tongue. Subjects who do not speak the language of the examiner present a special set of problems! Incidentally a discrepancy between pure-tone and speech thresholds, and particularly a discrepancy that varies from day to day, is a strong hint of pseudohypoacusis, or feigning, although the combination may occur in sense-organ impairment also.

After the routine speech audiometry the audiologist must decide whether further tests are needed. Perhaps the diagnosis is clear at this point. Perhaps a final test would be the test of tolerance, to determine the power of a hearing aid that might be recommended.

The diagnostic analysis should continue, however, if the "cochlear reserve" (speech discrimination) is not good, if the patient complains of the poor quality of the sounds he hears, or if there are any suggestions of a central neurological or motivational problem.

Inner-ear (sensorineural) impairment The impairments of the inner ear and auditory nerve comprise three major classes that can be distinguished fairly well by history, interview, and auditory tests, and which present very different problems of therapy and management. The first class includes noise-induced hearing loss, presbycusis, and most congenital defects of the inner ear. The second class is the type of sense-organ impairment that is encountered in Menière's syndrome. The third class is compression of the auditory nerve by a neurinoma. The classes may be combined, however, and the last two present rather difficult but important problems of differential diagnosis.

The common features of the first class, from the point of view of the results of simple auditory tests, are: (1) elevated thresholds for pure tones by both air and bone conduction; (2) some elevation of speech-reception threshold and reduction of PB max, but no more than might be predicted from the pure-tone audiogram; and (3) no particular complaint about poor quality or "noisiness" of pure tones or speech. The absence of distortion of musical tones and speech makes the auditory impairment of this first class rather like a conductive impairment, and we have pointed out in Chapter 4 that inefficient mechanical (acoustical) action in the inner ear, particularly in the organ of Corti, may be one of the basic difficulties in many congenital defects and in presbycusis.

Clinically there is usually no difficulty in distinguishing among the three members of this first class. Presbycusis occurs in elderly people, congenital defects are nearly always noticed in childhood, and noise-induced hearing loss appears in late adolescence or adulthood with a clear history of habitual noise exposure or an episode of acoustic trauma. We place here, with congenital defects, the abrupt high-tone hearing loss described in Chapter 4. This condition is identified by the air and bone audiograms. The chief diagnostic difficulty with this first class appears when presbycusis is superimposed on noise-induced loss or a congenital defect or when inner-ear impairments similar to those of congenital defects appear following or during an illness or suddenly with no apparent cause.

Noise-induced hearing loss represents an impairment of the organ of Corti. It is not certain to what extent sensory units (described in Chapters 3 and 4) are destroyed in whole or in part or else may simply have their thresholds permanently elevated. Whatever the pathology may be, one characteristic sign is the configuration of the audiogram with a high-frequency loss that is greatest at 4000 Hz (or sometimes 3000 or 6000 Hz). Even more characteristic is the presence of loudness recruitment accompanied by good discrimination for speech. Loudness recruitment is almost always associated with impairment of the sense organ, and so also quite frequently is dysacusis, manifested by poor quality of tones and poor articulation scores. We emphasize again, however, that recruitment and dysacusis do not always appear together, as illustrated in noise-induced hearing loss.

Loudness recruitment Loudness recruitment is a very valuable sign because of its strong association with the sense organ. It is *not* produced by conductive impairment, either of the middle or of the inner ear; it is not encountered in central dysacusis; and it is relatively infrequent (not over 25 percent of cases) in acoustic neurinomas. We use the term in Fowler's original sense, referring to a more rapid than normal increase in loudness as the intensity of the test tone is increased (see Chapter 4). It is measured by the method of loudness balance. Unfortunately, as mentioned earlier, it is not always easy to test for it. In the alternate binaural loudness-balance test, when one ear is normal or nearly so, a series of comparisons are made, at one or two or even at three frequencies, of the hearing levels on the audiometer that sound equally loud to the two ears. Many audiometers designed for diagnostic purposes are equipped with two separate oscillators and attenuators to make loudness balancing easier. The results are usually plotted in either of the two forms illustrated in Figures 8-6, 8-7, and 8-8. In Figure 8-6 the key feature that shows recruitment is the change from the sloping lines near threshold (that connect equally loud settings) to horizontal lines at high intensities. In Figures 8-7 and 8-8 the corresponding feature is the approach of the observed points closer and closer to the diagonal line that is the locus of equal loudness in two normal ears.

A binaural loudness balance is more difficult for the subject than a simple threshold test, but with a little practice most subjects are able to do it quite well, even though they may protest that the job is difficult and that they have little confidence in their loudness matches. A monaural balance, in which a high tone is balanced against a low tone, is more difficult, but it can be done by intelligent and cooperative patients.

Monaural loudness balance depends in principle on assuming that hearing is more abnormal at one frequency than at another. The "more abnormal" is identified by its higher hearing level and sometimes by its poor quality. A monaural loudness balance can show recruitment clearly only if there is a difference in threshold levels of 25 dB or so between the two frequencies that are compared. And sometimes there is recruitment even at the least abnormal frequency.

There is a strong tendency for binaural recruitment curves, when plotted in the form of Figures 8-7 and 8-8, to converge with the normal diagonal and with one another at the hearing level of 90 dB (Hood). The significance of this trend or of individual deviations from it is not clear, however.

Other tests for loudness recruitment Some patients are not able to make reliable loudness balances, and sometimes there is no frequency at which hearing is within normal limits in either ear that can be used as the comparison tone. We must sometimes, therefore, infer the presence of loudness recruitment from tests other than loudness balance. These tests are useful qualitatively, but they are not quantitative.

The test of *tolerance for loud sound* may give a clear qualitative indication of recruitment if the threshold for a particular frequency is elevated, but its tolerance level is low. If the tolerance level is high, some recruitment may still be present, and at high sound levels the discomfort may arise in the middle ear and not simply because the sounds become uncomfortably loud.

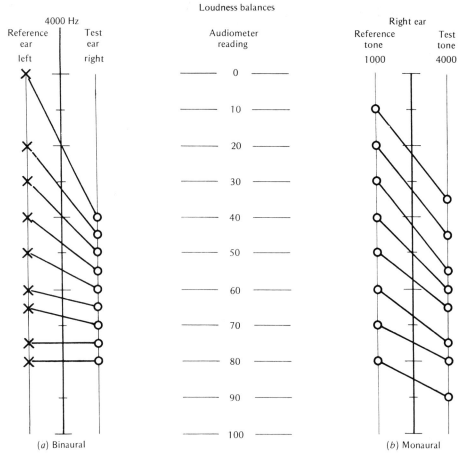

Loudness balances

Figure 8-6 *8-6a:* The results of binaural loudness balances at a given frequency are often plotted in this way *(Fowler).* One advantage of this form is that is can be superimposed on the regular audiogram. To do this, the values for the loudness balances are plotted about half an octave above and below the line corresponding to the frequency at which the balances are made and are joined by the straight lines. The conventional symbols for right and left are employed.

8-6b: The results of monaural loudness balances at two different frequencies may be plotted as shown here or in the form of Figure 8-7. The hypothetical case illustrated shows "delayed" partial recruitment at 4000 Hz. The monaural balance must be used when the losses in the two ears are substantially symmetrical. The lower of the two frequencies, usually 500 to 1000 Hz, should show a better hearing-threshold level than the frequency to be tested.

An extension of the test of tolerance is to determine the *range of comfortable listening.* The patient judges or selects the level, at each frequency, at which he would be willing to listen to the radio for a long time. The range of acceptable values may be quite narrow in the presence of recruitment, and it may lie quite close to the threshold of discomfort. Determination of the range of comfortable listening is obviously important in

assessing a patient for possible use of a hearing aid.

Another threshold that seems to be associated with the loudness of a sound is the activation of the *acoustic (intra-aural) reflex.* In humans this means practically the contraction of the stapedius muscle (see Chapter 3), although at very high levels the tensor tympani muscle may contract also. The response is bilateral. The best way to detect the contraction is by the resulting change in acoustic impedance-admittance. The appropriate methods are described in an earlier section. The air pressure in the ear canal is adjusted to give the minimum impedance (maximum admittance), and the sensitivity of the instrument is increased if necessary. The indicator is a *change* in impedance or admittance associated with an acoustic stimulus, usually presented to the contralateral ear. The threshold depends somewhat on the frequency of the test tone, but in general is between 70 and 90 dB HL. It may be 10 to 20 dB lower for noise. A positive response to a tone at 20 or 30 dB SL in an ear with threshold at 60 dB HL or higher is strong evidence of loudness recruitment. Of course the reflex

is absent if the reflex arc is interrupted, either centrally or peripherally, or if the stapes in the responding ear is fixed by otosclerosis. The intra-aural reflex, studied by this method, is currently attracting much attention. An excellent summary will be found in Dr. Feldman's chapter, listed among the references (Bradford, 1975).

The *Békésy audiogram* yields a simple sign that is often associated with loudness recruitment. The excursions of the tracing become shorter, meaning that the interval in decibels between "hear" and "don't hear" become smaller. In other words, the crossing of the threshold becomes more abrupt. Some narrowing of the excursions at the higher frequencies is normal, as in Figure 8-9. Further

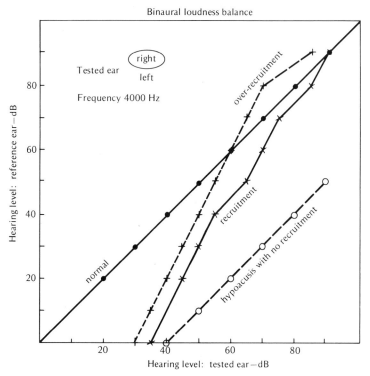

Figure 8-7   The results of binaural loudness balances at a given frequency may be plotted in this way *(Steinberg and Gardiner)*. If, as in the ideal normal case, the audiometer readings (hearing levels) are equal for every intensity setting, the points (solid circles) fall along the diagonal line labeled normal. A conductive hearing impairment shifts all the points to the right by an equal amount (open circles), and the line through them is parallel to the normal line. A hypothetical case of sensorineural impairment with recruitment (x, solid line) is shown and also a hypothetical case with overrecruitment (+, broken line).

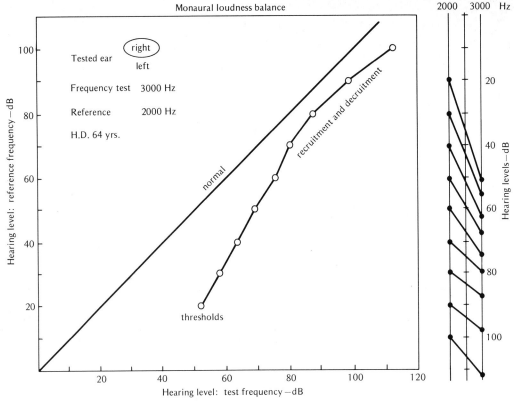

Figure 8-8 The monaural loudness balances between 3000 Hz and 2000 Hz show partial recruitment followed, at high intensity, by "decruitment" or negative recruitment. The loudness that could be elicited by 3000 Hz in this ear seemed to approach a maximum at high intensity. These are actual data obtained from an ear with abrupt high-frequency hearing loss, illustrated in Figure 7-7.

The results of an actual monaural bifrequency loudness-balance test in a case of abrupt high-tone hearing loss are plotted in both the expanded and the compact form. There is recruitment at moderate intensities and "decruitment" at the highest levels. Note that the threshold for the reference tone (2000 Hz) is slightly elevated, at 20 dB (ISO), and some recruitment may be present at this frequency also. The test actually shows the difference in recruitment at the two frequencies. The complete audiogram for this ear is shown in Figure 7-7 (seven years later).

narrowing, as in Figure 8-10, suggests that loudness recruitment is present and would be revealed by a direct loudness-balance test. This sign gives a partial indication of recruitment at threshold but does not test the upper part of the auditory area.

The *difference limen for intensity* is a test that theoretically should relate closely to loudness recruitment. It is the counterpart, at sound levels well above threshold, of the narrowed threshold trace of the Békésy audiogram. A pure tone at the desired level is presented to the subject, and small increases of intensity are introduced. The smallest increase that is detected with reasonable certainty is the subject's difference limen for intensity. A patient's difference limen is compared with values obtained with the particular instrument on a group of otologically normal subjects. The normal values vary as a function of both frequency and sensation level.

This type of test was introduced about 1950 by Lüscher and Zwislocki: it was modified by Denes and Naunton and later (1953) by Jerger. The best known modification is known as the *short-increment sensitivity index (SISI test)*. The principle in all variations is the same: The ear with loudness recruitment can detect smaller changes in intensity than the normal ear, and this reduced difference limen is a sign of sensorineural involvement. In the SISI test the patient listens to a tone 20 dB above his threshold for two minutes. An increment of 1 dB is introduced 20 times at approximately 5-second intervals. The increment lasts 200 milliseconds (ms) and has rise and fall times of 50 ms. The patient signals whenever he detects an increase in loudness. The SISI score is given in terms of percentage of increments detected. Two or more frequencies may be tested. Patients with conductive or retrocochlear lesions make low scores; those with sense-or-

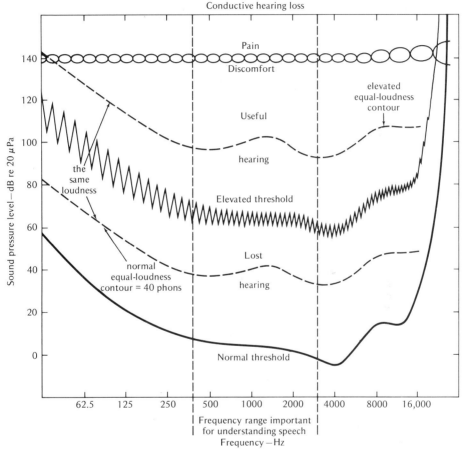

Figure 8-9 Reduced auditory area in pure conductive hearing loss. The normal threshold zone and threshold for pain are shown as in Figure 2-4. The threshold for pain is uncertain above 4000 Hz. The elevated threshold represents a hearing loss of about 60 dB at all frequencies, a so-called flat loss, produced by a severe but purely conductive lesion such as otosclerosis. This is the greatest possible purely conductive loss. The case is theoretical because a conductive hearing loss is rarely perfectly flat, and usually there is some high-tone sensorineural loss associated with it. The equal-loudness contours are raised without distortion. Nothing sounds very loud. The high equal-loudness contours have been elevated above the threshold of pain. The threshold of pain is not elevated, although the zone of discomfort may rise somewhat. The elevated threshold is a monaural free-field threshold. It is represented as a zigzag line that can be interpreted as showing the individual variability in successive measurements or else as the tracing that might be shown on a recording patient-controlled (Békésy) audiometer as in Figure 7-7.

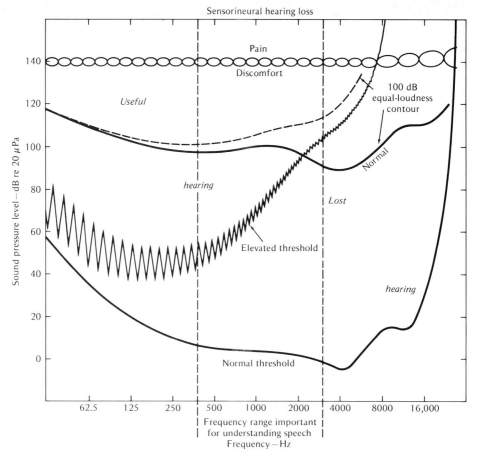

Figure 8-10 Reduced auditory area in a hypothetical case of sensorineural hearing loss. The normal free field, binaural threshold zone, and the threshold for pain are shown as in Figure 2-4. The threshold for pain is uncertain above 4000 Hz. The hearing loss is of the "gradual" high-tone type and is accompanied by strong "recruitment." The 100-dB equal-loudness contour is distorted but is only slightly displaced upward. High-level sounds are nearly as loud as for a normal ear. The threshold of discomfort is unchanged. The zigzag line, representing the elevated threshold as it might be shown by a patient-controlled (Békésy) type of automatic audiometer, covers a wide zone of uncertainty at low frequencies but a very narrow zone where the hearing levels are elevated and recruitment is present.

gan involvement tend to make high scores. This test has become fairly well established as a useful clinical test.

Tests for pitch and tone quality Tests of *diplacusis* have been proposed, based on binaural pitch matching or on the difference limen for frequency. These are not so much tests for diplacusis as measures of the degree of diplacusis, and they are not widely used.

The patient's description of the nature of his difficulty is usually sufficient, and it is not easy for him to match tones that are rough, complex, and noisy in one ear with pure tones presented to the other ear. The performance of the abnormal ear may fluctuate considerably. It is not the numerical values that are obtained in such attempts that are important but the degree of difficulty that the patient has in the attempt to make matches or fine pitch discriminations. Much the same considerations apply to attempts to measure *tinnitus*. Yet these disorders of discrimination are closely related to certain disorders of the sense organ and impairment of discrimination for speech.

Tests involving auditory fatigue or adaptation Gradually, since 1950, it has become evident that the threshold in some abnormal ears is not stable but rises more or less rapidly during auditory stimulation. The terms *auditory fatigue, fast adaptation,* and *tone decay* have all been used to describe this effect. The names of Dix, Hood, de Maré, Carhart, Miskolezy-Fodor, and Huizing are all associated with these early studies.

For some time there has been considerable confusion in the evaluation of various tests based on difference limens because the importance of adaptation was not recognized. Also validation was often in terms only of conductive versus normal versus sensorineural, or else as a predictor of "recruitment." Now it appears that we may be able to make a very important generalization. *Fast adaptation is a strong indication of involvement of the auditory nerve, particularly by a rapidly growing acoustic neurinoma, but loudness recruitment, and also poor tone quality, and low speech discrimination strongly suggest impairment of the sense organ. None of these signs or symptoms is produced by conductive impairment.* Certain qualifications and limitations of these generalizations will be or have already been noted, but they are good guides and emphasize the importance of tests of adaptation in audiological diagnostic strategy.

Tone-decay tests. A simple test of fast adaptation at threshold is the threshold tone-decay test. A sustained tone is presented to the subject at his threshold level, and the subject keeps his finger raised as long as he hears the tone. If he continues to hear it for a minute, he has no significant adaptation.

A modification of this test is to present the tone 5 dB above the threshold level and then, when the tone is no longer heard, to raise the level 5 dB to make it audible again, and to continue making such increases until the tone is heard for some specified length of time, such as 30 seconds, or decays completely. A Békésy-type of audiometer with fixed frequencies is the most convenient instrument to use.

Continuous-tone versus pulsed-tone threshold audiometry Subject-controlled automatic (Békésy type) audiometry may be carried out either with a continuous tone of slowly increasing frequency or with an interrupted tone. The interruptions may be at the rate of 2 or 3 per second, and a duty cycle with 50 percent "on" time is usually employed. The normal ear yields tracings that are completely (type I) or very nearly (type II) superimposable regardless of the interruptions. The Békésy type II audiogram shows a slightly better threshold for the interrupted tone, and both tracings may show the narrowing of the excursions mentioned as a "sign of recruitment." In the Békésy type III audiogram the continuous tone falls very rapidly below the tracing for the interrupted tone. In the Békésy type IV audiogram the continuous tone falls consistently below the interrupted tracing, usually without the narrowing of the excursions that is often present in type II. The amount of divergence depends somewhat on the rate of change of frequency in octaves per minute. The type III and type IV tracings are associated particularly with acoustic neuromas.

The gap between a continuous tone and the usual rate of interruption with intervals of about 200 ms can be explored by using shorter and shorter intervals. A *critical interval* appears for subjects with neural impairments at one or more frequencies. The threshold rises abruptly, as with a continuous tone, when the intervals are made too short. This test has not been widely exploited as yet (1976).

Tests of vestibular function A final item in diagnostic strategy, when the issue is a decision concerning sense organ versus neural impairment, is a test of vestibular function. The test most widely employed is the caloric test. In a common version the external ear canal is irrigated with known quantities of water at two definite temperatures, one above and the other below body temperature. Such caloric stimulation induces rhythmic side-to-side movements of the eyes, known as *nystagmus*. The movements may be observed visually, or electric potentials related to the movements may be amplified and recorded on a moving tape. The duration in seconds of the nystagmus is observed for each ear and for each temperature.

From the durations of nystagmus and from its amplitude and speed a judgment can be made of normality, hyperactivity, or hypoactivity of each labyrinth. We purposely omit all details concerning the technique of these (and other) tests of labyrinthine function since they are outside the scope of this book. Such tests are in the province of otology rather than audiology, and they figure prominently in the special area of neuro-otology. They do assist in audiological diagnosis, however, because of the prominence of labyrinthine involvement in Menière's disease and the occasional encroachment of acoustic neuromas on the labyrinthine as well as on the cochlear portion of the eighth cranial nerve.

Final Evaluation of Sensorineural Impairment

We repeat a primary principle of audiological and, in fact, of all medical diagnosis: *a diagnosis is not based on any single sign, symptom, or test.* All of the available evidence, including the history and interview, are considered, and the diagnosis, therapy, management, and perhaps additional tests are determined accordingly.

Some differential diagnoses are more difficult and also more important than others, particularly those that involve possible acoustic neuromas. One reason for the difficulty is that the symptoms and the test results may be quite different for a very slowly growing tumor from those caused by more rapidly increasing pressure. The sensory units that are impaired but still active seem to be those that cause the tone decay, the poor speech discrimination, and so on. The same principles apply in Menière's disease. The picture is quite different during an acute episode as opposed to the quiet period between episodes. The nervous system seems to adapt to the complete and stable loss of some sensory units rather well. Particularly confusing is the simultaneous involvement of sense organ and nerve when the tumor compresses the cochlear artery as well as the nerve.

The general pattern or profile of audiometric test results in advancing nerve involvement is (1) absence of recruitment, (2) total tone decay, (3) type III or type IV Békésy tracings, (4) low SISI scores, (5) hearing-threshold levels only slightly elevated below 2000 Hz but more elevated for high tones, (6) speech-reception threshold in agreement with pure-tone levels, but (7) speech discrimination usually somewhat reduced, particularly at high intensities.

FEIGNING: FUNCTIONAL OR NONORGANIC HEARING LOSS

In all of our discussions of tests of hearing, whether for pure-tone thresholds, speech thresholds, recruitment, or tone decay, we have assumed full cooperation by the patient. At worst, as in the case of babies or older autistic children, we assume indifference but not active deception. But when economic gain, "saving of face," or escape from danger is at stake, as in compensation for injury to hearing or discharge from military service, we may encounter a reversed motivation. The subject may not only make no real effort to hear; he may pretend not to hear at all or to hear much less than he really does. If the motivation to deceive for gain or safety is clear, this behavior is called *malingering*. If we are not sure of the motive, we call it *feigning*.

Two more general terms are also in widespread use: *functional* or *nonorganic* hearing loss. These terms describe hearing losses that cannot be ascribed to any "organic involvement." A more elaborate definition, given by Ventry and Chaiklin (1965), is: "Functional hearing loss is the appropriate diagnosis when there are audiometric discrepancies and/or discrepancies between observed behavior and audiometric findings and when no apparent organic condition can be found to account for the discrepancies." The terms cover a wide range, from deliberate malingering to true psychogenic deafness. In Chapter 4 we gave our reasons for preferring the more neutral terms "feigning" and "pseudohypoacusis" to malingering.

We are particularly concerned here with tests or tricks to detect feigning and to determine the "true" threshold of hearing in spite of more or less conscious and deliberate efforts of the subject to deceive the tester. Many devices have been developed to catch off guard the man who is suspected of feigning. One consists of imparting to him in a rather low tone of voice some information that is interesting or important to him and observing whether he reacts to it. Typically the "test" is made outside of what appears to the subject to be the test situation. The giving of the information is made to appear unintentional. The basic principle for success of such tests is very simple: *The tester must be smarter than the subject, and a better actor.*

Not all audiologists are good actors, and more sophisticated tests take advantage of psychoacoustic principles that are probably unknown to the subject or make it very difficult for him to control his behavior appropriately. Most of the formal tests to be described below are usually performed with a two-channel electric audiometer, but actually several of them are old tests that were originally carried out with tuning forks.

Feigning of Monaural Impairment

Stenger test The Stenger test depends on confusing the subject with respect to which ear is being stimulated. It is based on the fact that if two equally sensitive ears are stimulated simultaneously with an identical stimulus, the sound will be localized somewhere near the center of the head. If the stimulus is made more intense at one ear, then the listener will report that he hears sound only in that ear. He will not be aware of the weaker sound in the other ear. The threshold is determined on each ear for a tone of a particular frequency. The tone is then presented to the good ear alone at about 5 or 10 dB above its threshold. The patient will localize the sound to that ear. The tone is also presented to the supposedly bad ear the same number of decibels above its threshold. If the bad ear is as bad as the patient claims, he will probably localize the sound somewhere near the center of his head. If threshold is better in his bad ear than what he claims for it, the tone will sound louder in that ear and will be localized there. If the patient admits that he hears the sound in his bad ear, then this is a confession that he exaggerated the loss in that ear during the threshold measurement. Rather than admit that he hears in the bad ear he may claim that he hears no sound. In this case the tester gradually lowers the intensity of the sound in the bad ear until it is less loud than the sound in the good ear, which has been constant all this time. If the patient now says that he hears the sound in his good ear, this is an admission that previously the sound in his bad ear had been strong enough to obscure the sound in the good ear. By this procedure a close estimate can be made of the actual threshold in the supposedly bad ear. The Stenger test can be modified for use with speech instead of with pure tones.

Swinging voice test   One's monitoring of which ear is being stimulated can also be disrupted by the swinging voice test (sometimes called the shifting voice test). If speech is fed alternately (for example, every half second) to one ear and then to the other, the speech will be very intelligible if both ears are stimulated at about the same sensation level. The listener is hardly aware that his ears are being stimulated alternately. If one ear is bad, however, the speech will lose much of its intelligibility. If a person claims a unilateral loss and still shows normal understanding of speech in this test, he can be suspected of feigning.

One modification of the swinging voice test is to present a prepared story to the listener, switching back and forth from the good ear, to both ears, to the poor ear. The story is presented at a level 20 to 30 dB above the threshold of the good ear and is written so that if the loss is unilateral, it still is perceived as a sensible story to the listener. The test is positive if the listener repeats the part of the story presented to the poor ear. If he does this, the threshold in his poor ear must be *better* than the level at which the story was presented. If he claims that he could not understand the story, even after several presentations, this should arouse the tester's suspicions. This test does not give a threshold measurement but simply an indication that the listener is not giving a true threshold.

Binaural or Monaural Feigning

Lombard test   The Lombard test is based on the "voice reflex." In the presence of noise someone who is talking or reading aloud tends to raise his voice enough to hear himself speaking. We do this unconsciously when an automobile passes an open window or an airplane flies overhead. In the test, masking noise is introduced to both of the subject's ears while he is reading aloud. If he raises his voice when the noise is below his feigned threshold he gives himself away. The Lombard test can be used to detect feigned unilateral impairment by appropriately manipulating the noise levels at the two ears.

Delayed side-tone test   A different type of disruption of reading is used in the delayed side-tone test. The patient reads aloud into a microphone, which delivers the speech to a tape recorder. The recorded speech is played back, with a delay of about 0.2 second, to earphones on the patient's ears. The delay corresponds to about one syllable. So long as the delayed sound is softer than the sound of the patient's speech within his own head, his reading will not be disturbed. As the delayed speech is made louder, the patient will stutter or stumble, drag out his words, and usually raise his voice. With this test one can usually detect rather easily the feigning of a large hearing loss, but detection of small losses and the measurement of threshold are quite difficult.

Doerfler-Stewart test   One of the most extensively used quantitative tests for feigning has been the Doerfler-Stewart test and its modifications. This test depends on the interference by noise with the understanding of speech. The noise, however, must be at least as intense as the speech, and usually 10 to 15 dB greater, to make speech completely unintelligible. A person who is feigning may remember the loudness at which he pretends to begin understanding speech, but his monitor for loudness can be disrupted by the presence of noise. Both speech and noise, given to the same ear, are systematically varied in such a way that the person who is feigning cannot effectively retain the constant ratio of noise to speech expected from a cooperative patient and still remember at what level he is to stop "understanding." The details of the procedure are somewhat complicated, but a skilled examiner can manipulate the level of the test words, usually a spondee word list, and the masking noise in such a way as to arrive at a fairly accurate measurement of the "true" speech-reception threshold. The subject is concerned with the relation between the noise and the test words and pays little attention to the actual loudness of the words. He does not realize that a noise that just masks a test word sounds much louder than the test word.

Békésy tracings in feigned hearing loss Sometimes the tracings obtained with a Békésy type of recording audiometer reveal curious inconsistencies that assist in the identification of feigning or "functional hearing loss." Sometimes the thresholds are simply inconsistent with conventional pure-tone audiometry or with the speech-reception threshold. Particularly revealing, however, are Békésy tracings that regularly show better hearing for a continuous than an interrupted tone.

Feigned total deafness On the whole, it is usually easy to catch the person who pretends to be totally deaf. Feigned deafness in one ear is fairly easy to detect and so is a pretended very large loss. The deception most difficult to detect is the addition of some 10 or 15 dB to a genuine hearing loss of between 15 and 30 dB. This, like a psychogenic overlay, can easily pass undetected and even unsuspected; yet it may make quite a difference in relation to military discharge or to the amount of workmen's compensation award.

Signs and suggestions of feigning There are a number of signs or bits of behavior that should suggest the possibility of feigning to an alert audiologist. Prominent among these are (1) variations in thresholds on repeated trials, (2) incompatibility of different types of threshold, (3) bone conduction poorer than air conduction, (4) lack of agreement of speech with pure-tone hearing-threshold levels, or either of these with the history or with the clinical impression, (5) slow and deliberate responses, (6) partial (half-word) responses to spondee words, and (7) failure to respond to spondees at any level.

Tests of Psychogenic Overlay

Narcosynthesis, hypnosis, and suggestion At this point, for logical completeness, we refer to the method of narcosynthesis, described in Chapter 4, and the related methods of hypnosis and suggestion. These are methods of treatment rather than diagnostic tests, but the diagnosis of psychogenic deafness or overlay, as distinct from deliberate feigning, can hardly be made except in retrospect following a cure by one of these psychiatric methods. As a matter of diagnostic strategy, feigning rather than psychogenic deafness should be assumed until the evidence to the contrary is overwhelming. As we noted in Chapter 4, psychogenic deafness is apparently very rare in the United States at the present time (1976). The diagnosis must be made by a psychiatrist.

Physiological audiometry Physiological audiometry, to be described in the next section, particularly electroencephalic audiometry, may be very helpful in detecting and measuring the extent of a feigned or a psychogenic overlay, but it cannot distinguish between the two types. Only a few cases have been reported of electroencephalic testing in psychogenic deafness, but apparently the electrical responses of the brain are present with normal thresholds.

The principal methods of physiological audiometry depend on electrical responses from either the skin (electrodermal audiometry) or the brain (electroencephalic audiometry or "evoked-response" audiometry). In principle the physiological methods require only the passive cooperation of the patient, and they yield audiometric thresholds that are very close to the thresholds obtained by conventional clinical audiometry. The difficulties and limitations of the methods will be described in connection with their use in testing the hearing of children, but the Veterans Administration for a number of years required an electrodermal test of threshold, at least at 1000 Hz in each ear, as part of the evaluation of claimants for compensation for service-connected hearing loss. If the threshold by either method of physiological audiometry is 10 dB or more better than his behavioral threshold, the subject is suspected of feigning an overlay during the behavioral tests.

The electrodermal response, as used by the Veterans Administration, is one component in the famous battery of the "lie detector" test. This fact is known rather widely, and this knowledge tends to discourage feigning in audiometric tests.

TESTS OF HEARING FOR YOUNG CHILDREN

Most children who are 4 years old or older and some 3-year-olds can be tested by conventional behavioral audiometry. They can be instructed to raise a finger when they hear a tone and to lower it when they do not. The attention span is shorter in young children than in older children, but with encouragement and praise for correct responses 4-year-olds usually give quite reliable end points. Sometimes it requires two testing sessions to obtain complete pure-tone audiograms. The tester must be alert, however, for false positive responses by a child who is anxious to please, and therefore he must carefully avoid falling into a regular rhythm in the presentation of the test tones. It is usually easy to sense when the child understands what is expected of him and is cooperating well.

The real problems in testing the hearing of children arise when the child does not seem to understand or does not wish to cooperate. The children who require special testing methods are those (1) who are too young to understand, (2) who are mentally retarded, (3) who cannot make appropriate responses because of cerebral palsy even though they may hear something, (4) who are emotionally disturbed, (5) who respond only erratically or not at all to any stimuli (so-called autism or childhood schizophrenia), or (6) who may suffer from congenital or early acquired hearing loss so severe that they have failed to learn to pay any attention to whatever sounds they may be able to hear. As we shall see, it appears to be quite important that children with early hearing impairment be given the benefit of amplified sound during their first two or three years of life in order to avoid this kind of "habitual disregard" of hearing.

The tests that are appropriate for young children may be divided into three classes. Some tests are effective for children of 2 to 4 years who are able and willing to respond. They are really devices to increase the child's motivation and keep him interested in the test. Tests of the second class depend on unconscious, inborn reflex responses to sound, such as startle movements, eye blinks, or changes in respiration or heart rate. The third class takes advantage of the electrical responses of the brain or auditory nerve or the "electrodermal" response of the sweat glands. These are the physiological tests mentioned in the previous section in connection with feigned hearing loss or pseudohypoacusis.

Methods Based on Increased Motivation

Play audiometry Most children over 2½ years of age who are of normal mentality and without emotional disturbances can be taught to "play a game" with the tester. An auditory signal is used to tell the child that he may put a peg in a pegboard, turn over the leaf of a picture book, or do whatever is likely to interest a child of his age. Loud sounds are used at first until the child understands what he is expected to do; once this is accomplished, a pure-tone audiogram can be obtained. Perhaps the number of frequencies and intensities tested must be restricted or the testing spread over two or more sessions, but if the central processes of being able to attach meaning to a sound and of being able to keep attention concentrated are normal, it is just a matter of time to map out a peripheral hearing loss. The signals need not be pure tones. Valuable information can be obtained from a few clear responses to speech, to broadband noise, or to the sounds of selected noisemakers. Unfortunately, some children are very erratic on this and other tests, and some do not seem to be aware at any intensity of the auditory signals to which we wish them to respond. If the child is mentally retarded or shows negativistic "autistic" behavior, or has neurological difficulties, it may be very difficult to decide whether or not he also has impaired hearing. Such children simply do not learn to play this particular game.

The peep show This test is basically a formalization and standardization of the informal "play-a-game" type of test just discussed. Both types, incidentally, can employ either earphones or an acoustic field. The older the child, the fewer objections to earphones, and with earphones the ears can be tested separately.

In one form of the peep show the child looks into an illuminated box at a picture. Then the light goes out. When a small signal light goes on the child can illuminate the box again and see a new picture by pushing a button, but he must wait until the signal light goes on. When he has mastered the idea, which most children over 3 years do quite easily, an auditory signal, usually a rather loud pure tone, is sounded along with the signal light. After several combined trials the signal light is omitted. If the child responds correctly by pushing the button when the tone is sounded alone, he obviously "hears" usefully, and his hearing can be mapped out in the same way that it is by the play-a-game method.

The numerical results and their significance are practically identical for these two methods. In each the consistency of response and the ability of the child to understand what he is expected to do are as important for interpretation as the hearing levels in decibels.

The peep-show type of test, and there are many variations, was obviously inspired by the concept of the conditioned reflex. The subject responds correctly to a stimulus and receives a reward, like a monkey or rat pressing a lever for food. It has been customary to speak of "conditioning" the child and to describe a failure of the test by saying that the child "failed to condition." The same vocabulary is often applied to play-a-game audiometry in order to preserve an objective attitude and not seem to draw inferences as to "understanding" or "insight."

The peep show has gradually declined in

popularity during the last decade. Most clinics now rely chiefly on play audiometry and on their reflex, startle, and orienting responses described in the next section.

Physiological Audiometry for Children

The following tests, including those using electrical responses, are sometimes called "objective" audiometry because they do not require a subjective judgment or decision by the child. We prefer the term "physiological audiometry."

The simplest variety of physiological test depends on simple inborn reflexes such as startle, waking from sleep, blinking (the auropalpebral reflex), or looking toward the source of sound (the orienting reflex). For these responses the child does not need to be "conditioned." The tests are appropriate for young babies, and they will be considered in the order of the age at which they are most effective.

Reflex tests are given in an open acoustic field, and only the orienting reflex makes any differentiation as to which ear may be most severely impaired. The reflex tests are relatively crude with respect to both frequency and intensity, but they are very useful indeed as screening methods to identify the babies who need follow-up tests and perhaps the immediate special management discussed in Chapter 17.

Startle reactions The earliest startle response to a loud sudden sound is present at full-term birth and in many premature infants. At this stage it is known as the "Moro reflex," and consists of overall movements of face, body, and limbs, and strong closing of the eyes. The full classical picture of the Moro reflex fades out during the first weeks of life, but clearly defined movements, blinking or grimacing, often with some turning toward the side from which the sound comes, persist and are the best reflex indicators of hearing up to the age of "play audiometry."

Considerable attention has been given to the best type of sounds with which to elicit startle reactions or orienting (turning) reactions. Sudden sounds are more effective than those with gradual onset. Any particular sound may elicit a clear startle response on the first one or two trials but then become ineffective. (The popular word here is "habituation.") Many audiologists believe that familiar sounds are more effective than unfamiliar sounds and that noises are more effective than pure tones. Much work has been devoted to selecting the best battery of noise-makers, such as "clackers," rustling paper, squeaking dolls, spoon hitting cup, and so on, and to standardize their intensity in order to gain the most information on the character and severity of the hearing impairment. We shall not attempt to summarize these efforts. Perhaps more attention should be given to narrow-band or "peaked-spectrum" noise. Noise seems to be clearly more effective than pure tones in eliciting reflex responses from infants or awakening them from sleep.

Other reactions Many tests of hearing for neonates and young infants are essentially screening tests. In this context any movement of the body, a limb, or the face that seems clearly correlated with the stimulus may be used as an indicator. A change in the breathing rhythm or a momentary pause if the child is crying are among the many reactions to a sudden noise.

Awakening from sleep Awakening from sleep is another well-defined response, particularly useful for neonates. Here there seems to be some preference for a high-frequency pure tone, usually 3000 Hz, or for white noise delivered from a small loudspeaker held by hand close to the child at one or two standard sound-pressure levels. The lower level is intended to be one which will awaken an infant with normal hearing within one minute. Failure to wake does not prove a hearing loss, but it does indicate the necessity for further trials or careful observation by parents in the home surroundings. It is sometimes difficult to control the depth of sleep of the infant under test.

An infant who awakens in response to a loud noise does not necessarily have normal hearing. Particularly deceptive in this respect are children who have fairly good hearing for very high tones or very low tones, or both, but poor hearing for the important speech frequencies. They may respond to many everyday noises and to voice sounds but not hear well enough to learn speech and language spontaneously. Reflex audiometry has many pitfalls.

Orienting reaction More informative than simple awakening from sleep or a startle reaction to a sudden noise is the reflex turning of the head and perhaps the body also toward the side from which a new sound comes. This orienting response is usually well developed by the age of 6 months, when the child is able to sit on its mother's lap. It gradually becomes less clear after the first birthday and finally becomes submerged in general spontaneous movements and exploratory reactions. A skillful team can make a very good assessment of hearing on the basis of head-turning in response to noisemakers of various sorts, but great care must be taken to first attract the child's attention in the proper direction (forward), but not to attract it too much, and to avoid unwanted visual clues or air currents. Of course, the stimuli can be delivered by loudspeakers and can be standardized or calibrated in various ways. There are many variations on this theme and many different choices as to the best noise-makers, but the key to success is careful handling of the child and well-planned presentation of the stimuli, and above all careful observation. Habituation to sounds that were originally interesting presents one of the greatest difficulties.

Orienting reflexes are probably the best single method of reflex audiometry, and they have the advantage that they are at their best in the critical period from 6 to 12 months of age, when identification and approximate assessment of impaired hearing is so important.

A test based on conditioning a *visual* orienting response is closely related to the peep show (Suzuki and Ogiba). A strange visual stimulus, such as an illuminated doll, is presented to one side or the other of the child. The child looks toward the doll. This simple visual orienting response is now conditioned to a pure tone, as will be described below for the electrodermal response. As long as the tone is above threshold, the child turns his head *before* the doll is illuminated. This method is very simple and is one of the most reliable for children from 1 to 3 years old.

Electrophysiological Tests of Hearing

Simple observation of children's behavior, supplemented by reflex audiometry, can be very effective in identifying for closer attention and study the young children with impaired hearing, but nevertheless it is common for the first recognition of impairment to be the failure of the child to learn to talk by the usual age of 18 to 24 months. In any case, and particularly if there are complicating circumstances such as possible mental retardation, cerebral palsy, emotional disturbance, and so on, there is need for a more definitive test of hearing suitable for children of all ages and particularly from 6 months to 3 years. The most successful, definitive tests so far are based on the electrophysiological responses of the auditory nerve, the brain, or the sweat glands or else on changes in heart rate or the respiratory pattern. All of them require fairly elaborate and rather expensive equipment, and they should be considered as definitive tests to be used in major hearing clinics—not as screening methods.

Respiratory and cardiac audiometry Changes in respiration often form part of larger startle patterns and can be detected by direct observation, as in neonatal screening tests. More sensitive and more sophisticated methods, based on objective recording of respiratory activity, have been developed as definitive hearing tests. These methods have been well described (Bradford, 1975) but they have not yet been adequately validated. The instrumentation is simpler than for the more fully tested electrophysiological methods, and, if the latter prove to be too unreliable or expensive, respiratory audiometry for infants may be more widely exploited. (This writer confesses to a considerable bias toward electroencephalic audiometry.)

The same comments apply equally to cardiac audiometry. The response here is a complex acceleration followed by deceleration, or the reverse, immediately after an acoustic stimulus. The changes are rapid and subtle and require a method of measuring by computer the duration of the intervals between beats in the electrocardiogram and averaging them and displaying the trends in rate before and after the stimulus. The cardiac rhythms in infants are quite labile, and it is not yet clear whether the method can be made reliable enough for general use; for a good description, see Eisenberg (Bradford, 1975).

Electrodermal Audiometry (EDA)

The first electrophysiological method to be perfected is known as *electrodermal audiometry*. The response that is recorded is sometimes called the ''skin galvanic response'' or the ''psychogalvanic skin response'' (PGSR). The response is an activation of the sweat glands through the autonomic nervous system. It is detected by measuring the resulting change in electrical resistance (the Féré effect) or electric potential (the Tarchanoff effect), or both, usually between the palm and the back of the hand. Usually it is the change of resistance that is detected. Electrically the subject's hand constitutes part of one arm of a Wheatstone bridge. Any change in the resistance of the subject is recorded by a pen on a moving strip of paper. Another pen indicates when electric shocks or sounds are given.

A very loud unexpected sound may elicit the electrodermal response, but a mild electric shock is a much more effective and reliable stimulus. This response tends to become less effective with repetition, however, and seems to represent an alerting or ''orienting'' reaction. The electrodermal response is made useful for audiometry by forming a conditioned reflex with sound (the audiometric test tone) as the conditioned stimulus. The conditioning shocks are applied through separate electrodes. Tones are sounded from time to time, and shocks are given following some or all of them. The best interval between tone and shock is 0.6 second.

Some subjects do not even require any conditioning, but unfortunately there are other subjects who fail to establish a conditioned reflex even after repeated trials with strong shocks. If the subject does respond satisfactorily, it helps to reinforce the tones from time to time by giving the electric shock as well. With sensitive subjects who respond consistently, the threshold of hearing can be mapped out as well by EDA as by the usual behavioral methods of clinical pure tone audiometry, and the absolute thresholds may be within a few decibels of each other. The advantage of this type of test is that it does not involve conscious response to the tones. It is therefore suitable for either children or adults who cannot or will not respond voluntarily in conventional behavioral audiometry.

EDA has been employed and enjoyed a period of considerable popularity, but now because of various difficulties and uncertainties, it is falling into disfavor for use with children. It is not suitable for young children in any case because of the disturbing effects of electric shocks. It cannot be applied during sleep, and even mild tranquilizers seem to reduce the responses and interfere with the necessary conditioning. The very children who are uncertain and erratic in their responses to the peep-show or the "play-the-game" testing are the ones who are most likely to be erratic in their electrodermal responses.

Either with children or with adults a positive response means that the sound has stimulated the ear successfully, and the nerve impulses have reached at least the brain stem and have triggered off a response in the autonomic nervous system. Failure to respond, however, does not prove that there is a peripheral hearing loss, and even with a favorable subject it is often difficult to decide whether a given deflection of the pen is actually an electrodermal response or not.

In spite of its shortcomings, the electrodermal response is relatively simple and does not require a computer.

Electroencephalic Audiometry (EEA)

Another form of electrophysiological audiometry is *electroencephalic audiometry.* The brain is continually active, and in its activity it generates electric potentials like those in nerves and muscles. These potentials can be recorded by placing electrodes on a nerve or a muscle, or even in the general neighborhood of a nerve or muscle if the original signals are strong enough. The electro-

cardiogram is a familiar example of the distant recording of the electrical activity of a muscle, in this case the heart. The electroencephalogram (EEG) is to the brain what the electrocardiogram is to the heart. The electric potentials generated by the brain are strong enough to be detected by electrodes placed on the outside of the skull and even on the outside of the scalp. The potentials must be amplified, but the final patterns can be recorded by pens on a moving paper very much as the electrocardiogram or the electrodermogram is recorded.

The pattern of electrical changes shows very well whether the subject is awake or asleep, and whether his eyes are opened or closed. It so happens that the change in the EEG pattern between waking and sleeping is a rather striking one and, furthermore, that a person who is lightly asleep shows rather dramatic transient changes in his EEG pattern (the "K-complex" and other changes) in response to sounds. The changes are in the direction of waking up, although the subject usually does not fully awaken but sinks back to the previous level of sleep. The K-complex and other electroencephalic responses do not have to be learned. They are inborn patterns just like the electrodermal response to electric shocks.

The recognition of EER to measured auditory stimuli in sleep seemed to be a very promising tool for physiological audiometry. Now, however, with the advent of computer techniques that allow us to look at specific evoked potentials instead of merely the background indicators of arousal or the depth of sleep, attention has shifted entirely to electric response audiometry (ERA) and electrocochleography (ECochG).

Electric Response Audiometry (ERA)

Electric response audiometry is now the general term for all audiometry that uses as an end point any one of a considerable number of electric responses that can be evoked from various parts of the auditory system by acoustic stimulation. The term *evoked-response audiometry* is sometimes used, but here the word "evoked" is redundant and "electric" is more informative. The responses are all of them very small, and for recognition they require repetitive stimulation and the summation of many responses by means of some sort of *average-response computer*. The responses, which are time-locked to the stimuli, add in the memory of the computer, whereas the more or less random background activity of brain and muscles largely cancels itself out and its sum increases much less rapidly. The result is a great improvement in the signal-to-noise ratio. The ratio can be further improved by appropriate band-pass filtering of the electrical input, and particularly by obtaining good muscular relaxation of the subject.

Three major classes of electric response from different parts of the auditory system have been explored quite fully as audiometric indicators, and each seems to have found a particular area of application. One response is that of the cerebral cortex, probably quite closely related to the spontaneous electroencephalogram. Another is generated in the brain stem, and the third in the auditory nerve. Commercial instruments are now (1977) available and clinical experience with each method is increasing rapidly. We shall consider the three in a historical rather than an anatomical sequence. We shall not go into details of technique of recording the responses or into the electrophysiological problems of how and where they are generated. These problems and a systematic overview of ERA are treated in a recent monograph (Davis, 1976). We shall concentrate on the particular advantages and limitations of each method. A disadvantage shared by all three is the expense of the equipment and the expertise required to use it effectively. The methods are not suited to an otological office or to most hearing clinics. They belong in major medical or audiological centers to which dif-

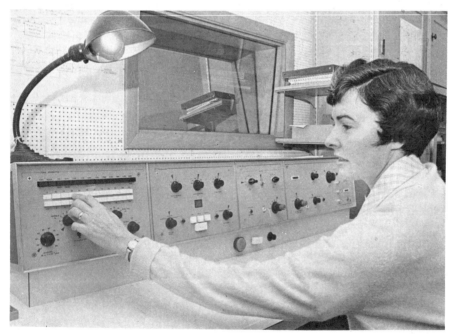

Figure 8-11 Evoked-response audiometer system (Princeton Applied Research Corp.). The operator is selecting the test tone. The records shown in Figure 8-13 were obtained with this instrument at Central Institute for the Deaf. *(Photo courtesy St. Louis Post-Dispatch)*

ficult cases can be referred when simpler methods do not yield definitive results.

Cortical ERA

The cortical class of electric response audiometry is usually understood when the abbreviation ERA is used without qualification. A slow cortical response was the first evoked potential to be identified. It was actually first seen without averaging in the ongoing electroencephalogram of some subjects in response to fairly strong, widely spaced stimuli in either the auditory, the visual, or the tactile modality (see Figure 8-11). In any normal subject only 30 to 60 responses need to be summed to identify this response clearly. The position of the electrodes on the head is not very critical, but, by a series of anatomical coincidences, the vertex (top of the head) is optimal or near optimal for all three modalities. (For this reason the response has been called the *vertex* [or *V*] *potential*). A reference electrode is placed on earlobe(s), mastoid(s), or elsewhere around the base of the skull, and a ground electrode is placed on the forehead. Standard EEG disk or cup electrodes are employed (see Figure 8-12). No discomfort or invasion is involved beyond cutting a small patch of hair and rubbing the skin with electrode paste.

The pattern of the auditory V-potential response is a series of waves of progressively longer periods. The latency to peak of the first really clear (vertex-negative) wave is about 100 ms, the second peak (vertex-positive) is about 180 ms, and the third (vertex-negative) is about 300 to 400 ms (see Figure 8-13). (The tactile and particularly the visual latencies are a little longer.) Actually the K-complex in sleep seems to be a member of the V-potential family, but the waves have long latencies and are probably generated in different neural structures with different an-

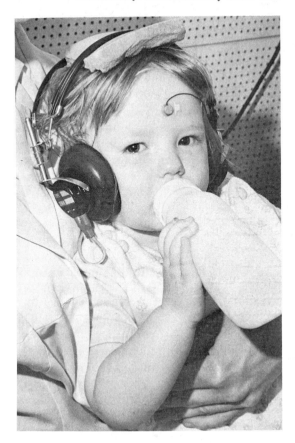

Figure 8-12 Evoked-response audiometry. The child, held by its mother, wears standard earphones. The electrode on the forehead is the ground lead. The "active" electrode is under the sponge rubber pad, and the reference electrode is behind the right ear. *(Central Institute for the Deaf; photo by Harold Ferman)*

atomical distributions. The V-potentials are generated rather diffusely in the auditory, the somatosensory or the visual areas. In sleep the responding area is even more widespread. The negative wave at 100 ms is not the first response of the cortex but probably of the third order and later. It is modified significantly by the alertness and attentiveness of the subject and is reduced in drowsiness.

The audiometric signals used in ERA are pulsed tones with durations of perhaps 200 ms and rise times of 10 to 20 ms. They are

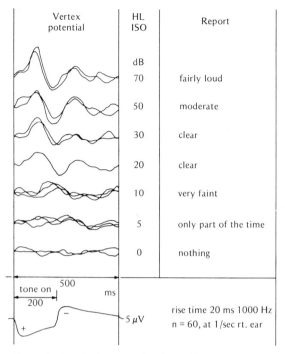

Vertex potential	HL ISO	Report
	dB	
	70	fairly loud
	50	moderate
	30	clear
	20	clear
	10	very faint
	5	only part of the time
	0	nothing

tone on 500 ms
200

rise time 20 ms 1000 Hz
n = 60, at 1/sec rt. ear

−5 μV

Figure 8-13 The form, amplitude, and latency of the vertex (V) potential in response to 1000-Hz tone bursts at various hearing levels are shown in the tracings in the left column. The corresponding reports of the subject are given on the right. The subject, an adult who was a practiced listener with well-formed V potentials, was reading and paying no special attention to the audiometric signals except at the 5 and 0 dB hearing levels. For these she stopped reading and listened. Her reports were very consistent, and from them her behavioral audiometric threshold was estimated at 5 dB ISO. Duration of the tone bursts, time constants of the equipment, and so on, are shown by the calibration tracing at the bottom. *(Test conducted with a Princeton Applied Research evoked-response audiometer, Model 140)*

delivered either by earphones or, for infants, by loudspeaker. Actually the V potential is an "on" effect, and only the first 30 ms or so of each tone burst is really important. The pulses must not follow one another too rapidly. Intervals of 10 seconds or more are needed for maximum amplitude of response, and the responses become very small if the interval is less than half a second. The most efficient rate to get the largest summed response within a minute is one per second if

the subject is awake or one every 2 seconds if he is asleep.

In nearly all alert, cooperative subjects the N_{100}-P_{180} response can be identified with good confidence at the 20-dB sensation level (see Figure 8-13), and usually at the 10-dB sensation level, as determined by behavioral methods. By using a well-chosen sequence of intensities following the strategy of the game of "twenty questions," and interpolating or extrapolating the final threshold of detectability it is usually possible to determine three thresholds in each ear in a total testing time of about 45 minutes. The three frequencies preferred by the writer for children with impaired hearing are 250, 1000, and 3000 Hz.

The ERA method as described is excellent for adults who are suspected of psychogenic deafness, malingering, or feigning and for cooperative mentally retarded, autistic, or multiple handicapped children.

Some young children with short attention spans who give erratic behavioral responses can be amused by pictures, puppets, and a variety of toys. An assistant skilled in the art of amusing children is an essential member of the ERA team, but hyperactive children, emotionally disturbed children, and most normal babies under 2 years of age are difficult or impossible to test by ERA while awake. The older and cooperative children can usually be tested quite reliably by behavioral "play" audiometry.

It was hoped for several years that with sedation the active, uncooperative children and infants could be tested by ERA using the slow (P_{200}-N_{350}) response of sleep. Unfortunately these responses are strong only in deep sleep and then only with rather strong (40 dB SL and higher) stimuli, and false positives are frequent. Responses are small and often erratic in drowsiness and light sleep. For these reasons the use of cortical ERA for infants and hyperactive children did not gain widespread popularity, yet it is exactly this group of subjects for whom a reliable physiological method is most needed.

The Electrocochleogram (ECochG)

In 1968, independently and almost simultaneously in Japan, Israel, and France, the action potentials of the auditory nerve were recorded from humans by the method of average evoked potentials. The potentials are much smaller than the V potentials, but the responses have very brief recovery periods, and stimulation rates of 20 clicks per second are quite practical. About 1000 responses can be summed in less than a minute. The latency of the response is very short, from about 1 to 4 ms. A major problem has been the placement of the "active" electrode. Yoshie and his associates put a needle subcutaneously in the external auditory canal near the tympanic membrane. Sohmer and associates used two surface electrodes outside but near the ear. Aran, Portmann, and others boldy passed a needle through the tympanic membrane to make contact with the promontory. They were rewarded with a tenfold increase in voltage, and at the present time the transtympanic approach is the method of choice in a majority, but not all, of the clinics where ECochG is performed.

Worldwide experience with thousands of cases has demonstrated the safety of the transtympanic electrode as far as otitis media or a permanent perforation are concerned. Two major drawbacks of the method are that the placement of the electrode is a surgical procedure that requires the participation of an otologist, and for children general anesthesia is necessary. The latter requires the continuing presence of an anesthetist. The procedure is suitable for a department of otology in a hospital but not for a hearing clinic. Adults and some older children may be tested with only local anesthesia and

perhaps a tranquilizer, but each ear tested in this way requires the surgical placement of the electrode.

The second disadvantage of the method is that the frequency selectivity of the acoustical test is poor, particularly for frequencies below 1000 Hz. When first introduced, the stimuli were simple clicks produced by a loudspeaker activated by rectangular electric pulses. The objective was not to derive an audiogram but simply to determine whether the ear was functional and whether its threshold for a broadband stimulus (a click) was normal or grossly elevated. This the method can do, and the threshold for detection of the auditory action potential is not far from the behavioral threshold of normal-hearing subjects.

The electrocochleogram (see Figures 8-14 and 8-15) yielded something new, however: the waveform of the action potential of the auditory nerve and the relations of its amplitude and its latency to the intensity of the stimulus. The response is clearly double. Near threshold the latency is long, about 4 ms, and the waveform rounded. With stronger stimuli the latency decreases while the amplitude increases slowly. At about 50 dB SL a new wave with shorter latency appears. It grows much more rapidly than the low-intensity wave and soon obscures the latter, but its latency of a little over 1 ms does not change appreciably. Sometimes the amplitude and the latency function, either or both, show clear breaks or abrupt changes of slope as the early high-threshold response becomes dominant over the later one.

Much speculation has ensued and still continues over the interpretation of the double character of the ECochG response. The earliest interpretation attributed the low-threshold long-latency response to the outer hair cells and the high-threshold short-latency response to the inner hair cells, and for many workers this interpretation has merit.

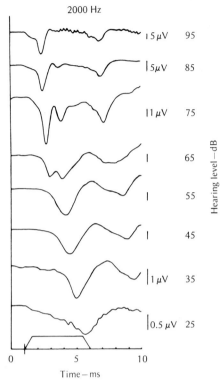

2000 Hz

| 5 µV   95
| 5µV   85
| 1 µV   75
| 65
| 55
| 45
| 1 µV   35
| 0.5 µV 25

Hearing level—dB

0   5   10

Time—ms

Figure 8-14 Electrocochleograms in response to 2000-Hz tone bursts of form shown at bottom. Transtympanic electrode on the promontory of a normal-hearing adult. Stimuli were delivered (by loudspeaker) in alternating polarity to cancel the CM. Downward deflection means promontory-negative. Note the double peaks at 75 and 65 dB HL and also the negative summating potential (SP) that starts with the stimulus before the action potential and continues throughout the tone burst. Note the differences in calibration for the very strong and very weak tones. (Eggermont, et al., Ann. Otol., Suppl. 28; 1976; by permission)

It is powerfully reinforced by the absence of the long-latency part of the curve from the response of ears with high-frequency sensorineural hearing loss of the type associated with recruitment of loudness. The high threshold and the rapid growth of amplitude of the action potential in these ears roughly parallels the subjective loudness; and in these ears the outer hair cells are thought to be abnormal or missing.

The story became more complicated, however, as it was finally realized that the acoustic signal delivered to the cochlea was complex, with a high-frequency component and a middle-frequency component (and perhaps others), depending on the resonances of the loudspeakers and of the ear itself. One component is usually centered near 2000 Hz or somewhat lower and the other above 4000 Hz. For the lower frequency, which is responsible for stimulating the ear near threshold, the traveling-wave delay in the cochlea gives its response a longer latency than that of the high-frequency component, which appears at higher levels.

Much experimentation—involving the use of acoustically simpler stimuli such as tone pips (filtered clicks), in which a single band of frequencies (about half an octave wide) dominates, and the use of filtered high-pass noise as a masker—has shown that the two-place interpretation is correct in principle but that it cannot explain the complexities of the input-output functions completely. On the other hand, a relatively pure low-frequency tone pip (such as 500 Hz) will, at a rather moderate intensity of about 50 dB SL, begin to stimulate extensively the high-frequency region of the basal turn. An additional complexity is the appearance in the ECochG at high intensities of the summating potential, described in Chapter 3.

At the present time (1977) much interest centers on the correlations being established empirically in the clinic between conditions such as ototoxic damage by drugs, permanent threshold shift from noise, Menière's disease, acoustic neuroma, and other pathological conditions, and in the laboratory on attempts to reconcile the paradoxes discussed in Chapter 3 that arise from the curious innervation pattern of the ear, the sharp tuning of acoustic sensory units, and the modifications of the shape of the tuning curves by drugs or other injury. These problems are discussed at some length in the Davis (1976)

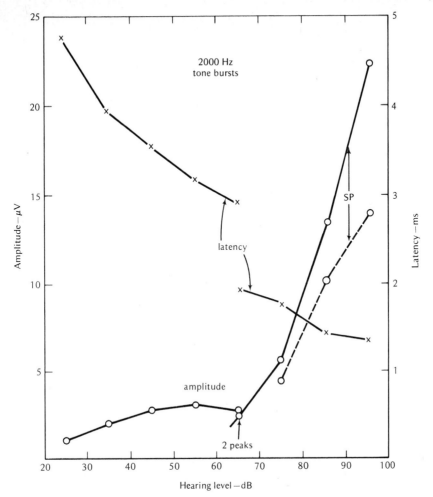

Figure 8-15 Latencies and amplitudes, measured from the tracings in Figure 8-14, plotted as functions of hearing level. The amplitude is measured to the largest peak (or to both peaks at 65 dB) from the baseline before stimulation. The amplitude is also measured from the SP at the foot of the AP (at 75, 85, and 95 dB) and plotted as open circles. The SP, the difference between these two measurements, evidently contributes significantly to the overall amplitude at high stimulus levels. (*Ann. Otol., Suppl. 28; 1976; by permission*)

monograph on ERA mentioned earlier and will not be considered further here.

The overall situation with respect to clinical ECochG can be summarized as follows: (1) it is a surgical procedure that requires hospital facilities and personnel; (2) the response is reliable and sensitive, best with the transtympanic electrode; (3) it yields excellent information concerning the state of the basal turn of the cochlea (frequencies 2000 Hz and above) but progressively less for the more apical regions; (4) *its greatest usefulness will presumably be for the analysis and diagnosis of sensorineural disorders in adults and particularly, in combination with other methods, in distinguishing sense-organ impairment from acoustic neuroma;* (5) it should not be employed for the assessment of hearing impairment in young children because the closely related brain-stem responses, to be described in the next section, give equally valid and sensitive indications with a simpler and less invasive technique. In short, electrocochleography seems to be, like impedance-admittance measurements, a very promising method for otological diagnosis but not a method of choice for audiometry as a measure of hearing.

Brain Stem Response Audiometry (BSRA)

The third family of electric responses that is useful for audiometry are the responses generated in the nuclei of the auditory system in the brain stem. These structures include the cochlear nucleus, the trapezoid body, the superior olivary complex, the nucleus of the lateral lemniscus, and the inferior colliculus. Their responses follow that of the auditory nerve in rapid sequence and, if the incoming volley of impulses is well synchronized, they constitute a series of waves at about 1-ms intervals that can be recorded in the "far field" from an electrode on the vertex with reference to the earlobe, mastoid, or neck. The sequence in humans was first clearly described in 1971 by Jewett and Williston, and Jewett's name and nomenclature are often used to designate them. We prefer a more generalized nomenclature that uses N or P to show vertex-negative and vertex-positive respectively and a numerical subscript to show the most characteristic latency for a 60 dB SL stimulus in a normal-hearing adult. In this terminology the most prominent, stable, and sensitive wave is P_6. It is almost certainly generated chiefly in the inferior colliculus, although waves P_3, P_5, and P_6 all probably arise from two or more nuclei that discharge almost simultaneously.

The brain stem responses are very small, with maximum voltage of the order of 1 μV,

but their recovery period is brief and stimulation rates of 20 to 30 tone pips per second can be used. Thus 2000 responses can be collected in less than two minutes. An important electronic adjunct is an artifact-rejection circuit, which rejects any sample that contains a wave of more than a modest preset maximum voltage. This protects the memory from being flooded by an occasional outburst of muscle potentials. Even so, *good muscular relaxation is essential, and for young children this means sedation.* Secobarbital, valium, and chloral hydrate are all popular choices. These can be administered orally or rectally by paramedical personnel in a hearing clinic on a physician's prescription.

The external scalp electrode and the use of sedation instead of anesthesia are the two major advantages of BSRA over ECochG. A minor advantage is the longer latency of the response, which greatly reduces interference from electrical stimulus artifacts. Ordinary audiometric earphones can be used, without special precautions, instead of a loudspeaker. Wave P_6 follows P_1 like a shadow, almost exactly 4 ms later. P_1 is the action potential of the auditory nerve. Thus the information gained from the BSR almost duplicates that from ECochG except that we do not see either cochlear microphonic or the summating potential or the changes in waveform of the ECochG that are reported in the presence of an acoustic neuroma. Wave P_6 does show the same complex relations of amplitude and latency to intensity as are seen in ECochG. A sequence of responses related to hearing level is shown in Figure 8-16. The figure also illustrates the sensitivity of BSR. Near-threshold responses are identified by their increased latency, up to 9.0 ms for a 4000-Hz tone pip, as well as by their reduced amplitude. The clarity of responses at low levels is due in large part to the higher thresholds for some of the components other than those from the inferior colliculus. At

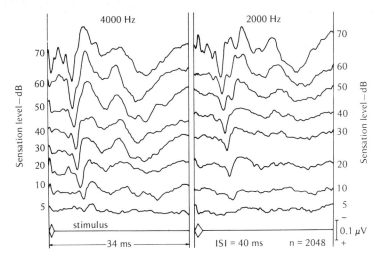

Figure 8-16   Brain stem electric responses P₆ of a young adult to tone pips at 4000 Hz and 2000 Hz. Electrodes on vertex and earlobe. Upward indicates vertex more negative. Sensation level of stimulus at right and left. Timing and approximate envelope of electric tone pips to earphones shown at bottom. (Ann. Otol., *Suppl. 28; 1976; by permission*)

higher levels the other components are normally not quite in phase with P_6 proper and tend to distort or obscure it.

The relations of BSR to frequency are the same as those of ECochG. The most effective stimulus is a "raw" unfiltered click, which is rich in high frequencies. Responses are also good to tone pips (see Figure 8-17) at 4000 and 2000 Hz. At 1000 Hz and below each sound wave becomes a separate stimulus, and the resulting patterns of action potentials become more and more confused. This is doubly true if, as is usual, the stimuli are presented in alternating polarity. The opposing polarities cause any stimulus artifacts and also the cochlear microphonic to cancel out. The action potentials do not cancel, but they shift in latency by half a period of the sound. This shift is serious at 1000 Hz because the resulting composite wave is rounded and cannot be identified below about 10 or 15 dB SL.

The usefulness and precision of BSR for audiometry depends largely on the nature of the information that is desired. Is it the *threshold for any response* to a particular

acoustic frequency, or is it the *integrity of a particular portion* of the cochlea? These questions are not the same because at sensation levels of 40 and upward, low tones, such as 500 Hz, stimulate the basal as well as the apical parts of the cochlea. The basal extension of excitation from the most sensitive region begins just above threshold. As pointed out in Chapter 3, this extension does not alter the subjective pitch, but it does contribute to loudness. The responses near threshold at 1000 Hz and at 500 Hz have a significantly longer latency than those to 4000 or 8000 Hz because of the travel time of the Békésy wave on the basilar membrane. The delay is a little over one full cycle of the frequency of the stimulus. The travel time is practically negligible at 4000 Hz and above. The latency in normal ears following strong stimuli is nearly the same for all frequencies, however, because the low frequencies now stimulate the basal turn without a traveling wave delay. The basal-turn response is larger and better synchronized than the apical-turn response and it obscures the latter. Actually in both ECochG and BSRA it is difficult to

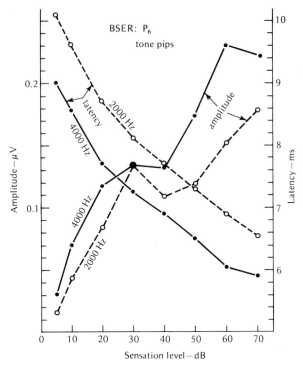

Figure 8-17   Latency and amplitudes of the responses shown in Figure 8-16, plotted as functions of sensation level. The latency for 2000 Hz is systematically longer than for 4000 Hz by about 0.8 ms at each sensation level. The amplitude is less for 2000 Hz at most levels. The plateaus (or reversals) in the amplitude functions resemble the breaks in the ECochG functions in Figure 8-16. Amplitude of P_6 is average of the differences between P_6 and the negative peaks about 1.5 ms before and 3.0 ms after it. Band-pass filters with slopes of about 30 dB per octave were used to generate the tone pips. The high-pass and low-pass sections were set to the same nominal cutoff frequency. (Ann. Otol., *Suppl. 28; 1976; by permission*)

identify in normal ears the response to 500 Hz that arises near the apex. The response may be revealed clearly, however, in the presence of high-tone hearing loss or of high-pass-filtered masking noise.

A real audiometric ambiguity arises when there is impairment of the apical portion of the cochlea but a normal basal portion. This can occur in Menière's syndrome. The threshold for 500 Hz is elevated by only 40 dB or less, but the responses are now those of the basal turn alone, and subjectively the sound is rough and buzzing. The pitch of the sensation is *periodicity pitch alone*. The pitch is vague and the tone quality very bad (dysacusis). The ECochG response is sharp and clear, however—a series of responses

corresponding to the individual low-frequency sound waves. The interpretation depends on the exact question that is asked, and it is important to note that *for apical impairment behavioral pure-tone audiometry is equally ambiguous* unless tonal quality is taken into account or *selective high-frequency ipsilateral masking* is employed.

Even in the most favorable situations the frequency selectivity of the ECochG and BSRA cannot be as sharp as with pure-tone audiometry. The reason is that these early responses are strictly "on" effects. In Chapter 2 the principle is outlined that very brief acoustic stimuli must have relatively broad spectra. Stimulation occurs with the first rarefaction wave of all frequencies from 2000

Hz downward, whether it be the ramp onset for a long tone burst or merely a tone pip. At high frequencies there may be temporal integration of two or more cycles, and the effective acoustic spectrum is somewhat narrower. For lower tones each sound wave is a separate stimulus, and the effective acoustic spectrum for each is broad and more difficult to define. The first response is the usual indicator of threshold, however, and for it the effective stimulus must be at least half an octave wide. The measured spectra of several *complete* tone pips are shown in Figure 8-18. The *effective* spectra must be still broader. *Nevertheless, the frequency selectivity realized with these tone pips is good enough for most clinical purposes.* A really abrupt high-frequency hearing loss will appear less abrupt than by behavioral audiometry with pure tones, but a steep downward trend will be evident.

Other Electric Responses

Two other electric responses offer some hope for improved sensitivity and selectivity at low frequencies. One of these is the *middle* set, with latencies from 12 to 50 ms.

These waves are probably generated in the midbrain and as the primary response of the cortex. Very brief tone bursts that are fairly frequency-selective are appropriate stimuli. A major difficulty has been interference from muscle potentials, which unfortunately lie in the same band of frequencies.

The other possible indicator is the frequency-following response, which is a complex response of the brain stem to a continuous tone. Actually 500 Hz is the most favorable frequency. Neither the middle responses nor the frequency-following response have as yet been well enough validated in the clinic to warrant further discussion here.

In summary, concerning ERA the writer considers the *slow cortical response* in waking subjects to be the most satisfactory if the subject is sufficiently cooperative. For young and otherwise difficult-to-test children sedation is needed, and with it the *brain-stem response* is the method of choice and is very satisfactory for frequencies of 1000 Hz and higher. The *electrocochleogram* offers unique diagnostic advantages for use with adults in whom an acoustic neuroma is suspected.

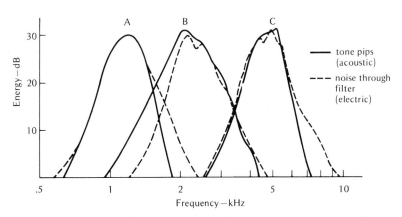

Figure 8-18 Acoustic energy spectra (smoothed) of tone pips and of white noise passed through the same filters. In A and C the filter was excited by a single sine wave of the same frequency as the center of the passband; in B by a rectangular wave of duration of half a cycle. *(Ann. Otol., Suppl. 28; 1976; by permission)*

AUDITORY SCREENING OF INFANTS

The audiometric screening of schoolchildren in the interest of conservation of hearing has been discussed in the previous chapter. It has served its purpose well and has stimulated the development of both puretone and speech audiometry, but such conventional behavioral methods cannot be applied to infants.

With the realization of the importance of early use of amplification for hearing-impaired children and with the advent of electric response audiometry as a reasonably accurate and reliable (although elaborate and expensive) method of measuring the hearing of infants, efforts were redoubled to develop a quick and inexpensive but reliable screening method to identify the infants who should be given special tests. The strategic point at which to install such a screening procedure seemed to be the maternity hospital. A larger percentage of the preschool population passes through this gateway than any other, and by school age the advantages of early use of amplification are lost.

In principle each infant must give a positive response to an appropriate test sound in the nursery or be tested more fully in an audiometric unit. The responses available are essentially the arousal responses described in an earlier section. One or more observers watch for any one of several movements, changes in breathing, or other indication of arousal. The stimuli have varied from clackers, bells, and the crumpling of paper to carefully calibrated bands of noise from portable acoustic sources. Unfortunately this type of testing did not prove sufficiently reliable. In several careful large-scale trials there were too many misses in addition to numerous false positives. The number of hearing-impaired infants was small: less than one in a thousand. The low rate of detections made it difficult for the observers to maintain their vigilance, and the economic cost in total testing time was considerable in relation to the number of infants correctly identified as deaf.

In 1970 the American Speech and Hearing Association asked the American Academy of Ophthalmology and Otolaryngology and the American Academy of Pediatrics to join with it to form a National Joint Committee on Infant Hearing Screening. This committee, chaired by Marion Downs, has reviewed data from many studies and has issued guidelines for hearing screening programs. The Joint Committee's first statement (1970) concludes with the words:

. . . and despite the committee's recognition of the urgent need for early detection of hearing impairment, we urge increased research efforts but cannot recommend routine screening of newborn infants for hearing impairment.

The next major step was a conference on Newborn Hearing Screening, held in San Francisco in 1971. The Joint Committee then issued a supplementary statement that included a condensed list of criteria for identifying a neonate as being *at risk* for hearing impairment. (This list is discussed in detail below.) Another major concern was to define satisfactory behavioral auditory screening techniques. A subsequent conference on Early Identification of Hearing Loss was held in Halifax, Nova Scotia, in 1974. The proceedings have been edited by George Mencher, and we rely heavily on this material for the following sections.

The High-Risk Register

A practical procedure that is nearly as effective as total screening in the nursery is to concentrate attention on those infants who have a higher than average risk of impaired hearing. The obvious examples are the infants known to be at risk for congenital deafness because of a positive history of familial deafness.

The original concept of the high-risk register was actually a list, to be kept by some public health authority, of high-risk infants and the administration of periodic follow-up hearing tests at well-baby clinics or elsewhere until the infant's hearing status could be established. This concept has gradually been modified so that now the "register" seems to refer equally to a list of infants at risk and a list of the conditions that cause an infant to be at risk. We should more accurately speak of the *high-risk factors,* and reserve the term "register" for the list of infants under observation.

The high-risk factors should be in the minds of doctors, nurses, and public health personnel alike, and even of parents, so that they may direct special attention to the hearing of these infants until normality is assured. A major present objective is to alert the medical and paramedical professions to the importance of early identification of hearing-impaired children. The high-risk register of 1964 enumerated 25 conditions that are statistically associated with juvenile impairment of hearing. Practical experience has now broadened some of the categories and omitted some of those with relatively low risk.

The list of high-risk factors recommended by the Joint Committee, but extended (items 6 and 7) as recommended by Feinmesser and Tell, is as follows:

1. Familial deafness (congenital sensorineural hearing loss in first cousin or closer)
2. Bilirubin level: 20 mg/100 ml of serum or over
3. Rubella (or other nonbacterial intrauterine infection such as cytomegalovirus) during pregnancy
4. Congenital malformations of ear, nose, or throat (any first-arch syndrome)
5. Birth weight 1500 grams or less
6. Apnea and cyanosis (apgar score 1–4)
7. Severe infection (neonatal)

A mnemonic device based on the shorter list is "*ABCDs to HEAR*": "**A**ffected family; **B**ilirubin level; **C**ongenital rubella syndrome; **D**efects of ear, noise, or throat; **S**mall at birth." The items to be assessed at follow-up are: "**H**earing concern? **E**ar test normal? **A**waken to sound? **R**esponses in the developmental and communication scale?"

The infants identified by these high-risk factors comprise about 7 percent of the newborn population. Not more than one-third of the children who ultimately have a serious hearing handicap should escape detection. These estimates are based on the results of very careful and important validation studies of the high-risk register conducted on a total of 27,000 babies in Jerusalem by Feinmesser and Tell (1971) and in Haifa by Altman (1969) and 10,000 more in Nebraska by Mencher (1972). The studies differed in experimental design, but the estimates of effectiveness were very much the same.

Whatever the details of high-risk factors and the register are, the general outline and the consensus seem to be clear. The factors identify the infants whose hearing should be tested with care, over a period of months if necessary—in addition, of course, to children without any of these factors who do not develop speech by the age of 2 years.

Behavioral Testing of Neonates

The concept of high-risk factors for hearing impairment merely concentrates our attention on a smaller population that deserves close observation. The problem of a satisfactory test still remains. So far the major recommendation of the Joint Committee is the *arousal test.* Arousal is currently defined as "any generalized body movement which involves more than one limb and which is accompanied by some form of eye movement." Such arousal is regularly elicited in normal infants by a narrow-band noise (3000 Hz) or white noise presented at 90 or 100 db SPL for a duration of 2 seconds. More precise details should be developed in the near future.

An automated method of detecting such arousal movements is the "crib-o-gram," which in 1973 was already undergoing extensive practical tests. It is well suited for screening infants, who may or may not be at risk, in the wards of maternity hospitals. The principle here is to make the detection of a response objective and automatic by delicate sensors attached to a set of specially supported cribs. The test stimuli are delivered to an entire ward of the nursery at hourly intervals throughout the day and night. The movements of all cribs are recorded on a multichannel writeout. The computer that controls the stimuli correlates the movements with the stimuli. The expense of operation is relatively small and the equipment is relatively simple. The preliminary results are encouraging, but there may still be practical administrative difficulties in incorporating this type of screening audiometry into overall hospital routine.

OTONEUROLOGY

Audiometry refers to the measurement of various aspects of hearing, with the implicit purposes of understanding the operation of the auditory system and diagnosing its disorders. It has been evident, however, that certain auditory tests may assist the neurologist or neurosurgeon toward a diagnosis or the localization of a lesion that only incidentally involves the auditory systems. Examples of such conditions are multiple sclerosis or tumors of the pontine region. Closely

related is the differential diagnosis of an acoustic neuroma. This application of auditory or labyrinthine tests is known as otoneurology.

The tests of labyrinthine function, particularly the caloric tests mentioned briefly in a previous section, are much more advanced and useful for otoneurology than auditory tests, but the brain-stem responses, described in a previous section, offer a very promising new opportunity for the development of auditory electrophysiological tests for lesions of the tracts and nuclei of the brain stem. Also the combination of these tests with the electrocochleogram should improve the detection of acoustic neuromas.

CENTRAL DYSACUSIS

In this section we return to disorders of the auditory system and the audiometric tests appropriate to their detection and diagnosis. A common question for the audiologist or otologist is whether a demonstrated impairment of auditory function is adequately explained on the basis of sensorineural impairment or whether a central impairment is indicated.

Within the cranial cavity we shall subdivide the auditory system into only three parts: the auditory nerve, the brain stem, and the cerebral hemispheres or cortex. Tests appropriate to impairments of the auditory nerve have been considered under sensorineural impairment. Someday we should be able to subdivide the brain stem into thalamic and infrathalamic levels, but we cannot do so usefully at present in terms of test results.

Tests for Brain-Stem Lesions

In general the disturbances of the brain stem rather resemble those of sense organ and nerve and may be explored by quite similar tests. For example, a test of the change of threshold for a brief tone as a function of its duration has been proposed. We know that the normal ear becomes less sensitive by some 10 dB as the duration is reduced from 200 msec to 10 msec. Theoretically we believe that the "temporal integration" of loudness takes place in the brain stem, probably in or not far above the cochlear nucleus. So far clinical experience has not supported this prediction very well as the integration seems to be disturbed by Menière's disease but not by acoustic neuromas. This type of test may well be developed usefully in the future.

We must expect that the effects of brain-stem lesions will not be clearly predictable and will often be quite bizarre. This very feature may distinguish lesions of such a small, compact, but complicated piece of nervous tissue in which so many neurophysiological functions are carried out.

The first interaction between the inputs to right and left ears takes place low in the brain stem (see Figure 3-20). Such an interaction must be the basis for *lateralization* of the source of sound. Studies of the disturbance of this function have been carried out, but we shall not describe details or attempt to evaluate them.

Another binaural effect is the *masking level difference.* A pure tone between about 200 and 500 Hz or speech is presented to both ears simultaneously, mixed with masking noise. The masked threshold varies, depending on whether the tones in the two ears and also the noise in the two ears are in phase or out of phase with each other. With a certain combination of phases a masking level difference of as much as 15 dB can be produced by simply reversing the phase in one ear of the tone or of the masker. A test of brain-stem function based on this phenomenon has been tried, but the results reported so far with patients are difficult to in-

terpret. Here, as with all other diagnostic tests, it is important to have trials on a large number of verified cases of relevant clinical conditions and a high correlation between the test results and the established diagnoses. A theoretical prediction that a particular result should be obtained is not enough.

Tests for Auditory Cortical Function

In animal experiments the removal of the entire auditory cortex bilaterally causes two clear deficits. One is the inability to form a conditioned reflex (learn) to respond to a particular *sequence* of tones of different frequency. The deficit is in the temporal frame of reference and seems to involve short-term memory. The other defect is an inability to be guided by the *position* of a sound source. Here the animal does not move until the sound has ceased. Short-term memory and perhaps the frame of reference of auditory space are apparently disturbed here also. These phenomena should suggest possible auditory tests of cortical function, but no tests of this nature are now available.

By far the most revealing and successful tests of human cortical auditory function are based on modifications of speech audiometry. The recognition of speech, which is learned and not inborn, has a large cortical component. On the other hand, good speech is quite redundant, and a word spoken poorly or heard incompletely may still be recognized quite effectively, particularly if the number of possible choices, that is, the vocabulary, is small.

The most sensitive tests for cortical impairment are not the monosyllabic words, although they too are useful, but garbled or *filtered speech* or *speech in noise.* The task which is difficult for the normal listener becomes extremely difficult or impossible for the impaired listener. A very effective way of modifying speech is to pass it through a low-pass filter with the cutoff at about 1200 Hz. Another is to mix it with either white noise or with a babble of other voices or with a competing message. All of these require a synthesis of a whole word or sentence from fragments. The task requires a good short-term memory and also nimbleness of wit.

Still another form of stress is to *speed up speech* by methods that systematically eliminate small bits from a recorded sample, shortening not only the pauses but the vowels and other sustained phonemes as well. This method preserves the original pitch of the sounds, and a doubling of the usual speed of talk does not usually reduce intelligibility.

It is no accident that the several types of stress that we have mentioned are exactly those that proverbially plague the elderly. Failure to discriminate speech in noise or in multiple conversation or to follow rapid speech are characteristic of the central-nervous-system component of presbycusis. When severe enough to affect word intelligibility in the quiet, it is "phonemic regression." But senile changes affect all parts of the brain, and no problem of localization is involved.

Unilateral cortical lesions that affect hearing do follow one important general rule. *The performance on any test by modified speech is worse when the material is presented to the ear opposite the affected hemisphere.* Of course, it is assumed that the ears are normal or at least symmetrical by simple audiometric tests. Pure-tone thresholds and speech thresholds are *not* affected by the cortical lesion. The PB max *may* be relatively reduced for the contralateral ear, even without garbling or noise.

Note that in the above generalization the brain is symmetrical. There is no suggestion of a dominant left hemisphere. The task of simple *recognition* of words is evidently quite different from the *language* function

that is impaired in aphasia. Also, even after hemispherectomy the contralateral ear does not become deaf. This is undoubtedly due to the rich crossing of auditory pathways in the brain stem.

Another interesting modification of speech is to give part of the input to one ear and part to the other. In this case the brain must integrate the inputs. Perhaps one ear receives high-pass and the other low-pass filtered speech. Perhaps alternate samples of various duration (from a tenth of a second upward) are given first to the right and next to the left ear. Still another is to overlap spondee words in the two ears so that the first syllable to the right ear comes at the same time as the second syllable of the word to the left ear, or vice versa. This is called the *staggered spondaic word (SSW) test.*

All of these tests have shown promise, but none is fully standardized and validated. Validation will be slow because suitable cases for test with proved lesions that are both sufficiently extensive and sufficiently discrete are rather exceptional, and the number per year in any one clinic is small. We have, therefore, simply mentioned several types of test that seem to hold good promise for successful validation. We must note, however, the credit due to two Italian otologists, E. Bocca and C. Calearo, who in about 1955 pointed out clearly the possibilities of modified speech audiometry and stimulated much of the subsequent activity in this area.

The physiological significance of the *evoked cortical V potentials* is not known. The potentials do seem to be generated by the primary projection areas and perhaps also by the immediately adjacent areas, and their presence implies integrity of the entire pathway through the thalamus from sense organ to cortex. We may hope that, with further understanding, they may help us to evaluate brain injuries, congenital defects, and so forth, but as yet this is not possible.

Aphasia

We shall not be concerned with the disturbances of the language function that are caused by certain lesions of the cerebral cortex. The impairment is a disturbance of the ability to communicate by speech, and it is related to injury of certain areas of the cerebral hemisphere that are "dominant" for speech, usually the left hemisphere (see Chapter 4). The impairment of function is obvious, although its exact description may be difficult. The neurosurgeon tries to avoid as far as possible any injury to the "speech areas" in the dominant hemisphere. Our present point is that the audiologist has little to offer in the diagnosis or description of aphasia. The sensitivity for pure tones is normal or nearly so, not only in aphasia but in lesions of the cerebral cortex in general, as long as the patient can understand and respond adequately to the test.

We have discussed also in Chapter 4 the conditon that has been called "congenital aphasia" and have pointed out that the condition is better described as a language disability or, better, a difficulty in learning language. We suggested the term "dysmathia" (difficulty in learning) or "dyslogomathia" (difficulty in learning language) as more appropriate terms. The reason for the difficulty in learning is not necessarily an organic brain lesion. The audiogram may be within normal limits, or it may show moderate or severe hearing loss. Such loss is due to peripheral organic impairment, usually in the inner ear, and not to any abnormality of the central nervous system. This situation reveals the complexity of problems of the central nervous system—to distinguish the organic from developmental, and from strictly functional or psychological difficulties, and to separate these from peripheral impairments that may also be present. The latter may seriously limit the input to the central nervous system and therefore its performance. In this situation it is probably best to think of a difficulty in *hearing*, which is an audiological problem, and a second difficulty in *understanding* or in *learning*, which is not.

SUGGESTED READINGS AND REFERENCES

Bocca, E., and C. Calearo. "Central Hearing Processes," in *Modern Developments in Audiology*, J. Jerger (ed.). New York: Academic Press, 1963.

A useful review of speech tests in otoneurology from the point of view of the Italian innovators.

Bradford, L. J. (ed.). *Physiological Measures of the Audio-Vestibular System.* New York: Academic Press, 1975.

The chapter titles and authors are: (1) "Audio-Vestibular System: Yesterday, Today, and Tomorrow," L. J. Bradford; (2) "Otologic Assessments," S. P. Lee and W. D. Chasin; (3) "Electronystagmography," A. C. Coats; (4) "Acoustic Impedance-Admittance Measurements," A. S. Feldman; (5) "Electrocochleography," F. B. Simmons and T. J. Glattke; (6) "Reflex and Conditioning Audiometry," W. G. Hardy; (7) "Conditioned Galvanic Skin Response Audiometry," I. M. Ventry; (8) "Respiration Audiometry," L. J. Bradford; (9) "Cardiotachometry," R. B. Eisenberg; (10) "Evoked Cortical Response Audiometry," D. C. Hood.

Davis H. "Principles of Electric Response Audiometry," *Ann. Otol.*, Suppl. 28, 85:1–96 (1976).

A useful overview.

Davis, H. (ed.). "The Young Deaf Child: Identification and Management," *Acta Otolaryng. (Stockholm)*, Supplement 206 (1965).

Proceedings of a conference held in Toronto, Canada, October 8-9, 1964. (Organized by Percy E. Ireland.) Includes a survey and assessment of both screening and definitive tests of hearing in young children.

Feinmesser, M., and L. Tell. *Evaluation of Methods for Detecting Hearing Impairment in Infancy and Early Childhood.* Project No. 06-480-2 Washington, D.C.: Maternal and Child Health Service, U.S. Department of Health, Education and Welfare.

A careful, thorough clinical trial of the high-risk register.

Grason-Stadler Company. *Otoadmittance Handbook 2*, 1973.

A clearly written, well-illustrated guide for users of the 1720 Otoadmittance Meter. Available from the Grason-Stadler Company, 56 Winthrop Street, Concord, Mass. 01740.

Jerger, J. (ed.). *Modern Developments in Audiology.* New York: Academic Press, 1963.

The chapter titles and authors are: (1) "The Measurement of Hearing by Bone Conduction," R. F. Naunton; (2) "Automatic Audiometry," W. Rudmose; (3) "Functional Hearing Loss," J. B. Chaiklin and I. M. Ventry; (4) "Measurement of Hearing in Children," D. R. Frisina; (5) "Electrophysiologic Audiometry," R. Goldstein; (6) "Middle-ear Muscle Reflexes in Man," O. Jepsen; (7) "Auditory Fatigue and Masking," W. D. Ward; (8) "Auditory Adaptation," A. M. Small, Jr.; (9) "Central Hearing Processes," E. Bocca and C. Calearo; (10) "The Theory of Signal Detectability and the Measurement of Hearing," F. R. Clarke and R. C. Bilger; (11) "Research Frontiers in Audiology," J. D. Harris. Many of these chapters are excellent, and all are pertinent.

——, Clinical Experience with Impedance Audiometry. *Arch. Otolaryng. (Chicago)*, 92:311–324, 1970.

——, and T. Tillman. "A New Method for the Clinical Determination of Sensori-neural Acuity Level (SAL)." *Arch. Otolaryng.*, 71:948–953 (1960).

Katz, J. "The SSW Test: An Interim Report," *J. Speech Hearing Dis.*, 33:132–146 (1968).

Some details of experience with the staggered spondaic word test.

——, R. A. Basil, and J. M. Smith. "A Staggered Spondaic Word Test for Detecting Central Auditory Lesions," *Ann. Otol.*, 72:908–918 (1963).

This is the original description of this test.

Mencher, G. T. (ed.). *Early Identification of Hearing Loss.* New York: S. Karger, 1976.

The proceedings of the Nova Scotia Conference on Early Identification of Hearing Loss held in Halifax, N.S., Canada, September 8–11, 1974. An excellent survey.

Northern, J. L., and M. P. Downs. *Hearing in Children*. Baltimore: Williams & Wilkins Company, 1974.

Detailed and up to date as of 1973.

O'Neill, J. J., and H. J. Oyer. *Applied Audiometry*. New York: Dodd, Mead & Company, 1966.

Up to date, well organized, well written and illustrated; probably the best available reference book for technical details of audiometric tests.

Ventry, I. M., and J. B. Chaiklin (eds.). "Multidiscipline Study of Functional Hearing Loss," *J. Aud. Res.*, 5:179–262 (1965).

This will probably be the classic in its field for many years.

Zwislocki, J. "Acoustic Measurement of the Middle-Ear Function," *Ann. Otol.*, 70:599–606 (1961).

This article is a clear statement of the principles involved in measurements based on acoustic impedance. Illustrative reactance curves are given.

HALLOWELL DAVIS, M.D.

9

Hearing Handicap, Standards for Hearing, and Medicolegal Rules

AUDIOMETRIC EVALUATION

Audiometry serves two major purposes that are quite different from one another. One of these is to assist in medical diagnosis. Here the pure-tone audiometer is the first instrument of choice. It is highly analytical, and the relations of hearing sensitivity to frequency that it reveals are often of considerable diagnostic significance. This has been discussed in Chapters 4 and 7, and various other diagnostic tests were reviewed in Chapter 8.

The other major purpose of audiometry is to assess the hearing of an individual in relation to the requirements of everyday life, of special tasks or occupations, or of his education. For such assessment it is very desirable to rate the individual in terms of a single number and to write various rules, standards, and requirements in such terms. Speech audiometry yields such a single number, namely, the speech reception threshold, which is very closely related to hearing handicap, and we shall see that most of the rules and standards are in principle related to or derived from the threshold for speech. We shall also see that the difficulties of standardizing speech audiometry have led to the practice of estimating the threshold for speech by calculating the average pure-tone hearing-threshold level for what we shall call the "central speech frequencies," namely 500, 1000, and 2000 Hz. The assessment of handicap or of everyday hearing ability by rules based on this single measure is very satisfactory for individuals who have reasonably flat audiograms and no special problems of poor discrimination for speech. In short, it is very satisfactory for the majority of individuals, for statistical surveys, and for general standards and regulations. No single number or simple rule can suffice, however, for the exceptional cases of steep audiograms or of sense-organ or central dysacusis.

MILITARY, ECONOMIC, AND SOCIAL COMPETENCE

In 1949 a very broad scale of hearing was prepared by the Committee on Hearing of the National Research Council for possible incorporation in a set of physical standards appropriate to the peacetime needs of the army and the navy, to partial mobilization, or to total mobilization. The general principles of this broad original scale are reflected in the more recent and more detailed military standards.

In 1965 the Committee on Conservation of Hearing of the American Academy of Ophthalmology and Otolaryngology published a "Guide for the Classification and Evaluation of Hearing Handicap," which contains this scale in slightly modified form and expressed in terms of the ISO audiometric reference zero level. We quote the first two sections of that guide, including the table (Table 9-1) that gives the classes of hearing handicap.

INTRODUCTION
(References at end of chapter: 2.1 through 2.6 and 3.1 through 3.5)

During the past several years the Committee on Conservation of Hearing has from time to time issued recommendations and approved for publication several articles dealing with the classification of hearing handicaps, the evaluation of hearing impairment, and the International Standard Audiometric Zero Level. These topics are interrelated and now, with the widespread adoption of the new International Reference Zero Level for Pure-Tone Audiometers, it becomes appropriate to restate and combine the recommendations and explanations with particular attention to the implications of the new audiometric scale.

CLASSES OF HEARING HANDICAP
(2.3, 2.4)

Many persons, both children and adults, suffer from impaired hearing. The handicaps that arise from this are economic, educational, and, above all, social. These persons need help, both medical and educational.

In order to plan facilities for the medical treatment, for the rehabilitation and for the special education required by those with impaired hearing, we must know how many persons with hearing problems there are in various age groups and in various communities. In addition we must know the severity of their handicaps. Those who are profoundly deaf or have a severe handicap must be distinguished from those who are moderately hard of hearing, and these must all be distinguished from those who suffer only from the inconvenience of a minor handicap.

The first step in making such distinctions is to divide hearing impairment into categories of handicap. The Committee on Conservation of Hearing of the American Academy of Ophthalmology and Otolaryngology recommends the division of the handicap of hearing into classes or grades, according to the accompanying table. The overall handicap of impaired hearing is best estimated in terms of ability to hear everyday speech well enough to understand it, but for statistical purposes the more precise measurements of pure-tone audiometry are preferable. This table defines each category in terms of pure-tone audiometric measurements such as are regularly made in surveys and tests of hearing, since it is possible to estimate a person's threshold of hear-

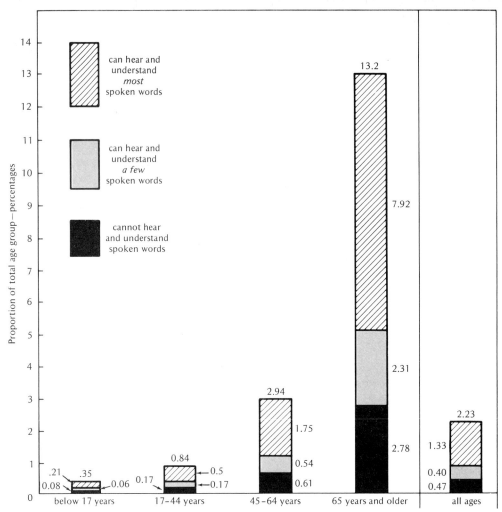

Figure 9-1 Binaural hearing impairment by age groups, based on response to supplementary questionnaire of the Health Interview Survey (Public Health Service), United States, July 1962–June 1963. Ability is estimated *without the use of a hearing aid.* The percentages are shown separately for each of four age groups and for the entire population. The data for the age group below 17 years are based on the responses of parents. Those who were reported to have impaired hearing in the first interview, often by another member of the family, but who did not respond to the supplementary questionnaire, are excluded. If they are included, the percentage of binaural hearing impairment for all ages becomes 2.7 percent, as in Table 9-3, instead of 2.23 percent. The percentage impaired is appreciably greater for males than for females in the two older age groups. *(National Center for Health Statistics, Series 10, Number 35)*

ing for speech reasonably well from pure-tone measurements.

Specifically, each class in the table is defined in terms of the average hearing threshold level for three audiometric frequencies that are important for the understanding of speech. The numbers represent the simple average of the hearing threshold levels in decibels (dB) at the frequencies 500, 1000, and 2000 Hz, obtained with an audiometer that is calibrated according to the International Organization for Standardization's (ISO) Recommendation of 1964 (1.9).

The present classification is intended primarily for statistical purposes. It is not related to the problem of medical diagnosis. Deviations from audiometric zero within the limits of Class A [Table 9-1], or at frequencies above or below those that enter into the average, may be of medical significance for diagnosis or prognosis but they are not needed to estimate the hearing handicap as indicated in the table. Neither can the present table legitimately be used to classify individuals for educational purposes or for employment except as this classification is modified by the other considerations which are pertinent. These other considerations may sometimes completely supersede the present table. The classes of hearing handicap as defined here indicate, however, the usual handicap of the average individual under the varying circumstances of everyday life.

With a given audiometric hearing threshold level some persons will understand speech more easily and accurately, and others less easily and accurately, than is indicated in the table. Intelligence, quickness of perception, special training, general education, language background, motivation, ability to understand and time of onset all contribute to the degree of an actual handicap. Any impairment of the central nervous system may greatly complicate the situation. Any one of several of these various factors may be vital in determining a person's overall economic or educational potentialities.

Social Adequacy Index for Hearing

An attempt was made in 1948 to develop an index for the adequacy of a person's hearing on the basis of his threshold for speech (spondee words) and his discrimination for speech (phonetically balanced (PB) monosyllables). The central concept was that although everyday speech is a dynamic fluctuating affair and is heard at various sound-pressure levels and in various acoustic environments, there is, nevertheless, a broad statistical average of speech levels and conditions.

Otologists have been well aware of the concept of "social hearing." They know that a high-tone hearing loss at 4000 Hz and above does not really impair listening except for hi-fi music, and that there is so much noise in everyday living that a hearing level for speech of 30 dB is often adequate and an excellent result for a fenestration operation. Even up to 40 dB hearing level for speech a person can "get by," most but not all the time, and only with some difficulty. Above the 40-dB hearing level for speech he definitely needs help, enough to have an operation or wear a hearing aid. On the average we hear speech at about 65 to 70 dB SPL (sound-pressure level) (see Figure 7-4). However, sometimes it is down to 45 dB, and sometimes, as in a noisy subway or at a cocktail party, it is as high as 90 dB or more at ears. A man with a conductive hearing loss who has a hearing level for speech of 45 dB does beautifully at the cocktail party but may hear nothing at a lecture or in church. With effort, he might be able to "get by" with everyday conversation about half of the time. If his hearing level is up to 55 dB, he probably will hear only in noisy places or when people really speak up for him, perhaps a third or a quarter of the time. People begin to leave him out of the conversation, or he must rely on speechreading. His hearing is now about at the threshold of social adequacy.

These relations are summarized in Table 9-1 in terms of hearing-threshold levels for speech. The social-adequacy index provided a continuous scale of handicap and took into account the two dimensions of the hearing of speech, namely, sensitivity and discrimination. If a man's speech discrimination and his threshold for speech are normal, he will hear everyday speech, with its rich context, correctly nearly all the time. If his threshold for speech is elevated, he may be listening to speech somewhere on the rising slope of his *articulation* curve, as described in Chapter 7. He will have more or less difficulty with everyday speech. He will also have difficulty if his articulation curve reaches its maximum well below 100 percent, even if his threshold for speech is normal, because he will never hear certain words correctly.

The social-adequacy index of hearing was conceived as the probability of hearing correctly a word of everyday speech, averaged across all words and all conditions. A table was constructed to express the trade-off between sensitivity and maximum discrimination score. The threshold of social adequacy of hearing was estimated to be at 55 dB HL (ANSI) if discrimination was perfect and at a PB (Hughes) articulation score of 35 if the threshold level for spondees was 10 dB or better. We do not give the details because in practice the idea did not work out very well. One reason is that the PB recordings never have been standardized well enough to measure a man's discrimination with anything like the accuracy with which we measure his threshold level. Also, we do not yet seem to know enough about the relation of the hearing and understanding of connected speech in words and sentences to its component frequencies, phonemes, and syllables.

Probably another dimension related to the speed of understanding should be added and perhaps still others. But the index was already as elaborate as it could well be for practical use. Our chief objective here has been to present the concept of a series of thresholds of various degrees of social adequacy of hearing. The various standards for hearing that will be presented below are based on such thresholds, but they are expressed simply in terms of threshold levels without regard for discrimination score.

The Prevalence of Hearing Handicap

Six categories of hearing handicap are defined in Table 9-1. In Table 9-2 is given the estimated percentage of the adult population of the United States that falls in the four most severe categories. The table is taken from "Characteristics of Persons with Impaired Hearing," based on data from the 1960–1962 National Health Survey. The age range included is 18 to 79 years. Note that the hearing-threshold levels are measured, as in Table 9-1, as the average hearing-threshold level for 500, 1000, and 2000 Hz in the better ear. These are audiometric measurements of a demographic sample of the population of the United States.

In Table 9-3, from the same source, are given the percentages of responses to direct questions concerning the extent of hearing deficiency, addressed to all those persons reported as having some deficiency of hearing in the continuing nationwide household interview survey conducted by the Division of Health Interview Statistics of the National Center for Health Statistics. If a family reported that a member or members had "deafness or serious trouble hearing with one or both ears," a supplementary questionnaire concerning its extent and other details was mailed. About 90 percent of those addressed replied, or a parent or guardian replied for them.

Three questions asked in the follow-up correspond broadly to the degrees of impairment *assumed* to be associated with particular audiometric hearing-threshold levels in Table 9-2. The actual individuals questioned were not the same ones as those represented in Table 9-2, and the methods of collecting the data were quite different. Nevertheless the estimates of prevalence of hearing impairment are almost identical in Tables 9-2 and 9-3. The agreement gives added confidence to the estimate of 2.7 percent of adults who have "serious trouble with hearing" and also to the designation of classes of handicap in Table 9-2.

The data of Table 9-3 are broken down by age groups in Figure 9-1. The increase in in-

TABLE 9-1
CLASSES OF HEARING HANDICAP

Hearing Threshold Level dB (ISO)	Class	Degree of Handicap	Average Hearing Threshold Level for 500, 1000, and 2000 Hz in the Better Ear[a]		Ability to Understand Speech
			More Than	Not More than	
	A	Not significant		25 dB (ISO)	No significant difficulty with faint speech
25					
	B	Slight handicap	25 dB (ISO)	40 dB	Difficulty only with faint speech
40					
	C	Mild handicap	40 dB	55 dB	Frequent difficulty with normal speech
55					
	D	Marked handicap	55 dB	70 dB	Frequent difficulty with loud speech
70					
	E	Severe handicap	70 dB	90 dB	Can understand only shouted or amplified speech
90					
	F	Extreme handicap	90 dB		Usually cannot understand even amplified speech

[a] Whenever the average for the poorer ear is 25 dB or more greater than that of the better ear in this frequency range, 5 dB is added to the average for the better ear. This adjusted average determines the degree and class of handicap. For example, if a person's average hearing-threshold level for 500, 1000, and 2000 Hz is 37 dB in one ear and 62 dB or more in the other his adjusted average hearing-threshold level is 42 dB and his handicap is Class C instead of Class B.

cidence of hearing impairment with age is obvious.

The agreement between the two surveys, audiometric and interview, is not so close when we try to estimate the total number of individuals in the United States who have a hearing handicap. The figure given in the 1960–1962 audiometric survey (National Center for Health Statistics, Series 11, number 11) for adults who have an average hearing level for 500, 1000, and 2000 Hz in the better ear of 26 dB (ANSI) or worse is "about 8 percent or 9.2 million persons." The figure given for the interview survey, 1962–1963, is about 8 million persons re-

ported to have impaired hearing in one or both ears, but of these only about 4 million were finally determined, by follow-up, to have impaired hearing in both ears. Obviously the criterion of impairment used by the respondents in the interview was more rigid than the one given in Table 9-1 for beginning handicap.

Military Physical Standards for Hearing

Military service requires that a person be physically fit to perform certain required tasks and duties. Of course, there are some

TABLE 9-2

Average Hearing Threshold Level for 500, 1000, and 2000 Hz in the Better Ear	Presumed Ability to Understand Speech	Percentage
Total, above 40 dB (ANSI) C + D + E + F		**2.7**
41–55 dB C	Frequent difficulty with normal speech	**1.6**
56–79 dB D	Frequent difficulty with loud speech	
79–90 dB E	Understands only shouted or amplified speech	**1.1**
over 90 dB F	Usually cannot understand even amplified speech	

military duties that can be performed quite successfully by a man with a minor handicap, but a missing trigger finger, fallen arches, a leaky heart valve, a perforated eardrum, or dependence on a hearing aid quite properly disqualifies a man for unlimited service. For unlimited service a man must pass a whole series of screening tests. Failure on any one of these disqualifies him. The set of minimum requirements is known as the "physical standards." Hearing is one of the items in military physical standards.

Most of these physical standards could more aptly be called biological standards. They actually take their name from the doctor's "physical examination," in which he looks, feels, listens, and also measures with physical instruments such as scales, meter sticks, and blood-pressure apparatus. The audiometer is now one of these "physical" instruments.

Actually there is not just one set of physical standards but many. The military standards, however, are typical of the minimum requirements set up for their own purposes by various organizations—police and fire departments, commercial airlines, and many other groups.

There is a whole series of military physical standards. The primary set is for "unlimited" service. Then there are the more rigorous requirements for various special branches or activities such as aircraft pilot, submariner, or paratrooper. Sometimes a very specialized duty, such as sonar listening, may require the passing of special tests of hearing or other aptitude. More lenient standards are set for admission to limited

TABLE 9-3
PERCENTAGE OF PERSONS, 18 TO 79 YEARS OLD, WITH SPECIFIED SPEECH COMPREHENSION, BASED ON RESPONSE TO HEARING SCALE

Total	Percentage 2.7
Can hear and understand most spoken words	1.7
Can hear and understand a few spoken words	
Cannot hear and understand spoken words	1.0

duty. Still another set of standards concerns dismissal from duty entirely or from a special category. For obvious reasons a higher standard is required for admission to a particular duty status than is set for mandatory separation. Experience, the investment in special training, morale, natural deterioration to be expected from aging—all of these enter the picture. The setting of initial physical standards is a difficult task of judgment, but separation involves many more conflicting interests and is even more difficult.

For many years the military physical standards for hearing were based entirely on the voice test, the whisper test, and sometimes the watch tick or the coin click (see Chapter 7). These old tests still survive in the regulations of many states and municipalities, but for military standards they now are used only as preliminary tests. The standards are based on pure-tone audiometry.

The hearing levels adopted by the armed forces represent what amount to *screening levels of hearing*. Different screening levels are needed for different purposes and situations. The sets of hearing levels or "profiles" given below are of general significance because they represent a large background of practical experience.

Hearing profiles for service The Armed Forces have now modified their hearing profiles for service to include the ISO-ANSI levels as well as the original ASA-1951 levels, using the approximate formula given in a later section of this chapter. The profiles given in Table 9-4 are adapted from Army Regulations AR 40-501, using the ANSI values. Notice that in this table only four audiometric frequencies are considered and that in many cases it is the average level for the three major frequencies most important for the understanding of speech that determines the adequacy of hearing. Notice the differences in hearing levels that are related to the purpose of the screen, whether it is for

capability for general unlimited military duty or merely for limited duty, and whether for enlistment in peacetime or for general mobilization. The standards for medical and dental registrants are included to illustrate the very different requirements set for a special highly trained group.

The *medical fitness standard for retention, promotion, and separation* deserves special attention as a standard appropriate to trained personnel at middle age or beyond. We quote from AR 40-501:

Trained and experienced personnel will not be categorically disqualified if they are capable of effective performance of duty with a hearing aid. Ordinarily a hearing defect will not be considered sufficient reason for initiating disability separation or retirement processing. Most individuals having a hearing defect can be returned to duty with appropriate assignment limitations. The following is a guide in referring individuals with hearing defects for physical disability separation or retirement processing:

a. When a member is being evaluated for disability separation or retirement because of other impairments, the hearing defect will be carefully evaluated and considered in computing the total disability.

b. A member may be considered for physical disability separation or retirement if, at the time he is being considered for separation or retirement for some other administrative reason, the medical examination discloses a substantial hearing defect. This refers particularly to cases requiring hearing aids and those having hearing levels which may be rateable at 30 to 40 percent or more in accordance with the Veterans Administration Schedule for Rating Disabilities. It should be further noted that past performance of duty does not, per se, preclude separation or retirement because of physical disability caused by a hearing defect.

The guidance given in this excerpt is vague, presumably to allow the decision to be made by a medical officer on the basis of all aspects of each individual case.

The foregoing military standards have

TABLE 9-4
ACCEPTABLE AUDIOMETRIC HEARING LEVELS (ANSI SCALE)

A. *For appointment, enlistment, and induction*

	500	1000	2000	4000 Hz
(a) Both ears	average of these three frequencies not over 30 dB with no one of them over 35 dB			55
or				
(b) Better ear	30	25	25	35
Worse ear		no requirement		

B. *Physical profile functional capacity guide*

Profile serial		500	1000	2000	4000 Hz
1	Each ear	average not over 25 dB			not over 45
2	Both ears	average not over 30 dB			not over 55
	Better ear	average not over 25 dB			not over 35
3		may have hearing level at 30 dB with hearing aid by speech-reception score			
4		below retention standard (see text)			

C. *Medical fitness standard for mobilization*
  Hearing: Uncorrected hearing, average level at 500, 1000, and 2000 Hz, of 40 dB or more is
       unfitting for service

D. *Medicodental registrants*
  Hearing: Hearing which cannot be improved in one ear with a hearing aid to an average hearing
       level of 30 dB or less in the speech-reception range is a cause of medical unfitness;
       unilateral deafness is not disqualifying

been presented in some detail because they are probably the most realistic standards available. Many corresponding standards for civilian employment in state or municipal departments are still phrased in terms of voice tests, watch tick, and so on, and many of them are highly restrictive.

THE PROBLEM OF MONITOR LIMITS

The object of monitoring audiometry (see Chapter 7) is to detect, by routine periodic tests of hearing, the individuals who show signs of incurring a significant noise-induced (or other) hearing loss. The specific rules and criteria for taking action must be evolved to fit the particular circumstances. "Monitor limits," appropriate in a military installation, may be quite different from those suitable for a textile mill.

Monitoring audiometry singles out those who are already in difficulty, as shown by a hearing level that is beyond some arbitrary monitor limit, and also those who are *threatened* with handicap even though their hearing levels are still below the monitor limits. This is possible if *changes for the worse* are observed, judged by comparison of the most recent monitor audiogram with a reference audiogram previously established for that individual. The practical problem is to evolve a set of rules that is effective in picking up such changes for the worse but eliminates spurious changes due to temporary threshold shift, transient middle-ear infections, and the like.

MEDICAL RATING OF PHYSICAL IMPAIRMENT

We shall not attempt to write a history of the legal recognition of noise-induced hearing loss as an industrial disease that entitles a worker to compensation under workmen's compensation laws. The social wisdom of the laws and the legal justice of court decisions are irrelevant to the otologist and the audiologist in their professional capacities, but the otologist is called upon to assess or "rate" hearing for the purposes of payment of compensation. He is also asked to diagnose the type of hearing loss that a workman has so that a reasonable "causal relation" to noise exposure can be affirmed or denied. His advice may also be asked as to the appropriate rules that should be followed by industrial commissions or even courts and legislatures in dealing with such cases, but more and more states are adopting explicit rules or codes.

Questions of the evaluation of permanent impairment, of causal relation, and the like, have been considered carefully and extensively by several groups and committees, however, and a consensus now seems to be emerging on most of the controversial points. Certain confusing terms, nobably "disability" and "hearing loss," have been or are being redefined with more restricted meanings. This should greatly improve communication between the medical and legal professions. The issues, and also the responsibilities, involved in the evaluation or rating of impairment and of disability have been clearly stated.

We have already commented on the term "hearing loss" and the clarification that is made possible by adding the term "hearing level" to our vocabulary (Chapter 4). A term that has caused particular difficulty over the entire medicolegal field is "disability." The physician has used it as almost a synonym for impairment or handicap. But *to the lawyer the term "disability" means that a person's ability to engage in gainful activity has been reduced.* In other words, disability in the legal sense is not a purely medical condition. Physicians and their affiliates, such as audiologists, should carefully respect this legal usage of the term.

We now quote again from the "Guide for the Classification and Evaluation of Hearing Handicap."

IMPAIRMENT, HANDICAP AND DISABILITY
(2.2, 2.3, 2.4, 2.7, 2.8, 2.9)

In various statements approved by the Committee on Conservation of Hearing, the terms *hearing handicap*, *hearing disability*, and *hearing impairment* have all been employed, usually with the intention of conveying substantially the same meaning, but some confusion exists because of connotations that are attached to each of the terms.

In the section on Classes of Hearing Handicap the meaning of *hearing handicap* has been stated once more. This definition of handicap is now almost identical with the definition of "impairment" that appears in the American Medical Association "Guides for the Evaluation of Permanent Impairment" (2.8), namely, "a medical condition that affects one's personal efficiency in the activities of daily living." It is further noted in the same guide that *disability*, as used in various workmen's compensation laws, involves nonmedical factors, such as may be related to actual or presumed reduction in ability to remain employed at full wages. "Permanent *impairment*" is therefore a contributing factor to, but not necessarily an indication of the extent of a patient's permanent *disability* within the meaning of the workmen's compensation laws. In other contexts, however, impairment does not imply a significant handicap but is used in a more general sense to denote any deviation from "normal." The impairment may be anatomical, or we may speak of an impaired function. The term is so useful in this very broad sense that *we are now departing from our previous usage and using "handicap" rather than "impairment" to make clear that we mean an impairment sufficient to "affect one's personal efficiency in the activities of daily living."* We shall thus speak of "percentage of hearing handicap" where formerly it was "percentage impairment of hearing," and at a still earlier date "percent hearing loss."

In summary, in this paper our definitions will be as follows:

Disability: actual or presumed inability to remain employed at full wages.

Impairment: a deviation or a change for the worse in either structure or function, usually outside of the range of normal.

Handicap: the disadvantage imposed by an impairment sufficient to affect one's personal efficiency in the activities of daily living.

HEARING LEVEL VS. HEARING LOSS
(4.1, 3.2, 3.3, 3.4, 3.5)

The term *hearing-threshold level* is the complete and accurate designation for the measurement of an individual's hearing threshold by means of an audiometer. The shorter term *hearing level* may be used when we refer to the intensity of the sound produced by an audiometer at a particular setting of its intensity dial, just as in psychoacoustics we speak of *sensation level* when we mean a sound pressure level that is a given number of decibels above the threshold of a particular subject.

The term *hearing loss* should never be used when speaking of a particular number of decibels. It is properly used in referring to a general medical condition such as "conductive hearing loss" or "a noise-induced hearing loss." It emphasizes the impairment of function. It is illogical and very confusing, however, to speak of a hearing loss of 20 dB (ISO), for example, because this value lies

well within the range of normal. It is very difficult to explain this fact to a layman. He automatically thinks of a hearing loss as an impairment and often as a handicap.

Throughout this document we have employed the term *hearing level* or *hearing-threshold level* to indicate the readings obtained on an audiometer. More precisely, hearing-threshold level means the number of decibels that the threshold of an individual's hearing lies above the reference zero level of the audiometer. . . .

NORMAL HEARING AND THE THRESHOLD OF HANDICAP

Healthy young adults differ from one another with respect to the sensitivity of their hearing just as they differ with respect to height, weight, blood pressure, basal metabolism and many other anatomical and physiological characteristics. The sensitivity of hearing also changes systematically with age, slowly at first through adolescence and early adulthood, a little more rapidly through middle age, and much more rapidly beyond 60 years of age. This is part of the normal expectation of aging. *Normal sensitivity of hearing, even for young adults who have not yet suffered much decline, is a range and not a single hearing-threshold level.* This range is generally considered to extend from the least intensity available on an audiometer to about 23 dB [HL (ANSI)]. Hearing-threshold levels near either extreme may be considered unusual but not abnormal, although the occurrence of changes of sensitivity within the range of normal may have some diagnostic significance, particularly in children and adolescents.

The values chosen for the International Standard Reference Zero for Pure-Tone Audiometers were obtained by combining the hearing-threshold values measured on 15 different groups of young adults who had been screened to eliminate any who had visible signs or a history of otological disease. The average hearing thresholds are not a standard of normal hearing in a medical sense, but the values do represent the central tendency of the range of normal and are therefore the most logical selection for the reference zero. . . .

The important point with respect to the evaluation of hearing handicap is that . . . the [ANSI] audiometric reference zero value [does not] correspond to the threshold of handicap. Actually, *handicap is generally conceded to begin at about the upper edge of the range of normal, and more specifically at 27 dB* [HL (ANSI)]. We refer here to the average hearing-threshold level for the three frequencies 500, 1000, and 2000 Hz. *The percentage handicap is not proportional to the number of decibels that an individual's hearing threshold lies above the audiometric zero nor does it depend in any way on which audiometric zero is used to describe that threshold.* This is true because handicap depends upon the relation of an individual's threshold of hearing to the physical intensity of the everyday speech which he hears. There must be no confusion between the reference zero levels for audiometers and the hearing-threshold level at which hearing handicap begins.

RULES FOR THE EVALUATION OF HEARING HANDICAP
(2.2., 2.6, 2.7, 2.9, 3.1, 4.2)

Ideally, hearing handicap should be evaluated in terms of ability to hear everyday speech under everyday conditions. The ability to hear sentences and repeat them correctly in a quiet environment is taken as satisfactory evidence of correct hearing for everyday speech. However, because of present limitations of speech audiometry, the preferred procedure is to *estimate the hearing-threshold level for speech from air-conduction measurements made with a pure-tone audiometer.* For this estimate the Committee on Conservation of Hearing recommends *the simple average of the hearing-threshold levels (in decibels) at the three frequencies 500, 1000, and 2000 Hz.*

In order to evaluate the hearing handicap it must be recognized that the range of partial hearing handicap, comprising classes B, C, D, and E in the accompanying table, is not nearly as wide as the total dynamic range of human hearing. The audiometric reference zero level recommended by the International Standards Organization represents the average sensitivity of healthy young adults who have no indication of present or previous otologic disease. Thus, zero hearing-threshold level on the audiometer obviously represents

very good hearing; it is not the point at which handicap begins. Actually, if the average hearing-threshold level at 500, 1000, and 2000 Hz is 26 dB (ANSI) or less, usually no handicap exists in the ability to hear everyday speech under everyday conditions. At the other extreme, if the average hearing-threshold level at 500, 1000, and 2000 Hz is over 93 dB, the handicap for hearing everyday speech should be considered total. The possibility of utilizing any residual hearing beyond 93 dB [HL] by means of a hearing aid is not taken into account in this evaluation. *For every decibel that the estimated hearing-threshold level for speech exceeds 26 dB . . . , allow one-and-one-half percent in handicap of hearing, up to the maximum of 100 percent.* This maximum is reached at 93 dB. . . .

The Committee further recommends that any method for the evaluation of hearing handicap should include an appropriate forumla for binaural hearing which will be based on the hearing-threshold levels in each ear tested separately. Specifically, the Committee recommends the following formula: The percentage of handicap of hearing in the better ear is multiplied by five (5). The resulting figure is added to the percentage of handicap of hearing in the poorer ear, and the sum is divided by six (6). The final percentage represents the binaural evaluation of hearing handicap.

The Committee also recommends that in the calculation of the percentage of handicap of hearing from the results of audiometric measurements no correction or allowance should be made for age.

PROBLEMS OF CAUSAL RELATIONS
(2.7, 3.1)

Often in evaluating a case of impaired hearing for purposes of compensation, an otologist will recognize two or more causes of the condition, perhaps acting simultaneously like aging and noise-exposure, or perhaps in sequence like chronic otitis media and an automobile accident. And sometimes, by virtue of pre-employment audiograms or periodic hearing tests for other purposes, the contribution from each cause may be estimated fairly accurately. If liability or compensation are involved, the question arises as to how to evaluate the various causal relations.

In some situations the various liabilities and the rules for calculating them are established by law or by administrative rules and interpretations. In other situations, and notably in circumstances where workmen's compensation laws and rules do not apply, the otologist must exercise his independent judgment. The proper division of liability in proportion to the contributions from two or more different causes is not easy, however. It is particularly difficult when discrimination loss or central dysacusis of any sort is combined with loss of auditory sensitivity. Even if the combined impairment is only a loss of sensitivity, the logic of the situation is complicated because, as noted in an earlier section, handicap does not begin at the zero of the audiometric scale. It is therefore necessary to *estimate first the extent of the total over-all hearing handicap and then, by an entirely independent calculation or estimate, apportion the liability according to the various contributing causes.*

An obvious simple example of difficulty in apportionment is the evaluation of binaural as opposed to monaural deafness. Monaural deafness is not half as handicapping as binaural, but it does involve half of the *peripheral* auditory apparatus. A less obvious example is the superposition of a mild otitis media on a hearing loss from industrial noise that was just below the level at which handicap and compensation begin. Neither condition alone is bad enough to cause a handicap but together they do. In some of these situations there are specific legal rules or precedents, but more often there are not.

Stabilization of Hearing Thresholds

The guide from which we have quoted does not mention the necessity of assuring that the individual's hearing is stable before evaluating it for workmen's compensation or other monetary award. The usual practice is to make audiograms on three or more days, preferably spaced a week or so apart, to show that there is no progressive improvement of hearing, and to accept the best overall audio-

grams as the basis for evaluation. Opinions and practice differ as to the minimum "waiting period" that should (or must by administrative rule) be allowed after the last hazardous noise exposure or after an accident to allow full recovery from temporary threshold shifts. Two weeks is probably sufficient for industrial noise-induced hearing loss, but at least six months should be allowed after an accident or a sudden acoustic trauma. And, of course, whenever there may be a monetary award, the audiologist must be alert for the possibility of feigning.

PRINCIPLES OF EVALUATION OF IMPAIRMENT

The rules for calculating the percentage of handicap (or impairment) of hearing, as recommended by the American Academy of Ophthalmology and Otolaryngology and endorsed by the American Medical Association, have been stated in the foregoing section. Many of the principles on which these rules are based have been discussed in this or in previous chapters, but some of the rules are quite arbitrary. We summarize several of these principles as follows:

1. The threshold of handicap is related to the average intensity of everyday speech. It is in no way related to the range of normal hearing or to the reference zero levels of the audiometer (see Figure 7-4). The value of this threshold is at a speech-reception threshold of about 25 dB (ANSI). This value was based originally on the clinical experience of otologists, but it has been confirmed in the National Health Survey. The threshold of handicap lies about 10 dB above the most rigorous of the military standards for hearing.

2. In principle the evaluation of hearing handicap should be based on the speech-reception threshold measured by direct speech

audiometry, using samples of everyday speech. This is not feasible, however, because no suitable samples of everyday speech have been standardized. Such standardization is not likely because of difficulties related to vocabulary and to regional dialects and the specifications for an "average talker." The threshold for speech is therefore *estimated* by taking the average hearing-threshold level for the frequencies 500, 1000, and 2000 Hz. (In California the frequency 3000 is included also.)

3. The ceiling (100 percent) of hearing handicap is related to the power of the average human voice and to such social amenities as the distance from talker to listener and the acceptable loudness for group conversation. It is less clearly defined than the threshold of handicap and has been set, somewhat arbitrarily, at 93 dB HL. The exact value was chosen because it is reached by going up from the threshold according to the simple rule of 1.5 percent per decibel.

4. The simple linear relation stated above between percentage handicap and decibels is arbitrary. It has the great advantage of extreme simplicity (see Figure 9-2).

5. The evaluation of percent hearing handicap can be made equally well on the ISO (ANSI) or the ASA-1951 scale of hearing level. Only the numerical values of the threshold and the ceiling are different.

6. The ratio of 5 to 1 in favor of the better ear in calculating the binaural handicap is arbitrary, but it is based on clinical observation and judgment.

7. No consideration is given to the possible benefits from a hearing aid or to known difficulty in obtaining such benefits. Thus many individuals whose handicap is rated as total (100 percent) for statistical purposes or for workmen's compensation are able to communicate quite effectively with the help of a hearing aid, but others cannot.

8. No consideration is given to poor discrimination for speech, to tinnitus or other forms of dysacusis, or to any special importance of hearing to the individual because of his profession or employment. The rules as stated above were developed to meet the needs of workmen's compensation and of Veterans Administration rating of disabilities. Here the major types of hearing loss are conductive or noise-induced. For many other types of hearing loss the rules will considerably underestimate the actual degree of handicap.

9. No consideration is given to age and presbycusis. This rather arbitrary exclusion will be discussed below.

Previous Rules for Evaluation

Before the formulation of the AAOO rules for calculating percent handicap from pure-tone audiometric thresholds, two other rules had been employed. The first of these, known as the "Fletcher point eight" rule, is almost as old as the electric audiometer itself, but it was never intended to be used as a measure of handicap! Harvey Fletcher, who was largely responsible for the early development of the audiometer at the Bell Telephone Laboratories, recognized early that an overall evaluation of a hearing loss with a single number would be very desirable. For many purposes the audiogram is too analytical. He proposed the *percentage of normal hearing that had been lost*. He realized that the hearing of speech was the most important single function of hearing, and that the central frequencies, 512, 1024, and 2048 Hz, were the most important for this. He took the average hearing level, or hearing loss as it was then called, for these three frequencies. The dynamic range of the early audiometers at these frequencies was 120 dB. To convert the decibels of hearing loss to percentage of the total range he therefore multiplied the loss by five-sixths. This

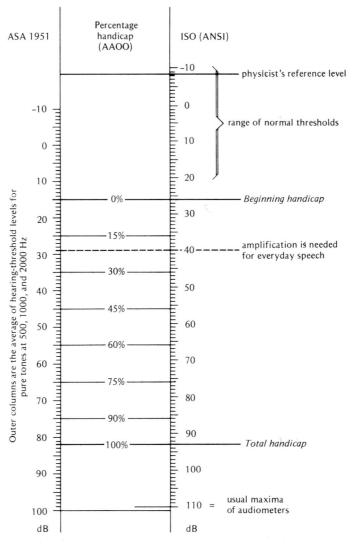

Figure 9-2. The center column represents percentage handicap of hearing, calculated according to the rule originally formulated by the Subcommittee on Noise in 1958 and adopted by the AAOO in 1959 for use in cases involving compensation. "ISO (ANSI)" refers to the reference zero levels for pure-tone audiometers, recommended by the International Organization for Standardization and subsequently adopted by the American National Standards Institute (S3.6-1969). "ASA 1951" refers to the audiometric scale defined in the American Standard for Audiometers for General Diagnostic Purposes, Z24.5-1951. (After Davis and Kranz)

ratio was later approximated to 0.8 ("zero point eight"), which gave the name to the rule. The result was the percentage of originally available "auditory area" (in the speech range) that had been "lost," that is, the "percent hearing loss."

The rule is simple and easy to remember, and it effectively rank-orders hearing losses. It is not satisfactory for calculating disability or insurance claims, however, because it disregards the concept of a threshold of handicap below which it is illogical to claim disability. It opened the door to many small claims, even on the basis of audiograms within the range of normal. On the other hand, it penalized those with severe hearing losses because 100 percent was not reached as long as any response to the audiometer was obtained in the speech range.

The second set of rules was issued by the American Medical Association's Council on Physical Medicine in 1947. It was prepared by Drs. E. P. Fowler and Paul E. Sabine. This method employed the four frequencies 512, 1024, 2048, and 4096 Hz but weighted them differently: 2048 = 40 percent, 1024 = 30 percent, and 512 and 4096 = 15 percent each. It made the important advance of introducing a threshold and a ceiling. These were near the present AAOO threshold and ceiling, respectively. The increase in percent hearing loss was not linear as a function of decibels. The calculation of the overall percentage required a chart that included a separate scale for each frequency. Probably it was because of the complexity that the method never became very popular. It was, however, the direct ancestor of the AAOO rules, which differ from it chiefly in their much greater simplicity and their total rejection of 4000 Hz from the calculation.

Since 1970, when the Occupational Safety and Health Act (OSHA) set criteria for industrial noise, there has been much discussion of the AAOO rule, with only three frequencies (500, 1000, and 2000 Hz) and its rather high threshold of beginning handicap (27 dB HL). Frequencies above 2000 Hz certainly assist the understanding of speech, particularly in noisy situations. Sentiment more and more favors the inclusion of 4000 Hz or at least 3000 Hz in the calculations, but opinion is divided as to which frequency it should be and whether it should be given full weight in the average. Sentiment also favors lowering the threshold of handicap, but such a change carries with it the implica-

tion that the protective levels for noise exposure (such as OSHA and EPA) should be recalculated to lower the permissible exposure levels. The economic consequences of this could be very great indeed.

Here we call attention to item 8 (in the previous section) in the list of the principles on which the AAOO rules were based originally. The rules were developed to meet the particular needs of workmen's compensation and of Veterans Administration rating of disabilities. Here the major types of hearing loss are conductive or noise-induced. *For other types of hearing loss, which involve tinnitus or dysacusis, the rules will considerably underestimate the actual degree of handicap.*

THE PROBLEM OF NORMAL HEARING

We have discussed the question of the "normal" threshold of hearing in Chapters 2 and 7 in relation to the choice of the reference zero levels of pure-tone audiometers. "Normal" should not be interpreted as meaning "the very best," but rather as the median or mode of a distribution, because even ears that are entirely free of disease differ significantly in sensitivity. The standard deviations as well as the medians of thresholds of one group of healthy young men are shown in Figures 2-4 and 2-5. We repeat from Chapters 2 and 7 that there is not a *single* "normal" threshold but instead a *range of normal thresholds.* Even so, it is still necessary to specify the age and sex of the subject and the psychoacoustic procedure by which the threshold is determined if we are to judge whether a particular threshold is within its appropriate range of normal or not.

More serious confusion arises from the implication that normal means free of disease and that "abnormal" or "outside the range of normal" means disease or injury. The decision as to whether an ear is "abnormal" or not in this sense is a medical decision, involving much more than the determination of pure-tone thresholds.

The concept of a range of normal is very familiar to the physician, yet he always hesitates to draw a sharp line and say, "This is the limit. Anything beyond this limit is abnormal," because to him and to most laymen "abnormal" implies disease or defect—that is, something wrong. The 5 percent of subjects with the very best hearing lie outside the range of two standard deviations. Should we call their hearing "abnormally good"? On the other hand, the physician knows that as hearing gets poorer and poorer, the more likely he is to find *on closer examination* a disease or defect, such as otitis media or otosclerosis, that is responsible. But the significance of a hearing-threshold level of 30 dB will depend on the age and the sex of the subject, among other things. And even if there is a considerable deviation, he is not likely to say, "Your hearing is abnormal." He will say, "Your hearing is below average for your age. I shall try to find the cause [that is, make a diagnosis]."

The statistician, however, finds another way out. From the number and scatter of the original measurements he can calculate the limits within which any given percentage of new cases can be expected to fall. One common convention is arbitrarily to take two "standard deviations" as the range of normal, which practically means that we agree to call the most deviant 5 percent "abnormal" (without inquiring into cause) and to consider the other 95 percent as "within normal limits." This is illustrated in Figures 2-4 and 2-5. (For these data the distributions were symmetrical about the median.) The situation is more complicated when, as in the National Health Survey, the deviations are greater in the direction of poorer hearing than of better hearing. Then the percentiles are a better way to express the deviations, as in Figure 9-3.

Incidentally, it was in very nearly this way that the limits of normal for the 4C Group Hearing Test, described in Chapter 7, were established. A small but definite percentage of thresholds lay beyond the arbitrary cutoff point, and these were therefore automatically considered "abnormal." It later came as a shock to some people to learn that calculations from the results of the test, as applied

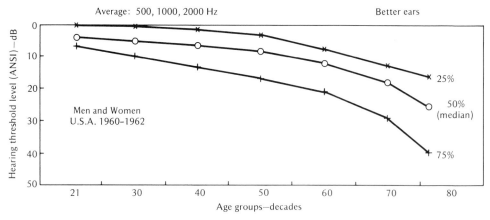

Figure 9-3 Medians and quartiles of hearing-threshold levels by age groups for the better ears of men and women, average of values for 500, 1000, and 2000 Hz. (*Data from National Health Survey, United States, 1960–1962, corrected to ANSI reference level*)

to New York schoolchildren, showed that there must have been 3,000,000 hard-of-hearing children of school age in the United States. This result had been built into the test by statistical definition at the start.

Above all *it must not be thought that the choice of a standard reference zero level for audiometry establishes a standard of normal in any legal sense.* It is true that the ANSI levels do correspond closely to the mean or median threshold levels of otologically normal young adults. The ears tested had no detectable disease or history of it. Their hearing thresholds are convenient values for an arbitrary single reference level at each frequency, but this does not mean that there is necessarily anything wrong with ears that are somewhat less sensitive. This should be obvious, but it is possible that some people who do not understand that the threshold of handicap is quite independent of the threshold of hearing may be misled by a careless statement that "the zero of the audiometer is the normal hearing threshold." They might think that therefore any poorer sensitivity, that is, a "hearing loss" in the old sense of the term, represents abnormality and injury and therefore automatically deserves compensation or payment for injury if any plausible causal relation can be established. This argument has actually been advanced in court in the past, particularly in connection with the "Fletcher point eight" rule, and it might be tried again in the future.

"Actuarial" Hearing Thresholds

In 1966 this writer introduced the term *actuarial hearing thresholds* to mean the average expectation of hearing according to age and sex. In a sense these are normal thresholds, inasmuch as it is normal for the tissues of the body to change their characteristics with age (see Chapter 3) and for hearing to be very sensitive in childhood and less so in old age.

The National Health Survey of 1960–1962, to which we have referred repeatedly, has given us actuarial hearing thresholds for the United States for the age range 18 to 79, and separately for children in the range 6 to 11 years. The data have been analyzed and presented in many ways, according not only to age and sex, but with respect to race, region, area of residence, educational attainment, and many other factors, so that the average expectation (and for many items the interquartile range also) for almost any group can be stated with reasonable confidence. Figure 9-3 shows the overall trend with age for men and women combined for the average of 500, 1000, and 2000 Hz (see also Figure 9-1).

SUMMARY OF REFERENCE LEVELS, SCREENING LEVELS, AND STANDARDS

For convenience we assemble here, in ascending order of physical intensity, the various reference levels, screening levels, and physical standards that we have mentioned in this and other chapters. We shall refer to the average of values at 500, 1000, and 2000 Hz as the "central speech range." There are minor discrepancies between these numbers and certain graphs (for example, Figures 2-4 and 7-4) because ANSI pressures are coupler pressure and some others are free field. All HL values are ANSI levels. These reference levels are as follows:

1. The physicist's reference level for sound pressure (SPL), which is 0.0002 μbar per cm² or 2×10^{-5} newtons per square meter (N/m²), or 20 micropascals (μPa), independent of frequency.
2. The ninetieth percentile of thresholds of hearing for young adults at the best frequencies. Corresponds quite closely to the physicist's reference level.
3. ANSI reference zero levels for pure-tone

audiometers. The median threshold of hearing for otologically normal young adults under laboratory conditions. A function of frequency. About 9.5 dB SPL (coupler pressure) across the central speech range (Figure 2-5).

4. U.S. National Health Survey (1960–1962) median for 18- to 24-year age group. Central speech range = 3.5 dB HL. (For other age groups see Figure 9-3.)

5. ASA-1951 reference zero levels for pure-tone audiometers, based on USPHS survey of 1936. A function of frequency. Central speech range = 11 dB HL or about 20 db SPL (coupler pressure). See also Figure 7-4.

6. ANSI reference zero level for speech audiometers. Calibration tone 1000 Hz = 20 dB SPL (coupler pressure) or 12.5 db HL.

7. Screening for schoolchildren. Central speech range = 25 dB HL.

8. The most rigorous U.S. military physical standard (for appointment, enlistment, and induction). Better ear, central speech range = 26 dB HL (Table 9-2).

9. Threshold of hearing handicap, AAOO rule. Central speech range = 27 dB HL.

10. More lenient U.S. military standards, such as profile 2. Central speech range = 31 dB HL (Table 9-2).

11. Practical limit of hearing without amplification. Central speech range = 40 dB HL (see Figure 9-3).

12. Usual level for recommendation of special management of children. Central speech range = 41 dB HL.

13. "Unfitting for military service" (mobilization) if uncorrected by hearing aid. Central speech range = 41 dB HL.

14. Beginning of marked handicap, AAOO classification. Central speech range = 55 dB HL.

15. Comfortable listening level. A range centering about 65 dB SPL (free field).

16. EPA (1972) threshold for detectable permanent threshold shift at 4000 Hz after cumulative habitual noise exposure of 10 years = 75 dBA SPL (free field). See Chapter 5.

17. EPA (1972) threshold for detectable noise-induced permanent threshold shift for central speech range = 85 dBA SPL (free field).

18. OSHA (1970) level for mandatory hearing conservation program if noise exposure is habitual = 90 dBA SPL (free field). See Chapter 5.

19. Total (100 percent) handicap, AAOO rule. Central speech range = 93 dB (HL).

20. Threshold of discomfort. Almost independent of frequency. About 120 dB SPL or about 110 dB HL (see Figure 2-5).

21. Threshold of tickle. Almost independent of frequency. About 130 dB SPL or about 120 dB HL.

22. Threshold of pain. Almost independent of frequency. About 140 dB SPL or about 130 dB HL.

THE PROBLEM OF MULTIPLE CAUSES

Among the most difficult problems relating to handicap and insurance claims are those that concern "causal relation," particularly when two or more causes of the hearing impairment can be identified.

One classical case is that of *second injury*, in which a worker incurs some noise-induced hearing loss under one employer and then leaves to work for another employer. His hearing levels may be known when he terminates the first employment, and a preemployment audiogram may define them again a little later. Exposures in both employments contribute to the final impairment and handicap. Who should pay the workmen's compensation insurance claim, or in what proportion? In several states this situation is handled by special provisions in statutes or rules, and in some of them, for example in Missouri, a clear principle of *proportional liability* emerges. The situation is very unclear, however, when there is no record of the hearing of the employee at the start of his first employment. In any case it is difficult because handicap is proportional to decibels of hearing level *above a certain threshold,* 26 dB HL. The employee's original hearing was presumably better than this. He worked for some time in his first employment, losing hearing but without passing the threshold of handicap. To what extent, if any, should the first employer be liable for the subsequent handicap?

The other classical problem is *presbycusis combined with noise-induced hearing loss.* Here the two causes, noise and aging, act simultaneously and in parallel. Perhaps neither one *alone* would have caused a handicap by the time a worker retired, but together they have done so. What proportion of the liability does the employer bear? The AAOO rule says "all of it." Some states reduce the award by an arbitrary percentage related to age. Missouri requires a correction for age in terms of a certain number of decibels per year of age that are subtracted from the hearing levels before applying the AAOO rule. This procedure penalizes the worker very heavily. It seems to this writer that the most equitable solution is found according to the principle of proportional liability, making use of the actuarial thresholds that are now available. In 1966 this writer wrote as follows:

The actuarial threshold will become increasingly important if the principle of proportional liability is more generally utilized in medico-legal situations. Here is an example to illustrate the principle. An elderly patient who has been injured in an automobile accident complains of impaired hearing since that time. No previous audiograms are available. An otologist is called upon to decide what proportion of the impairment should be assumed due to natural causes, particularly his age. His present audiogram shows an average hearing level for 500, 1000 and 2000 Hz of 50 dB. The otologist may reason thus: "It is fair to assume that as a young man the subject had a hearing threshold level for the major speech frequencies at 500, 1000, 2000 Hz equal to the median value given for the 20-year age group in the statistical tables of the 1960–1962 National Health Survey. This value, his original actuarial threshold, is 3.5 dB. The subject is now 70 years of age. The actuarial hearing-threshold level for this age and for the same frequencies is 17.5 dB. The total shift of his speech threshold since he was 20 years old is from 3 to 50, or 47 dB. The shift that can be ascribed to aging alone, i.e., the difference in the actuarial threshold is, from 3.5 to 17.5, or 14 dB. The amount to be attributed to the accident is therefore 47 − 14, or 33 dB. The proportion of the liability for the subject's hearing impairment that should be ascribed to the accident is 33/47 or 70 per cent."

Notice that this calculation of proportional liability or "percentage responsibility" is completely independent of the threshold of handicap and of the calculation of the percentage handicap and the appropriate monetary award. Those other calculations tell how big the pie is. The principle of proportional liability tells how the pie should be cut. Notice that a hearing impairment may be the sum of two or three separate impairments, each with a different cause. No one of the separate impairments need be severe enough to cause a hearing handicap alone, yet they may combine to give a very significant handicap. It does not seem fair or logical to place all of the responsibility on either one of the impairments, particularly when two impairments may develop slowly and concurrently, like aging and noise-induced hearing loss. It would seem fairer to assume, as the otologist did in the above example, that the responsibility should be divided according to the number of decibels threshold shift that can reasonably be ascribed to each cause. The actuarial thresholds provide a very reasonable basis for estimating the average effect of aging, including the everyday noise exposure of the general population. It also provides a starting point from which to reckon the threshold shifts in case no previous audiograms are available.

PROBLEMS OF INDUSTRIAL AUDIOMETRY

In 1964, it was proposed in the United States of America Standards Institute to adopt the ISO reference zero levels for pure-tone audiometers in a revision of the old ASA standard of 1951. This proposal was opposed vigorously by many users of audiometers, notably organizations composed of industrial users engaged in hearing conservation in industry. By 1969 the objections had been met by appropriate wording of the proposed standard, the inclusion of explanatory material, and the simultaneous rewriting of the standard for audiometric booths, and the ISO reference levels were adopted. It is worthwhile, however, to examine some of the more substantial objections raised during this debate.

The objections centered on the overall average difference in level of about 10 dB between the ISO and the ASA-1951 contours (see Figure 7-4). It was explained that the adoption of ISO values would not alter the actual sound pressures specified in existing rules and standards, although the numbers used to express them would differ. The objection was tacitly withdrawn when various state and national bodies, notably several workmen's compensation boards or commissions, amended their rules to include explicitly the equivalent ISO values.

A quite different argument was that the ASA-1951 standard actually expresses better than the ISO standard the average expected hearing of the young people who become industrial workers as opposed to college students or the usual laboratory subjects. No published data were available to support this claim, however, and the thresholds for all young adults found in the recent National Health Survey are closer to the ISO zero than to the ASA-1951 zero.

The probable basis for the difference be-tween the ASA and the ISO standards was revealed in a report by Dr. Aram Glorig of two normal hearing studies conducted in successive years, 1954 and 1955, at the Wisconsin State Fair. Each year volunteer subjects were obtained, questioned, and examined otologically in the same way to obtain comparable groups of "otologically normal young adults." The audiometers and the audiometric environment were similar and fully adequate. In 1954 each subject was tested "only once, by the conventional manual procedure." The resulting average hearing thresholds at 500, 1000, and 2000 Hz corresponded almost exactly to those of the USPHS data of 1935–1936, which were the basis of the ASA-1951 audiometric reference levels.

In 1955 the procedure was made more deliberate. At least three threshold crossings in each direction were made at each frequency. Also the audiometers had been provided with attenuators with 2.5 dB steps. The overall test required 30 to 45 minutes. This was a laboratory atmosphere. The subjects became interested and tried hard. The data from this 1955 study agree very well with those of Dadson and King in England (see Chapter 2) and are about 10 dB more sensitive than the 1954 Wisconsin State Fair thresholds. (Actually both the Dadson and King and the 1955 Wisconsin State Fair data are among the 15 studies on which the ISO reference levels are based.)

The factor that seems to differentiate the 1954 and the 1955 Wisconsin State Fair studies most clearly is the more deliberate pace and repeated trials in 1955 and the resulting improved understanding and motivation of the subjects. Glorig calls this factor the "test-subject relationship."

It seems reasonable to assume that patients who come to a clinic or doctor's office because of difficulty with hearing are well motivated, and a good audiometric technician does not rush the patient but establishes an atmosphere like that of the laboratory. The patients have come for help, and they try hard. It seems clear that the ISO standard is appropriate in this situation. It is worth noting that in all of the studies on which the ISO standard is based, the pace was deliberate. It is unfortunate if systematic differences in psychoacoustic method, notably the tempo of the test, and perhaps in the motivation of the subjects, crept in and caused a separation between industrial audiometry and medically oriented audiometry. The difference seems to be of the order of 10 dB for the expected initial threshold. However, if the difference depends on a rapid as compared with a deliberate routine, the divergences in results should be less marked if the subject has suffered some noise-induced threshold shift. Then his thresholds become much sharper, due to recruitment.

Industrial audiometry serves a very useful purpose in the conservation of hearing, and it is probably most important for its purposes that its procedures should be *consistent* in order to reveal reliably any changes in hearing-threshold levels. It is of less concern whether the average of the thresholds of new young workers in their first tests matches exactly the thresholds that are consistently obtained in the more relaxed laboratory or medical atmosphere.

TRANSITION FROM ASA-1951 TO THE ISO-ANSI SCALE

We are now (1977) near the end of the period of transition from the ASA-1951 scale for pure-tone audiometers to the ISO-ANSI scale. Old audiometers have been recalibrated, but it will be a wise precaution for another decade to label audiogram blanks specifically as ANSI (or ISO) and to reassure readers of journals and reports by a specific statement that all hearing levels in the report are actually ANSI. Even so there is still the problem of handling old audiometric data that are based on the ASA-1951 scale.

Recommendations to facilitate this transition in the Armed Forces were prepared (1967) by a Working Group of the NAS-NRC Committee on Hearing, Bioacoustics, and Biomechanics ("CHABA"). We quote those that still seem of general interest.

1. To translate "ASA-1951" audiometric data to ISO values
   a. The following *exact formula* may be employed for statistical, research, or special clinical purposes at the discretion of the individual user.

At	250	500	1000	2000	Hz
Add to ASA-1951	15	14	10	8.5	dB
At	3000	4000	6000	8000	Hz
Add	8.5	6	9.5	11.5	dB

   b. Use the following *approximate formula* when translating individual audiograms from ASA-1951 in order to compare them with more recent ISO audiograms or to apply one of the regulations.

At	250	500	1000	2000	3000	Hz
Add to ASA-1951		15	10			dB
At	4000		6000	8000		Hz
Add	5		10			dB

   The average correction for 500, 1000, and 2000 Hz, sometimes called "the speech range," is 10 dB.

The exact translation formula represents the differences between the ASA-1951 values and the ISO values, rounded to the nearest half decibel. These exact differences are appropriate for certain statistical, research, and perhaps special clinical purposes. For translations for other purposes the approximate formula is a sufficiently close approximation and far simpler in application and results. The approximations are all exact multiples of 5, appropriate to the 5 dB steps in which pure-tone audiometers are calibrated.

The greatest deviation from the exact values is 1.5 dB, which is within the tolerances allowed in the ANSI standard for audiometers. The average deviation for the three frequencies 500, 1000, and 2000 Hz is 10.8 dB, and for the four frequencies 500, 1000, 2000, and 3000 Hz it is 10.25 dB. The rounding errors are negligible for all practical purposes.

2. Prepare revisions of all regulations relating to hearing levels and the recording of audiometric data, including screening levels, physical standards, physical disability, and audiometric forms, using the approximate formula of paragraph 1. Consider minor modifications of the resulting requirements and criteria in order to simplify the resulting regulations. A blanket adjustment of 10 dB at all frequencies instead of application of the approximate translation formula will provide more uniform and more easily applied rules and regulations without changing the absolute sound pressure levels to a clinically significant degree.

3. The present range of screening and monitoring audiometers, in terms of sound pressure levels, is satisfactory. These sound pressure levels will not be altered significantly by the recalibration, although the numbers that designate them will be different.

SUGGESTED READINGS AND REFERENCES

Army Regulations. *AR 40-501, Medical Service—Standards of Medical Fitness.* Washington, D.C.: Headquarters, Department of the Army, December 1969.

Davis, H. "The Articulation Area and the Social Adequacy Index for Hearing," *Laryngoscope,* 58:761–778 (1948).

The articulation curves are based on the Rush Hughes recording and should be revised. The ideas may be of theoretical interest.

Davis, H. (assisted by the Subcommittee on Hearing in Adults for the Committee on Conservation of Hearing of the American Academy of Ophthalmology and Otolaryngology). "Guide for the Classification and Evaluation of Hearing Handicap in Relation to the International Audiometric Zero." *Trans. Amer. Acad. Ophthal. Otolaryng.,* 69:740–751 (1965).

This is the article from which the extensive quotations in the text have been taken. The following list of other guides, standards, and approved articles is taken from the same source, with additions and updating.

1. *Standards*
   1.1 AMA Council on Physical Medicine. "Minimum Requirements for Acceptable Audiometers," *JAMA,* 127:520–521 (1945).
   1.2 AMA Council on Physical Medicine and Rehabilitation. "Minimum Requirements for Acceptable Pure Tone Audiometers for Diagnostic Purposes." *JAMA,* 146:255–257 (1951).
   1.3 AMA Council on Physical Medicine and Rehabilitation. "Minimal Requirements for Acceptable Pure Tone Audiometers for Screening Purposes," *JAMA,* 144:465 (1950).
   1.4 ANSI S.3-1969. *Specifications for Audiometers.*
   1.5 IEC Publication 177 (1965). *Pure Tone Audiometers for General Diagnostic Purposes.*
   1.6 IEC Publication 178 (1965). *Pure Tone Screening Audiometers.*

1.7 ISO Standard 389-1975. *Audiometry—Standard Reference Zero for the Calibration of Pure Tone Audiometers.*
(Publications of the International Electrotechnical Commission and International Organization for Standardization, Items 1.5-1.7, are available from the American National Standards Institute, 1430 Broadway, New York, N.Y. 10018.)

2. *Committee Reports and Guides*

2.1 AAOO Committee on Conservation of Hearing. "The Listing of Audiometers," *Trans. Amer. Acad. Ophthal. Otolaryng.*, 62:247–249 (1958).

2.2 AAOO Committee on Conservation of Hearing (Subcommittee on Noise in Industry). "Guide for the Evaluation of Hearing Impairment." *Trans. Amer. Acad. Ophthal. Otolaryng.*, 63:236–238 (1959).

2.3 AAOO Committee on Conservation of Hearing. (Subcommittee on Noise). *Guide for the Conservation of Hearing in Noise.* Revised 1969. Supplement to *Trans. Amer. Acad. Ophthal. Otolaryng.*

2.4 AAOO Committee on Hearing and Equilibrium. (Subcommittee on Conservation of Hearing). *Guide for the Conservation of Hearing in Noise.* Revised 1973. Supplement to *Trans. Amer. Acad. Ophthal. Otolaryng.*

2.5 L. R. Boies et al. (AAOO Committee on Conservation of Hearing). *Guide to the Care of Adults with Hearing Loss.* Rochester, Minn.: American Academy of Ophthalmology and Otolaryngology, 1966.

2.6 AAOO Committee on Conservation of Hearing (Subcommittee on Noise). "The Relation of Presbycusis to Hearing Impairment Induced by Noise," *Trans. Amer. Acad. Ophthal. Otolaryng.*, 68:695–696 (1964).

2.7 AMA Council on Physical Medicine and Rehabilitation. "Principles for Evaluating Hearing Loss," *Trans. Amer. Acad. Ophthal. Otolaryng.*, 59:550–552 (1955).

2.8 AMA Committee on Medical Rating of Physical Impairment. "Guides to the Evaluation of Permanent Impairment," *JAMA*, 168:475 (1958).

2.9 AMA Committee on Medical Rating of Physical Impairment. "Guide to the Evaluation of Permanent Impairment; Ear, Nose, Throat and Related Structures, *JAMA*, 177:489–501 (1961).

3. *Approved Articles*

3.1 Davis, H. "Missouri Senate Bill No. 167 Concerning Industrial Hearing Loss: An Interpretation," *Arch. Otolaryng. (Chicago)* 72:87–95 (1960).

3.2 Davis, H., and Kranz, F. W. "The International Standard Reference Zero for Pure Tone Audiometers and Its Relation to the Evaluation of Impairment of Hearing," *J. Speech Hearing Res.*, 7:7–16 (1964). Also *Trans. Amer. Acad. Ophthal. Otolaryng.*, 68:484–492 (1964).

3.3 Davis, H., and Kranz, F. W. "The International Audiometric Zero," *J. Acoust. Soc. Amer.*, 36:1450–1454 (1964). Also *Amer. Industr. Hyg. Ass. J.*, 25:354–358 (1964), and *Ann. Otol.*, 73:807–815 (1964).

3.4 Davis, H. "The ISO Zero Reference Level for Audiometers," *Arch. Otolaryng.* 81:145–149 (1965).

3.5 Davis, H. "International Standard Reference Zero for Pure Tone Audiometry. *Trans. Amer. Acad. Ophthal. Otolaryng.*, 69:112–118 (1965).

Davis, H. "Reference Levels and Hearing Levels in Otology," *Ann. Otol.*, 75:808–818 (1966).

A review article that also serves to introduce the "actuarial threshold."

———, G. D. Hoople, and H. O. Parrack. "Hearing Level, Hearing Loss and

Threshold Shift," *J. Acoust. Soc. Amer.,* 30:478 (Letter to the Editor).

This is the original proposal to distinguish hearing level from hearing loss.

Glorig, A. "A Report of Two Normal Hearing Studies," *Ann. Otol.,* 67:93–112 (1958).

Jerger, J. F., R. Carhart, T. W. Tillman, and J. L. Peterson. "Some Relations between Normal Hearing for Pure Tones and Speech," *J. Speech Hearing Dis.,* 2:126–140 (1959).

National Center for Health Statistics

   Series 11, number 11: "Hearing Levels of Adults by Age and Sex: United States 1960–1962," A. Glorig and J. Roberts (eds.)

   Series 11, number 26: "Hearing Levels of Adults by Race, Region and Area of Residence: United States 1960–1962," J. Roberts and D. Bayliss (eds.).

   Series 10, number 35: "Characteristics of Persons with Impaired Hearing: United States July 1962–June 1963," A. Gentile, J. D. Schein, and K. Haase (eds.).

   Series 11, number 31: "Hearing Levels of Adults by Education, Income, and Occupation: United States 1960–1962," J. Roberts and J. Cohrssen (eds.).

   Series 11, number 32: "Hearing Status and Ear Examination Findings Among Adults: United States 1960–1962," J. Roberts (ed.).

   Series 11, number 102: "Hearing Levels of Children by Age and Sex: United States 1963–1965," J. Roberts and P. Huber (eds.).

   Series 1, number 5: "Plan, Operation, and Response Results of a Program of Children's Examination: United States 1967," Public Health Service Publication No. 1000, Series 1, No. 5.

   The data are from the National Health Survey, Public Health Service, U.S. Department of Health, Education and Welfare. These very informative pamphlets are for sale by the Superintendent of Documents, U.S. Government Printing Office, Washington, D.C. 20402.

Schmidt, P. H., "Presbycusis: The Present Status," *Int. Audiol.,* Supplement 1, 1967.

   An excellent review.

Tillman, T. W. and J. F. Jerger. "Some Factors Affecting the Spondee Threshold in Normal-hearing Subjects," *J. Speech Hearing Dis.,* 2:141–146 (1959).

Weissler, P. G. "International Standard Reference Zero for Audiometers," *J. Acoust. Soc. Amer.,* 44:264–275 (1968).

   This is a detailed report on the technical activities of ISO's Technical Committee on Acoustics No. 43, Working Group on Threshold of Hearing, which led to the ISO Recommendation R389, Standard Reference Zero for the Calibration of Pure-Tone Audiometers, November 1964.

Part IV

REHABILITATION FOR HEARING LOSS

Arthur F. Niemoeller, Sc. D.

10

Hearing Aids

A hearing aid is any instrument that brings sound more effectively to the listener's ear. It may simply collect more sound energy from the air, it may prevent the scattering of sound during transmission, or it may provide additional energy, usually from the battery of an electronic amplifier.

The first objective of a hearing aid is to make speech intelligible. The "quality" or naturalness of the speech may be sacrificed if necessary. Little thought was given to quality by those who used the old ear trumpets. They were well enough satisfied if only speech could be made loud enough to be intelligible. Even with early electric instruments, the chief difficulty was still to deliver enough energy, and any necessary compromises were acceptable as long as speech could be understood. Now, however, the arts of electronic amplification and electroacoustic engineering have made it possible to deliver as much sound as the ear can tolerate. We can therefore raise our sights and say that a hearing aid should deliver sounds loudly enough to be heard easily, but without discomfort. The listener's hearing loss should be overcome and his auditory nerve stimulated in a pattern as nearly normal as possible. Of course, the instrument should not add new "internal" noises. Distortion of the original pattern of sound should be introduced only to the extent that it assists in bringing to the listener speech that is intelligible, comfortable, and of a pleasing quality.

ACOUSTIC HEARING AIDS

The simplest hearing aid, used since man became civilized enough to grow old and become hard of hearing, is the hand cupped behind the ear. The hand

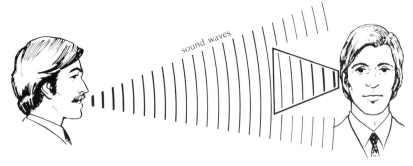

Figure 10-1 Ear trumpet. Collects sound energy, but has no batteries or amplifier.

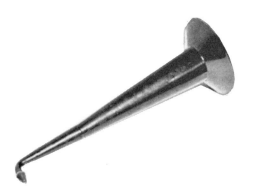

Figure 10-2 An old ear trumpet. *(Goldstein Collection, Central Institute for the Deaf)*

intercepts more of the oncoming sound wave than does the ear alone and deflects more of its energy into the external canal. The larger the scoop, the more the energy that can be collected. The efficiency of the scoop can be improved if it is shaped to favor the delivery of the energy into the ear canal. The broad principle of the ear trumpet is illustrated in Figure 10-1.

The ear trumpet took many forms in efforts to compromise between effectiveness, con-

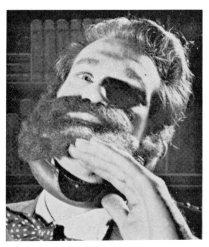

Figure 10-3 Concealment by a beard of a large nonelectric hearing aid. *(Goldstein Collection, Central Institute for the Deaf; photo by St. Louis* Post-Dispatch*)*

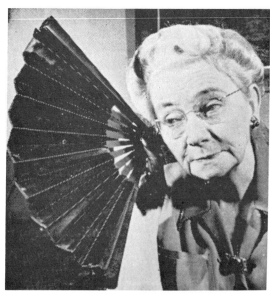

Figure 10-4 An acoustic fan. *(Goldstein Collection, Central Institute for the Deaf; photo by St. Louis* Post-Dispatch*)*

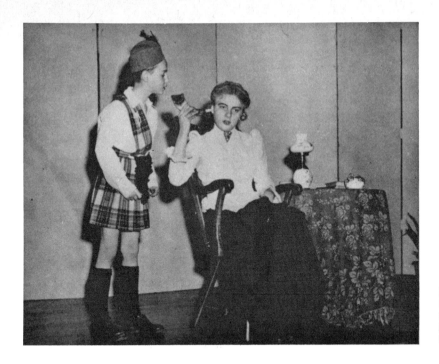

Figure 10-5 Deaf children reenact the story of Alexander Graham Bell. *(Goldstein Collection, Central Institute for the Deaf)*

venience, and the user's vanity. Some of the varieties of shape and style are shown in Figures 10-2 through 10-5, photographs of the Goldstein Collection of nonelectric hearing aids at the Central Institute for the Deaf. Some instruments were small and convenient, but not very effective. Others were built into cane heads, ear ornaments, or vases. Nearly all the instruments in the collection are black, probably to be as inconspicuous as possible, and all have in common a large surface or opening to catch the sound. Some also extend toward the speaker, where his voice is louder, and carry the sound to the ear in a tube without allowing it to scatter. When we recall that the intensity of sound in open air falls off rapidly with the distance the sound travels, we can see that much more energy can be collected if the ear trumpet reaches well out toward the speaker's mouth.

The acoustic gains provided by the head and external ear, the cupped hand behind the ear, and the ear trumpet (of Figure 10-2) in the ear canal are shown in Figure 10-6. These curves were measured using a manikin that was developed specifically for research on hearing aids and related devices.

Most of the old-fashioned ear trumpets were more than mere scoops to collect acoustic energy. They were also "resonators," tuned broadly to frequencies in the speech range. Sound pressures build up to higher levels at and near the resonant frequencies of the instrument, and at these frequencies the energy delivered to the ear may sometimes be increased in this way by as much as 10 to 20 dB. The external ear canal deals with sounds at frequencies between 2000 and 4000 Hz in the same way. The tube of the trumpet is larger and longer than the ear canal and is thus "tuned" to a lower band of frequencies.

By empirically combining the principles of resonance and sound conduction, the ear trumpet or the speaking tube can be a fairly

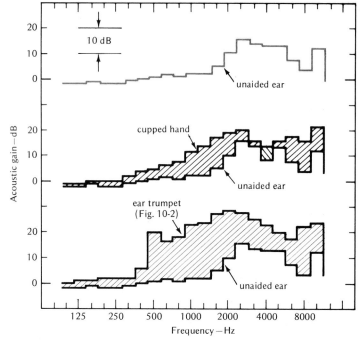

Figure 10-6 Frequency response of some acoustic hearing aids as measured on a KEMAR manikin in a plane-progressive sound field of pink noise (equal energy per band), measured in third-octave bands. The shaded areas indicate acoustic gain relative to the gain of the unaided ear. All curves were measured with the sound source directed toward and normal to the face of the manikin. *(KEMAR: trademark for an acoustic research manikin manufactured by Knowles Electronics, Inc.)*

effective hearing aid. Those instruments are very simple and easy to use, and should not be forgotten in this electronic era. The gain for speech provided by an ear trumpet is likely to be about 10 to 20 dB. Even the cupped hand behind the ear gives us 5 to 10 dB. As we all know, this may make just the difference between understanding and not understanding a lecture or a sermon.

"Louder, Please!"

The cupped hand at the ear also politely tells the speaker that the listener is having difficulty hearing him, and almost always, so universally is the sign understood, the speaker will raise his voice. An extra 10 dB of voice means only a little extra effort for most speakers. We instinctively and often

unconsciously raise our voices this much in noisy surroundings when we begin to have a little difficulty hearing ourselves. The intensity of the voice is increased at the source, and the hard-of-hearing listener gets the benefit.

In the Psycho-Acoustic Laboratory the wartime project dealing with hearing aids was nicknamed "Louder, Please."

Early Bone-Conduction Devices

Among the hearing aids of the nineteenth century it is interesting to find one, the acoustic fan, which took advantage of bone conduction. A sheet of metal or hard rubber, shaped and decorated like a fan, was held with one corner against the teeth. The vibrations of the metal were transmitted through the teeth to the bones of the skull and thus to the inner ear. More recently, men have used devices resembling pipes that employ the same principle. Bone conduction can, as we have seen, bypass a conductive deafness. The acoustic fan or pipe is unable, however, to collect enough energy from the air to be a very effective aid to hearing.

Devices Within the Ear

Formerly some otologists employed a "prosthesis," usually a bit of tissue paper to cover a perforation in the tympanic membrane or a wisp of cotton within the middle ear and touching the stapes, to improve the transmission of acoustic energy. Suitable cases were few, the improvements were only moderate at best, and the prosthesis had to be replaced frequently. The use of such devices in the middle ear has now been given up almost entirely in favor of the operations of myringoplasty or tympanoplasty, described in Chapter 6. The occasional temporary success of such simple prostheses nevertheless lent a glow of plausibility to a host of devices that were and probably still are advertised by unscrupulous individuals in uncritical newspapers and periodicals.

Complete restoration of hearing with a simple, inexpensive, but miraculous gadget that fits comfortably within the ear canal is the dream of everyone who is hard of hearing. Even the most sober and rational of us dream and wish. We are not very far removed from the days when the right ear of a lion was believed to be a cure for deafness or when we bought "snake oil" from the Indian medicine man. There are still enough wishful and gullible people to keep in business a few who are willing to promise enough at not too high a price. A thousand-to-one chance that the wonderful gadget may be a tenth as good as it is claimed to be seems to be worth a few dollars to many people. But

actually there is no such chance. Claims of restoring hearing by "resonance" are a pseudoscientific smoke screen. Very rarely, it is true, something pushed blindly into the ear canal might open a passageway through or around a plug of wax. This might cause a real improvement; but, except for such cases, we may be quite sure that those who believed themselves benefited by mysterious nonelectrical within-the-ear gadgets were honestly self-deluded one way or another.

One of the most rigid laws of physics (although apparently not of human society) says, in effect, "You can't get something for nothing." What the hard-of-hearing man must get in order to hear is *more energy*. He may induce the speaker to provide it by saying, "Louder, please"; he may move closer to the speaker to intercept more of it; he may collect more energy in an ear trumpet or a speaking tube and bring it more efficiently to his ear; or he may provide it from the battery of an electric hearing aid.

Now, with the extreme miniaturization of modern electronic circuits, electroacoustic hearing aids of moderate power can actually be worn within the ear, but they are not simple or inexpensive gadgets.

ELECTROACOUSTIC HEARING AIDS

An electroacoustic hearing aid is a miniature telephone. It differs fundamentally from the acoustic aids we have just described in that *its batteries, and not the human voice, supply the energy of the sound that the listener finally hears.* The voice of the speaker merely serves to control the flow of electric current in the wires to the earpiece and gives it the pattern of the voice sounds. The receiver in the listener's ear, like the telephone receiver at the end of the line, converts the electric current back into sound. The point is that the sound generated in the earpiece, like the sound from a public-address system, may be made much louder than the sound that falls upon the microphone (transmitter) because its energy comes from the battery. A telephone is designed to produce at a distance a sound nearly as loud as the original voice. Electric energy is required to overcome the losses in the long wires. A hearing aid is designed to produce a louder sound from a very small receiver at the end of a short wire. Thus the energy of the battery serves to overcome the hearing loss of the listener.

Types of Electroacoustic Hearing Aids

Electroacoustic hearing aids are of three general types: wearable, portable or desk types, and group.

Comfort, convenience, desire to conceal the instrument, and individual acoustic needs have all contributed to the development of a variety of types of wearable hearing aids. Some types are more popular than others, depending on what the user considers most important to him. Later in this chapter we shall comment on the relative ef-

fectiveness of the different types in various listening situations.

Wearable instruments differ mainly in where they are worn on the body and in whether there is a receiver in one ear or in both ears. The following types are commercially available:

1. Monaural body-worn or pocket aid: one instrument (microphone, amplifier, battery) carried usually on the chest, either in a pocket or special cloth carrier, and connected with a cord to an insert receiver which is plugged into the earmold.
2. Monaural head-mounted: one instrument, housed in the temple of a pair of spectacles or in a case worn behind the ear and connected by plastic tubing to the earmold. The device also can be fashioned to be located entirely within the ear, usually with the shape of an earmold.
3. Pseudobinaural or Y-cord: one body-worn instrument with a cord connected to two receivers, one for each ear.
4. Binaural body-worn: two separate instruments worn on the chest about 8 inches apart. They can also be packaged within one case, each with its own microphone,

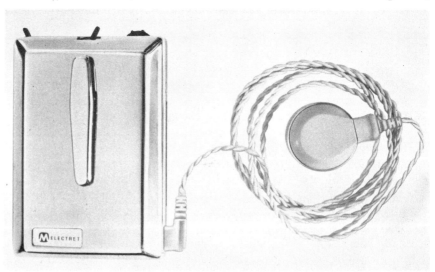

Figure 10-7 A body-worn monaural hearing aid. (*Maico Hearing Instruments, Inc.*)

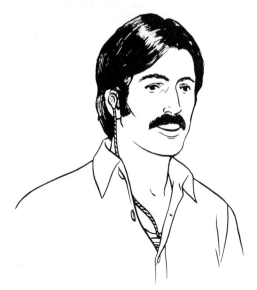

Figure 10-8 Use of a body-worn monaural hearing aid. Men may wear the instrument in a pouch suspended from the neck under the shirt or they may clip it in a shirt, vest, or coat pocket. Women may clip the instrument to the bra or slip or they may tuck it in a pouch and pin the pouch to a bra strap. *(Adapted from an illustration by Sonotone Corp.)*

amplifier, volume and tone control, cord, and receiver.

5. Binaural head-mounted: two separate instruments, packaged in the temples of spectacles, in behind-the-ear cases or within-the-ear.

6. CROS (contralateral routing of signals) aids: one microphone placed over one ear, either in the eye-glass frame or within a dummy behind-the-ear case, and connected across the head to an amplifier and receiver placed over or within the opposite ear. If a second microphone is added to the system and located over the stimulated ear, the configuration is called "BICROS."

These wearable types of hearing aids are illustrated in Figures 10-7 through 10-14.

The portable or desk type of instrument can be used by a single hard-of-hearing lis-tener who spends much of his time in one place. It may deliver more power with better quality than wearable instruments do, and it draws its power from a wall socket as a radio does. It does not require an insert receiver and frequently has two "over-the-ear" receivers. The portable hearing aid (Figure 10-15) may have multiple outlets, an advantageous feature for an itinerant teacher who wants to use the instrument with two or three children.

A group hearing aid (Figure 10-16) consists of one or more microphones, an amplifier, and as many as ten pairs of over-the-ear or insert receivers. Frequently a turntable is included for playing recorded speech, music, or sound effects. The effect of a group hearing aid may now be achieved with in-

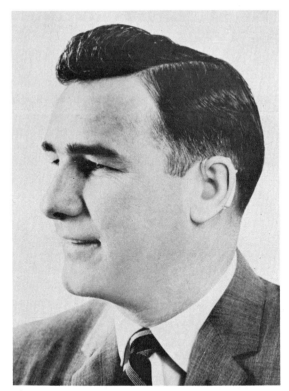

Figure 10-9 Wearing a "behind-the-ear" instrument. It is held in place by the tube around the auricle. *(Maico Hearing Instruments, Inc.)*

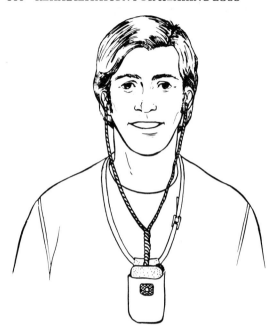

Figure 10-10   A Y-cord hearing aid. Note the single instrument, with a receiver in each ear.

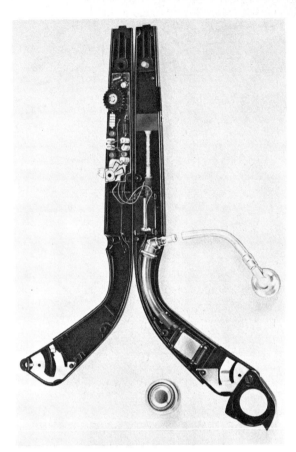

Figure 10-12   Eyeglass hearing aid opened to show components. *(Zenith Hearing Instrument Corp.)*

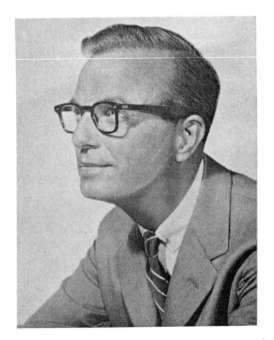

Figure 10-11   Wearing an eyeglass-type hearing aid. *(Sonotone Corp.)*

dividual wearable instruments without connecting wires from the amplifier to the listeners. This is done by using electromagnetic transmission. One method uses an "induction loop," a loop of wire around the classroom that receives electric energy from the amplifier of the group aid. The magnetic field created by the loop current is sensed by a "telephone pickup," a small coil of wire in each of the personal aids worn by the listeners. Movement of the listeners within the room is not limited by wires. For best signal-to-noise ratio, the speaker normally wears or carries a microphone held close to the lips.

Rooms equipped with induction loops

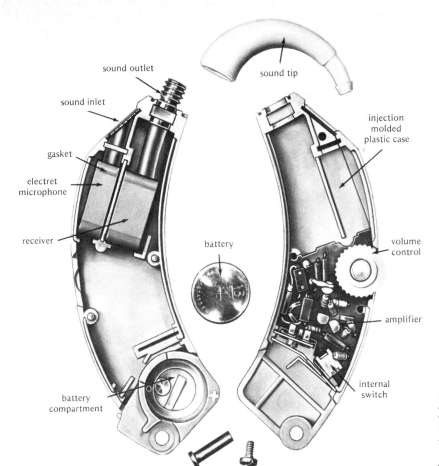

Figure 10-13 Enlarged cutaway view of components within a behind-the-ear hearing aid. The actual height of the instrument is a little over 1 inch. *(Zenith Hearing Instrument Corp.)*

must be sufficiently far from each other to prevent excessive "crosstalk" from the loop of one aid to the listeners of another. Such crosstalk can be greatly reduced by using radio-frequency (RF) transmission, in which the speaker's voice is used to modulate a "carrier" signal. The modulated carrier is "broadcast" through the loop to small radio receivers that are carried by each of the listeners and are tuned to the transmitted carrier signal. Adjacent rooms operate on different carrier frequencies, and receivers tuned to one carrier will reject all others. Two rooms with sufficient distance between them can operate on the same carrier frequency. In

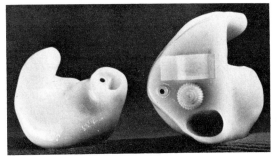

Figure 10-14 Two views of a within-the-ear hearing aid. Note the large vent, the smaller microphone opening, the volume control, and the battery drawer. The aid is custom-molded to a particular individual's ear. The components are chosen to control gain, output, and frequency response and may include compression circuitry. *(Zenith Hearing Instrument Corp.)*

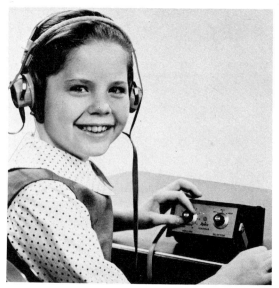

Figure 10-15 Using a desk-model hearing aid. *(Maico Hearing Instruments, Inc.)*

recent years, group hearing aids using radio-frequency carriers have almost completely replaced the magnetic loop systems when wireless transmission is required.

More recently, group hearing aids have been introduced that use modulated infrared rather than radio-frequency radiation. Since infrared energy is easily contained in a room made of conventional building materials, crosstalk between rooms is minimal, and the need for different carrier frequencies in each room is eliminated.

In some group hearing aids both teacher and students are free from wires. This is accomplished by using a "wireless microphone," actually a small portable radio transmitter worn by the teacher that transmits to small portable radio receivers worn by the students (Figure 10-16). The radio re-

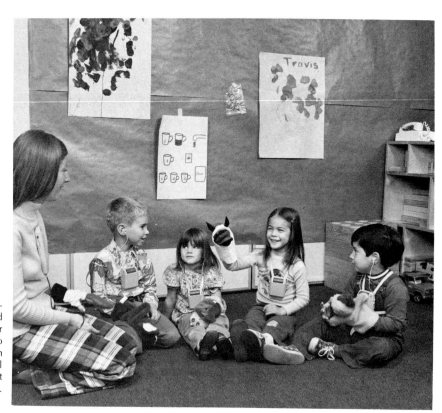

Figure 10-16 A wireless group-hearing-aid system. The teacher wears a small radio transmitter and each student wears a small radio receiver that drives insert earphones. *(HC Electronics, Inc.)*

ceiver must be sophisticated, having tracking capabilities to enable it to follow the frequency drift in the less stable "wireless microphone." Consequently, at present, totally wireless systems are generally the most expensive.

Group hearing aids are used primarily in schools for the deaf and hard-of-hearing, in churches, in meeting halls, and in theaters. Binaural features are now being increasingly incorporated in these instruments.

Basic Components of Electroacoustic Hearing Aids

The electroacoustic hearing aid is quite like a telephone or public-address system. Each is an electronic system interposed between talker and listener to increase the acoustic signal at the listener to a level sufficiently above his "threshold" to make it intelligible. The threshold of the listener is controlled either by his aural sensitivity or by his noise environment, or perhaps by some combination of these. Although the transmission properties of the telephone, public-address, and hearing-aid systems are usually quite different, their basic components are the same. Each has a microphone that transforms the acoustic signal from the talker into an equivalent electric signal, an amplifier that increases the power level of

that signal, and an output transducer that transforms the electric signal back into acoustic energy. Figure 10-17 illustrates the basic components of a hearing aid. The characteristics of each, as they are related to the overall performance of the hearing aid, will be examined.

Microphones

Hearing-aid microphones have a number of distinctive requirements and features that make them unique. In a hearing aid the microphone should be acoustically sensitive but mechanically and environmentally insensitive, and it should be compact, rugged, and inexpensive. In addition, the hearing-aid microphone often must emphasize certain frequencies and deemphasize others. It is noteworthy that with present technology these often conflicting requirements and distinctive features can be and usually are achieved to the degree that the microphone seldom imposes an unwanted constraint on either the design or use of the aid in which it is placed.

In recent years three types of microphones —the magnetic, the ceramic, and the electret —have been used in hearing aids, and each type has certain advantages and disadvantages. Since the "state of the art" of electronic circuitry and packaging is changing so

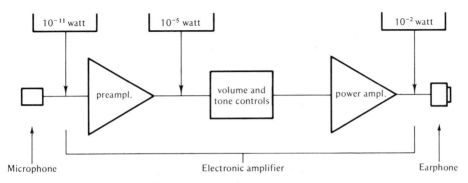

Figure 10-17 Block diagram of a possible electronic hearing aid.

rapidly and since microphones are described in detail in other texts, only an outline of the characteristics and principles of operation of each type that is used in hearing aids will be presented. Each microphone has a diaphragm that is set into motion under the influence of an acoustic pressure wave; the diaphragm is a mechanoacoustic transducer that transforms acoustic energy into mechanical energy. The diaphragm motion, in turn, is transformed into a voltage at the electrical terminals of the transducer. The method by which the mechanical energy is transformed into electric energy is principally what distinguishes one type of microphone from another.

The magnetic microphone   The magnetic microphone has a low electrical source impedance that matches the low impedance of many solid-state hearing-aid amplifiers. The principal parts of a balanced-armature magnetic microphone are shown in Figure 10-18.

Fluctuations of sound pressure cause corresponding motion of the diaphragm, which is coupled through the rigid drive pin to the armature. The armature is a thin strip of soft magnetic metal and is positioned within a coil having turns of very fine wire. As the armature moves, the magnetic flux in the armature changes, and a voltage proportional to the rate of change of flux is induced in the coil.

The magnetic microphone is subject to damage when exposed to excessive mechanical shock but is relatively insensitive to normal changes of heat and humidity. Its inherent electrical noise is low because of its low electrical impedance. Because of the improved frequency response of ceramic and electret condenser microphones, they have almost completely replaced magnetic microphones in hearing aids of recent manufacture.

The ceramic microphone   With the development of inexpensive, low-noise, low voltage field-effect transistors (FETs), microphones with ceramic piezoelectric elements became feasible for use in hearing aids. Ceramic elements, such as lead zirconate-titanate, are

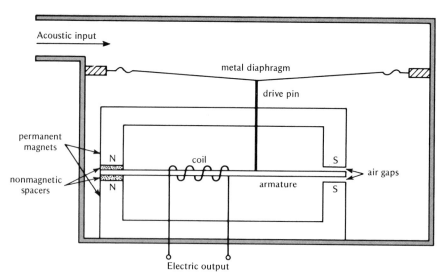

Figure 10-18   Schematic diagram of a balanced-armature microphone.

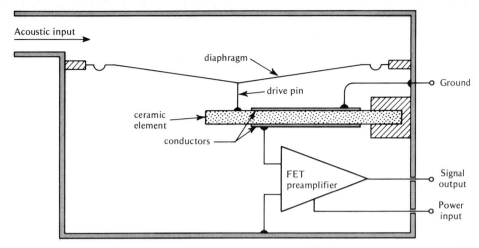

Figure 10-19 Schematic diagram of a ceramic microphone with field-effect transistor (FET) preamplifier.

called *piezoelectric* if a mechanical deformation of the material produces an electric potential across a pair of opposing faces. Thus, when a piezoelectric ceramic bar is anchored at one end, the other end is connected to the microphone diaphragm, and conducting surfaces are deposited on the faces as shown in Figure 10-19, the electric voltage output at the ceramic faces is proportional to the acoustic pressure input to the diaphragm. However, the high electrical impedance of the piezoelectric ceramic is poorly suited for directly driving the lower input impedances of the solid-state amplifiers used in present hearing aids. Therefore, an FET preamplifier is interposed both to amplify the electric signal and to provide the necessary impedance match. To minimize pickup from external electrostatic fields, the FET preamplifier is located within the metal microphone case.

The ceramic microphone is mechanically rugged, and it is insensitive to changes in temperature and humidity. Compared to the magnetic microphone, the ceramic microphone has much wider bandwith, it has greater sensitivity to low-frequency vibration but is less sensitive to high-frequency vibration, and it has about 5 dB greater inter-

nal electrical noise when referred to its equivalent acoustical input. The ceramic microphone with FET preamplifier has three electrical connections: one for power, one for signal, and a common "ground" for power supply and signal.

The electret condenser microphone A magnet and an electret can be viewed as analogous devices. A magnet is made from a special material that permanently retains a *magnetic* polarization that is applied during manufacture. An electret is made from a special material that permanently retains an *electric* polarization or "charge" that is applied during manufacture. Although the concepts of electret microphones are not new, realization of these concepts in a subminiature microphone for hearing aids had to wait for development of both miniature FET preamplifiers and fluorocarbon plastic electret films. It was not until the early 1970s that electret microphones became commercially available for use in hearing aids. These microphones have all of the desirable features of the ceramic microphone and, in addition, are significantly less sensitive to vibration. Thus, with the use of electret microphones in hearing aids, problems from structure-borne feedback and from thump transmitted by walking were significantly reduced.

In the electret microphone, an electric capacitor or "condenser" is formed by the conducting surfaces of the diaphragm and backplate, as shown in Figure 10-20. The electret film that is bonded to the backplate establishes an electrostatic field and resultant polarization voltage in the air gap to the diaphragm. As the diaphragm moves under the influence of the acoustic input sound pressure, the electrostatic field, and hence the diaphragm-to-backplate voltage, will change proportionally to the diaphragm motion so long as only negligible charge flows between diaphragm and backplate. The very high impedance of the FET preamplifier ensures this. In addition, the preamplifier lowers the impedance and amplifies the level of the signal, and with the shielding provided by the microphone case, these functions are accomplished with minimal pickup of extraneous electrostatic fields.

Directional microphones A directional microphone is more sensitive to sound coming from one direction than from other directions. Such microphones have been used in broadcasting, recording, and sound-reinforcement systems for many years, but only since the introduction of the ceramic and electret microphones has it been possible to make directional microphones small enough for use in hearing aids. Any hearing aid is given a directional preference by the acoustic shadows cast by the head or body, depending on where it is worn. A directional microphone enhances this phenomenon and improves the wearer's ability to separate desired sound, which usually comes from a particular direction, from undesired sound or noise, which in rooms usually comes from many directions. Thus, the signal-to-noise ratio can be increased, with proper use of a hearing aid, by use of a directional microphone.

Whereas a nondirectional microphone has one sound port that leads to one side of the microphone diaphragm, a directional microphone has two ports, one leading to each side of the diaphragm. The two ports are spatially separated, with one at the front of the microphone and the other at the rear. As the sound wave passes the microphone, sound

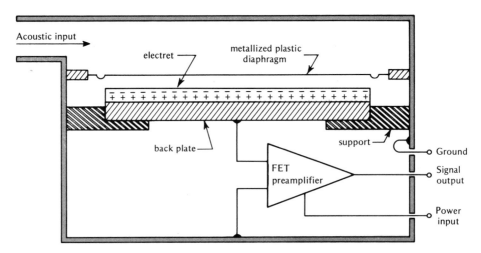

Figure 10-20 Schematic diagram of an electret microphone with field-effect transistor (FET) preamplifier.

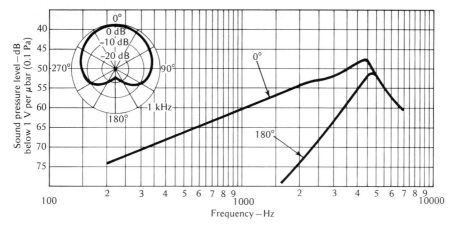

Figure 10-21   Frequency and polar responses of a directional electret condenser microphone for hearing aids. Frequency responses are shown for both 0° and 180° sound incidence. The polar responses, upper left, are the responses at 1000 Hz as a function of angle of incidence of the sound waves. (An extension of 8-mm tubing, 2 mm in diameter, is added to the front port of the microphone.) *(Knowles Electronics, Inc.)*

entering one port is delayed relative to sound entering the other. The amount of delay depends on the distance between the ports and their orientation relative to the direction of sound. Another delay is produced within the microphone by an acoustical network between the rear port and the back side of the diaphragm. With the ports lined up along the direction of sound propagation, the amount of internal delay from rear port to diaphragm is set equal to the delay between ports outside of the microphone. Thus for sound arriving from the rear the delays to, and hence the pressures on, each side of the diaphragm will be equal, there will be no net force to move the diaphragm, and the microphone output will be zero. Conversely, when sound arrives directly from the front, one side of the diaphragm is exposed directly to the pressure at the front port while the other side receives the pressure delayed once as the sound moves from front to rear ports and again by an equal amount through the internal delay network. The resultant pressure differential across the diaphragm, over the frequency range where the distance between ports is small compared to a wave-

length, varies directly with frequency. Indeed, the distance between ports is small over the useful range of most hearing aids and the frequency response of their directional microphones rises 6 dB per octave. When equalization of this rising characteristic is required, it is easily done in the amplifier. The frequency and polar response curves on a directional hearing-aid microphone are shown in Figure 10-21.

Amplifiers

The history of electronic amplifiers in hearing aids began in the early 1930s when a ·carbon amplifier was used to modulate battery power to a receiver. In the late 1930s the first vacuum tube aids were manufactured and used until the early 1950s when the first transistor aids appeared. By the mid-1960s integrated-circuit amplifiers were being used, particularly in the "ear-level" and "in-the-ear" hearing-aids, where space is so important.

It has been possible, since the time of the vacuum tube aids, to build amplifiers of high quality. However, the tradeoff between electronic excellence and cost, size, and ruggedness must be considered seriously by the manufacturer. Advances in the electronics and hearing-aid industries have led to more efficient, rugged, and linear aids, which are becoming smaller and smaller without significant increase in price.

The amplifier of a modern hearing aid is a system of transistors, diodes, resistors, and capacitors interconnected in such a way that, when supplied with electric energy from a battery or other source, the level or amplitude of the output signal exceeds the level at the input. If designed and used properly, the amplifier will be linear over a wide range of input levels, and its self-noise will be low. The amount that the signal level increases as it passes through the amplifier is called the "gain." Hearing-aid gain is manually controlled by the "volume control." Often it is automatically controlled to give relatively constant output for a wide range of input levels, and typically the gain, by design, is nonuniform over its useful frequency bandwidth. Amplifier stages located just after the microphone where the signal levels are very small are called "preamplifiers," and those high-level stages just preceding the earphone are usually referred to as "power amplifiers."

An amplifier *stage* typically consists of a transistor with some resistors and capaci-

tors, and the combination is supplied with electric energy from a battery as shown in Figure 10-22. The n-p-n transistor (shown in the figure) is formed by a thin p-type semiconductor (the base) between two n-type semiconductors (the collector and the emitter). In the n-p-n transistor, current of positive charges will flow from base to emitter and from collector to emitter. With a p-n-p transistor an n-type semiconductor is sandwiched between p-type materials, the symbol is changed to have the emitter arrow pointing toward the base, and current will flow from emitter to base and from emitter to collector. The transistor acts as an electronic valve for current in the sense that a small change in input current to the base causes a much larger change in output current to the collector. Input current changes arise from the output voltage from a microphone or from a preceding amplifier stage. Output current and resultant voltage changes are passed on to an earphone or a succeeding amplifier stage.

In the circuit of Figure 10-22, with no signal input, the transistor acts to hold the base-to-emitter voltage to about 0.5 volt independent of base current. Thus, with the 1.5-volt battery, 1 volt will be across the 1-megohm (1 MΩ) resistance, and a current of 1 microampere (1 μA) will flow from base to emitter. Each 1 μA of base-to-emitter current,

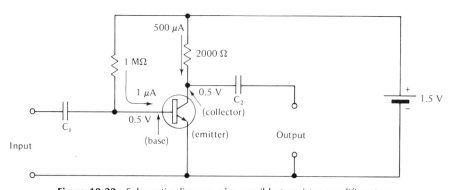

Figure 10-22   Schematic diagram of a possible transistor amplifier stage.

due to the valve action of the transistor, controls 500 μA flowing from collector to emitter through the 2000-ohm (2 kΩ) resistor. Thus, with 1.5 volts supplied by the battery, 1 volt (0.0005 $\times$ 2000) is dropped across the collector resistor to give 0.5 volt across the transistor from collector to emitter. These "bias" currents exist in the transistor with no signal input.

Suppose now that an electric signal input to this stage causes the base-to-emitter current to fluctuate by 0.1 μA. This change is amplified 500 times to give 50-μA fluctuations in collector-to-emitter current and 0.1-volt (0.00005 $\times$ 2000) fluctuations across the 2000-ohm resistor in the collector circuit at the output. The capacitors at the input and output simply serve to pass the alternating-current (ac) components of the voltages while blocking the direct-current (dc) or constant components. With these capacitors, the bias currents, so essential for proper operation of the transistor, are relatively unaffected by the manner in which the stage is driven or loaded.

The complete hearing-aid amplifier normally has many amplification stages. Sometimes they are made of discrete components that are mounted on printed-circuit boards. However, it is becoming increasingly common to use integrated circuits or hybrid circuits. The integrated-circuit amplifier has all transistors, resistors, and diodes produced on a silicon chip only about 0.07 inch square. Development costs of integrated circuits are quite high, production costs after development are relatively low, and modifications are very difficult. Thus integrated circuits are appropriately used in aids where large numbers of a fixed design are expected to be produced. In the hybrid-circuit amplifier, a conductive wiring pattern is printed and fired or vacuum-deposited onto a thin ceramic plate. Then resistors are deposited and trimmed, and chips containing transistors, integrated circuits, capacitors, and diodes are soldered to the wiring pattern. Development costs of hybrid circuits are not so high as those of integrated circuits, but production costs are higher. Generally, hybrid circuits are larger than integrated circuits, and hybrid designs can be modified if necessary. Thus hybrid circuits are used when expected production numbers are not so large and when modifications are anticipated.

The volume control A volume control, or "gain control," makes it possible to adjust the overall gain of a hearing aid to intermediate values. The volume control is usually a resistance that is provided with a sliding contact. It is usually located between stages of the electronic amplifier. The full strength of the signal from the first stage is applied to the resistance, and the slider takes off and passes on to the next stage more or less of the signal according to its position.

The tone control The tone control is usually an arrangement of capacitors and resistors. It may be placed ahead of the first stage or between stages; and the circuits actually employed in different instruments vary considerably.

The tone control changes the relative strength of the high- and low-frequency tones in the signals that pass through it (see Figure 10-17). To obtain "high-tone emphasis," a combination of capacitors and resistors is chosen that transmits high frequencies efficiently and low frequencies inefficiently. The low frequencies are reduced in strength, or "attenuated," more than the high, and thus a *relative high-tone emphasis* is obtained. High-tone emphasis may really be only *low-tone suppression*; but as long as plenty of gain is available, it makes no difference. The wearer simply pushes up the volume control, thereby increasing the strength of all frequencies equally, and the net result is an increase in the high frequencies with no loss in the middle or low range.

Low-tone emphasis is obtained by other combinations of capacitors and/or resistors chosen to suppress the high frequencies.

Some makes of instrument do not have an adjustable tone control, but instead offer several models, each with its own particular emphasis of high tones, low tones, or middle tones. The purchaser then selects the model that best suits his particular needs. Other instruments have an internal adjustment for tone, which is set by the dealer when he sells the instrument; thus he "fits" the device to the purchaser's individual requirements. Still other instruments are "fitted" by selection of the appropriate receiver.

Earphones

An earphone provides the inverse function of a microphone; that is, it transforms an electric input from the hearing-aid amplifier to an acoustic output.

Output transducers for hearing aids are of two general kinds: air conduction and bone conduction.

Air-conduction earphones Air conduction earphones for body-worn electroacoustic hearing aids are worn in the ear; they are supported by an earmold of molded plastic. Even smaller than these are the type built into eyeglass hearing aids and the other tiny aids worn in or behind the ear. With the eyeglass and behind-the-ear types, the sound from the self-contained earphone is carried into the ear canal through a transparent plastic tube that terminates in the earmold. These tiny earphones represent one of the most difficult bits of electroacoustic engineering in the hearing aid. They must transform electric energy efficiently into sound, and at the same time they must avoid exces-

sive mechanical resonance, which would emphasize some frequencies too much. All this is difficult to accomplish in such a small size, but it is being approached more and more closely.

Earphones with very good acoustical characteristics, such as those used for audiometers and professional sound systems, are too large to be practical for wearable hearing aids. They are, however, included in many portable and group hearing aids.

The most common type of earphone used on larger, body-worn hearing aids is the *moving-iron magnetic* earphone. A thin diaphragm of magnetic material is mounted close to a permanent magnet, as shown in Figure 10-23. The electric current from the amplifier passes through coils that are wound on cores of special magnetic material fastened to the permanent magnet. According to the strength and direction of the current through the coils, the magnet becomes stronger or weaker. The magnet thus pulls

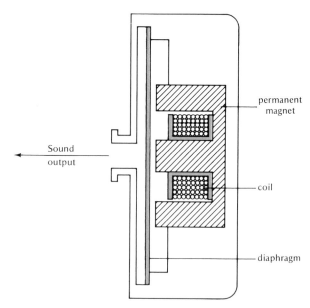

Figure 10-23 Diagram of a moving-iron magnetic receiver.

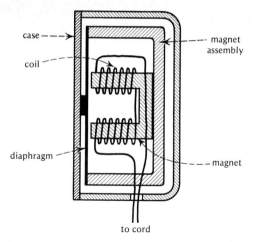

case

coil

diaphragm

magnet
assembly

magnet

to cord

Figure 10-24   Diagram of a bone-conduction vibrator.

more or less strongly on the diaphragm. The diaphragm vibrates and sets up sound waves in the air.

The *balanced-armature magnetic* earphone that is used in many miniature headworn aids is physically quite like the balanced-armature magnetic microphone. Current through the coil causes the armature to move by changing the magnetic forces on it, and sound waves are produced by rigidly coupling the armature to a diaphragm.

Bone-conduction vibrators   The most common type of *bone-conduction vibrator* is magnetic. It is designed to vibrate its case instead of setting up sound waves in the ear (Figure 10-24). Its diaphragm is attached rigidly to a plastic case shaped to fit comfortably against the mastoid bone behind the ear. The magnetic system is supported by the edge of the diaphragm. The pull of the magnet varies with the changes in the flow of electric current through the coil, and both magnet and case move in relation to one another. The inertia of the magnet is considerable, however, and therefore the case, and with it the mastoid bone, vibrates appreciably. The case moves less than does the

diaphragm of an air-conduction earphone, but it moves with considerable force and can therefore set up an adequate vibration in the skull. The vibrator is held in snug contact against the mastoid by means of a light spring headband, as shown in Figures 10-25 and 10-26.

Partly because of the way in which skin and bone transmit sound, it is difficult to design a bone-conduction vibrator that will deliver high frequencies to the inner ear as efficiently as it does some of the lower frequencies, but its range compares very favorably with the range of many air-conduction earphones.

Comparison of bone conduction and air conduction   In the chapter on the medical aspects of deafness, the principle of bone con-

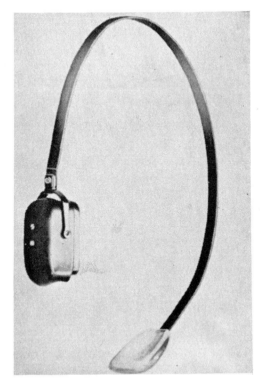

Figure 10-25   A bone-conduction vibrator with its spring headband. *(Sonotone Corp.)*

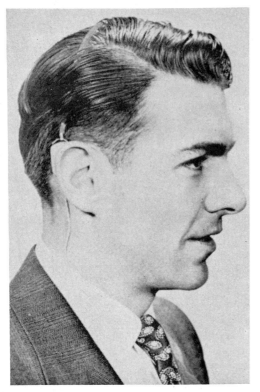

Figure 10-26 A bone-conduction vibrator in place behind the ear. *(Sonotone Corp.)*

duction was discussed. It will be recalled that bone conduction is definitely preferable to air conduction when, for any medical reason, the wearer cannot safely or comfortably use an earmold. Bone conduction is most successful when the hearing loss is primarily conductive and the inner ear is still normal. We shall return to the problem of bone as compared with air in connection with the selection of a hearing aid; but it is worth noting that recent technical developments have favored air conduction somewhat more than bone conduction.

Thanks to the individual earmold, a small in-the-ear air-conduction earphone can deliver into the ear more sound of good quality than was formerly possible. A considerable fraction of the sound that reaches the inner ear from an air-conduction receiver may actually arrive by way of the bone. The faithfulness of reproduction by a good air-conduction earphone is generally better, particularly for high frequencies, than by a bone-conduction vibrator. When the bone-conduction vibrator was first introduced, it was often preferred because it was less conspicuous and perhaps more comfortable than large, over-the-ear air-conduction earphones. Some wearers still prefer bone-conduction vibrators for the same reasons and find them perfectly adequate; but with the increased efficiency of small and less conspicuous air-conduction earphones that require no headband, the choice is based more and more often on the combination of greater convenience and simple effectiveness, and the majority of the hard-of-hearing prefer air conduction.

The Cords and the Case

The cords of a body-worn hearing aid are obviously nothing more than light, flexible, insulated wires that carry the current from the amplifier to the earphone.

The problem with cords is to make them light and flexible and yet mechanically strong, durable, and electrically insulated. Furthermore, the covering must not generate static electricity or make a noise when it rubs on clothing, for noise carried mechanically by cords to the amplifier case and microphone can be a source of great annoyance. In addition, the covering of a cord must keep its insulating properties when moistened by perspiration.

The case deserves mention because it, too, must be strong, light, and durable. The shape of the case and its smoothness, as well as the material of which it is made, must be carefully planned and chosen to reduce as much as possible the noise made by the friction of clothing.

THE CUSTOM EARMOLD

An important accessory to all air-conduction hearing aids is the individually cast earmold (Figure 10-27; also Figure 10-14). The earmold is a molded plastic device that fits snugly into the wearer's ear. A small hole in the earmold serves to conduct sound from the earphone to the eardrum. With body-worn hearing aids, the earphone snaps directly onto the earmold. For head-worn aids, the earphone is contained in the hearing-aid case, and transmission from earphone to earmold is accomplished with a small plastic tube.

The first step in making an earmold is to take an impression of the ear with a special elastic plastic. Dealers in hearing aids usually provide this service. They make the impressions and send them to a special laboratory, where the actual earmolds are made according to the patterns.

Occasionally acoustic leaks are deliberately introduced in the earmold to "roll off" low frequencies. Usually, however, the earmold is made to fit the ear snugly and pre-vent escape of sound around it. The close fit makes the action of the earphone more efficient, as no energy is then lost through leakage. If there is a leak, the sounds reaching the eardrum will be weakened, particularly in the low frequencies.

Squeal If a loud sound is delivered within the ear, it is important that as little as possible should escape around the earmold. If sound escapes, it may reach the microphone of the hearing aid and be picked up and amplified. The result will be a "squeal," resulting from what is known as *acoustic feedback*. Not only is the "squeal" unpleasant; it may also drown out the sounds that the wearer wishes to hear. The development of the custom earmold was an important advance. A hearing aid can deliver to the ear much louder sounds without squeal if the earmold fits well than if it does not. However, even with a well-fitted earmold, the gain of hearing aids worn at the ear is limited by acoustic feedback.

The designer of a hearing aid must sacrifice some sensitivity if an instrument is to

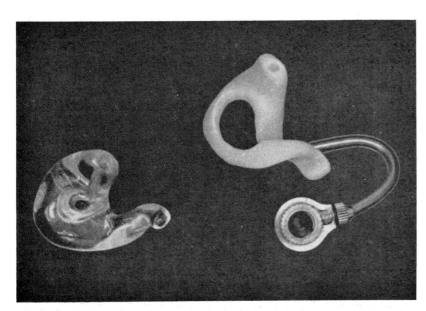

Figure 10-27 Molded plastic eartips. At left, a conventional eartip. In the "hideaway" type at right the receiver may be concealed with only the eartip visible. The size and shape of the couplers that connect receivers to eartips are standardized for all hearing aids. *(Central Institute for the Deaf)*

have a high acoustic output. He cannot rely on *all* the output staying within the ear. Even if the earmold fits well, *some* sound inevitably escapes through the back of the earphone. A very sensitive, high-gain instrument may squeal too easily to take advantage of its available gain.

Some *possible* ways of avoiding squeal are:

Improve the fit of the earmold to the ear (and of the earphone to the earmold)
Reduce the gain of the hearing aid
Move the microphone farther away from the earphone
Adjust the tone control for the best practical compromise

Unfortunately, these strategies often cannot be implemented because reduction of gain and adjustment of the tone control may seriously reduce the effectiveness of the hearing aid and because the distance from microphone to earphone may be fixed, as it is in almost all head-worn aids. Under these conditions abatement of feedback squeal may be feasible only with a hearing aid having different response characteristics or with a new earmold that fits better.

The Telephone Pickup

A telephone pickup is a feature of many of the more elaborate models of hearing aids. An inductive pickup coil is mounted within the case. A switch allows the user to substitute it for the microphone as the input to the hearing-aid amplifier. Thus when the telephone pickup is in use, there is no interference from the acoustic noise of the surroundings. The user simply throws the switch to the "telephone" position and holds the telephone receiver against the case of his instrument.

Batteries

A battery is a reservoir of energy. The energy is stored in the chemical state and is transformed into electric energy through electrochemical conversion when called upon. The *rate* at which energy is used by a hearing aid, that is its *power* consumption, is of the order of milliwatts and is determined by the amount of acoustic power that is required at the receivers and by the output and the efficiency of the microphone, electronic amplifier, and earphone. One of the most significant improvements of the solid-state hearing aid over the vacuum-tube instrument is the increased efficiency of the amplifier and the resultant decrease in the cost and size of batteries.

The term "battery" is used to mean a group of electric cells that are interconnected to provide electric power, with the proper voltage and current, to the amplifier. Each cell has a voltage between its terminals of approximately 1.5 volts, the exact value being determined by the type of cell and the amount of energy that it has already given up. Cells can be rated according to their capacities for energy storage, measured in milliwatthours. However, since electric power (milliwatts) is the product of voltage (volts) and current (milliamperes), the cell normally is rated in milliampere-hours, which, given a constant output voltage, also represent a measure of the stored energy. A 350-milliampere-hour, 1.5-volt cell, for example, could be expected to provide 5 milliamperes of current for 70 hours (525 milliwatthours). Two such cells when connected in series would give a 3-volt, 350-milliampere-hour (1050 milliwatthour) battery, and when connected in parallel would give a 1.5-volt, 700 milliampere-hour (1050 milliwatthour) battery.

Carbon-zinc cells   In a carbon-zinc, or Leclanché, cell a carbon rod is suspended within a zinc case and the space between them contains a black mix of manganese dioxide and an electrolyte paste of ammonium and zinc chlorides and water. The output voltage of this cell, with constant current drain, decreases rather uniformly with time, as shown in Figure 10-28. If the cell is drained with intermittent periods of rest, some of the voltage is regained after each rest period, and the battery life is prolonged. If the cell is drained beyond its normal limit, it may leak fluid and damage the hearing aid.

Other types of cells are not so susceptible to fluid leakage, have a relatively constant output voltage when drained over normal working periods, are not affected by adverse temperature and humidity, and store more energy per unit volume. For these reasons, carbon cells are not widely used in present (1977) hearing aids.

Mercury cells The mercury cell operates on the same principle as the carbon cell, but typically one electrode is mercuric oxide, the other is a zinc-mercury amalgam, and the electrolyte is a solution of potassium hydroxide and zinc oxide. The cell container is a corrosionproof, nickel-plated metal, so designed as to inhibit leakage. The energy density of these cells is quite high. They are not adversely affected by normal heat and humidity, and they maintain rather constant voltage (see Figure 10-28) over their useful life. Nominal voltage for these cells is 1.3 volts.

Silver-oxide cells This type of cell has the greatest energy of those used in hearing aids. One electrode (anode) is zinc and the other (cathode) is silver oxide, with an alkaline electrolyte of potassium hydroxide between them. The nominal voltage of 1.5 volts remains relatively constant over the life of the cell, as shown in Figure 10-28.

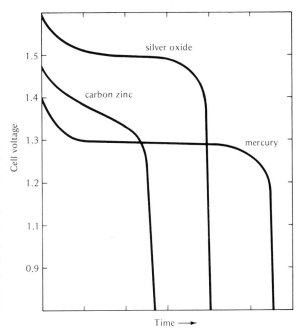

Figure 10-28 Approximate voltage decay characteristics of three kinds of cells. The curves are drawn assuming constant current drain of cells of similar size. When the voltage falls below 0.9 volt, the cell is no longer useful.

FUNCTIONAL GAIN

The gain of a hearing aid usually is defined by the difference (in decibels) between its output and input sound-pressure levels. The output is measured in a standard coupler or artificial ear, and the input is measured at the hearing-aid microphone. Although this *output/input gain* is very useful to those who design hearing aids, it can be misleading in estimating the *functional gain* realized with actual use of an aid. The functional gain of a hearing aid is the difference (in decibels) between sound pressure levels at the eardrum with and without the hearing aid.

Because of differences among individuals in the anatomical configuration of the body, head, and external ear, functional gain of an aid will vary from one person to another.

Therefore, in judging performance of an aid for a particular individual, functional gain is best measured using audiologic procedures with the aid on that person. However, it is often sufficient to know the functional gain when the aid is used on a typical listener. Then the hearing aid is placed on a manikin whose anatomical properties are typical of the population on which the aid will be worn. The manikin has an artificial ear at the end of its ear canal whose acoustical impedances simulate those of the average real ear and whose microphone produces an output signal that corresponds to sound pressure level at the eardrum of a typical listener. Such a manikin is manufactured and sold by Knowles Electronics, Inc., under the trade-

mark KEMAR. Measurements of the electroacoustic properties of a hearing aid on a KEMAR manikin and on a typical or average person presumably are the same within reasonable measurement error. Experimental evidence available at present (1977) suggests that this presumption is valid. However, for scientific completeness and because this manikin is a relatively new device, measurements using it should be appropriately labeled, and caution should be exercised in inferring real-ear performance from data derived from the manikin.

Without a hearing aid, the body, the head, and particularly the external ear reflect and diffract incident sound waves so that in the frequency range between about 2000 and

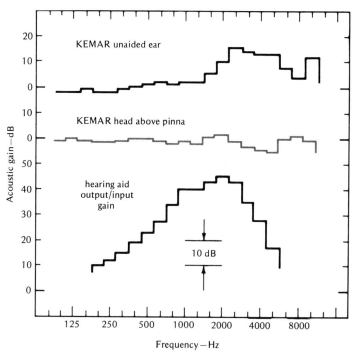

Figure 10-29 Acoustic gain curves of a KEMAR manikin and of a hearing aid using a source of plane-progressive sound waves of pink noise and measured in third-octave bands. For the upper two curves, the sound source was directed toward and normal (perpendicular) to the manikin's face. The gain of the manikin's unaided ear is shown in the top curve. The gain of the head and body, with the measurement microphone located just above the ear at the location of the microphone of a phantom behind-the-ear hearing aid, is shown in the center curve. The lower curve is the output/input gain of a behind-the-ear hearing aid with the aid suspended in a free field and with the output measured in a Zwislocki coupler. *(KEMAR: trademark for an acoustic research manikin manufactured by Knowles Electronics, Inc.)*

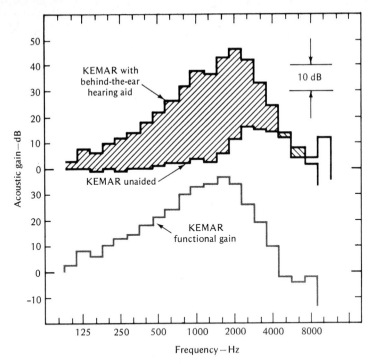

Figure 10-30   Acoustic gain curves of a KEMAR manikin with and without a behind-the-ear hearing aid: upper two curves. Resultant KEMAR manikin functional gain: lower curve. The upper curves were obtained using a source of pink noise directed toward and normal (perpendicular) to the manikin's face in a free field, and responses were mea-sured in third-octave bands. A KEMAR manikin uses a Zwislocki coupler. The differences between the upper curves, indicated by the shaded area, and the lower curve are each measures of functional gain of the hearing aid on the manikin. *(KEMAR: trademark for an acoustic research manikin manufactured by Knowles Electronics, Inc.)*

5000 Hz the sound-pressure levels are en-hanced by as much as 15 to 20 dB depending on the frequency and angle of incidence. This is shown in Figure 10-6 and again in Figure 10-29 for sound waves of third-octave bands of noise directed toward and normal (perpendicular) to the plane of the KEMAR's face.

When a hearing aid is worn, the sound that is sensed depends on the location of the hearing-aid microphone. Perturbations of the sound field by the head and body at the location of the microphone seldom exceed 15 dB, but their effects can be significant de-pending on how they aid or oppose the peaks and dips in the output/input gains curve of the hearing aid. The middle curve in Figure 10-29 shows the perturbations in the

sound field caused by the head and body of the KEMAR manikin just above the ear at the location of the microphone of a behind-the-ear hearing aid. The lower curve in Figure 10-29 is the output/input gain characteristic of the aid.

With the hearing aid on a KEMAR mani-kin, the sound-pressure level in his artificial ear relative to the level of the incident sound wave is shown in the upper curve of Figure 10-30. Within measurement error this is pre-dicted by the perturbations caused by body and head (the center curve of Figure 10-29) plus the output/input curve of the aid (the lower curve of Figure 10-29). The KEMAR manikin's functional gain is shown in the lower curve of Figure 10-30. This curve rep-resents the simple difference in decibels between the upper two gain curves (the shaded area) of the manikin aided and unaided. Although the general shapes of the output/input gain curve of Figure 10-29 and the KEMAR functional gain curve of Figure 10-30 are similar, comparison of the curves show that for frequencies above 800 Hz the output/input gain of the hearing aid is significantly greater (4 to 15 dB) than the KEMAR manikin's functional gain.

The above discussion of output/input gain and functional gain using a KEMAR manikin and a signal source of pink noise is not in accordance with current (1976) American National Standards and International Standards for specification and measurement of hearing-aid characteristics. However, use of a manikin is being considered by standards-writing groups. Also, these characteristics and measurement procedures have some pedagogical advantages, and therefore they were included in this chapter.

FREQUENCY RESPONSE

Between the input and output of a hearing aid the factors that affect the frequency response include an acoustical network that may precede the microphone, the microphone itself, the amplifier with tone controls, the earphone, and another acoustical network that follows the earphone.

The frequency response of the microphone

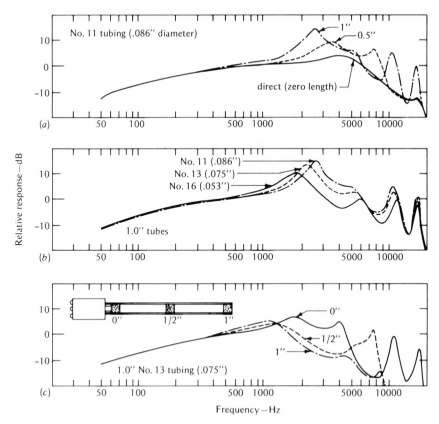

Figure 10-31 Frequency response of an electret condenser hearing-aid microphone with a plastic tube on the sound port showing *(a)* effects of tube length, *(b)* effects of tube diameter, *(c)* effects of acoustical damping plug at different locations in the tube. *(Data courtesy of Knowles Electronics, Inc.)*

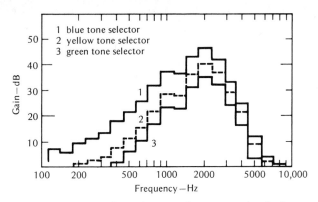

Figure 10-32 Effect of "tone selectors" on the third-octave noise-band response of a behind-the-ear hearing aid on a KEMAR manikin. *(KEMAR: trademark for an acoustic research manikin manufactured by Knowles Electronics, Inc.)*

can be changed by adding acoustic tubes and resistors to the input sound port. These elements react somewhat differently with each type of microphone, but generally a tube will enhance the amplitude of peaks in the response and shift them downward in frequency. The amplitude will be enhanced more with tubes of larger diameter and resonant peaks will shift to lower frequencies with longer tubes. These effects are shown in Figure 10-31. Acoustic resistors, in the form of cylindrical plugs of metal particles that are sintered together, serve to smooth the peaks in the microphone response, particularly when they are inserted at the open or sound-access end of the tube. This effect is shown also in Figure 10-31.

The response of magnetic hearing-aid microphones typically "rolls off" or attenuates low frequencies. The frequency at which the roll-off begins is usually lower for larger microphones, but even the largest magnetic microphones do not respond well to frequencies below 200 or 300 Hz. Ceramic and electret microphones do not have this limitation, although they are often designed to gently roll off low frequencies, at which room and environmental noises are more likely to dominate and the information content in speech is relatively low. Microphones

typically are designed so that response peaks are located between 1500 and 4000 Hz. In this range the information content in speech is relatively high and functional gain often suffers because of the loss of signal enhancement that would be provided by the unaided external ear.

Modifications of frequency response in the amplifier usually are accomplished with simple electronic circuits in which elements are changed to attenuate either high or low frequencies preferentially. Tone controls are marked to indicate high-frequency emphasis when low frequencies are attenuated and they indicate low-frequency emphasis when high frequencies are attenuated. Any loss in signal level that results with adjustment of the tone control is easily recovered by adjusting the volume control. Although some hearing aids have tone-control switches that can be operated with the finger tip according to changes in the acoustical environment about the user, the tone adjustments in most hearing aids are made with a jeweler's screwdriver, and such adjustments are usually made by the hearing-aid dealer or the audiologist. The curves of Figure 10-32 show the effects of tone adjustment in a behind-the-ear hearing aid on a KEMAR manikin.

The frequency response of a hearing aid usually is very strongly influenced by the response of the earphone. With the exception of some body-worn aids for which several earphones may be available to the user, hearing-aid earphones are selected by the designer. As with microphones, resonant peaks in the response of hearing-aid earphones are often located in the 1000–4000-Hz frequency range, wherein the information content in speech is relatively high and functional gain may be low because of the loss of signal enhancement by the external ear. The low-frequency response of the magnetic earphone can be made uniform, but more often it is rolled off intentionally to reduce effects of

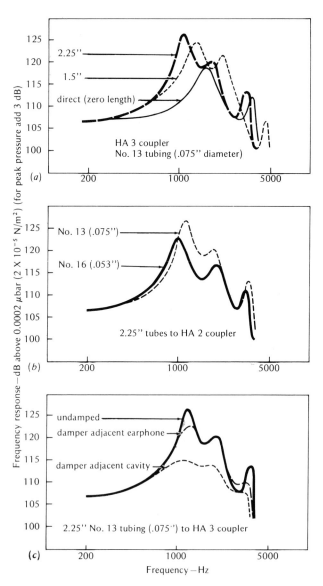

Figure 10-33 Frequency response of a hearing-aid earphone with a plastic tube showing (a) effects of tube length, (b) effects of tube diameter, (c) effects of acoustical damping plug at different locations in the tube. (Data from Knowles Technical Bulletin, "Effects of Source Impedance and Acoustical Termination upon BK Receiver Response," Knowles Electronics, Inc.)

environmental noise. Because of limitations imposed by constraints on size, efficiency, and smoothness of response, the magnetic earphone usually controls the upper frequency limit of a hearing aid. For both body and head-worn aids, basic earphone designs have not changed in recent years, although the range of sizes and responses has increased.

The acoustical tubes and resistors or dampers between the earphone of the hearing aid and the eardrum generally affect the peaks in the earphone response by increasing their amplitude and shifting them downward in frequency. Tubes of larger diameter give peaks of greater amplitude, and longer tubes give greater frequency shifts. Acoustical resistors of lamb's wool or sintered metal are often inserted in the tubes to smooth the frequency response. The effects of tube length, tube diameter, and damping resistors on the response of a magnetic earphone are shown in Figure 10-33.

A hole in the earmold conducts sound from either the earphone or the sound tube to a cavity in front of the eardrum. The size and shape of the earmold hole, the acoustical impedances of the cavity, and the impedance of the eardrum all affect hearing-aid response. Sometimes the earmold hole is specially shaped, and acoustic resistors or dampers are inserted to affect frequency response. More commonly, however, particularly in recent years, frequency response is altered by venting the cavity between earmold tip and eardrum. This is accomplished with a second hole in the earmold from the tip to the outside. A very small hole (less than 0.8 mm) will not affect frequency response significantly, but it will relieve excess static pressure at the eardrum. With vent holes of increasingly larger diameter, low-frequency sound from the earphone will be increasingly shunted away from the eardrum by the vent. The vent then forms a low-impedance path for sound back to the hearing-aid microphone. This, in turn, restricts available acoustic gain before feedback. Other features of the earmold vent, in addition to the obvious comfort factor, are that a direct sound path is provided from the source to the eardrum, at least for low frequencies, and that some of the desirable enhancement that is related to the external ear may be regained in the 2000–5000-Hz frequency range.

DIRECTIONAL RESPONSE

Because of the physical size and configuration of the head and ears, the human hearing system is relatively nondirectional for frequencies below 1000 Hz. The directivity of that system—that is, the degree to which it preferentially receives sounds from one direction at the expense of reception sensitivity from other directions—increases for increasing frequencies. This is shown in Figure 10-34a, which shows the third-octave noise-band directivity patterns for a KEMAR manikin unaided at frequencies of 500 and 4000 Hz. With a KEMAR manikin unaided or with a nondirectional behind-the-ear aid (see Figure 10-34b), reception of sound is rather nondirectional at 500 Hz. At 4000 Hz, sound is received best from angles between 30 and 60 degrees off an axis drawn normal (perpendicular) to the plane of the face. With a directional behind-the-ear hearing aid on a KEMAR manikin, the directional response at 4000 Hz, as shown in Figure 10-34c, is almost unchanged. However, the response at 500 Hz is significantly more directional when compared with either the unaided (Figure 10-34a) or nondirectionally aided (Figure 10-34b) conditions. Hence, with this directional hearing aid, a KEMAR manikin is significantly more sensitive to sounds coming from 30 to 60 degrees off axis at *all* fre-

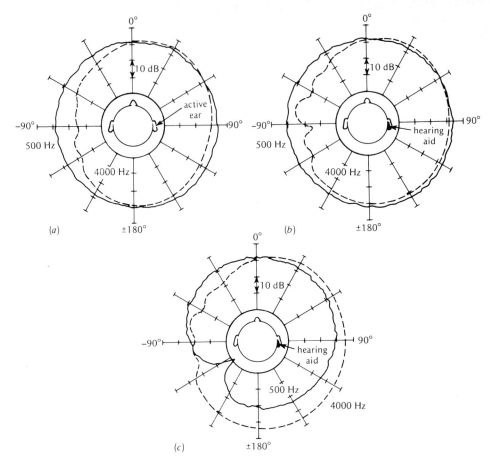

Figure 10-34 Directional responses of a KEMAR manikin to third-octave noise bands at 500 Hz and 4000 Hz. *a:* Unaided response. *b:* Response with a nondirectional behind-the-ear hearing aid. *c:* Response with a directional behind-the-ear hearing aid. *(KEMAR: trademark for an acoustic research manikin manufactured by Knowles Electronics, Inc.)*

quencies. At low frequencies this results from the directional properties of the hearing-aid microphone; at high frequencies it is caused by the directional properties of the head and external ear.

By facing the source of sound, a person wearing a directional hearing aid can enhance the level of that sound relative to unwanted sound coming from other directions. This can be particularly advantageous indoors since the effects of reverberation and room noise can be reduced significantly.

THE OVERALL PERFORMANCE OF HEARING AIDS

The objective of hearing-aid design is to amplify speech without undue distortion and at the same time to protect the user against discomfort from too loud an output. The speech sounds are "packaged" for delivery to an elevated and more or less restricted auditory area (compare Figures 8-9 and 8-10). In addition, the frequency bands above and below the important speech range are often deliberately suppressed so that noise in these bands will not annoy or distract the user.

The performance of a hearing aid is illustrated in Figures 10-35 and 10-36. Here the acoustic area of conversational speech ex-

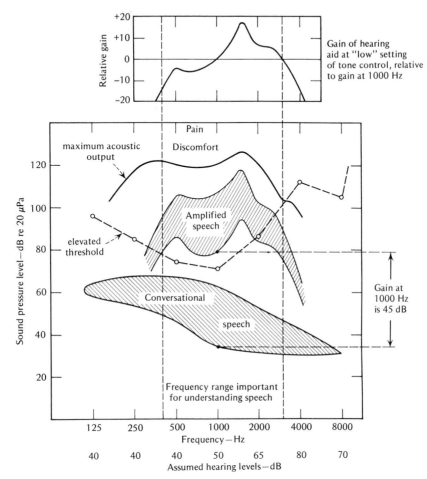

Figure 10-35 Amplification of speech by a hearing aid without peak limiting. The area of conversational speech, as measured in a free acoustic field, is shown here with arbitrary sharp boundaries (see Figure 2-6). The upper boundary represents the level above which the peaks of speech, at that frequency, very seldom rise. The speech elements below the lower boundary contribute very little to intelligibility and can be disregarded. All of the measurements of output are made in a 2-cm³ coupler. The *gain of a hearing aid* at 1000 Hz is the difference between the sound-pressure level measured in the field before the hearing aid is introduced and the sound-pressure level measured in the 2-cm³ coupler. The *area of amplified speech* in this figure was found by moving the speech area upward by 45 dB at

1000 Hz and then modifying the shape of the area according to the overall frequency characteristic of the hearing aid, as drawn above. This is the curve shown for the "low" setting of the tone control. The shape of the curve of *maximum acoustic output* is determined by the receiver. The level of maximum acoustic output is measured at 1000 Hz and is here assumed to be 120 dB SPL, measured in a 2-cm³ coupler. This is close to the usual threshold of discomfort. Only occasional peaks of pressure at the frequencies near 1500 Hz reach this level. The limited auditory area for a hypothetical case of mixed hearing loss is shown. The amplified speech is delivered efficiently and with a minimum of distortion to this reduced "target area."

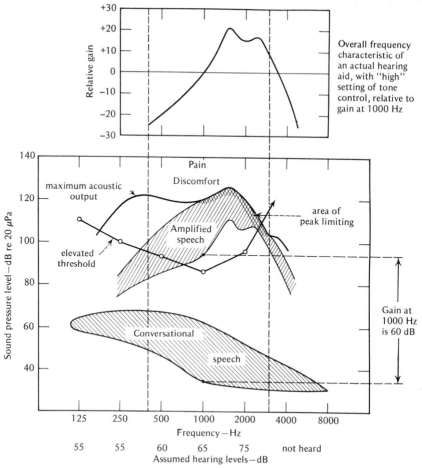

Figure 10-36 Amplified speech with peak limiting. The hearing aid is now set for maximum volume, assumed to be 60-dB gain at 1000 Hz, and for *high* tone control. The hypothetical hearing levels, shown below, leave only a small target area below the threshold of discomfort. The maximum acoustic output is 120 dB at 1000 Hz. The amplified speech (shaded area) is delivered efficiently to the target area. Peak limiting occurs at frequencies above 1000 Hz, but not below. This holds distortion to a minimum. This result is achieved by the sharply rising frequency characteristic of the microphone-amplifier combination. The input is assumed to be ordinary conversational speech. Of course, with loud speech there would be more peak limiting.

tends from about 100 to about 8000 Hz, while the range important for good understanding of speech extends from about 400 to 6000 Hz. The sound pressure levels of conversational speech extend from a maximum of 66 dB in the lower frequencies to 30 dB or so in the high frequencies. The available auditory area of a user who has the common type of mixed hearing loss, that is, an overall conductive loss plus some high-tone sensorineural loss, lies largely above this area. His threshold of discomfort is assumed to lie at 120 dB, which is a likely level (Figure 10-35).

The frequency characteristic of a hearing aid is shown at the top of Figure 10-35. Its breadth measures the frequency range. The gain is negligible at very high and very low frequencies. The whole curve is moved up and down by changing the volume-control setting. The acoustic "gain" of a hearing aid is measured by comparing the sound-pressure level developed in a 2-cm³ coupler with the sound-pressure level (at 1000 Hz) measured in a free field before the hearing aid is introduced into it. The gain at 1000 Hz measured in this way may be 60 dB or more. (It is worth noting that the "gain for speech," measured as the difference in the threshold for speech of a hard-of-hearing listener with and without the hearing aid, is often considerably less than the laboratory measurement of gain.)

There is, however, a maximum acoustic output beyond which the instrument cannot go, regardless of the setting of the volume control or the strength of the input signal. The frequency characteristic at maximum output (Figure 10-35) is flatter than it is in the normal operating range, but it has one or more maxima because of the resonant peaks of the magnetic receiver. The position of this limiting maximum acoustic output curve describes the maximum "power" of the instrument.

In Figure 10-35 we see how the "area" of conversational speech is elevated and modified in shape by a hearing aid set to moderate gain and "low" tone control. Nearly all of the speech sounds now fall in the auditory area of the listener, but they do not encroach on his threshold of discomfort.

In Figure 10-36 we see how the distribution of the sounds of conversational speech would be modified by using a higher volume-control setting and at the same time altering the frequency characteristic to "high" by means of the tone control. The stronger low tones of speech are now deliberately amplified less than the weaker higher tones. The fidelity of the output is not as good as in the first example, but the speech may be easier for this particular listener to understand because another kind of acoustic distortion

(which will be described below and which occurs when the maximum acoustic output is approached) is minimized.

In terms of these measures of performance —frequency response and frequency range, gain, and maximum power output—we can judge the performance of present-day hearing aids.

HEARING AIDS CANNOT DO EVERYTHING

No hearing aid can ever compensate completely for a hearing loss. Everyone who is thinking of getting a hearing aid should realize at the outset that there are limits to what *any* hearing aid can possibly do. Some limits are imposed by the ear and others by the nature of the sounds that we wish to hear. There are practical limits also, set by size, weight, and expense, to what can be built into a wearable hearing aid at the present time.

For example, an ear with sensorineural deafness may be unable to hear high tones no matter how much they are amplified. If *all* the nerve fibers that are normally stimulated by tones above 3000 Hz have degenerated, then no conceivable hearing aid can ever make sounds above 3000 Hz audible again except by transforming them to some lower frequency. This is the fundamental reason why hearing aids are usually of little or no assistance in the "abrupt" type of high-tone sensorineural deafness.

Until about 1940 a practical limit of performance was set by the inability to provide enough amplification without undue distortion. Now, however, a powerful instrument can deliver a sound as loud as most wearers are willing to tolerate even after they have become accustomed to loud sounds. The limit of useful power is now set by the ear. A good hearing aid must, of course, bring sound above the threshold of audibility, but its output must never exceed the listener's threshold of discomfort or be a possible cause of acoustic trauma.

In the hard-of-hearing ear the thresholds of discomfort and pain usually stay near the normal levels, so that *the range (in decibels) between the faintest audible tone and the loudest tolerable tone is diminished.* Now if we amplify all sounds equally, the strong sounds may become intolerable before the weak sounds are powerful enough to be heard. *Some suppression of the strong sounds may therefore be necessary if the weak ones are to be made audible.*

Speech is a mixture of sounds of different intensities, and the weakest sounds may be as much as 30 dB below the strongest (see Figure 10-35). If the range between audibility and discomfort is less (as it may be with a severe hearing loss), it may be possible to make speech audible and intelligible as well as tolerable, but only at the sacrifice of some "naturalness" or "quality." Fortunately, however, this compromise is necessary only when the hearing loss is very severe.

Input/Output Limitations

Any sound amplification system necessarily imposes restrictions on the levels of signals that can be accepted at the input and can be delivered at the output. When the system is properly designed and used, these restrictions are of little consequence; when it is not, signals may be noticeably distorted, and noise may be objectionable. To better define the input/output limitations for a hearing aid, at least in a heuristic way, consider the input/output graph of Figure 10-37, where any input level to and corresponding output level from a hearing aid is represented by an operating point. Since the scales are in decibels, the output sound-pressure level is simply the input sound-pressure level plus the gain of the aid. By defin-

ing those limitations that the aid imposes on the input and output levels, the range of locations of acceptable operating points becomes evident.

For definiteness, assume that the hearing aid can be represented schematically, as shown in Figure 10-17, by the cascade of a microphone at the input, a preamplifier, volume and tone controls, a power amplifier, and an earphone at the output. Minimum acceptable *input signals* are limited by the effective input noise level of the microphone and preamplifier since signals of lower levels will be contaminated by this noise. Maximum levels of input signals are limited by the saturation or clipping level of these input stages. These upper and lower bounds on the range of acceptable input levels are indicated by vertical lines in Figure 10-37. In like manner, upper and lower bounds on the range of acceptable *output levels* that are imposed by the hearing-aid output stages are indicated by horizontal lines in Figure 10-37. The minimum level is due to the effective output noise level of the power amplifier, and the maximum level results from saturation or clipping in the power amplifier and/or the earphone. The effective output noise level of a magnetic earphone is very low compared to noise from preceding amplifier stages.

For a particular value of hearing-aid gain, the locus of all operating points on the graph of Figure 10-37 will be a diagonal line. If the gain is increased, this diagonal line or "operating curve" is raised vertically, and if the gain is lowered, the curve is lowered. As a practical matter, there are very real restrictions on gain that further limit the range of acceptable operating levels. The condition where output levels are less than input levels, which leads to negative gain in decibels, is seldom of value. Thus, 0-dB gain can be considered a practical minimum. Maximum gain is controlled by the gain of the aid before feedback. Thus, even though additional

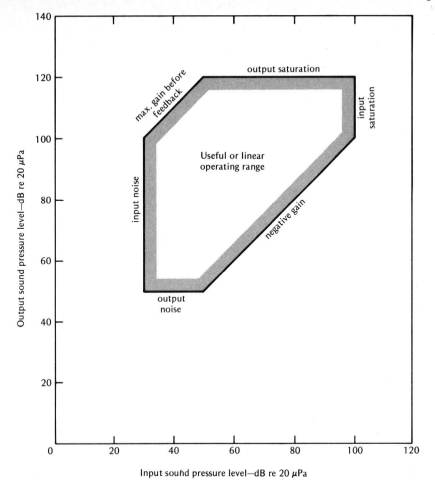

Figure 10-37 Possible range of useful input and output signals in an electronic hearing aid.

electronic gain may be available, the gain before feedback defines a practical maximum. Limitations on gain are indicated by the diagonal lines in Figure 10-37.

The range of acceptable operating levels usually is still further restricted (1) by environmental acoustic noise, which may increase the effective input noise level of the aid, (2) by the hearing loss of the listener, which may increase the minimum acceptable output level, and (3) by the tolerance level of the listener, which may decrease the maximum acceptable output level of the aid. To further complicate matters, limitations imposed by the hearing-aid system, the environment, and the listener are frequency-dependent, and many of the factors that control these limitations can vary in the course of a day.

Distortion in Hearing Aids

Whenever the output of a system is not some constant times its input, then the system is said to distort the signal. Since all physically realizable systems are power limited and have finite bandwidth, they are necessarily linear only for certain classes of sig-

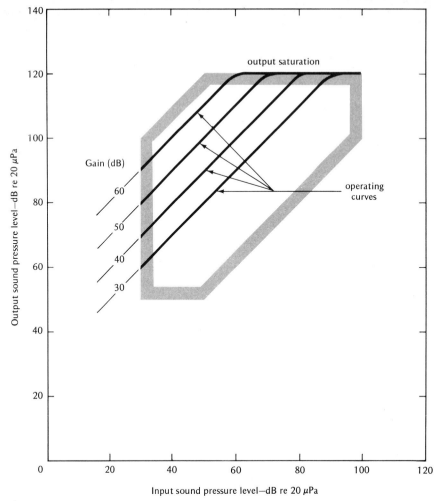

Figure 10-38 Operating curves of a hearing aid, showing the linear range (diagonal line), partial saturation (knee), and complete saturation (horizontal line) at the output for various values of hearing-aid gain.

nals. If the input signals are members of this class, the system is linear; if not, the system is nonlinear, and distortion results. Although this concept is simple, methods of accurately defining distortion are not. The reason is that so far as a listener is concerned, some kinds of distortion are completely tolerable or even desirable, but other kinds will completely destroy his ability to receive information. For this reason there are many different measures of distortion,

and it is up to the designer and user of the system (for example, a hearing aid) to decide which one best describes the nonlinearity of his system with respect to the expected signals in the system and the capabilities of the listener at its output. The relation between various measures of distortion in a hearing aid and the ability of an impaired listener to receive information is not fully understood. The problem is too complicated; there are too many kinds of signals of interest, too many kinds of nonlinearity, and too many kinds of hearing impairment. Nonetheless, there are some combinations of signals, nonlinearities, and listeners that are of special interest.

"Limiting" of Output

The necessary protection against discomfort can be provided automatically. We have pointed out that an amplifier can deliver only just so much power from its last stage even when the "valve" is open wide. *One of the fundamental principles of selecting a hearing aid is to pick an instrument that has enough amplification but also has a maximum output that will be both tolerable and safe.*

When a hearing aid is used near its saturation output, as may be necessary if the hearing loss is severe, the strongest peaks of the electric waves will reach the saturation level of the instrument. We may think of the saturation output as a ceiling, as shown in Figure 10-38. For a fixed gain of the hearing aid, the operating curve follows the diagonal constant-gain curve for low input levels, but then for greater input levels it bends and follows the "ceiling" defined by the horizontal line of output saturation. So long as the input signal is sufficiently low that the operating point lies on the diagonal part of the operating curve, amplification is linear and the output signal is an amplified replication of the input. For a greater input signal, when the operating point falls on the bend of the operating curve, at least some of the peaks of the signal will bump against the ceiling and will be "clipped." For even greater input signals, when the operating point falls on the horizontal output saturation line, almost all of the peaks of the output signal will be clipped. The effects of these limiting conditions on the output signal are shown in Figure 10-39. The clipped waves shown in this figure are obviously distorted in shape. That is why the quality of the sound suffers.

Effects of Peak Clipping

Fortunately a considerable amount of simple peak clipping does not greatly reduce the intelligibility of speech, even though it may make the voice sound harsh, rough, and unnatural. Ordinarily the low frequencies of vowel sounds, which are the most powerful of the speech sounds, as indicated in Figures 10-35 and 10-36, reach the limiting maximum acoustic output first and consequently suffer from peak clipping. The change of quality in the speech is most noticeable in these vowel sounds. It is actually rather surprising, however, to see on an oscilloscope how severely the speech waves may be squared off and distorted by simple peak clipping before the speech becomes really difficult to understand.

In order to reduce or avoid the distortion

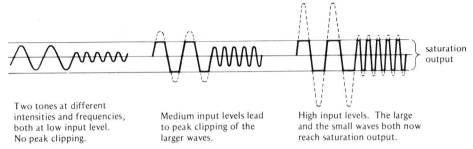

saturation output

Two tones at different intensities and frequencies, both at low input level. No peak clipping.

Medium input levels lead to peak clipping of the larger waves.

High input levels. The large and the small waves both now reach saturation output.

Figure 10-39 Diagram showing various degrees of output "peak clipping" with different levels of input signals.

and loss of quality introduced by peak clipping it is desirable to amplify the higher frequencies of speech more than the lower frequencies, so that both the high frequencies and the low frequencies reach the limit of maximum acoustic output together. Such "high-tone emphasis" is introduced by reducing the amplification of low tones, as shown in Figure 10-32. This moderate high-tone emphasis allows for the use of the greatest gain before the clipping level is reached. It uses most efficiently the restricted auditory area of most hard-of-hearing listeners, as illustrated in Figure 10-36.

One reason that the intelligibility of speech suffers so much more from peak clipping of the low tones than from corresponding clipping of the high tones is that some of the harmonics that are introduced by the peak clipping of low frequencies are clearly audible, and for high frequencies most of the harmonics lie above the range of speech frequencies and are very inefficiently transmitted by the receiver of the hearing aid. If the listener has a high-tone hearing loss, these high-frequency distortion products are doubly excluded and of no consequence.

With the proper combination of high-tone preemphasis and appropriate limiting of the output by peak clipping, plenty of amplification can be used in a hearing aid to make faint sounds audible while at the same time the ear is protected against discomfort and overexposure. Intelligibility is effectively, although not completely, preserved. There is some deterioration of quality when the peak clipping becomes severe. We must pay for the protection, so to speak, but the price in quality need not be very high. The high-tone emphasis must be introduced *before* the peaks are clipped, as said in the Harvard Report (Davis, et al., 1947). That is why we speak of high-tone *preemphasis*. No additional high-tone or low-tone emphasis should be put in by the receiver *after* the clipping.

In order to get the best combination of protection and intelligibility, an earphone with good acoustic characteristics must be used. Some hearing aid earphones are too "resonant," meaning that they respond too well to one particular band of frequencies. After the amplifier has clipped the peaks of the waves electronically, the earphone should deliver all parts of the speech spectrum to the ear at about the same maximum level, a little below the threshold of tolerance.

An earphone that has a resonant peak will amplify not only that frequency of the input but also the second, the third, or even the fourth harmonics that are introduced by the peak clipping of lower frequencies. Not only may the resulting high peak pressures reach the threshold of discomfort; they also cause a further deterioration of the intelligibility of certain vowel sounds, to say nothing of the unpleasant ringing quality that it introduces. For example, an earphone with a resonant peak at 1500 Hz gives a strong response at this frequency to inputs in the neighborhood of 750, of 500, and of 375 Hz when these are strong enough to reach the clipping level. The output waveforms are shown in Figure 10-40.

Compression Amplification

Another way of limiting the output of a hearing aid is by *compression amplification.* Whereas simple clipping through output saturation limits the average output of a hearing aid by clipping the peaks of the signal, compression amplification limits the average output by automatically adjusting electronic gain in the aid. Since peaks are not clipped with compression amplificaiton, distortion is significantly reduced. The intent in using compression amplification is to provide a distortion-free signal to the ear in the restricted range between a level that is sufficiently intense to be heard and the level that will cause discomfort. Compression amplifi-

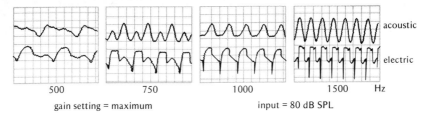

500 750 1000 1500 Hz

gain setting = maximum   input = 80 dB SPL

Figure 10-40 Electric waves recorded at the output of a hearing aid across the terminals of the earphone. The peak clipping in this instrument is unsymmetrical, and a sharp transient peak is introduced by the output transformer. The receiver has a resonant peak at 1500 Hz. It smooths out the sharp irregularities of the electric waves, but it accentuates the first two or three harmonics of frequencies that are an octave or more below its resonant peak. (For these oscillograms: input, 80 dB SPL; gain setting, maximum; tone control, "low.") *(Courtesy of J. R. Cox, Jr.)*

cation is particularly useful when the range between threshold and discomfort is so small that the typical range of input signal levels cannot be accommodated without excessive distortion when conventional linear amplifiers with output saturation are used. Hearing aids with compression amplification are becoming increasingly popular.

Compression amplification can take many basic forms, and each form can have its refinements and adjustments to better accommodate tolerance and hearing-level requirements. A typical form of compression amplification in a hearing aid is shown in the block diagram of Figure 10-41. A *feedback circuit* and *compression amplifier* have been added to the basic hearing-aid system of Figure 10-17. In Figure 10-41 the feedback circuit senses the electric output of the hearing aid and provides to the compression amplifier a signal that is roughly proportional to the *average value* of the output signal. This average-value signal is then used to control the gain of the compression amplifier. For example, as the average value of the output increases because of increased input level, the increased signal level from the feedback circuit will decrease the gain of the compression amplifier. Thus, for each 2-dB increase in input sound level the output level may increase only 1 dB. The *compression ratio* gives a measure of the degree of compression and is the ratio of input change to output change, where each is expressed in decibels.

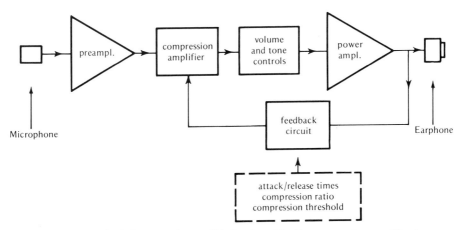

Figure 10-41 Block diagram of a possible hearing aid with compression amplification.

In the above example, the compression ratio would be two-to-one (2/1). The output level at which the operating curve departs from the 45-degree line of conventional nonadaptive linear amplification is the *compression threshold* level. The compression ratio in some hearing aids is not constant over the range of compression, and sometimes the compression threshold occurs at a fixed input level (independent of gain) rather than at a fixed output level.

A certain amount of time is required for the feedback circuit to sense a change in input level and cause an appropriate change in gain of the compressor amplifier. The time to respond to an increasing signal level before decreasing gain is the *attack time*, and conversely, the response time to a decreasing signal level before increasing gain is the *release time*. Attack times typically are chosen between 5 and 100 ms and release times between 50 and 150 ms. With improper choice of attack and release times speech intelligibility will suffer, and a "flutter" or "thump" may be heard.

Usually compression ratio, compression threshold, attack and release times, and saturation output are fixed and not easily changed once the instrument leaves the factory. However, it is becoming increasingly common to make one or more of these parameters adjustable, usually with a jeweler's screwdriver.

A possible set of operating curves for the hearing aid of Figure 10-41 is shown in Figure 10-42. Each curve relates to a different setting of the volume or gain control. Below compression threshold, all operating curves have 45-degree slopes that are implied when a 1-dB change at the input produces a 1-dB change at the output. Between compression threshold and output saturation, the slopes will be less than 45 degrees and equal to the reciprocal of the compression ratio. When saturation is controlled in the output stages, all operating curves are asymptotic to the saturation output level for sufficiently large input.

Harmonic Distortion

If a pure tone of frequency f_0 is applied to a linear hearing aid, the only signal that will appear at its output will be a pure tone of frequency f_0. At most, the amplitude and phase at the output will be different from those at the input. If the hearing aid is nonlinear, harmonics of the input frequency f_0, namely $2f_0$, $3f_0$, . . ., will appear in the output. The ratio of the power in the harmonics to the power in the fundamental frequency f_0 gives a measure of "harmonic distortion." The harmonics, either singly or in combination, are easily measured, and for this reason harmonic distortion is often used to specify distortion in a hearing aid. The amount of harmonic distortion in a system varies with the fundamental frequency; low frequencies will have many harmonics that fall within the system passband and higher frequencies will have fewer.

Intermodulation Distortion

Most input signals to hearing aids, even relatively "steady" signals, are not pure tones; they contain many frequencies. Therefore, it can justifiably be argued that perhaps a more valid measure of system distortion is *intermodulation distortion*. A linear system with input frequencies f_1 and f_2 will have only those two frequencies in its output. A nonlinear system will have the two input frequencies plus their harmonics, plus the sums and differences of the input frequencies and their harmonics. The measure of intermodulation distortion of the system is the ratio of the power of the output signal at frequencies other than the applied frequencies relative to the output signal power at the ap-

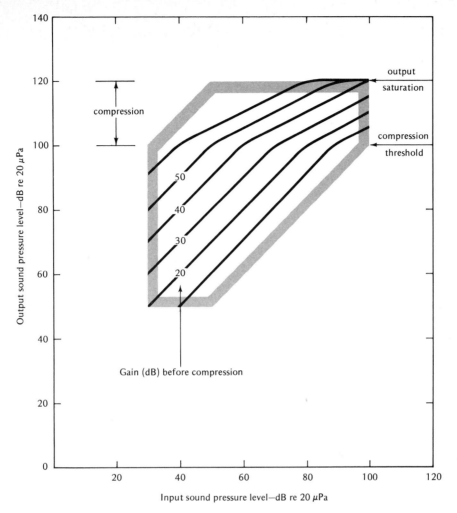

Figure 10-42 Operating curves of a hearing aid with compression amplification. The compression ratio of this hearing aid is 2:1; the compression threshold is 100 dB output sound pressure level.

plied frequencies. There are several methods for measuring intermodulation distortion. They differ in the kinds of input signals that are used and the kinds of output signals that are measured. All methods attempt to give an estimate of power at distortion frequencies relative to the power at applied frequencies, and in practice none is easily implemented.

Ringing

Speech is inherently a transient kind of signal; bursts of energy are often followed by periods of relative silence. If speech is applied to any band-pass system and to hearing aids in particular, we notice that the response of the system lags behind the excitation. In particular, the output will continue for a short time after the input has been abruptly turned off, much as a bell will continue to ring after being struck. This kind of distortion is called "ringing." The measure of ringing that is often used is the time required for decay at the output when a pure-tone input has been abruptly squelched. Like other forms of distortion, ringing is frequency-dependent. Unlike other forms, ringing occurs in *linear* as well as in nonlinear systems. Ringing in the earphone of a modern hearing aid is shown in Figure 10-43.

Use of Hearing Aids in Noisy Environments

The use of hearing aids in noisy environments is perhaps best understood by considering an example. Suppose that two people are trying to communicate in a noisy environment. One has impaired hearing and uses a hearing aid. In many situations, both indoors and out, ambient noise levels are relatively constant over a region in which two people are talking. This is assumed for the example.

In relatively echo-free spaces the noise and speech levels at the microphone of the hearing aid might appear as shown in the lower two curves of Figure 10-44 when

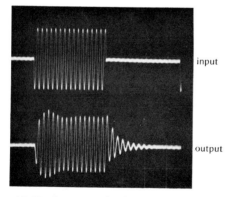

Figure 10-43 Response of a hearing-aid earphone to a 2000-Hz tone burst. The output builds up gradually and does not terminate immediately or abruptly.

plotted as a function of distance to the talker. Notice that the signal-to-noise ratio (the difference in decibels between speech and noise levels) decreases as the distance from talker to listener increases. Six inches from the talker's lips the S/N ratio is large (24 dB), and 8 feet away the signal and noise levels are equal. *Speech intelligibility will decrease as the S/N ratio decreases* independent of whether or not the listener uses a hearing aid. Therefore for good communication the talker and listener should be close together. In this respect the person with a hearing aid even has an advantage over the person with normal hearing, since it may be possible to put the hearing-aid microphone quite close to the talker's lips.

In regions that are more reverberant, where the speech levels do not decrease, as shown in Figure 10-44, the case for minimizing the distance between talker and listener can still be made. As the distance between talker and listener increases in a reverberant space, the ratio of *direct* to *reverberant* speech levels will decrease even though the *total* speech level does not decrease appreciably. For a given total speech level, intelligibility decreases as the ratio of direct to reverberant energy decreases.

If the listener adjusts his hearing aid so that at any distance the speech level of the output remains the same (see Figure 10-44), then the required acoustic gain must increase as the speech-level input decreases. That is, the hearing-aid user would want to increase the gain as he backs away from the talker. With respect to the hearing aid, high gain is undesirable because the self-noise, which arises within the hearing aid itself, generally will be higher for higher gains. In addition, and perhaps more important, when the high gain is accompanied by poor signal-to-noise ratio at the input, the *total* power that must be supplied by the aid must be greater in order to achieve a given output speech level because the aid must supply

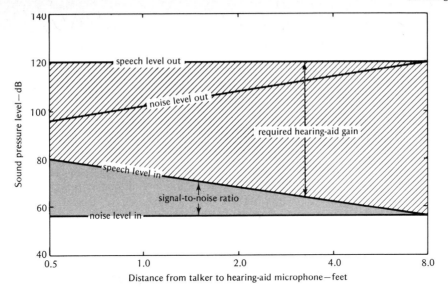

Figure 10-44 Effects of distance between talker and hearing-aid microphone on the signal-to-noise ratio and required hearing-aid gain.

power for both the amplified speech *and* the amplified noise. If the noise is comparable in level to the speech, a considerable portion of the available power from the aid must then be used to amplify the noise.

A final argument can be advanced in favor of low gain and high speech-input level by observing that the impaired listener will hear his own voice through his hearing aid at a comfortable level only if his voice level and the speech level from the person with whom he is communicating are equivalent at the hearing-aid microphone. If the aid is worn on the head or body, this means that two people must be close together so that the speech levels from both persons will be high compared to the noise, and the hearing-aid gain can be low.

OUTLOOK

There is little doubt about the improvement in speech perception and production that often occurs with the proper use of a

hearing aid, and there is little doubt about the numerous advances in hearing-aid technology that have increased the effectiveness and acceptability of hearing aids. Still there is a significant segment of the hearing-impaired population that does not or cannot benefit from a modern hearing aid, and the relative size of this segment has not been dramatically reduced even with advances in technology. In *basic theory and design*, hearing aids have changed little over the years.

With knowledge of technological advances of the recent past, it is reasonable to predict that hearing aids of the future will probably be smaller, more rugged, particularly those for children, and easier to operate by the elderly. They probably will have more available gain before feedback, have less internal noise, have wider bandwidth, and have greater efficiency. Moreover, the relative number of hearing-aid users will probably increase. Still this increase is not likely to be dramatic unless the measurable features of hearing impairment can be more dramatically and precisely related to the measurable features of hearing aids. Establishment of such relations will be difficult and must involve the joint efforts not only of engineers and physicists but also of audiologists, otologists, psychologists, and physiologists.

SUGGESTED READINGS AND REFERENCES

American National Standards Institute, Inc., 1430 Broadway, New York, N.Y. 10018:
ANSI S3.8-1967 (R 1971). *Method of Expressing Hearing Aid Performance.*
ANSI S3.22-1976. *Specification of Hearing Aid Characteristics.*

Anon. "Effects of Sound Inlet Variations on Microphone Response," *Knowles Technical Bulletin.*

Anon. "Effects of Source Impedance and Acoustical Termination on BK Receiver Response," *Knowles Technical Bulletin.*
These two papers are available from Knowles Electronics, Inc., 3100 North Mannheim Road, Franklin Park, Ill. The first discusses the effects of tubes and damping resistance at the input to microphones for hearing aids. The second discusses the effects of the impedance of the electrical source and of the acoustical load on the response of receivers used in miniature hearing aids.

Burkhard, M. D. "KEMAR, A Tool for Hearing Aid Evaluation," *Audecibel Mag.,* 25(3): (1976).
Describes the design and development of the KEMAR manikin for measuring the electroacoustic characteristics of hearing aids.

Carlson, E. V. and Killion, M. C. "Subminiature Directional Microphones," *J. Audio Eng. Soc.,* 22(2):92–96 (1974).
Methods of design and use of directional microphones in hearing aids are outlined.

Dalsgaard, S. C. (ed.). "Earmoulds and Associated Problems," Seventh Danavox Symposium, G1. Avernaes, Denmark. Distributed by the Almgvist & Wiksell Periodical Company, Stockholm, Sweden (1975)
The design of earmolds and their effects on hearing-aid response are discussed.

Davis, H., et al. *Hearing Aids: An Experimental Study of Design Objectives.* Cambridge, Mass.: Harvard University Press, 1947.
This is a technical report of experiments conducted at the Psycho-Acoustic Laboratory under contract with the Office of Scientific Research and Development, frequently referred to as the "Harvard Report."

―――. "The Selection of Hearing Aids," *Laryngoscope,* 56:85–115, 135–163 (1946).
A reprinting in full of report "PNR-7" issued December 31, 1945, by the Psycho-Acoustic Laboratory, Harvard University, Cambridge, Mass.

Hirsh, I. J. "Use of Amplification in Educating Deaf Children," *Amer. Ann. Deaf.,* 113:1046–1055 (1968).

Various kinds of wired and wireless group hearing aids are discussed, along with their advantages and disadvantages.

Killion, M. C. and Carlson, E. V. "A Subminiature Electret-Condenser Microphone of New Design," *J. Audio Eng. Soc.*, 22(4):237–243 (May 1974).
The technical aspects leading to the development of electret-condenser microphones for hearing aids are reviewed.

Lybarger, S. F. "Personal Hearing Aids," *Volta Rev.*, 78(4):113–120 (May 1976).
Improvements in hearing-aid technology during the period 1965–1975 are reviewed.

Nielsen, T. E. "Various Methods of Output Limitation," *Oticongress 2*, Oticon A/S, Copenhagen (1972).
A thorough treatment is presented on various methods of hearing-aid output limitation in terms of input/output functions and distortion.

Olsen, W. O. and Matkin, N. D. "Comments on Modern Auditory Training Systems and Their Use," *Bull. Educ. Hearing Impaired*, 1:7–15 (1971).
Various types of auditory training systems, their limitations, and suggestions for their effective utilization are presented.

Pollack, M. C. (ed.). *Amplification for the Hearing Impaired.* New York: Grune and Stratton, Inc.
Historical, technical, audiologic, and pedagogical aspects of hearing aids are reviewed by experts at a professional level.

Rubin, M. (ed.). *Hearing Aids.* Baltimore: University Park Press, 1976.
Audiologists discuss the problems of hearing-aid use, manufacture, recommendation, and delivery.

Silverman, S. R. "Tolerance for Pure Tones and Speech in Normal and Defective Hearing," *Ann. Otol.* 56:658–678 (1947).
A summary of investigations at Central Institute for the Deaf, under contract with the Office of Scientific Research and Development, dealing with the mapping of thresholds of discomfort and pain in listening to loud sounds.

Topholm, C. *Hearing Aids, Basic Theory*, Widex Hearing Aid Company, Inc., Topholm & Westermann, Denmark, 1973.
The technical aspects of hearing-aid design are presented at an elementary level for audiologists, hearing-aid dealers, and hearing-aid technicians.

S. Richard Silverman, Ph.D.
David P. Pascoe, Ph.D.

11

Counseling About Hearing Aids

The major responsibilities of the audiologist who is considering a hearing aid for his client are to take account of the overall performance of hearing aids, as described in Chapter 10, in order to have a basis for his recommendations, and to give advice about selection of and adjustment to instruments. This chapter deals with the questions about hearing aids that are likely to occur to a prospective user, particularly to a first-time user. In a sense, the suggested "friend" referred to in the chapter may well be the audiologist counseling his client. This is the point of view of the chapter.

A hearing aid may be ridiculed as a "tin ear." It may be thought to detract from a person's appearance or suggest premature old age. But the man or woman whose hearing is failing should want so earnestly to hear that he will not worry about such real or imaginary trifles. His friends will welcome his use of a hearing aid because it spares them the painful necessity of having to shout and repeat for him. In fact, *it shows lack of consideration for his family and friends when the hard-of-hearing person does not wear a hearing aid if he can possibly do so and benefit by it.* Moreover, his hearing aid opens to him a broad vista of enriched social experiences that every person, hard of hearing or otherwise, needs for a happy adjustment to our complex world. Let it not be said of the hard-of-hearing, "Vanity, vanity, all is vanity."

TABLE 11-1
NUMBER AND PERCENT DISTRIBUTION OF PERSONS WITH A BINAURAL HEARING IMPAIRMENT WHO HAVE EVER USED A HEARING AID, BY BASIS FOR SELECTING AID AND ACCORDING TO SPEECH COMPREHENSION GROUP: UNITED STATES, JULY 1962 –JUNE 1963

Basis for Selecting Aid	Persons Who Have Ever Used an Aid			
	Total[a,b]	Cannot hear and understand spoken words	Can hear and understand a few spoken words	Can hear and understand most spoken words
	Number of Persons in Thousands			
All persons	1214	468	294	444
	Percent Distribution			
All bases.......................	100.0	100.0	100.0	100.0
Prescribed by doctor	12.9	16.7	*10.5	*11.0
Prescribed by clinic..................	18.1	15.8	21.4	18.2
Advised by dealer	33.7	29.9	35.7	36.5
Saw it advertised	7.8	*7.1	*7.1	*9.2
Recommended by friend or relative	11.9	13.0	*10.5	11.5
Other and unknown	15.7	17.5	*14.3	13.5

[a] Includes persons whose functional degree of hearing impairment was unknown.
[b] Without the use of a hearing aid.
* This figure is approximate.
(Data from Table 11, "Characteristics of Persons with Impaired Hearing." U.S. Department of Health, Education, and Welfare, Public Health Service Publication No. 1000—Series 10–No. 35, April 1967)

TO WEAR OR NOT TO WEAR A HEARING AID

According to Table 11-1, which was taken from the National Health Survey, approximately 1,214,000 persons had ever used a hearing aid at that time (1963). The survey also indicated that 882,000 were using them in the period from July 1962 to June 1963. From the point of view of this chapter it is interesting to note, from Table 11-1, the basis for selection of an aid, with dealer advice predominating. From Table 11-2 we find that the degree of satisfaction from the use of a hearing aid varies, with more than half of the users either very satisfied or fairly satisfied.

It is interesting to estimate the proportion of satisfied users as related to age. In Figure 11-1 we present our rough guess of this relation. As our criterion of those who can be "helped" by a hearing aid, we have chosen a hearing-threshold level of 40 dB or more at one end of the scale and the ability to receive communication satisfactorily (socially) at the other end. We note that the greatest percentage of people who need help fall between the ages of 20 and 60. Statistics from the National Health Survey bear this out. In the top portion of the figure we have attempted to indicate when certain conditions related to hearing impairment manifest themselves. This information essentially leads us to the rationale of the graph.

We do not mean to imply that all individuals with such conditions as noise-induced hearing loss and presbycusis can be helped substantially by hearing aids, but we believe that it is important to keep in mind the prevalence of these circumstances in arriving at estimates of the distribution of potential users.

Whoever has difficulty with his hearing in *everyday conversations should think seriously of getting a hearing aid.* The difficulty may vary with different situations, depending on the distance from the source of sound, the surrounding noises, the clarity of the speech or music, the lighting (which may help or interfere with speechreading), and many other factors. For example, someone with a mild hearing loss may not need amplification for ordinary conversation but may need it for lectures, sound movies, and church, and in social gatherings where there

TABLE 11-2
NUMBER AND PERCENT DISTRIBUTION OF PERSONS WITH A BINAURAL HEARING IMPAIRMENT WHO HAVE EVER USED A HEARING AID, BY DEGREE OF SATISFACTION WITH THE AID AND ACCORDING TO SEX AND SPEECH COMPREHENSION GROUP: UNITED STATES, JULY 1962 –JUNE 1963

Sex and Degree of Satisfaction with Hearing Aid	Persons Who Have Ever Used an Aid			
	Total[a,b]	Cannot hear and understand spoken words	Can hear and understand a few spoken words	Can hear and understand most spoken words
	Number of Persons in Thousands			
Both sexes	1214	468	294	444
Male	625	210	134	274
Female	590	258	160	170
	Percent Distribution			
All degrees.....................	100.0	100.0	100.0	100.0
Very satisfied	32.5	37.6	28.6	30.0
Fairly satisfied	29.0	30.3	32.3	25.7
Not satisfied	9.1	8.3[c]	9.9[c]	9.7[c]
Not currently using aid...............	27.4	21.8	28.2	32.4
Unknown	2.1[c]	1.7[c]	1.4[c]	2.3[c]

[a] Includes persons whose functional degree of hearing impairment was unknown.
[b] Without the use of a hearing aid.
[c] This figure is approximate.
Data are based on household interviews and a follow-up mail supplement and refer to the living, civilian, noninstitutional population.
(Data from Table 13, "Characteristics of Persons with Impaired Hearing," U.S. Department of Health, Education, and Welfare, Public Health Service Publication No. 1000—Series 10–No. 35, April 1967)

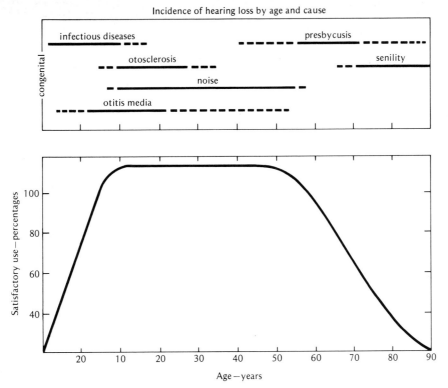

Figure 11-1   Estimated degree of satisfaction of users of hearing aids related to ages of users and causes of hearing loss.

is likely to be a background of many voices. Also, obviously, the accurate understanding of speech is more important for some than for others. The businessman who must know exactly what goes on in conferences needs it more than the elderly person who merely wishes to hear the radio, the television, or casual conversation more easily. In the long run, each person must decide for himself whether his hearing loss makes him socially (or economically) inadequate.

If a person is in doubt as to the need for a hearing aid, the audiogram is a very helpful guide. Generally, *if the hearing level for speech in the better ear is worse than 40 dB, a hearing aid is needed.* But the prospective user must realize that, in spite of optimistic advertisements, a hearing aid is not a perfect instrument. It does not provide complete compensation for hearing impairment. It will benefit the wearer only in proportion to his willingness to accept it, short of unattainable perfection, and to his patience and effort in learning to make the most of it.

Some types of hearing loss are less likely than others to benefit from a hearing aid. For example, a man's audiogram may show a slight impairment (20 to 30 dB) in the low frequencies and a precipitate drop beginning at 1000 Hz. He will probably complain, "I hear, but I can't make out what you are saying." This is understandable, since the frequencies above 1000 Hz convey sounds that are very important for the intelligibility of speech. For example, "fin" may sound the same as "thin" or "sin." Ordinarily, a hearing aid alone is of little value in overcoming this difficulty. However, even in such a case a proper hearing aid, *supplemented by a program of intensive auditory training* in discrimination of the sounds that make up speech, can be of great assistance. This is true even if the auditory training and instruction in speechreading turn out to be more helpful than the hearing aid! It is well, however, to repeat that in addition to whatever reduction in dynamic range and frequency response the user must learn to tolerate, he must also accept the fact that he will suffer many extra listening failures, brought on by reduced signal-to-noise ratios, in workaday situations *even after full auditory training and full acclimatization to his instrument.* Acceptance of these limitations in hearing-aid use can lead to greater satisfaction in the benefits it does bring. These benefits are likely to increase with the current available coupling of the hearing aid and a simple tube that eliminates the earmold and preserves the natural acoustics of the outer ear.

Hearing Aids for the Aged

The use of hearing aids by elderly people is likely to present another special problem. Their deafness is usually of the sensorineural type. Their ability to hear high frequencies decreases with advancing age. As we have just pointed out, such a pattern of hearing loss often results in imperfect discrimination. In younger people intensive auditory training and constant use of an instrument help the listener learn to make use of all auditory clues.

When the other problems of advancing age are added to deafness, the situation becomes still more difficult. We must frequently reckon with poor health and gradual failure of other faculties, particularly of vision, which is so helpful as a supplement to hearing. Not only do old people often become very dependent on others; they may also find themselves unable to "keep up with the times." In addition, many of them live alone or with children who "have their own lives to lead." All these factors may lead to tensions, fears, and general nervousness, which are hardly conducive to the concentration essential for effective and comfortable use of a hearing aid. Nevertheless, we should be encouraged by the favorable reports of the Veterans Administration of its experience with elderly users of hearing aids.

Each elderly person should be evaluated in terms of his particular temperament and way of living. When there appears to be any possibility of benefit, we strongly suggest a trial period with a hearing aid during which the person is encouraged but not forced to use the instrument. If he himself then expresses a desire to have the hearing aid, it should be purchased.

Hearing Aids for Children

There is a great difference of opinion, again without much supporting evidence, on when a child is ready to wear a hearing aid. One point of view holds that the early years are the years in which the child learns the meaning of sounds, particularly speech, and hence he should wear a hearing aid at all times from the moment it is discovered that he is deaf. This appears to be the predominant point of view. On the other hand, some workers believe that the child must first be trained to some degree of awareness and discrimination of sound, since failure to benefit from the instrument will discourage its use. Furthermore, some young children may be frightened by the loud sound of an instrument and become conditioned against it. Some audiologists fear possible damage to an ear exposed to the high sound-pressure levels generated by a hearing aid. Although this possibility has not been clearly demonstrated, it suggests a cautious approach that involves careful and continuous monitoring of the child's hearing and appraisal of the maximum power output of the hearing aid. This is especially true when the child's hearing levels are not yet clearly established.

The various types of hearing aids that were described in Chapter 10 are available for children. Commonly used is the body or pocket-type aid because of its capacity to provide greater power with less feedback. Its ruggedness and ease of handling also commend it for use with children. However, there has been a recent trend to behind-the-ear aids probably because of their increased power output, improved earmold fitting, lower noise level, and better sound localization by head movement. Their cordless, low visibility, and general cosmetic features increase their appeal for children, especially for teenagers.

Group aids are generally used in classrooms. They are likely to produce a better quality of speech signal, due mainly to improved signal-to-noise ratio because the microphone is closer to the teacher's mouth, and have a lower probability of acoustic feedback because the microphone is farther from the earphones. They are also more rugged, and their components are more durable. Among their disadvantages are the limitation of use to school hours, and varying levels of signals originating in the child's own voice and the voices of the teacher and other children. Furthermore, the signal from a group aid may be markedly different from the signal obtained from an out-of-school wearable instrument.

Most group hearing aids use insert earphones instead of large over-the-ear earphones to achieve increased comfort and to reduce electric power level and thus increase battery life. Also, individual aids have been adapted to wireless systems to increase freedom of action and to ensure uniformity of signal. Suitable acoustical treatment of classrooms is recommended as an integral part of a hearing-aid system and is *essential* where individual hearing aids are used.

An underlying concept for preference of group aids over wearable ones is that the better signal of a group aid will help the child develop a greater appreciation of sound and that this will carry over to the use of his own wearable aid, which he can have with him at all times.

The selection of hearing aids for children has consisted primarily of the determination of needed gain and safe maximum power output. A significant advance has been the use of narrow bands of noise to determine the gain that the child receives at various frequencies. In this manner more can be known about the levels of sound he can perceive from the various portions of the speech spectrum. With this information more can be said about the suitability of a particular hearing aid or about the selection of volume-control and tone-control settings.

The insertion of appropriate filters to compensate the lack of balance between the high and low portions of the speech-frequency spectrum that accompanies auditory impairment has been suggested. The higher-frequency formants contributing to perceptibility may be "raised" to a level at which they may be audible. This principle may be useful for children whom we can expect to achieve refined auditory discrimination. The importance of an extended low-frequency response to aid in speech development, particularly of rhythmic patterns, in profoundly deaf children has also been suggested. The desirability of compression amplification (see Chapter 10) is generally recognized, but how restricted the dynamic range of the compressed signal should be is an open question.

Will a Hearing Aid Endanger Hearing?

The prospective user of a hearing aid often asks, "Will the use of a hearing aid destroy what is left of my hearing by overloading it?" An associated question is: "Will using a hearing aid help restore or at least maintain my hearing by keeping it in use?" A carefully chosen hearing aid should never overload and thereby injure an abnormal ear; neither can it alter or improve the status of impaired hearing. It merely enables the user to make better use of the hearing that he possesses and keeps his hearing in practice. He remains attentive to sound. If, however, the new hearing aid makes the wearer "nervous," he should break it in by using it for short periods daily, gradually increasing the length of each period of use. We have to repeat that we must be cautious when we are not sure of our assessment of hearing in a very young child.

Hearing Aids and Speechreading

There is little likelihood that the use of a hearing aid will diminish one's skill in speechreading. On the contrary, the hearing of speech may reinforce speechreading because auditory clues assist in the discrimination of words that look alike on the lips. For example, in the sentence, "The package is heavy," the word "baggage" might be substituted for "package." The context, which the speechreader ordinarily uses to distinguish words that look alike on the lips, is no help here, since both words fit the context. But a hearing aid might enable the speechreader to discriminate between the initial "p" and "b" and between the "k" and "g" in the two words. Of course we have chosen an extreme example, but long-time users of hearing aids generally report that *the continuous association of hearing and seeing speech is mutually advantageous.* Even in cases of extreme hearing loss, in which complete understanding of speech is not attainable, a hearing aid may furnish enough auditory clues, such as stress and intonational patterns, to supplement speechreading quite effectively.

Ear-Level or Body-Worn?

We have seen in Chapter 10 that hearing aids can be worn on the body or at ear level —either behind the ear, within the ear, or mounted in an eyeglass frame. Most users prefer an ear-level instrument because it is convenient, inconspicuous, and free of clothing noise. Furthermore, it enables the listener to turn his microphone easily to the source of sound. However, users with hearing-threshold levels over 60 dB (ANSI) require so much power that it may result in squealing in an ear-level hearing aid even with a perfectly fitting earmold. In cases of such severe loss, trials under a variety of conditions should precede the final decision.

Air Conduction and Bone Conduction Compared

Air- and bone-conduction hearing aids differ in the construction of their output transducers and in the pathways over which the amplified sound is delivered to the inner ear. The buttonlike air-conduction earphone, coupled to the external auditory canal by a fitted plastic earmold, delivers sound through the normal pathway. The bone-conduction vibrator, on the other hand, makes contact with the mastoid bone behind the ear, and its vibrations are transmitted by the bone directly to the inner ear (see also Chapter 10).

We might suppose that a bone-conduction instrument is indicated whenever the deafness is of the conductive middle-ear type. The obstruction that interferes with the passage of sound presumably can be bypassed by bone conduction, and the intact nerve endings can pick up the sound waves as they come, relatively unimpeded, directly through the bones of the skull. However, physical difficulties limit the performance of bone-conduction units. Bones and the skin that covers them vary in density and elasticity and therefore in their ability to transmit sound. It is more difficult to get efficient delivery of speech sounds by bone conduction than by air conduction. Full bone-conduction efficiency is difficult to achieve with ear-level aids. The bone vibration system has been incorporated in some eyeglass types of units, but the vibrator is then hard to isolate from other parts of the hearing aid, inducing feedback; and sufficient pressure against the skull is hard to maintain. Moreover, many good prospects for these units (persons with conductive loss) are good candidates for middle-ear surgery for improvement or restoration of their hearing. As a consequence, clinicians generally report that not more than 1 percent of their subjects can use bone conduction more satisfactorily than air conduction. This rather small percentage suggests that, if the prospective user of a hearing aid is still in doubt after listening by both air and bone conduction, unless he has competent advice to the contrary, he should choose air conduction.

Bone conduction is definitely preferable, however, when the user suffers from chronically discharging ears. Also, a few users who can hear over the telephone without a hearing aid, but who cannot quite follow face-to-face or group conversation, find it a great convenience to have the ear free for direct contact with the telephone receiver. However, a telephone pickup, described in Chapter 10, makes an air-conduction instrument also very convenient for telephone conversations.

Custom Earmolds

Anyone who expects to use an air-conduction hearing aid should have an earmold that has been fitted to the contours of his own external ear. An earmold that is not properly fitted may irritate the ear canal and may also interfere with the efficient transmission of sound. As was pointed out in the preceding chapter, a well-fitting individual earmold not only is more comfortable and more secure; it allows the hearing aid to deliver sounds as it is designed to deliver them, that is, with the greatest efficiency and fidelity. Even for the person who has not yet made his final selection of a hearing aid, be it body-worn or ear-level, a custom earmold is a good investment because it will fit almost any make of air-conduction earphone to which it is attached. For adults the fit is permanent, but growing children obviously require a periodic change of earmolds. It takes considerable instruction and practice to get the earmold in and out properly, and some modification for comfort may be critical for acceptance in the early days of use.

Monaural or Binaural?

Of great interest to hearing-aid users is the advent of the binaural hearing aid. As described in Chapter 10, the Y-cord hearing aid consists of one microphone and amplifier, with an earphone going to each ear; on the other hand, a binaural aid is made up of two complete instruments, one for each ear. Since the microphone is the new ear for the user, the binaural aid attempts to duplicate nature by providing two "ears." The conventional means of "packaging" the binaural aid is to house an instrument in each temple of a pair of spectacles as shown in Figures 10-11 and 10-12. Of course, individual aids of the type shown in Figure 10-9 can be worn behind the ears.

Research on binaural hearing aids has now progressed to the point where some conclusions can be drawn with high confidence. The first conclusion is that the major handicap imposed by using only one hearing aid (assuming an ear-level instrument) is that about half of the time this aid is on the wrong side of the head and is hence shadowed from the primary message. In such an event, a second hearing aid with its microphone on the favored side will yield much more efficient reception for the moment.

The second conclusion is that *binaural* help does occur. It gives secondary but real advantage to the aforementioned monaural reception. This advantage is equivalent to improving the speech-to-noise ratio about 3 dB. Such a modest benefit, however, is frequently obliterated, during which time binaural reception will be no better than monaural reception. Thus, it is unrealistic to expect a new dimension of intelligibility in everyday listening because of binaural interactions. Instead one should expect the second aid to be helpful because it combines a little binaural facilitation with more continuous favorable monaural reception (see Chapter 2).

The third conclusion is that the modest binaural facilitation of intelligibility is essentially independent of the binaural benefit to localization. When two hearing aids can recreate an auditory sense of space, the user achieves a sense of orientation, which may make him much more comfortable. For some people, this comfort is a reason in its own right for wearing a second instrument. However, the sense of comfort does not mean that intelligibility against competing sounds is improved more than the 3 dB mentioned above.

Right Ear or Left?

The audiogram is a useful guide to the choice of the ear on which to wear the hearing aid. If both ears show hearing levels for speech between 40 and 75 dB, the hearing aid should be worn on the *worse* ear. The better ear is left free, and it is still good enough to be of some use without a hearing aid. If, however, one ear or both ears have a hearing level worse (numerically greater) than 75 dB, the *better* ear should be fitted. If the level is worse than 75 dB, it is difficult enough to get good hearing with the better ear. There is usually a good deal of sensorineural hearing loss in such a case, and intelligibility may be poor even with a powerful instrument. Furthermore, the margin between the threshold of hearing and the threshold of discomfort begins to get rather narrow when the hearing level is worse than 75 dB. Of course, there are exceptions to these rules, but experience has shown this rule to be a guide in a majority of cases. If an audiogram is not available, the user should wear the aid on the worse ear if his hearing loss is only mild, but on the better ear if he is severely handicapped without any aid at all.

Hearing Aids for Unilateral Hearing Loss

A person with unilateral hearing loss may have difficulty in three ways: in hearing a person who addresses him from the side of his poor ear, in determining the location of the source of sound, and in hearing in the presence of a background noise. To deal with these difficulties Harford and his co-workers (1966) have suggested and demonstrated the value of Contralateral Routing of Signals (CROS) for certain cases of unilateral deafness.

Harford describes CROS as follows:

A behind-the-ear air-conduction hearing aid is mounted in a headband with a wire extending from the amplifier, across the headband, to a hearing-aid earphone mounted on the other end of the band. With this arrangement, signals originating on the side of the impaired ear are picked up by the hearing-aid microphone mounted near that ear, amplified slightly, and routed *electrically* across the head to the earphone mounted near the good ear. A plastic tube carries the acoustic signals from the earphone into the otherwise open canal of the good ear.

CROS can also be adapted to a standard eyeglass hearing-aid frame.

CROS offers the unilateral case (with normal hearing in one ear) escape from adverse head shadowing in noisy surroundings when the wanted sound is on his "bad" side. Furthermore, he is actually helped in this case by the imperfections of reproduction inherent in the contemporary ear-level hearing-aid, since these imperfections introduce a difference in the quality of the redirected signal. This quality difference helps him recognize the side from which the wanted sound is coming.

The use of CROS in cases of high-frequency loss is simply a way of restoring high-frequency components by retaining the normal resonances of the ear canal and by filtering out the lower frequencies. The advantage CROS offers here is to reduce the feedback problem. The most important thing is that the sound from the hearing aid is being fed into the ear via an open ear canal, so unaided sound can be received directly at the same time. This is a neat way to achieve selective amplification without plugging the ear.

Selective Amplification and Individual Fitting

We have deliberately spoken of "selecting" rather than "fitting" a hearing aid. "Fitting" suggests too strongly the fitting of a pair of eyeglasses or a suit of clothes. The differences among hearing aids are not as large and as obvious as they are among eyeglass lenses and suits of clothes, and it is difficult to judge with sufficient precision the success of the "fitting" of a hearing aid.

Selecting a suitable hearing aid is first a series of tests of adequacy in fundamentals, and then a series of judgments of intangibles or a series of compromises. There is usually no one best fit that is demonstrably best under all circumstances.

The idea of "fitting" a hearing aid was supported by the very plausible argument that a hearing aid should compensate for each person's particular hearing loss by amplifying some frequencies more than others. The audiogram was taken as the guide to show which frequencies needed "selective amplification." This principle seemed obvious but was not convincingly demonstrated by early investigators.

In a series of wartime studies at the Psycho-Acoustic Laboratory at Harvard University it was found that *an instrument with good overall characteristics and true square-top peak clipping that amplified a wide range of frequencies about evenly or with moderate emphasis of the high tones gave the best results.* Hard-of-hearing listeners made as good (or better) articulation scores with it and had more "elbow room" than they had with any other combination that was tried. This was true for all of the common types of hearing loss. Other "compensations" that were tried (but with no better results) included several that more nearly followed the principle of selective amplification. The details of these experiments are available in book form for the technical reader (see Davis, et al., page 336). In general, similar results were obtained by British investigators (1947) and these were made the basis of the design of the Medresco (Medical Research Council) hearing aid that is manufactured for, and distributed by, the British government.

Current clinical and commercial practice increasingly invokes the principle of "individual fitting." Conventionally, this means a specific relation between the audiogram and the frequency response of the aid. This approach disregards the important difference between these measurements. One involves measurement of hearing sensitivity to pure tones using supra-aural earphones and the other involves measurement without the listener in a coupler or artificial ear, and neither represents a true listening situation.

A promising approach to this situation supported by recent investigations (Pascoe, 1975) grows out of the concept of *functional gain*. Functional gain is simply the difference between unaided and aided *field* thresholds. It has been shown for many hearing-impaired listeners that only the use of functional gain measurements allow us to determine whether a true "mirroring" of the audiogram has been achieved. This correction enhances the clarity of speech, especially when listening is done in a background of noise.

However, this equalization to the normal pattern of hearing is not feasible in all cases. Those listeners that experience severe discomfort for levels of sound that are not much above their thresholds cannot accept this kind of amplification. Among such cases are the common noise-induced hearing losses. A recent study (Skinner, 1976) showed that for these cases word discrimination is best when the high portions of the speech spectrum are amplified just enough to be heard but not enough to cause discomfort. These cases may be helped by the use of selective compression.

Precise compensation for the audiogram has by and large not been tried. Most audiograms are irregular, and the frequency characteristics of a hearing aid are nearly always irregular also. Only by chance could an exact compensation at all frequencies ever be achieved. However, current technology now enables us to manipulate rather accurately the frequency response, bandwidth, gain, and maximum output of an instrument. Selective compression as a function of frequency is also within reach. Given these developments precise "fitting" may soon become a reality.

At present, however, the selection of hearing aids is based on important but limited information. The audiologist helps make the crucial decision on whether a hearing aid is indicated. He makes his decision on the basis of a careful case history, an interview, and conventional pure-tone and speech audiometry described in Chapter 7, in quiet and frequently in noise, in a context of competing messages or even in reverberant rooms. Despite their limitations, those tests, when they are properly administered and interpreted, are helpful in the selection of a hearing aid.

HOW TO CHOOSE A HEARING AID

The medical aspects of deafness have been discussed in Chapter 6. In summarizing these rules for the choice of hearing aids we assume that the prospective user has consulted his family physician or, better, an otologist, and that the medical profession has done all that it can do. The otologist will presumably make an audiogram for his records and to assist him in his diagnosis, and he will give advice as to whether a hearing aid is indicated.

We believe that a qualified audiologist should be consulted in all decisions about hearing aids for children. There are now many clinics that offer unbiased advice on the selection of hearing aids, whether for children or for adults. These problems are complicated, and it is difficult for even an expert audiologist to pick out objectively and scientifically the hearing aids that best "fit" each individual. Furthermore, many persons are forced to rely on themselves, their friends, and the distributors of hearing aids in making their selection (see Table 11-1). Otologists will continue to give assistance.

The hearing-aid dealer is obviously not a disinterested party except for assistance in the selection of the most suitable model from his own particular offerings. Most purchasers must rely very largely on their own judgment and be prepared to discount some of the claims for special methods of "fitting" put forward by competing manufacturers.

Now let us consider how a person who wants to buy a hearing aid may, without the benefit of expert advice or special apparatus, make a reasonably satisfactory selection from the makes and models of instruments that may be available in his community. Fortunately, the selection among the better instruments is no longer as critical as it once was or as is suggested by some advertisements. *Any one of several choices is likely to be a good one,* thanks to the great advances in recent years by the hearing-aid industry and its distributors.

Of course, a hearing aid should be as small, light, durable, and inexpensive as possible, and it should amplify sound without unnecessary impairment of quality. But when we use the terms "as possible" and "unnecessary," we admit that we are prepared to compromise. If he cannot have both, the user will sacrifice quality in order to obtain intelligibility. We have pointed out some of the features that make a hearing aid "good" in general, but exactly the same instrument may not be the best for everyone. People differ too much in their hearing losses and in the loudness of the sounds that they will tolerate, not to mention in the size of their pocketbooks! Different features will be more important for one man than for another.

Available Dealers

It is generally not wise to buy a hearing aid by mail if there is any practical alternative. Direct personal contact with the dealer is most desirable. The prospective user should find out first, therefore, which hearing-aid companies have local representatives in his district. His choice is practically restricted to the makes of instrument available to him for inspection and trial. Nearness to a dealer is also a great advantage for subsequent repair and replacement service.

Service, Batteries, and Earmolds

Specific inquiry should be made about the availability, quality, and cost of service, including the replacement of batteries. Hearing aids, like automobiles, must sometimes be repaired. If repair service is not immediately available, the user may be deprived of his instrument for long periods of time. Some dealers replace the entire hearing aid, others lend an instrument while an aid is at the factory for service, and others may be able to replace immediately such major parts as amplifier, microphone, or earphone. Unnecessary repairs at exorbitant prices are to be avoided, and the user is cautioned against being "high-pressured" into buying a new model of an instrument to substitute for an older model that happens to get out of order. It is wise to look into the company's policy regarding trade-in value of old instruments in the event that new models appear on the market.

For body-worn hearing aids spare cords should be purchased, particularly if the dealer is not easily reached. As a matter of fact, *we suggest a complete spare hearing aid if the cost is not prohibitive.*

Dealers in hearing aids arrange for the manufacture of the custom earmold. The contract of purchase should clearly indicate whether the cost of the earmold is included in the final price of the instrument.

Size, Cost, and Convenience

Even when expert advice is available, the decision on size, weight, cost, style, color, and convenience of the instrument is the user's own. Only he can strike the balance of his preferences. He must, however, weigh these items against the performance of the various instruments in overcoming his own particular hearing loss. There are three major items of expense in a hearing aid: the initial cost, repairs and replacements, and batteries. Low cost of one of these items does not necessarily mean low cost of the others. Issues related to pricing, trial periods, distribution, and servicing of hearing aids are now the subject of active investigation by government agencies. (See Chapter 16.)

Simple Tests of the Performance of a Hearing Aid

In general the prospective user may rely on the dealer to recommend the particular combination of amplifier, earphone, and tone-control setting that are most likely to be suitable for him. An audiogram will usually help the dealer arrive at his conclusions, and some dealers make their own audiometric tests. Each company that relies on the audiogram or other tests usually has a system or formula to show which of its several instruments or combinations is most likely to give satisfaction. The systems have been worked out with care, partly on theory and partly from the experience of actual users, and the choices based on them are usually rather good. It is advisable to try the first two or three combinations suggested by a dealer, but it is rarely necessary to try more.

No simple set of rules for self-selection will do for everyone, because some people are much more seriously handicapped than others. The following method should work well, however, for someone who is just becoming really hard of hearing but can still "get by" if people will only speak up loudly enough. If the rules we suggest do not fit your case, you can probably judge readily

enough what feature of a hearing aid is most important for you and how to test for it. The general principle is this: Test for the essentials; follow your preferences thereafter.

The features of performance that should be tested when a hearing aid is chosen are:

Tolerability
Intelligibility of ordinary speech
Intelligibility of faint speech
Intelligibility of difficult words
Freedom from internal noise
Aesthetic "quality"
Intelligibility under difficult conditions

It is impossible to test these items *accurately* without elaborate apparatus; but with the help of a friend it is not difficult to come to a useful opinion on most of them. The assistance of a friend is essential, however, because *the tests should all be made under similar conditions and with the same voice and the same set of words and sentences.*

The ideal arrangement is a loan or trial period with each of several instruments so that they may all be tested at leisure at home under the same conditions and in the same place, and the more promising ones tried in actual everyday situations. Trial periods are not generally encouraged by dealers because some unscrupulous "prospects" have no intention of purchasing the instrument and because others will not take responsibility for damage. A compromise can be worked out in most instances. Perhaps it may be possible to rent an instrument or to make a deposit for the trial period that will be applied to payment for the hearing aid if it is purchased, but otherwise will be sacrificed by the user.

If arrangements cannot be made for home testing, the prospective user should ask a friend to go with him to the various agencies and try to carry out the same trials and tests in each case under as nearly the same conditions as possible. The friend must have a good, normal voice and be willing to practice the trick of speaking test words and reading some selected passage from a book or magazine over and over in just the same tone and *with the same loudness.* If he can standardize three different voices—average, faint, and loud—so much the better. During the trials he must keep his distance with care. A distance of 5 feet, which is an average conversation distance, is good; but 3 feet is better if the room is small or if there is some unavoidable noise. For most of the tests a quiet room is very important.

The desirability of obtaining an individual earmold has been mentioned. For the very first trials one of the stock earmolds provided by the various companies will have to do. With them, however, it may not be possible to test the instruments at full gain, because, as has been explained, a hearing aid is more likely to "squeal" if the earmold does not fit snugly.

Each of the instruments should be worn as they are meant to be worn. They should not merely be held in the hand. The body reflects, absorbs, and distorts sound waves and is part of the acoustic system of the hearing aid when the instrument is actually in use. During the actual tests the friend should be faced, but the eyes should be closed to avoid unconscious speechreading.

Tolerability Although *tolerability* is very important, it is very difficult to test unless you are already an experienced user of a hearing aid. Sounds that are uncomfortably loud at first become tolerable with a little practice. The unfamiliar experience of hearing a really loud noise may be terrifying to someone who has been hard of hearing for a long time. Therefore, feel your way with a little care. Unless your hearing loss is quite severe, an instrument of only medium or low power may be better at first. However, with your friend, you should cautiously *try the maximum output of the instrument before the final choice is made.* But remember: *An otherwise satisfactory instrument should not be rejected simply because it is very loud, but only if it is really intolerable.* Unless your hearing loss is severe and you must use nearly full gain, you will rarely hear the loudest output except by accident, as when a door slams, and then only for a very short time.

Intelligibility Intelligibility of speech can be tested in three ways. First, your friend reads a selected passage from a book or newspaper in an ordinary, but even, voice. The same passage of connected speech should never be listened to more than once for purposes of judging intelligibility. Experiment with the volume control and the tone control *to be sure that you can find a combination that makes it easy to understand what he is reading.*

If more than one instrument makes ordinary speech easily intelligible to you, the test can be made more difficult. Let your friend read in a *very quiet voice.* This is, of course, equivalent to "hearing at a distance." It is important to vary the position or orientation of the hearing aid to the sound source. Most users can benefit from ear-level instruments. Care should be taken that the instrument is worn firmly and placed for best reception of sound with proper length of tubing and at the right angle. A higher setting of the volume control may be necessary, but be sure that you can find *some* setting that will do the job. Some instruments may fail on this test. Eliminate them from the competition, and center your attention on those that pass.

Now comes the test with difficult words. You should have prepared in advance a set of word lists, with each word written on a separate card. These can be prepared from the lists in the Appendix. Shuffle the cards each time they have been read. Prepare a number of such little packs with the words in each pack alike except for one sound. A series of words to test the vowels is *bat, bite, boot, beat, boat, bout, bit, bait, but, bet, bought.* For consonants, the following words can be used: *vie, by, high, thy, shy, why, thigh, die, lie, tie, rye, pie, fie, my, sigh, guy, nigh.* If you know that you have difficulty with certain kinds of sounds, it is easy enough to make up a list that is heavily loaded with just the words that you find most confusing.

Your friend should read the words in an ordinary voice and all at the same volume. It may help him to say "now" before each word to get his voice going smoothly. You should set the volume control so that the words come to you quite loudly, but not uncomfortably so. This is not a test of sensitivity of the instrument but a test of how well it enables you to discriminate among and to recognize correctly the sounds that ordinarily are difficult for you. Loud sounds are easier to discriminate than faint ones, so the instrument is "given a break" by being set so that words will not be missed simply because they are too faint.

It is a good plan to put some words two or three times over on the same list. The important points to keep in mind are these:

Use the same list, reshuffled each time, for all instruments.
Your friend must keep his voice, his distance, and all other conditions as nearly the same as possible.
Avoid speechreading.
Keep score systematically.

This test is about as elaborate and rigorous as is practicable without special apparatus. The remaining "tests" depend much more on your opinions and preferences, but your friend can be very helpful by making sure that all points are considered systematically and by noting your comments. Let him be

scorekeeper. Without some sort of scorecard, it is very difficult to compare the performance of one instrument heard in one shop with another heard somewhere else and perhaps on another day. Remember, as we have said previously, hearing aids cannot do everything.

Internal noise   By the time you have finished the test of intelligibility, you have probably formed some opinion of the "quality" of the instrument, that is, whether or not you "like its sound." If the instrument has any great internal noise, either electrical or from friction against your clothing, you will certainly have noticed it by this time and will have scored a black mark against that instrument.

Quality   As to "quality," it is well known that men and women who have heard high tones poorly for some time, as well as many with normal hearing, prefer the quality of a hearing aid (or radio) that does not emphasize—or may even suppress—high tones. They describe its sound as "smoother, more mellow, more comfortable, more pleasing." When the high tones are emphasized, or even merely restored to their normal strength, such listeners say the voice or music is harsh and unpleasant, even though words may be crisper and easier to understand. Remember, therefore, that if your hearing has been subnormal for some time, you are likely to prefer the instrument with the "full, smooth tone," even though the word test may show that you understand difficult words better with an instrument that emphasizes the high tones a bit. Your friend will probably remind you of the importance of understanding correctly. He represents your "talking public." Other people, too, are interested in having you understand them readily, and to them *your ability to understand is more important than how mellow* *their voices sound.* If the word tests do not show any great difference, then pick the instrument that "sounds best" by all means, but remember that *the quality preferences of those who have heard poorly for some time are notoriously misleading.* You may have forgotten how speech *should* sound.

As a final word of advice, when you are scoring an instrument on quality, lean toward the crisp rather than the mellow. You are likely to get the best results with it in the long run, even though some practice will probably be necessary before you realize the full benefits.

Difficult conditions But it is not enough to judge the quality of an instrument under good conditions only. An instrument may work very well when its volume control is set low or when your friend talks in an ordinary voice, but it may lose its clarity when the control is set high or when your friend suddenly raises his voice. The reasons for this were explained in the preceding chapter. The point to remember is this: Compare instruments for *loud* as well as for average voices *without moving the volume control from the position that makes the average voice easy to understand.* This test gives some idea of the leeway the instrument has before it either loses quality from "overloading" or else becomes intolerably loud. Plenty of leeway, technically called a "good operating range," is important for those whose auditory area has been much restricted by a severe hearing loss. But, in this test your friend should raise his voice by degrees. Don't invite someone with a distorted sense of humor to help on this one! It is particularly helpful to listen under different conditions of instrument orientation and noise to more than one person talking at the same time. This is known as a "competing message" test.

There is no very good way to find out without actual trial periods how different hearing aids sound in noisy places. Your friend may have a fairly standard voice, but he cannot carry a kit of sound effects with him. We have mentioned the desirability of a trial period if the dealer will consent. It is not necessary to make such trial of *every* available instrument. The tests that you and a friend can do on the spot should be enough to narrow the field down to two or three leading instruments.

It is an open question whether anyone who has not already had experience in wearing a hearing aid is really qualified to judge the performance of an instrument in noise. The novice is likely at first to suppress the high frequencies with the tone control, then turn down the gain control, and end by "throwing out the baby with the bath." If there is much noise around you, you must listen to noise if you are to hear voices also. Normal listeners must put up with the noise and often must struggle to understand. The tone control of a hearing aid may take some of the sting out of the noise, but no instrument can magically sort out speech from noise or one voice from another when both sounds occupy the same part of the frequency spectrum and come from the same direction. Here is where two hearing aids may be much better than one.

A trial period gives a better idea of the strong and the weak points of an instrument; but *play fair with the first instrument you try. Give it another trial after you have tried other instruments.* You are likely to do better in everyday situations with the second or third instrument and you may prefer them also because you are learning how to wear and use them. After you have gained this experience, a second trial of the first instrument may show that it is better than you thought.

Families and associates of hearing-aid users *should not shout* into the microphones.

It is better to speak naturally but distinctly and to face the listener so that he can take full advantage of speechreading. Slamming of doors and pounding, which are nerve-racking to most wearers of hearing aids, should be avoided.

If a hearing-aid user has difficulty hearing the radio or television clearly enough for his enjoyment, he should consider having the set equipped with a socket into which he can plug earphones. High-fidelity earphones are available, and they may reproduce music and voice more faithfully than can a hearing aid. It may be very helpful to avoid the unnecessary transformations, first into sound by the radio and then back into electrical signals by the hearing aid. All noises in the room are thus excluded. The arrangement should offer no difficulty for a good radio or television serviceman.

Some persons with a long-standing hearing loss may not like a hearing aid simply because it sounds "strange." They have often forgotten what it means to hear well, and therefore their judgment of how things should sound is not very reliable. They must be as patient with a hearing aid as they are with a new pair of shoes, and their families must be equally patient with them.

No one but an expert should ever open the case of a hearing-aid amplifier. Even opening and closing it may cause trouble, and to poke around inside may cause severe damage that will be expensive to repair. If you must satisfy your curiosity and see the inside, your dealer will be glad to show it to you. Remember, if you do damage through opening up the case (and don't think your dealer will fail to detect it), it is liable to void your service guarantee! As explained in the previous chapter, the miniaturized transistor amplifiers of many modern hearing aids cannot be repaired, even by an expert, but must be replaced as a unit in case of failure.

SELECTED CASES

We have pointed out some of the features that make a hearing aid "good" in general, but, we repeat, exactly the same instrument may not be the best for everyone. People differ too much in their hearing losses and in the loudness of the sounds that they will tolerate. Different features will be more important for one person than for another. Let us illustrate with a few examples.

John Peters is a young salesman who complains of frequent misunderstandings when talking to customers in shops, factories, and retail stores. His hearing for low frequencies is within the normal range, is borderline for 500 and 1000 Hz, and drops to 40 dB hearing-threshold level (HTL) at 2000 and 4000 Hz. His hearing level for speech is 25 dB HTL in both ears. Normal bone-conduction thresholds suggest no conductive components in the hearing loss.

Mr. Peters reports no problems when listening in quiet, one-to-one situations. He prefers to make contacts through the telephone because voices appear to be clearer. Usually, however, he has to talk in noisy surroundings, and words appear to lose their clarity.

If a hearing aid is to help Mr. Peters, it should have little or no gain in the low frequencies and it should have 15 to 20 dB more gain at 2000 and 4000 Hz than at 1000 Hz. This configuration of gains can be achieved with an "open-ear" fitting in which the ear canal is not occluded by the presence of an earmold. With this amount of gain, feedback should not be a problem. This "open-ear" condition would retain the unamplified sound in the low frequencies and would provide the natural acoustic effects for the higher ones, thus giving almost natural reproduction. The aid should have as low a maximum output as feasible, in order to protect Mr. Peters' substantial hearing. Such a maximum output should aim lower than 100 dB SPL. If Mr. Peters wishes to have the greatest chance for success, he should try two such aids, one for each ear. But even in this condition, he should be warned not to expect miraculous results. The conditions which he has trouble with are difficult even for one with perfect hearing. He can definitely profit by learning to use the visual clues that accompany speech. He should be helped to make an objective trial of these hearing aids, both at home and at work. And after this trial period, Mr. Peters should be encouraged either to reject or to purchase the aids, based upon his own personal experience.

Elizabeth Brown has a moderate conductive hearing loss with hearing-threshold levels at about 55 dB (ANSI) in the "speech range." The maximum intensity of average speech is about 65 dB (SPL). Faint speech becomes just intelligible to a person with 0-dB hearing-threshold levels at approximately 20 dB (SPL), but speech must be at about 75 dB for Ms. Brown to understand it. She may catch a word or two of average speech now and then but no more. But a hearing aid that provides 40 dB of amplification will raise all but the faintest sounds of average speech above her threshold. Since her loss is conductive in nature, and therefore without recruitment, the amplified speech will not sound particularly loud to her, but it should be fully intelligible. She will do well in ordinary social situations when there is not a confusion of many voices or other noise. This 40 dB of assistance is Ms. Brown's first requirement.

Ms. Brown's second requirement is that the amplified sound must not cause discomfort. Most persons, whether their hearing is normal or hypoacousic, do not feel discomfort until the peaks of speech reach at least

115 dB (SPL). If Ms. Brown's threshold of discomfort is at about 115 dB, she should select a hearing aid that has a maximum output just under 115 dB. There is no conflict between her two requirements. The 40 dB of amplification raises average speech peaks from about 75 dB to only 105 dB. There is still a margin of 10 dB before the hearing aid's maximum output of 115 dB is reached. This margin will allow Ms. Brown to hear loud speech naturally and without noticeable peak clipping. The distortion of peak clipping will seldom occur, and she is therefore not much concerned about how the instrument sounds when it is "overloaded." The limiting feature is for her merely an emergency protection that guards her against great discomfort from sudden unexpected noises. She should easily find an instrument that gives her practically perfect intelligibility whether the speaker talks loudly or softly.

Ms. Brown will probably find, if she shops around, that several different makes of instrument are about equally effective, clear-toned, and attractive. Certain models may not sound as pleasant as others, but two models or combinations of the same brand may very well differ more in "how they sound" than two similar models made by different companies.

Suppose that Ms. Brown goes to a laboratory and is tested with different hearing aids by elaborate and time-consuming speech tests. She would probably make a nearly perfect score with each of several instruments. Then even the expert who tested her would be unable to say with certainty that *one* instrument is better for her than any other. Ms. Brown is easy to "fit."

But consider George Jones, who has a really severe hearing loss. He has not been able to find an instrument that can "get through" to him without hurting his ears.

His audiogram shows about 90 dB HTL for low and middle frequencies, and he cannot hear 4000 Hz at all. He obviously needs a great deal of amplification. The critical point for him is to find an instrument that will provide this high gain and yet not be uncomfortably loud even when it is driven to its maximum output. The 65 dB or so of amplification that Mr. Jones requires, added to the original 65 dB of average speech, makes a total of 130 dB (SPL). This total is at least 10 dB more than the usual threshold of discomfort. The fact that Mr. Jones is hard of hearing does not mean that his ear is any "tougher" than normal. We shall assume that his threshold of discomfort is 120 dB. For comfort, therefore, Mr. Jones must be satisfied with less than the full amplification that he apparently needs. He must find a hearing aid with just the right maximum output. The instrument must "package" speech accurately by clipping its peaks or by compression, and it must deliver this speech into the very restricted range between his threshold of hearing and his threshold of discomfort. Success or failure may depend on whether the receiver is "flat" instead of "resonant" and on whether the tone control suppresses the low frequencies enough to keep speech intelligible when it is distorted by peak clipping. Mr. Jones is difficult to "fit."

If Mr. Jones has not used a powerful hearing aid before, he is likely to profit considerably by auditory training. Listening systematically to sound that is loud but not quite uncomfortable may increase his tolerance so that he can use an instrument with greater maximum output. Such an instrument will have more "elbow room" and will not clip the peaks of speech so heavily. Speech will then sound more natural and probably be more intelligible; but Mr. Jones' high-tone loss is severe, and he must not expect any instrument to give him a perfect articulation score.

Julia Smith is quite hard of hearing, but not to the degree that Mr. Jones is. She has hearing-threshold levels of 70 dB at 500 and 1000 Hz, increasing to 110 dB at 4000 Hz. Figure 10-35 shows this kind of a sensitivity curve and how a fairly powerful hearing aid should make speech loud enough for her. She can probably find several instruments that (1) are tolerable, even for loud speech when the gain control is well up; (2) make faint or distant conversation intelligible; (3) make nearly all words intelligible under good listening conditions; and (4) have a "quality" that is acceptable to her.

In making comparisons of instruments, Ms. Smith should listen at both low and high levels. Two hearing aids may sound very much alike at low levels; and yet one may be obviously superior to the other when loud sounds drive them to the limit of their output and force them to clip and distort some of the sound waves. On the whole, Ms. Smith will probably do best with an instrument that has a definite high-tone emphasis, but she may prefer the quality of an instrument without the high-tone emphasis. This compromise is probably best settled by Ms. Smith herself, but her decision is easier if she can choose an instrument that has an adjustable tone control. Then she can increase or decrease its high-tone emphasis according to the situation.

SUGGESTED READINGS AND REFERENCES

American Speech and Hearing Association. *A Conference on Hearing Aid Evaluation Procedures*, ASHA Reports, No. 2. Washington, D.C.: American Speech and Hearing Association, 1967.
Very useful discussions of the problem.

Committee on the Judiciary, United States Senate. *Hearings before the Subcommittee on Antitrust and Monopoly.* "Prices of Hearing Aids." Eighty-Seventh Congress. Washington D.C.: U.S. Government Printing Office, 1962.
Contains testimony from the hearing-aid industry, economists, audiologists, and others about issues related to the distribution of hearing aids.

Donnelly, K. (ed.). *Interpreting Hearing Aid Technology:* Springfield, Ill.: Charles C Thomas, 1974.
Particularly relevant are Chapters 5 and 6 on evaluation procedures for adults and for children.

Harford, E., and E. Dodds. "The Clinical Application of CROS: A Hearing Aid for Unilateral Deafness," *"Arch. Otolaryng. (Chicago)*, 83:455–464 (1966).

Katz, J. (ed.). *Handbook of Clinical Audiology.* Baltimore: Williams & Wilkins, 1972.
A textbook directed to professionals. Chapters 33 and 34 concern hearing-aid evaluation and counseling.

National Center for Health Statistics. "Characteristics of Persons with Impaired Hearing: United States, July 1962–June 1963," Series 10, No. 35, A. Gentile, J. D. Schein, and K. Haase (eds.).
Data from the National Health Survey, Public Health Service, U.S. Department of Health, Education and Welfare. (For sale by Superintendent of Documents, U.S. Government Printing Office, Washington, D.C. 20402. Price 45 cents.

Pascoe, D. P. "Frequency Responses of Hearing Aids and their Effects on the Speech Perception of Hearing-Impaired Subjects," *Ann. Otol.*, 84 (Suppl. 23): 1–40 (1975).

Shore, I., R. C. Bilger, and I. J. Hirsh. "Hearing Aid Evaluation: Reliability of Repeated Measurements," *J. Speech Hearing Dis.*, 25:152–170 (1960).

Shore, I., and J. C. Kramer. "A Comparison of Two Procedures for Hearing Aid Evaluation," *J. Speech Hearing Dis.*, 28:159–170 (1963).

Skinner, M. W. "Speech Intelligibility in Noise-Induced Hearing Loss: Effects of High Frequency Compensation." Unpublished Doctoral Dissertation, Washington University, St. Louis, Mo., 1976.

Victoreen, J. A. *Hearing Enhancement.* Springfield, Ill.: Charles C Thomas, 1969.
A popular presentation of principles and background of hearing aids.

Norman P. Erber, Ph.D.
Ira J. Hirsh, Ph.D.

12

Auditory Training

Babies with normal hearing accompanied by good intelligence *learn* to respond to, and to distinguish among, an enormous variety of sounds. They seem to differentiate the sounds of different persons approaching, to recognize speech from adults and from other children, and eventually to control their own production of speech through hearing (see Chapter 14). Furthermore, through their auditory reception of speech around them, they appear to acquire the rules for making words and sentences in their own language.

There are two special cases in which these normal steps of auditory learning are not sustained over long periods of time or are not taken at all. The first is the child or adult who once had normal hearing, who learned to speak and to use language properly, but who subsequently lost some of his hearing through disease or accident. The second is the child who was born with impaired hearing and whose original learning and experience therefore did not have the usual auditory components. In both cases the normal use of auditory cues and the normal course of learning must somehow be compensated for by special additional auditory learning or practice. The principles underlying this special training are the subject of this chapter.

HEARING AND AUDITORY PERCEPTION

When we speak of *hearing* we refer to any of the various ways in which human beings react to sound waves. When the clinician obtains an audiogram, he is reporting on only one facet of auditory response, namely, the sensitivity to very weak tones at different frequencies. In the course of testing hearing further, to know something about the nature of a hearing impairment, he may test still other functions, such as sensitivity to differences between intensities of different sounds heard at one or the other ear. In addition, when the clinician uses speech audiometry, he may be interested in the weakest levels of speech that a patient requires for a certain degree of intelligibility, or he may be interested in the percentage of speech items in a list that the patient can repeat correctly, sometimes in the quiet and sometimes when the speech is presented against a background of noise (see Chapter 7). These clinical tests of hearing represent only a small sample of the auditory functions that might be tested, and they rarely exhaust those that the listener actually uses in everyday life.

One of the most common uses of hearing is in communication by speech. In such a situation we know that the talker and listener must be able to distinguish sound from nonsound, speech sounds from nonspeech sounds, and particular speech sounds from other speech sounds. In addition to these rather simple auditory discriminations, the listener must have sufficient memory to hold a short string of received sounds in storage long enough to fit them into the pattern of a sentence, and he must have learned something about the rules of his language in order to use this auditory memory span appropriately for communication. In the sections that follow we shall try to separate the hearing function into what appear to be its most important components and then discuss how each of these parts is impaired by the loss or absence of hearing.

In Table 12-1, we have used a simple matrix to outline the variety of acoustic speech stimuli (for example, words, sentences) that a hearing-impaired person might encounter

TABLE 12-1
AN AUDITORY SKILLS MATRIX

	Stimulus					
Response Task	Speech elements	Syllables	Words	Phrases	Sentences	Connected discourse
Detection (presence/absence)						
Discrimination (same/different)						
Identification (recognition)						
Comprehension (understanding)						

The instructor describes the hearing-impaired individual's perceptual abilities for each level of stimulus-response complexity. These observations are used to specify goals for auditory training.

in his daily life and also the range of response tasks (detection, discrimination, identification, and comprehension) that he might be required to perform whenever these stimuli occur. Each box in this diagram describes the interaction between a particular type of stimulus and a manner of responding during conversation (for example, the listener may be required to *discriminate* between two *phrases*, such as "in the box" versus "on the box," or he may need to *comprehend* the *sentence* "What time is it?"). Nearly all auditory tasks can be broken down in this way. A person must be capable of success at a given level of task complexity before he will be able to perform well at the next higher level. For example, it is clear that a word first must be detected before it can be discriminated from another word. Brief descriptions of the four levels of response behavior are given below.

Detection is the basic process of determining whether sound is present or absent. This response normally results in the listener's orientation to the sound and establishes a setting for further acquisition of information from the source of sound. Detection helps the young child understand that some things produce sound and that others do not. It also is important in indicating the relation between objects or people and the sounds that they produce. Awareness of ongoing environmental sounds helps one to maintain contact with the acoustical world around him and alerts him to nearby activity. For the hearing-impaired person who depends partly on lipreading for communication, speech detection signals to him that someone is talking and that he should turn and face the speaker for additional information.

Detection responses are used by audiologists not only in pure-tone audiometry but also to establish minimal hearing-aid settings. That is, a hearing aid must be set to make speech at least audible to the listener. Hearing clinicians have used detection responses to determine which speech sounds

are available to a deaf child under particular acoustic conditions. Some phonemes may be clearly detectable, others reach the level of awareness only when strongly amplified, and still others are not detectable under even the best conditions.

Even if a person can respond to a large variety of sounds, by raising his hand or otherwise, his hearing has little utility unless he also can distinguish these sounds from one another. *Discrimination* allows the listener to perceive the differences between sounds; failure to discriminate yields perception of similarity. Discrimination allows the young child to perceive that different things produce different sounds, or that the same source (for example, a human being) may produce different sounds. Same-different discrimination and generalization of sounds into categories are complementary abilities. In order for one to describe several sounds as the "same," he must place them into a common category. Moreover, the concepts of "same" and "different" can be somewhat relative things, depending on the range of sounds presented. For example, the words *duck* and *duck* spoken by two different talkers may be described as different stimuli in one context, but these sound probably would be called "the same" if they were presented in contrast to several samples of the word *apple*.

Teachers of deaf children often use discrimination tasks remedially to check a child's auditory perception when he makes an error on a recognition task. For example, a child may identify the stimulus *running* as the word *run*. The teacher can present the stimulus and the incorrect response together to determine whether the child can hear the difference, that is, to find out whether the error is one of hearing the difference between the confused words or merely of knowing that the two sound patterns (words) are labeled differently.

Identification, or recognition, responses are simply labels for what the listener has heard. He indicates this by saying, pointing to, or writing the word or sentence that he has perceived. These all are forms of repetition response, in which the listener must recall the stimulus in some way.

Identification of speech stimuli is related to the child's developing awareness that objects have names and that these names can be represented acoustically. In addition, the child develops the concept that the sounds that things or people produce have names themselves (phonemes or words, for example) and that these are important for communication by speech. An identification response may be *specific*, in the sense that the listener describes the stimulus exactly (for example, he points to a dog when he hears the acoustic stimulus "dog"); or the response may be *categorical*, in the sense that he describes the general class of the stimulus without specifically naming it (for example, he indicates that he perceives one syllable when he hears the acoustic stimulus, "dog"). The latter sort of response, recognition of syllable number or stress rather than exact word identification, is typical of profoundly deaf children.

Teachers use identification tasks to determine how speech is perceived by their hearing-impaired pupils. If a child fails to answer a question or follow an instruction correctly, he may be asked to restate what the teacher said. The nature of his response may indicate whether the child's problem is in identifying (or remembering) the stimulus sentence or in understanding its meaning.

The most difficult auditory skill, *comprehension* of speech, requires that the listener understand the meaning of acoustic messages, usually on the basis of his knowledge of language. It also requires that he be able to acquire new information through his ears and act appropriately on this basis. A comprehension response differs from an identification response in that the listener cannot simply repeat what was said. Instead, he must indicate that he has understood the meaning of the acoustic message in a way that differs in content from the stimulus. In general terms, comprehension implies that the idea which the speaker encoded acoustically in his spoken message has been transmitted to the listener's brain. As an example, if an adult asks a young child "What is your name?" and the child responds similarly, "What is your name?" he has demonstrated only identification of the acoustic stimulus. But if the child responds with his name, "Robert," then he has demonstrated comprehension of the question.

Comprehension is a necessary requirement for genuine auditory communication to occur, as over the telephone. Teachers of hearing-impaired children often evaluate their pupils' auditory comprehension abilities by giving instructions or asking questions in the classroom under conditions of acoustic-only stimulation. In some facilities, telephone communication skills also are taught.

AUDITORY TRAINING IN REHABILITATION

In focusing on *rehabilitation* we mean to imply that our aim is to restore, as far as possible, functions that previously have been normal. The concept applies to children or adults who, as a result of sickness or accident, lose some of their ability to hear. The various kinds of hearing losses have been reviewed in Chapter 4, but we will recount some of the auditory symptoms that accompany such hearing loss, particularly those that affect the perception of speech.

Nature of the Problem

Consider a young adult who has sufficient intelligence and hearing abilities to have completed high school or perhaps college and to have obtained employment. He has learned his language well, can communicate easily with others in a variety of acoustic environments, enjoys listening to music, attends movies or theater, and enjoys programs on radio and television. He may attend church and meetings and can hear the speakers in such circumstances without difficulty. His first symptoms will be a noticeable increase in the effort with which he must attend and concentrate in order to understand the minister or lecturer, and his family members may begin to notice that he prefers to have the radio or the television sound at a higher level than is desired by others. Usually, except in cases of accident or in certain types of disease, the hearing loss will increase gradually over a period of months or years. Only rarely do auditory symptoms appear suddenly.

The particular problem will of course depend upon the type of hearing loss. In otosclerosis, for example, the impairment is almost purely conductive, and the primary problem is one of sensitivity, which deteriorates gradually over a period of years. Such a patient notices that he does not have great difficulty when people are talking loudly enough, in a noisy automobile, during a television program when he can turn up the volume, or in a noisy office or factory environment where everyone shouts because of the noisy background. If his loss in sensitivity cannot be alleviated through surgery, this kind of patient can be helped greatly by amplification. In stating that the essential problem is a loss of sensitivity, we mean to imply that if the sensitivity is restored surgically or is compensated for by amplification, then the other aspects of auditory perception, which are not affected by the disease, are still available for his use.

He will still have difficulty, however, if the surgical or prosthetic remedies were not called into play immediately. Several aspects of auditory perception contributing to discrimination, pattern recognition, and language, which had been used less frequently, must now be relearned. This important point means that even though the loss of sensitivity is the principal problem in a conductive impairment, the clinician cannot assume that everything else will become normal again as soon as the sensitivity is restored. Depending upon the severity of the loss, *rehabilitative procedures that focus on auditory training, speechreading, and improved monitoring and production of one's own speech often must accompany surgery or a hearing aid.*

Problems associated with sensorineural hearing impairment are somewhat more complicated. The individual's auditory sensitivity, his ability to detect weak sounds (for example, those described by the pure-tone audiogram) is reduced. For most persons with sensorineural hearing impairments, who have lost some of their hearing through noise exposure, disease, or the natural aging process, the hearing is poorer in the high than in the low frequencies. This loss of sensitivity for high frequencies adversely affects the person's ability to detect numerous speech sounds such as /s, sh, t, k/. In addition, sensorineural hearing loss often affects other auditory functions besides detection of weak sounds. One's ability to discriminate differences in frequency or intensity often is abnormal also. Many high-frequency consonants, although detectable when amplified through a speech audiometer or a hearing aid, are heard as distorted and often are indistinguishable from one another. For one with a typical high-frequency loss, most vowel sounds usually will remain detectable and distinguishable. Still, in some cases the individual's ability to make use of even these clearly audible sounds is reduced, and he scores poorly on clinical tests of word recognition.

In spite of these apparently severe limitations to speech perception, many hearing-impaired adults with sensorineural losses are able to function reasonably well in daily communication. They seem to be able to apply their knowledge of language to fill in those portions of words or sentences that they are not able to perceive acoustically. In some cases, however, comprehension is poor because the individual's auditory system reduces perception of important speech cues so severely, because the person does not know how to use his remaining speech-perception skills effectively, or because he lacks the confidence to respond to statements or questions that are directed to him.

In summary, the role of auditory training for the patient with a progressive conductive impairment, with or without surgery or a hearing aid, is to help him recall those listening rules, cues, and strategies that he used when his hearing was normal. The more complicated varieties of sensorineural hearing loss, unequal at the different frequencies, require rehabilitative procedures that not only reteach what was once known but also attempt to substitute other ways of listening. This includes development of communication strategies and supplementing listening with looking to substitute new visual cues for those acoustic cues that no longer are clearly perceived, even with a hearing aid.

AURAL REHABILITATION OF THE HEARING-IMPAIRED ADULT

Before beginning aural rehabilitation, the hearing clinician usually will estimate the extent of the person's auditory speech-perception loss, both through objective tests and through observation. Often this will include evaluation of his ability to detect certain speech sounds and also his ability to tell whether these sounds are the same or different. In most cases, his word-recognition ability also will be measured in the clinic with standard lists of one- or two-syllable words. In addition, during the case-history interview, the audiologist will estimate the individual's ability to comprehend spoken phrases or sentences. These preliminary tests and observations will provide a broad estimate of the hearing-impaired person's auditory speech communication abilities and will suggest to the audiologist specific perceptual areas where practice in certain speech-perception tasks may be beneficial.

After speech-perception testing is complete, hearing-aid evaluation is provided. In general, hearing-impaired adults require hearing aids that provide an increase in sound intensity throughout the frequency range considered important for speech perception (roughly 200–4000 Hz). These aids should not produce so much sound output that they are uncomfortable under conditions of high speech or noise input. Still, the most important selection criterion is that the hearing aid provide a level and quality of sound that results in optimal speech perception by the user. Adults with different types and degrees of hearing impairment naturally will require different kinds of hearing aids. The degree to which the aid provides good speech perception will be evaluated by the audiologist in quiet and in noise, with and without lipreading of the talker allowed. Although a hearing aid cannot correct or restore hearing (any more than eyeglasses can correct a retinal defect), it at least can make some speech sounds more audible and thus potentially usable to the listener in communication.

As we have seen in Chapters 10 and 11, the audiologist usually will determine the best frequency response, gain, and output power limitations for the hearing-impaired individual, who is advised to purchase a hearing aid with these general characteristics. The audiologist then will help the purchaser adapt to his new aid. He will explain how to adjust the controls, replace the battery, clean the earmold, provide routine maintenance, and use the aid in different acoustic conditions (Figure 12-1).

After hearing-aid orientation, the audiologist may recommend formal auditory training for his client. In many clinics, individual or group instruction in speech perception is available on a regular (for example, weekly) basis for new hearing-aid users. This may include experience in listening to vowel or consonant sounds in syllables or words. With instruction, the hearing-impaired person can learn to identify the unfamiliar speech sounds that now are available when amplified through the aid. Often a person is surprised that he can perceive speech cues that he has not heard for a long while. They may not sound the same as he remembers them, but he can learn to recognize them under the new conditions.

Even with his hearing aid, a severely hearing-impaired adult may perceive only portions of the acoustic speech signal. In most daily situations, the hearing-impaired person relies considerably on his knowledge of the sound and word sequences of language as an aid to recognition and comprehension of speech. He is able to communicate by piecing together those fragments of speech that he does hear by making ongoing predictions about the content of the message and by checking with the talker occasionally to determine whether these "guesses" are correct. If he is right most of the time, he will develop confidence in his ability to perceive speech acoustically through his hearing aid(s) and through his impaired ear(s). The act of reconstructing spoken messages from perceived fragments of speech is feasible, however, only under optimal conditions. The speech must be perceived in quiet surroundings, with a few distracting influences. The talker must speak slowly and clearly, using language that is not overly complicated.

Many hearing-impaired persons can benefit from special practice in predicting word sequences or language patterns and in making decisions about partially perceived spoken messages. The audiologist usually can

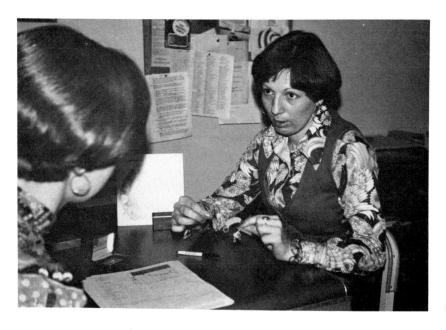

Figure 12-1 An audiologist describes the operation of an ear-level hearing aid to a hearing-impaired adult. *(Central Institute for the Deaf)*

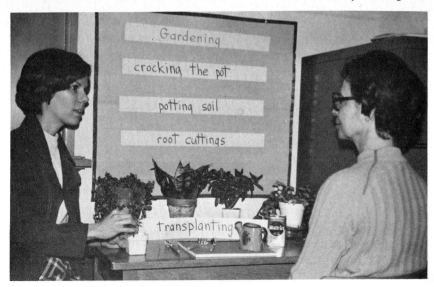

Figure 12-2 A hearing clinician uses "gardening" as a situational context for communication during therapy. *(Central Institute for the Deaf)*

demonstrate how the language context, the surrounding environment, or the conversational situation can help one to make reasonable guesses and also to recognize and correct misperceptions when they occur (Figure 12-2). For example, a hearing-impaired adult who has toured the zoo for several hours with his young grandchild may hear the tired child say something that sounds like "I walked home!" or possibly "I want to go home!" Under the circumstances, the latter message is the more likely of the two.

Most hearing-impaired adults complain of difficulty in understanding speech when they listen in noisy places, when the talker speaks rapidly or without precision, or when the vocabulary or language used is unfamiliar. Under these conditions, the fragments of speech that normally provide a contextual framework for "filling in" missing bits of information may themselves be misperceived or not perceived at all. Thus, the observer's impaired hearing cannot provide adequate input for successful communication. The audiologist can provide practice in listening under noisy conditions or can suggest other ways of overcoming these difficulties.

Many hearing clinicians combine much of their auditory training instruction with practice in *lipreading* (see Chapter 13). The purpose of such auditory-visual training is to show the hearing-impaired person how easily lipreading can enhance his auditory perception of speech. Many of the high-frequency sounds that a hearing-impaired person cannot identify reliably through listening alone become much more identifiable when he simultaneously watches the talker's face as he listens. For example, the words *fee* and *she* may be indistinguishable through ear alone but are easily identifiable when the hearing-impaired listener also attends to the talker's face.

The development of social strategies (although not *auditory* training in a strict sense) helps the hearing-impaired adult gain maximum benefit from his hearing aid in difficult listening situations. For example, the audiologist may show him that he can control the effects of environmental noise to an extent by decreasing the distance between himself and the speaker. This improves the signal-to-noise (and signal-to-reverberation) ratio and thus enhances his ability to understand spoken messages. Also, the hearing-impaired individual can develop a willingness to ask the speaker to repeat, clarify his message, or talk louder in order to improve his speech perception. These requests are especially important for telephone communication, where visual cues are not available and lipreading thus is not possible. A person with a hearing loss must not be passive about difficulties that he encounters in communication. Whenever possible, he should request that the speaker consider his problem and make it easier for him to understand.

The audiologist also may counsel the adult and his family regarding potential communication difficulties at home and at work. Those who communicate with a hearing-impaired person on a daily basis will help him considerably if they develop an understanding of his communication needs. They will learn that making their faces visible for lipreading, speaking clearly and slowly, and repeating when necessary contributes greatly to reducing many potential communication difficulties.

Auditory Training Program

Although it is not our intent to produce here a manual on auditory training, the rationale for the basic steps can be summarized.

It is not likely that the hard-of-hearing adult or older child needs to be taught again to be aware of sound. On the other hand, gradual loss of hearing will be accompanied by a failure to attend to those aspects of sound that have become more difficult to hear. Such patients, newly equipped with hearing aids, should not be sent out to unscramble for themselves the new buzzing confusion that they now encounter. Attention to weak, not recently heard sounds must be focused, and gross discrimination and recognition must be carefully retrained. With

higher frequencies again available, the telephone bell and the doorbell can be distinguished, but such discriminations may not be immediately obvious and therefore must be made part of a training program.

With respect to speech perception, several goals must be kept in view. Through audiometric testing, the clinician knows something of the character of a loss. This information plus the results of careful evaluation by hearing clinicians will show which auditory cues are available to the listener, which can be made available through training, and which are not likely to be available at all. The emphasis here, of course, is on the individualization of the program.

Drills and exercises are particularly useful for adults, especially when the items contain contrasting elements based on cues that the patient is to learn. Recognition based on such cases must be carefully trained through several stages. At first the cue may be used in isolation and slowly enough that the listener can succeed. Then speed becomes important, especially as the cue is introduced into syllable and word contexts, such as bed and red. Finally, the availability of the cue must be demonstrated and trained as it occurs in the rapid exchanges of conversation. Teachers in many fields find that proceeding from easy, rewarded steps to the finer, more difficult ones will produce better learning with less frustration than when the most difficult and challenging aspects of auditory perception are introduced early.

AUDITORY EDUCATION OF THE HEARING-IMPAIRED CHILD

As indicated earlier, the problems associated with congenital impairment of hearing are more complicated and more serious than those that follow an acquired impairment. The child or adult who becomes hard of hearing knew about sound, knows that a person talking influences another by the sounds he produces, knows that different kinds of sound produce different effects, and also has learned to talk while listening to the acoustic effects of his own speech and vocal activities. The deaf child has had no such incidental introduction to the world of sound.

The Nature of the Problem

A child with a 50-dB hearing-threshold level will hear either no speech at all or else only occasional loud bits, or perhaps some continuous speech from a mother who holds him close. Yet a 50-dB level is not uncommonly severe. It is more usual, as a result of maternal rubella or hereditary deafness, that babies will show much poorer thresholds. Children who are subsequently seen in nursery school or kindergartens for deaf children typically show thresholds as poor as 70 dB (hearing-threshold level) in the low frequencies and 100 dB or poorer at 1000 Hz and above.

When we point out that the speech of a talker a meter or so away will not be heard at all by these children, it is not only to comment on the difficulty that they will have in understanding the speech of others. It is rather to emphasize that they are deprived of all sources of acoustic stimulation out of which the awareness of sound, the awareness of the possibilities of communication, the basis of language, and the learning of speech are built. Left unattended, without a hearing aid, and without appropriate schooling, these children will become as if totally deaf, and their education, begun at a later time, will be difficult. They are likely to fall short of their maximum potential (see also Chapter 17).

Even the most optimistic teachers do not pretend that severe hearing losses can be completely compensated for, or that excellent training and the proper hearing aid will help the children to hear normally; but even the most pessimistic will recognize that carefully planned steps plus the use of amplification will prepare such children for an optimum educational opportunity to realize their individual capabilities.

AUDITORY TRAINING FOR CHILDREN

A child's awareness and acquisition of language is dependent upon his ability to hear the spoken messages of others as well as perceive his own attempts to imitate. A hearing loss in a young child hampers these processes and may delay or inhibit his language development. Most teachers and clinicians feel that the main habilitative goal in these cases is to help the hearing-impaired child develop an awareness of language and an ability to communicate through language. A delay in language development is such a serious problem that early diagnosis of the child's hearing loss, provision of a proper hearing aid, and educational assistance all are vitally important.

In general, the object of auditory training is to help the hearing-impaired child use his impaired auditory sense to the fullest capacity in language communication, regardless of the degree of damage to the auditory system. This includes his own speech production. In some cases the child eventually may be able to perceive speech very well through his ears alone, even over the telephone. In other cases, where the hearing loss is more serious, the child may learn to use acoustic cues for speech primarily as a supplement to communication through lipreading. It now is clear that nearly all hearing-impaired children show a sensitivity to sound that can be exploited by a skillful teacher, clinician, or parent to contribute significantly to the child's ability to communicate through speech.

Typically, the first step in any auditory training program is the selection and evaluation of an appropriate hearing aid (or aids) for the child. Without sufficient amplification of speech, auditory training cannot be very useful. At normal conversational levels, speech generally is not intense enough for most hearing-impaired children to understand what they perceive. Some may not hear anything at all at normal speech levels. Thus, a hearing aid is necessary. One must remember that a hearing aid only makes the sounds of speech louder, not necessarily clearer to the child. But without this increase in loudness of speech, the child has no chance of interpreting acoustic information for the purpose of communication.

Hearing-aid selection for young hearing-impaired children can be made difficult by the fact that they often have little language or vocabulary with which to describe their sensory impressions. They may not be able to tell the audiologist which of two hearing aids produces clearer speech or, for a specific hearing aid, whether one frequency response ("tone") or volume setting is better than another for speech perception. In spite of these limitations, audiologists are able to select aids and adjust control settings for young children with a reasonable degree of accuracy. It is not until the child is much older, however, that the audiologist is able to verify that the early decisions were appropriate.

Selection procedures that are used in these cases with a moderate degree of confidence are:

(1) Careful observation of the child's behavior. Both parents and clinicians watch the child at home and in the clinic as he uses different hearing aids adjusted to various settings. A judgment is made about optimum conditions for responsiveness and understanding of speech.

(2) Electroacoustic measurement. The aid's output is measured electroacoustically and is compared with the child's detection and discomfort thresholds. Settings are chosen that boost speech to a comfortable level above threshold but not so much that the intensity is unpleasant.

(3) Comparison with previous cases. Subjective judgments are made based on clinical experience with other children who exhibited similar hearing losses. An aid is chosen which has proven beneficial in speech perception for other, comparable children.

Because none of these procedures is exact, hearing-aid evaluation should be considered an ongoing process, often lasting throughout much of the child's educational life (see Chapters 11 and 17).

Both the child and his parents must be made aware of the importance of routine procedures to maintain a hearing aid. These include keeping the device in good working condition, replacing the batteries when necessary, and cleaning accumulated wax from the earmold.

In most preschool programs for hearing-impaired children the parents are urged to take an active part in their child's auditory development. They may attend lectures, demonstrations, or classes on the nature of hearing loss and course of language development. Most early education programs provide instruction to parents on how to capitalize on daily home experiences and how to communicate about them with their hearing-impaired child. Because a child is more likely to attempt to talk and listen if the topic is something that interests him, appropriate home activities are suggested. The parents also are shown how controlling noise in the home environment and speaking close to the child's hearing aid increases the clarity of the amplified speech signal.

Early auditory training may take several forms. Listening games can be played with the child, which require him to perceive certain speech sounds, words, or instructions in order to participate in the play activity. These introductory listening activities are quite useful in familiarizing both the child and his parents with the use of a hearing aid in auditory tasks. They also serve to introduce the parents to their role in auditory training. The listening games are motivating to most children and can be used to maintain their auditory attention for long periods of time.

To many teachers and hearing clinicians, the first goal in an auditory training program is to make the child aware of sounds, especially the sounds of speech. The child can be taught how to indicate that he detects sound in some specified way (such as looking up or pointing to his ears whenever he perceives sound in the immediate environment). Speech *detection* is particularly important because it alerts the child that someone is talking and suggests that he look around to see whether the spoken message is intended for him. Awareness of the onset of speech should be a cue to the child to prepare for further listening and also to locate and attend to the face of the speaker for useful lipreading cues.

Once the teacher is confident that the child is able to use his hearing aid to detect speech reliably, he may advance to more complicated listening tasks. A common activity involves the auditory *identification* of spoken sentences that describe a recent activity or experience. These sentences may be written and illustrated on a set of large cards or may be listed in the form of an "experience chart story" (Figure 12-3). The teacher usually gives the children practice in saying these sentences and in identifying them through combined auditory-visual cues first. Then he covers his mouth and requires the children to listen. When he presents only the acoustic cues for each sentence (the sentences are presented in random order), the children must determine which one was spoken. Most hearing-impaired children are able to perform this listening task, given sufficient practice. Even if their hearing ability is very poor, they often are able to identify the sentences on the basis of their characteristic acoustic time-intensity patterns.

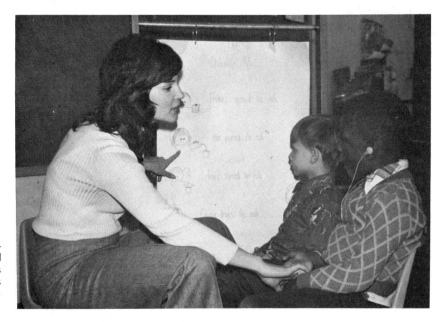

Figure 12-3 A teacher familiarizes hearing-impaired children with sentences that describe a recent class activity. *(Central Institute for the Deaf)*

Some teachers prefer to begin identification tasks with *words* as the speech material, in consideration of the difficulties some children have with remembering long strings of syllables. The early tasks may require the child to distinguish among a small set of words with different stress patterns (for example, *cat, turtle, hot dog, ice cream cone*). Later work of this sort might require the child to identify words among a set all having the same stress pattern, which is a more difficult task (for example, *dog, leaf, man*, or *airplane, baseball, popcorn*). Even more difficult listening practice would require the child to recognize words that are similar but for one or two vowels or consonants (for example, *knot, pot, pots* or *beet, bit, bet*).

If it seems that a child is having a great deal of difficulty with any of these recognition tasks, the teacher may decide that he needs special practice discriminating between certain words or sentences that differ in a particular way. *Same-different discrimination* tasks of this sort have been used as remedial activities in cases where children have a problem identifying (that is, labeling) specific speech stimuli. In a discrimination activity the teacher usually will pair two words, phrases, or sentences and ask the child if they sound the same or different (for example, *on the wall, in the hall*). In this way, both the teacher and the child can learn about the capabilities and limitations of the child's speech-perception ability and his hearing aid. In some cases the use of another hearing-aid volume setting may help the child make the desired discrimination. In other cases concentrated practice in attending to the minimal cues will help. In still other cases the child's auditory system may be so impaired that the distinction is not possible through audition alone, and he must use lipreading to achieve an awareness of the differences.

It should be mentioned that for profoundly deaf children, lipreading is the primary mode for the perception of speech. Acoustic cues serve mainly to supplement the visual mode. The pattern cues for speech that are provided by a hearing aid in these cases provide information about vowel articulation, consonant class, syllable number and stress, as well as gross cues for sentence structure (for example, pause and rate change). With instruction these cues all can become valuable supplements to the lipreader.

If the child's hearing capacities permit it, auditory *comprehension* of connected speech is the ultimate goal of any auditory training program. This skill involves the interchange of information through speech, and it requires more than simply pointing out or repeating the message that was received. The acoustic speech stimulus may stimulate the recall of images, develop associations, and elicit complicated behavioral responses in the child. Comprehension requires that the child understand the meaning of word sequences—that he develop an appreciation of acoustically encoded language.

This high degreee of appreciation of perceptual and cognitive complexity without benefit of visual cues (lipreading) can occur in some children only after many years of dedicated work by the child, his parents, and his clinician or teacher. Confidence in the child's ultimate success is important as well as hours of constant practice in receiving speech by piecing together messages from the distorted bits of information that the child perceives through his hearing aid(s). For a child with a severe hearing impairment, development of these skills requires familiarity with acoustic language patterns, established only with great effort. Even with speech comprehension ability sufficient to communicate over the telephone, most hearing-impaired children still need to depend on lipreading when the clarity of the message is reduced either by a careless speaker or by poor acoustic conditions.

The preceding paragraphs may seem to imply that auditory training should follow a quasi-developmental sequence of increasing complexity from detection of speech, through (remedial) discrimination, identification (recognition), and comprehension. This approach describes only a particular instructional point of view. A large number of teachers and hearing clinicians choose instead to employ connected speech first in auditory training, with expectations for the child's comprehension. In this approach, one communicates with the hearing-impaired child in approximately the same way as he would with a normal-hearing child. If difficulty in comprehension occurs, the instructor either may simplify the stimulus material, request a lower-level response from the child, or provide additional cues. For example, if the acoustically presented question "Does Steven's rabbit have long ears?" elicits no response from the child, then the parent or teacher might request auditory recognition of the single word "rabbit" to establish the situational context before attempting the original question again. This might be described as a "natural" approach with periodic remediation of observed difficulties.

COOPERATION OR COMPETITION AMONG THE SENSES

When acoustic conditions are poor, most people normally do not rely on hearing alone for understanding speech. In very noisy factories, even workers with normal hearing use lipreading in communication with one another. An unfamiliar language heard on radio or telephone often is more difficult to understand than it is in face-to-face speech. Even in the lecture hall, the student of a second language will understand much better if

he sits near the front so that he can watch the face of the speaker. Hearing-impaired people always are listening under less than optimum conditions, and they too must rely on visual information to support the auditory information. Numerous studies have shown that, regardless of one's hearing loss, his auditory-visual performance on a speech-perception test will be superior to his score when he either listens alone or lipreads alone. Chapter 13 treats the learning of lipreading. Here we are concerned with the interaction between lipreading and auditory perception.

The problem can be presented by means of an example. Suppose that a severely hearing-impaired student in auditory training has great difficulty hearing the distinction between the words *beet* and *boot*. The principal difference between these two words lies in the vowel, and one of the main differences between those two vowels is the presence of a second formant between 2000 and 3000 Hz for the vowel *ee* and the absence of such a high-frequency formant in the spectrum of the vowel *oo*. Let us suppose further that the student's hearing aid has adequate amplification in the frequency region between 2000 and 3000 Hz and that he also can detect sounds in this part of the spectrum. Because of his high-frequency loss, he may never have heard that high-frequency energy before he began using a hearing aid. We now must call his attention to its presence and train him in the distinction between these two vowels that will be based on perception of high-frequency sounds.

If the two confused words are *beet* and *boot*, however, even a listener with normal hearing can distinguish them perfectly well without any sound at all (through lipreading), because the shape of the lips is so different for the two vowels. Should auditory training be carried out under "real life" circumstances in which the student both hears and sees, or should we cover the mouth of the talker during such practice? And, conversely, if the instructor wants to clarify the visible difference between two speech sounds, should the student be permitted to listen to them at the same time that he is learning to distinguish them visually?

The answers to these questions depend considerably upon the intent of the spoken message. Both laboratory research and clinical experience have shown that nearly all hearing-impaired people understand speech optimally when they are able to lipread as well as listen through hearing aids. Thus, when communication of important information is the object of speech (at home or in the classroom), simultaneous attention to auditory and visual input is the best method to insure accurate perception of the message. For example, if a parent wants to explain for the first time how to build a birdhouse to his hearing-impaired child, he probably should do it through auditory-visual communication so that the child can comprehend the complicated instructions and new vocabulary.

When the goal, however, is to provide special practice for a hearing-impaired person in developing perceptual skills that are important for his speech communication, then concentrated effort in each sensory mode alone can be very beneficial. This is true even though most hearing-impaired persons usually combine audition and vision when they communicate, and for many with serious hearing impairments the acoustic input itself is not sufficient for comprehension. Clinicians often find it easier to direct the hearing-impaired person's attention to particular characteristics of words or phrases if the acoustic stimuli are presented in isolation from the visual speech cues that normally accompany them. And, of course, practice in auditory perception alone is necessary if one wishes to improve his communication by telephone.

The instructional strategy used by a clinician will depend partly on the auditory capacities of the hearing-impaired individual and also will be determined by the degree of success that the student has demonstrated in responding to acoustic input. For a person with a moderate-to-severe hearing impairment, a commonly used auditory training strategy is to present the speech material acoustically first. If the individual has difficulty with the auditory task, the clinician repeats or varies the stimulus several times *acoustically* before the listener finally is allowed to observe the talker's face for visual cues. This approach, which uses visual perception mainly for clarification or remedial work, is employed by clinicians who confidently expect their clients to learn to perceive speech through their ears. Directed acoustic-only stimulation of this sort can be very effective as an instructional method if it is used skillfully by an experienced teacher, clinician, or parent who knows how and when to introduce the visual input.

For an individual with a profound hearing impairment, many clinicians first will establish the language context audiovisually before attempting acoustic-only stimulation. This helps the client to associate his perception of certain gross acoustic patterns of speech with examples of previously learned language structures that are similarly patterned. Concentrated pattern-perception practice requiring detection, discrimination, and categorical identification of acoustic speech stimuli can be useful in helping the profoundly deaf client to recognize the occurrence of stressed words, prepositional phrases, or clause boundaries, all of which are important to successful auditory-visual comprehension of connected speech.

The question of whether to use an auditory-only or an auditory-visual approach becomes difficult when one considers auditory training in the education of the deaf infant or young child. It is clear that all children must learn to make many auditory-visual associations during their development, such as a dog and the sound of barking or a passing car and the sound of its engine. Such associations must be reinforced repeatedly for sound to become meaningful for an infant. The concern of hearing clinicians is whether vision should be excluded during speech communication with the child (the unisensory approach) or whether he should be allowed to lipread while listening to the speaker's voice (the multisensory approach). Those who advocate a unisensory method feel that if an infant with a serious hearing impairment is allowed and encouraged to use his unimpaired visual sensory system, he may never bother to attend to, and learn to use, those auditory cues that are extremely difficult for him. That is, if he is allowed to see the faces of talkers, he may not need to focus his attention on the sounds of speech. Those who support a multisensory approach feel that the infant should be allowed to take advantage of whatever auditory or visual cues for speech are available to him. The child should be allowed to develop an interactive organization of audition and vision for communication, using whatever speech information is accessible in each modality.

There is little evidence that clearly supports a choice between the unisensory and multisensory approaches. A direct comparison is difficult because strict application of either instructional method rarely is made. Teachers who prefer auditory-alone procedures tend to resort to auditory-visual input whenever the child has great difficulty perceiving speech acoustically, while the auditory-visual advocates often provide special listening activities when they are confident that the task will yield success. Both groups tend (perhaps unconsciously) to provide more acoustic stimulation to those children who seem to respond well to it and emphasize auditory-visual input with those children who appear to perform poorly acoustically. A more goal-directed approach for both groups might be to optimize each child's auditory and auditory-visual perceptual skills according to an evaluative/instructive outline like that shown in Table 12-1. With a clear description of a child's present abilities, a teacher or clinician could choose whatever system (auditory-only or auditory-visual) best meets the child's needs at the moment in order to bring the child to the desired goal in his perceptual development, regardless of the stated philosophy of the clinic or school. In addition to this sort of eclectic approach, an experimental attitude is desirable, in which the clinician or teacher would carefully observe and record the effects of particular therapies (based on certain philosophies) with a given child or group.

SUGGESTED READINGS AND REFERENCES

Erber, N. P. "Auditory-Visual Perception of Speech." *J. Speech Hearing Dis.*, 40:481–492 (1975).

——."The Use of Audio Tape-Cards in Auditory Training for Hearing-Impaired Children," *Volta Rev.*, 78:209–218 (1976).

——, and C. W. Greer. "Communication Strategies Used by Teachers at an Oral School for the Deaf." *Volta Rev.*, 75:480–485 (1973).

Fant, G. (ed.). *Speech Communication Ability and Profound Deafness.* Washington, D.C.: Alexander Graham Bell Association for the Deaf, 1972.

A collection of papers presented at a conference in Stockholm, Sweden, in

1972. Most of the research is concerned with the speech-perception abilities of hearing-impaired children and with recent developments in technical apparatus.

Hirsh, I. J. "Communication for the Deaf," in *Report of the Proceedings of the International Congress on the Education of the Deaf and of the Forty-First Meeting of the Convention of American Instructors of the Deaf.* U.S. Document No. 106. Washington, D.C.: U.S. Government Printing Office, 1964, pp. 164–183.

———. "Audition in Relation to Perception of Speech." In *Brain Function III: Speech, Language, and Communication,* E. C. Carterette (ed.). Berkeley: University of California Press, 1966, pp. 93–116.

Lowell, E. L., and M. Stoner. *Play It by Ear!* Los Angeles: John Tracy Clinic, 1960.

Simple materials and activities that parents and teachers can use in oral communication practice with young hearing-impaired children.

Pollack, D. *Educational Audiology for the Limited Hearing Infant.* Springfield, Ill.: Charles C Thomas, 1970.

A rationale for the "acoupedic" unisensory approach. Suggestions for auditory activities and case history information are included.

Ross, M. In *Amplification for the Hearing-Impaired,* M. C. Pollack (ed.). New York: Grune & Stratton, 1975.

Sanders, D. *Aural Rehabilitation.* Englewood Cliffs, N.J.: Prentice-Hall, 1971.

A text for teachers and rehabilitative personnel. The book discusses factors that affect speech perception by deaf children and describes several approaches to auditory training.

Simmons-Martin, A. A., *Chats with Johnny's Parents.* Washington, D.C.: Alexander Graham Bell Association for the Deaf, 1975.

A guide for parents of young hearing-impaired children. This booklet describes how to help a child develop oral communication skills through use of amplification and auditory experience.

Stark, R. E. (ed.). *Sensory Capabilities of Hearing-Impaired Children.* Baltimore: University Park Press, 1974.

Report of a conference held in Baltimore in 1973. New data on speech perception and language learning are presented and analyzed by researchers in a variety of fields.

Whetnall, E., and D. B. Fry. *The Deaf Child.* London: William Heinemman, Ltd., 1964.

A book for teachers and parents that describes speech acoustics, speech perception, and an auditory approach to development of communication in the deaf child.

Ann L. Perry, M.S.
S. Richard Silverman, Ph.D.

13

Speechreading

VISIBILITY OF SPEECH

Speechreading, or lipreading, is the skill that enables a person, regardless of whether his hearing is normal or impaired, to understand language by attentively observing the speaker. Spoken language is a rapid succession of some forty-odd phonemes, which have varying degrees of visibility; only about one-third of these are clearly visible. In general, the consonants are easier than vowels for the speechreader to see. As we see in Chapter 14, consonants are obstructed emissions of breath or voice, and it is the movement of articulators causing these obstructions that are visible to the speechreader. The vowels, particularly the short vowels, are extremely difficult for the speechreader to observe; they must be recognized by a fleeting mouth shape alone, and this shape varies with coarticulation. Fortunately, the vowel sounds, which are so difficult to see, are relatively easy to hear because they have more energy in the low and midfrequency range, where the majority of hearing-impaired people have useful residual hearing.

A speechreader must be able to recognize all the visible movements, and he must fill in those that are less visible. To help him fill in the gaps in what he hears and sees, he can learn to use the sensations that he imagines or actually feels in his own speech muscles as he watches the speaker. Even an expert speechreader, when puzzled, often silently imitates the movements he sees. This imitation helps him translate a visual image into a motor speech image,

The chapter on speechreading in the three earlier editions was contributed by Miriam Pauls Hardy, Ph.D. The editors are grateful for her review of this revision.

and usually with practice may increase its value as a cue.

The speechreader's identification of even the sounds he can see must always be tentative, however, because so many words are homophenous; that is, they look exactly like other words on the lips. The words *pair*, *bare*, and *mare*, for example, look identical to the speechreader. The visual pattern must be held in mind and automatically translated into meaningful language, but the speechreader must be ever ready to shift as he gets more information. From the context of the total message he will know which of a set of homophenous words "fits." This is not so very different from what all of us must do with words that sound alike, such as *their* and *there*, or *sow*, *so*, and *sew*. The speechreader simply has many more choices to make as well as blanks to fill.

The speechreader must be cognizant, too, of the rhythm and flow of connected speech. Each language has a characteristic rhythm, determined by its syntactical structure as well as by the pronunciation of specific words. An appreciation of this basic rhythm and syntactical order helps to fill in the many gaps in what is actually seen and heard. In addition, the stress patterns that reflect phrasing and emphasis markedly affect what the speechreader sees. Prolongation of certain syllables, and the pauses between syllables, carry important information. The same group of words said with different emphasis and phrasing has its meaning changed completely. Read aloud the following sentences, stressing the italicized word, and note the results. Then watch to see the difference in timing when someone else says them, and you will have a better appreciation of this point.

Good! By God, we're going to Kansas.
Goodbye, *God*. We're going to Kansas.
Goodbye. *God*, we're going to *Kansas*.

Even people with normal hearing do some speechreading. We have unconsciously learned that if we watch the speaker, we do not have to listen as intently. We get more information more readily when we can both see and hear the speaker. Most of us prefer to turn on the television, rather than the radio, to hear the President's address to the nation. We crane our necks to peer around a woman with a large hat or an elaborate coiffure sitting in front of us at a lecture. During a critical verbal exchange, we watch intently not only to concentrate on the spoken words, but also to take in facial expression, gestures, subtle changes of posture, and helpful situational cues. In noisy situations such as are found at large social gatherings, riding on the subway, or in industrial plants, we become even more dependent on visual cues.

There are wide variations in ability to speechread. Some people are "born speechreaders." The majority have reasonable facility in utilizing visual cues. But some find the speechreading process extremely difficult to learn. The factors that nurture the development of strong speechreading skills have been explored in various studies, which will be discussed later in the chapter. There is reason to suspect that not fully understood biological factors contribute to the process. The ability to speechread can be sharpened with instruction, determination, and practice, but individual differences in the overall level of performance seem to persist despite training, at least the kind of training commonly employed to date.

Because people with normal hearing are seldom in a situation in which they are dependent on speechreading, they are usually amazed, then intrigued, when it is demonstrated that they can and do speechread. On the other hand, the hearing-impaired individual is forced by the very nature of his handicap to utilize speechreading as a major support for diminished auditory information.

LANGUAGE AND SPEECHREADING

Language is one of man's highest achievements. It is a common symbol code. This code can be used to communicate in four different ways, or modalities. The receptive modalities, through which most people receive communication, are audition and reading. The expressive modalities, by which we communicate to others, are speech and writing. Because hearing impairment reduces a person's ability to receive speech information by audition, it becomes necessary to supplement listening with visual information obtained from watching the speaker. Speechreading and the various forms of manual communication may therefore be considered as additional receptive modalities. Similarly, manual communication may be a mode of expressive language for deaf persons who do not speak (see Chapter 15).

People with normal hearing learn oral language effortlessly as they listen to other people talk. Using auditory and kinesthetic feedback, they gradually refine their own vocalizations until they "sound like" the speech of others around them. This match of one person's speech to that of other speakers extends to the structural and lexical meaning he conveys, as well as the correct production of sounds and words. We internalize the linguistic rules of our native tongue to order, systematize, and give meaning to our sending and receiving of the common symbol code. It is a closely interlocked system as each input and output modality enhances the other.

The comprehension of language depends on rapid processing. From incoming bits of sequenced acoustic and visual events, language meanings must be derived within milliseconds. This requires good short-term memory as well as ready storage and retrieval from the long-term language memory bank.

For the reception of language, speechreading and reading are similar in some aspects. Both involve the association of visual symbols with spoken language. In learning either to speechread or to read there are two basic steps. The first step is decoding (recognizing) and holding in immediate memory a sequence of visual patterns. The second step is comprehending the decoded message by putting the pieces together meaningfully. Success in speechreading or reading depends on an adequate command of language. The adult who had language firmly established before acquiring a hearing loss has a problem very different from that of the child who has never heard or never heard well. Language is acquired slowly and painfully when the auditory system is defective. Unfamiliar language forms or vocabulary cannot be understood readily, either from the lips or from the printed page. Beyond these points, however, the analogy between speechreading and reading breaks down.

For many reasons, decoding spoken language (speechreading) is a more difficult process than reading the printed page. Fundamentally, they relate to control of the message. For the speechreader, the fleeting visual events which must be held in short-term memory are never fixed, and he cannot review unless the speaker repeats. The reader of printed words, in contrast, can proceed at his own pace and review as often as he likes. Speechreading is hindered by the wide variations in phoneme visibility. Furthermore, unlike in reading, there are variations in the visual patterns that are presented by different speakers even when speaking the same material. The speechreader is further affected by lighting, distance from the speaker, the angle at which he must speechread, and other factors that frequently cannot be controlled when speechreading. A major difficulty for many beginning speechreaders arises from confusion of speech sounds seen on the lips with the spelling patterns they are accustomed to reading. The difficulty is compounded when instructors use material for speechreading practice that is intended to be read. This is not appropriate, because the vocabulary and sentence structures of conversation are typically much simpler than those of written language beyond about a third grade reading level. Conversation is more redundant but less coherent than written language. And abrupt changes of topic and incomplete sentences are common problems for the speechreader in conversation, although they occur rarely in good writing. In talking, there are no pauses between words as there are on the printed page. For example, "plenty of potatoes" has the same number of syllables as "plenipotentiary." Both are said within the same time span, with no division between syllables. The division into words is an interpretive process that takes place in the mind. It is never seen on the lips or, for that matter, heard by the ear. In a sense there is no oral punctuation. A speechreader must also be aware that speakers often refer to the present situation and people or objects nearby, without naming them; in written material these are described and/or named. Use of situational cues, gestures, and body language are at least as important in speechreading as visual perception of the phonemes spoken. If there is any analogy to the reading process here, it would be that speechreading is something like reading a picture story, where at least as much information is obtained from the pictures as from the captions underneath, although both are necessary to complete understanding of the message.

Speechreading thus involves many processes similar to scanning the printed page. But it demands more in terms of visual perception, visual memory, and visual "fill-ins." Errors are inevitable for the speechreader, and good speechreaders have well-developed strategies for checking, or giving "feedback," to be sure they have put the pieces together correctly or to obtain the pieces they missed.

FACTORS IN SPEECHREADING

The factors that contribute to speechreading ability have been suggested by experienced teachers, by research investigators, and by speechreaders themselves. Research findings may be organized under two principal headings. The first is *perceptual efficiency,* which in this context refers to the ability to perceive speech elements rapidly. Associated skills are visual acuity, attention span, speed of focusing, and use of peripheral vision to get information from the entire face while focusing on the mouth. The second principal factor in speechreading is *synthetic ability,* by which the speechreader augments the words and phrases he can identify with whatever linguistic and situational cues are available, to discern the gist of the message. The concept of flexibility is one of the most important in this group of subskills, which are cognitive in nature. The quality of language learning, use of amplification, and certain other factors also contribute to synthetic speechreading ability.

Perceptual Factors

Experience has shown the importance of perceptual proficiency in speechreading. The visual perception of speech sounds and perceptual closure are probably the most important processes involved in the rapid and accurate identification of isolated speech sounds or words. This assumes good vision, and even minor deviations in visual acuity may result in lower speechreading scores. Visual memory is involved, but the extent and nature of its contribution to the speechreading task have not been determined. The peripheral cues of facial expressions and gestures seem to enhance speechreading performance if appropriate, but tend to decrease performance if inappropriate. Visual distractions or degree of facial exposure appear not to affect performance.

It is generally agreed that most speechreaders benefit from training in visual perception and visual memory early in a course of instruction. With or without auditory cues, the acquired ability to categorize speech sounds enhances speechreading performance. The improvement tends to plateau once all the categories have been introduced, however, and further development of speechreading skill seems to depend on synthetic ability, which requires longer periods of training before results become evident.

Synthetic and Linguistic Factors

Although there is disagreement about the contribution of perceptual proficiency to the total speechreading task, a reasonable estimate is about 40 percent. Because the cognitive and linguistic skills that comprise the other 60 percent are much harder to quantify, research data are scarce. It has been suggested that innate talent may be involved, making it easy for some people to learn speechreading, and difficult or impossible for others. Good speechreaders are also known to be highly flexible, revising tentative identification of a message whenever necessary.

Another aspect of synthetic ability may be knowledge of linguistic rules. For deaf children, language proficiency is highly correlated with speechreading ability. Although there appears to be no correlation between speechreading skill and general language ability among adults who already possessed adequate language when their hearing failed, it can be assumed that none of this group has deficient language competence that would inhibit understanding of ordinary spoken messages. The ability to fill in missing words that were not visually perceived also strengthens speechreading skill. This ability may well be a corollary of language competence.

Speechreading difficulty increases as a function of sentence length and structural complexity. Phrases are easier to speechread than single words or complete sentences. Most subjects obtain a better score with spondee stimulus words (for example, *baseball*), with equal accent on both syllables, than with other two-syllable words such as *pumpkin* (accent only on the first syllable) or *giraffe* (accent on the second syllable). All two-syllable words seem to be easier than monosyllables. Familiarity of the words and the number of response possibilities are thought to be important factors influencing the test results for any class of words, however.

When a speechreader encounters homophenous words, at least three types of linguistic clues are available to help him avoid errors. Verbal context (sequential redundancy) enables the speechreader to make a logical guess based on the language preceding and following homophenous words. In the case of *pair, bear,* and *mare,* for example, any of the three words might fit in the expression, "I looked at a ———." But as the speaker continues saying, "I looked at a ——— of shoes in the store window," only the word *pair* makes sense. The natural verbal redundancy, or circularity, of conversational speech gives the speechreader a "second chance" to perceive the same thought expressed in different words. The speaker in the example above might go on to say, "I hadn't decided what kind of shoes I wanted. But the pair on display caught my fancy." And finally, the speechreader may use an intuitive knowledge of the probability that a given word was spoken (distributional redundancy), based on its relative frequency in spoken English. Even without other clues, the speechreader is likely to perceive the word *pair,* rather than *bear* or *mare,* because people say *pair* more often. In the perception of single speech sounds, the speechreader's unconscious knowledge of linguistic constraints is also helpful; he will "see" only the phonemes that occur in his language.

Psycholinguistic Implications

Psycholinguistic studies have generated models for the developmental sequencing of language skills. Such studies have been an impetus for earlier and earlier intervention when language development does not meet expectations for chronological age. The concept that natural language skills are acquired in the first few months of life is now generally accepted. This has led to the movements for screening of hearing in newborns, for parent-infant programs, and for preschool classes. All such programs for the hearing-impaired must include attention to speechreading.

At the other end of the age continuum, an emerging body of literature and experience has significance for older speechreaders. Many investigators have questioned the stereotype of intellectual decline in the elderly, documenting that some cognitive functions may improve or even emerge in the seventh or eighth decade of life. But there is no question that older people are slowing down in psychomotor responses and in the processing of sensory information. They also give evidence of difficulty with divided attention (cannot do two things at once). Not only are they unable to react quickly, but decline of their senses, especially vision and hearing, limits the sensory information accessible at all. There is evidence that auditory, visual, and auditory-visual scores all decrease as

age of the subjects increases. As a group the elderly have more trouble learning than younger people but can probably remember equally well once the task is mastered. Of course, this varies with background and state of health. The task of geriatric aural rehabilitation in this country is growing. As of 1977 those over the age of 65 comprise about 10 percent of the population, and a substantial portion, if not all, have some degree of hearing loss. The "aging ear" constitutes a growing responsibility for audiology.

Looking and Listening

As we have said, speech sounds are not all equally visible. The traditional classification scheme of all English speech sounds into twelve consonant and four vowel visemes—that is, visually distinguishable categories—by nearly all the early teachers of lipreading is probably correct, although it has occasionally been challenged and modified. Perhaps the number of discernible categories varies from person to person or from one environment to another. In any case, there are far fewer visually distinctive speech sounds than the approximately twenty-four consonant and twelve vowel phonemes available to those with normal hearing. Sets of two or three phonemes represented by the same viseme result in homophenous words, which we discussed earlier.

Fortunately, most speechreaders are able to complement visual information with auditory cues. The homophenous consonants are identical in place of articulation (visual information) but not in manner (auditory information). Auditory training appears to help hearing-impaired people to distinguish among voiced, voiceless, and nasal consonants, and thus to distinguish among homophenous possibilities. For example, the listener may discriminate auditorially among the homophenous words *dune, tune,* and *noon* if he recognizes that the initial consonant is voiced for *dune,* unvoiced for *tune,* and nasalized for *noon.* The vowels are categorized by the relative amount and direction of mouth opening, and increments from one vowel to another in the same category are not easily discriminated. Ask a friend to stand on the other side of a closed door with a window, and to say softly the words *beat, bit, bet,* and *bat.* Now ask him to say *beat* and *bat* in random order; you will not find it hard to distinguish them. But ask your friend to say all four words in random order, and you will no doubt have difficulty. *Bit* will be confused with *beat* and with *bet; bet* will be confused with *bit* and *bat.* The speechreader who supplements visual information with auditory cues generally performs better. Turn on a radio, then repeat the experiment above with your friend in the same room as you and see how much better you do. Even normal-hearing listeners receive more information through combined auditory-visual input than through either alone, especially in noisy situations.

The precise influence of hearing level on speechreading has not been established, although hard-of-hearing subjects perform better on most tasks than the profoundly deaf —presumably because of the greater contribution their hearing makes in learning new language and in perceiving it through combined looking and listening. Intelligence, educational achievement, age of hearing loss onset, and personality factors show no consistent correlation with speechreading ability. When the research literature does not agree with the experience of teachers and clinicians, investigators must determine which cause-effect relationships are involved in the speechreading process, and which are artifacts of the research procedures. At least some of the discrepancies may be attributed to variations in definition of the speechreading task, training procedures and materials used, adequacy of controls, and selection of the experimental subjects.

METHODS OF TEACHING SPEECHREADING

Conventional Approaches for Adults

Before 1940 help for the hard-of-hearing adult was limited chiefly to a series of thirty or more speechreading lessons. A number of methods were developed by hard-of-hearing individuals who became interested in helping others after they themselves learned to speechread. There were few college courses on speechreading before World War II; the training for instructors tended to emphasize known approaches rather than underlying theory.

Anyone preparing to teach speechreading today should read the textbooks written by the pioneers, especially Bruhn, Nitchie, Kinzie, Bunger, and Ewing. They tend to be overly structured, and the materials and procedures they outline in detail are not always appropriate vehicles for the skills they propose to develop. But they do contain the distillation of years of experience and hard-earned wisdom that is not available elsewhere. Many people have learned to speechread by each of these methods. There is no evidence to date that one approach is more effective than another.

An eclectic approach that draws from each of the traditional methods to meet the individual needs of a student or group is the most common "method" used today. Careful review of the traditional methods reveals more similarities than differences. All stress the need for synthesis rather than too much analysis. In varying degrees they all stress the value of auditory and kinesthetic cues as adjuncts to visual cues. All systematically employ syllable drills using a particular movement or position, then provide practice using it in words, sentences, and stories; the major differences lie in the way the speech positions and movements are presented to the student so that he learns to recognize and discriminate among them on the lips. All but the Jena method proceed from the most visible to the least visible elements, and from simple to complex language forms in a sequence of lessons.

The Jena method is unique in its presentation of an overall introduction to phonetics in the first few lessons, followed by rhythmic syllable drills and talking-together exercises to enhance automatic recognition. Its proponents hold that this makes for the interlocking of speechreading with auditory training and speech production. Lessons are centered around topics rather than a single speech sound, as in the other methods.

Group and Individual Instruction

Cogent arguments can be made for both group and individual instruction. Group teaching is more efficient when professional services are limited, as well as being less expensive for the student. However, the students must all have about the same aptitude for the task so that the material can be challenging, but not overwhelming, for each member of the group.

Screening tests administered before instruction usually demonstrate that prospective students fall into three groups in facility for speechreading: excellent, average, and poor. Tests administered to these same individuals after a period of instruction show that, although each student demonstrates improvement, he tends to remain within the same relative groupings. This suggests that these differences are significant and should be respected.

Individual instruction has the advantage

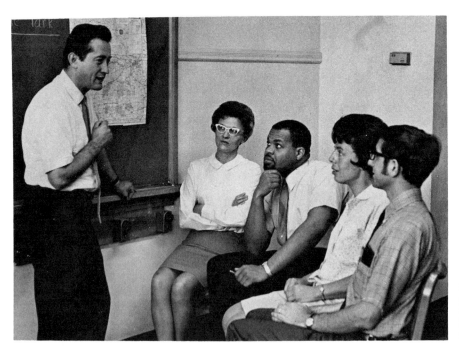

Figure 13-1 Group instruction in speechreading. *(Central Institute for the Deaf; photo by Harold Ferman)*

of being flexible to the immediate needs of each student. It is essential for those who have had their hearing suddenly wiped out by illness or trauma and are plunged into a silent world. This is a catastrophic experience that requires immediate expert management on a highly individualized basis.

The effectiveness of group instruction was demonstrated in the military hearing rehabilitation programs during World War II, where it was necessary, because of the pressure of numbers, to plan the most efficient and effective program for a large turnover of hospitalized patients with a limited staff. It required adapting old techniques and creating new ones. However, the advantages of well-planned group instruction were retained on their own merits. Results can often be obtained with a group that are difficult to achieve with individual instruction. The association with others, similarly handicapped, continually reminds the student that his case is not unique. He is less inclined to self-pity, and he profits by the successes, the observations, and even the errors of his classmates. The element of competition enters, and the interplay of personalities as well as the spontaneous comments of the group produce the easy natural atmosphere favorable for learning. These same comments develop the student's ability to anticipate, as well as the mental flexibility to deal with, abrupt changes of subject. It provides a rich experience with the speech patterns of the varied personalities within the group.

SPEECHREADING IN THE TOTAL PROCESS OF HEARING REHABILITATION

As we see throughout this book, advances in the medicine and the surgery of the ear and the emergence of clinical audiology as a professional field have done much to improve our understanding and management of auditory disorders. With the perfecting of the modern wearable aid, speechreading is no longer considered the only help. Nevertheless, it holds its own as an integral part of a total hearing rehabilitation program.

A careful diagnostic evaluation is the first step in any hearing rehabilitation program. For certain individuals, a complete physical examination, with various specialists contributing to the total picture, may be required. Any indicated medical or surgical treatment should be carried out, not only for improving hearing but for general health. The audiologic evaluation not only should measure the nature and degree of the hearing impairment, but, what is even more important, should assess the total communicative function of the individual and the communicative demands of his particular "world" and how he can be better prepared to meet them.

Detailed communicative evaluations as well as psychological appraisals are indicated for children. The psychological evaluation should be a sophisticated one that does not penalize the child for his language retardation and the effects of sensory deprivation, yet establishes a reasonable estimate of his intellectual potential and points up factors that interfere with learning. The objective is to describe as fully as possible the child's capabilities and limitations so that an effective program can be initiated. It must be recognized that a significant number of children with hearing impairment have multiple problems. In addition to the hearing loss, there may be a language disorder, other specific learning disabilities, attentional peculiarities, limited intelligence, or emotional problems to complicate the learning process. These must be identified if the child is to have an appropriate program to help him learn through and around his difficulties (see Chapter 17).

If otologic and audiologic findings indicate a hearing aid, its selection should be guided by the audiologist, and he should help the subject learn to use it as effectively as possible over a period of time (see Chapters 11 and 12). With this kind of management, it is possible to plan a training program that is hand-tailored to the needs of that individual. There are rarely two similar, much less identical, problems; one is dealing with people, not "ears."

The experience gained in the military rehabilitation programs during World War II laid the groundwork for current concepts of hearing rehabilitation. In a military organization one has complete control over the patient and his time. Thus it was possible to have concentrated daily instruction for four- to eight-week periods. Such a program is not practical for the average adult engaged in earning a living or managing a busy household. Thus most programs must be worked out in terms of feasibility as well as need. Such a concentrated program might profitably be considered, however, for hard-of-hearing children for whom little or no special help is available in their local community. With an intensive short-term program, even in a residential facility, many children who are now floundering could better maintain themselves in the regular educational stream (see Chapter 17). We need imaginative approaches, for the hard-of-hearing child is far too often a neglected youngster in our schools.

The major role of the itinerant speech and hearing clinician in the public schools is not just giving the child speechreading lessons or auditory training, or struggling to correct an off-pressure 's,' but ensuring that the child's vocabulary and language are expanding as rapidly as possible. As we see in Chapter 17 most hard-of-hearing children have mild-to-severe language handicaps, which contribute the major obstacle to their progress in the regular classroom. Curricular tu-

toring as indicated, as well as other kinds of imaginative supportive help, should make it possible for most hard-of-hearing children to keep up with their peer group.

Two basic approaches are required: First, the individual must understand the nature of his hearing impairment and face objectively the problems it poses, and he must be helped to assume responsibility for meeting them. It is profitable to instruct the members of the family so that they better understand the problem and learn how they can and must help. With schoolchildren, this information needs to be given to the classroom teacher as well as to the parents. Second, the three aspects of the communicative process —speechreading, auditory training, and speech conservation and correction—must be developed in a close-knit fashion, with emphasis on which aspect is most pertinent for the individual. There can be no "cookbook" approach.

Just as important as the initial otologic and audiologic evaluation is regular reassessment over the years by the otologist, the audiologist, and other specialists who may be needed. The physical status may change, the hearing loss may vary, and hearing aids may wear out. The nature of the problems that arise, particularly for children, shifts in the process of growth and maturation. The problems are not static, and there can be no single diagnosis that provides "the truth" for all time.

PRACTICAL ADVICE FOR THE SPEECHREADER

Speechreading is seldom easy, because so many critical factors cannot be controlled. A poorly lighted room that throws deep shadows on the speaker's face or a seating arrangement that forces the speechreader to look into a bright light are deleterious. The friend who attempts to help by buttonholing the speechreader merely presents an additional problem. At close range the speechreader cannot readily follow the speech, nor can he observe any situational cues. Approximately 6 feet has been found to be the most comfortable distance. Furthermore, it is well worth the speechreader's efforts to seek a position from which he can observe most comfortably all members of the group without facing the light. Confusing and disturbing movements and noises only serve to divert his attention and increase his fatigue.

As we have pointed out, the very character of speech itself presents a major problem. Ideas must be grasped in a fleeting instant, for speech is never static. Much of it is invisible, and every new combination of syllables produces minor changes in the individual sounds. No two mouths are alike; no two individuals' speech patterns are identical. Poor speakers impose a burden, for their articulation is careless and indistinct and therefore hard to see. *The greatest help is good quiet speech.* The well-intentioned person who shouts or exaggerates his speech pattern only increases the difficulties. One who covers his mouth or turns while talking, or has annoying mannerisms, presents similar problems. Likewise, it is well-nigh impossible to follow the speech of a man who has his teeth clamped on a pipe or has a cigarette dangling from his lips. An impassive, expressionless face is more difficult than a mobile one. The considerate speaker, however, can materially reduce all these problems.

The sociable person, keenly interested in people and events, usually makes rapid progress in speechreading, whereas the shy, reserved individual and the unimaginative, phlegmatic type are at a disadvantage. The secret of successful speechreading lies in the ability to grasp an idea intuitively and develop its meaning without attempting to follow every word. A too literal person, or one who clings tenaciously to a preconceived idea about where the conversation is headed, always has serious difficulties. An illuminating answer was given one of the authors by a relatively uneducated pupil. Pressed for an explanation of his unusual skill in speechreading, he replied "Well, Missy, I figures out where you're going and I beats you there!"

Essential as it is to be on the alert to catch significant trends and changes in a conversation, it is also true that undue tension and fatigue may cause a mental "block." Therefore the speechreader must strive to maintain a happy balance.

From the outset, a speechreader needs a sense of humor to help him surmount many failures. Speechreading can best be improved by constant practice in everyday living rather than by repeated returns to the classroom. The student's progress depends largely upon himself, for the teacher can only chart the way. The student's intelligence, application, and determination are vital factors in achieving success. It cannot be too strongly emphasized that a person with a hearing loss should frankly face this fact. The natural tendency is to ignore the hearing impairment or to attempt to conceal it. These efforts, even though partly successful for a time, lead to an increasing strain. Eventually both social and business life will be affected.

A handicap in hearing can be successfully overcome only by the efforts of the individual himself. Instruction and guidance will provide the groundwork. Continual practice of speechreading in daily contacts will usually develop the skill to carry on a normal life comfortably.

Anyone with a hearing loss should profit from the following suggestions.

1. Only the person with a hearing handicap can overcome it. Teachers and friends cannot do it for you; instruction and guidance merely point the way for your own application to the task.

2. Your continual practice of speechreading in daily contacts will help you develop the skill to carry on a normal life comfortably.

3. Remember that hearing is the natural and normal way to understand speech. Thus the hearing-impaired should learn to make the best use of an appropriate hearing aid.

4. Combine looking and listening to provide better understanding of speech, with less strain, than either used by itself.

5. Keep relaxed, but remain alert and tuned in.

6. Anticipate what may be said, but be ready to shift as the message develops.

7. Do not expect to get every word. Follow along with the speaker, and key words will enable you to put two and two together.

8. Develop a sense of humor so that inevitable mistakes are not regarded as setbacks.

9. Confront the fact of a hearing loss honestly and do not attempt to hide it from others. They will know that some problem exists, and it's better to tell them the truth than to leave them bewildered or to let them arrive at their own mistaken conclusions.

10. Inform others that their best way to help is by quiet natural speech. When they shout, exaggerate lip movements, cover their mouth, or talk to you from the next room, it is your responsibility to educate them; they are only trying to help, and have no idea they're actually making it harder for you.

11. Stage-manage situations to facilitate speechreading whenever you can. A good light on the speaker's face is important, but avoid facing a bright light yourself. Keep about 6 feet between you and the speaker so that you can observe the entire situation.

12. Consider the noise factor when choosing where you will carry on conversations. It is easier to hear in smaller rooms with upholstered furniture and sound-absorbing materials on the walls, ceiling, and floor. This is particularly true if you wear a hearing aid.

13. When joining a group, try to determine the topic of conversation immediately. Friends can be coached to give an unobtrusive lead, such as "We are discussing the housing problem."

14. Keep abreast of national and local current events. You will be a more interesting conversationalist and will be better able to follow the comments of others.

15. Remember that conversation is a two-way affair. Do not monopolize it in an effort to direct and control it.

SUGGESTED READINGS AND REFERENCES

Berger, Kenneth W. *Speechreading, Principles and Methods.* Baltimore: National Educational Press, 1972.
   A textbook emphasizing research findings and their application to the teaching of speechreading.
Black, J. W., P. P. O'Reilly, and L. Peck. "Self-Administered Training in Lipreading," *J. Speech Hearing Dis.,* 28:183–186 (1963).
Bruhn, M. A. *The Muller-Walle Method of Lip-Reading.* Lynn, Mass.: The Nichols Press, 1929.
Bunger, A. M. *Speech Reading—Jena Method.* Danville, Ill.: The Interstate Press, 1954.

Deland, F. *The Story of Lipreading*. Washington, D.C.: Volta Bureau, 1968.
> *An authoritative account of how lipreading instruction evolved, by a former superintendent of the Volta Bureau.*

Erber, N. P. "Auditory-Visual Perception of Speech," *J. Speech Hearing Dis.*, 40(4):481–492 (1975).

Farwell, R. M. "Speech Reading, a Research Review," *Amer. Ann. Deaf.*, 121(1):19–31 (1976).

Frisina, D. R. "Speechreading," *Report of the Proceedings of the International Congress on the Education of the Deaf and of the Forty-First Meeting of the Convention of American Instructors of the Deaf*. U.S. Document No. 106. Washington, D.C.: U.S. Government Printing Office, 1964, pp. 191–207.

Haspiel, G. S. *A Synthetic Approach to Lip Reading*. Magnolia, Mass.: Expression Company, 1964.
> *Graded lipreading lessons for hard-of-hearing children in elementary school, designed to focus the child's attention on ideas rather than on the speaker's lip movements per se.*

Jeffers, J. "The Process of Speechreading Viewed with Respect to a Theoretical Construct," *Proceedings of International Conference on Oral Education of the Deaf*. Washington, D.C.: Alexander Graham Bell Association for the Deaf, 1967, pp. 1530–1561.

———, and M. Barley. *Speechreading (Lipreading)*. Springfield, Ill: Charles C Thomas, 1971.
> *A comprehensive text dealing with historical background, visibility, principles, methods, practice material, and tests.*

Kinzie, C. E., and R. Kinzie. *Lip-Reading for the Deafened Adult*. Philadelphia: The John C. Winston Company, 1931.

Nielsen, H. B., and E. Kampp (eds.). "Visual and Audio-Visual Perception of Speech," *Scandinavian Audiology*. Supplementum 4, Stockholm, Sweden: The Almquist & Wiksell Periodical Company, 1974.

Nitchie, E. B. *New Lessons in Lip Reading*, Philadelphia: J. B. Lippincott Company, 1950.

O'Neill, J. J. "Frontiers of Research in Visual Communication," *Proceedings of International Conference on Oral Education of the Deaf*, Washington, D.C.: Alexander Graham Bell Association for the Deaf, 1967, pp. 1562–1571.

———, and H. J. Oyer. *Visual Communication for the Hard of Hearing, History, Research, and Methods*. Englewood Cliffs, N.J.: Prentice-Hall, Inc., 1961.
> *A textbook for prospective teachers of lipreading. Recommended for its overview of procedures and materials useful in testing lipreading performance and devising individualized programming.*

Sanders, D. A. *Aural Rehabilitation*, Englewood Cliffs, N.J.: Prentice-Hall, Inc., 1971.
> *A theoretical approach to rehabilitation measures for speech and hearing disorders, geared to advanced students in professional training programs. Cites pertinent research findings in linguistics, psychology, phonetics, communication theory, physics of sound, and education.*

S. Richard Silverman, Ph.D.
Donald R. Calvert, Ph.D.

14

Conservation and Development of Speech

Speech normally is controlled by the ear. Of course in this context when we speak of the ear we mean the ear-brain system. Nowhere is this more clearly shown than in the way a baby learns to talk. At first the baby can only cry. Some weeks after his birth he begins cooing, gurgling, and laughing. He then seems to enjoy lying in his crib and entertaining himself by listening to his queer noises. Without realizing it, he is building connections between his ear and his voice. As he listens to his own randomly produced sounds, he is beginning to learn muscular control of his speech mechanism. Before long he passes into the "parrot" stage, in which he amuses himself by repeating noises over and over. He keeps himself happy by saying trains of syllables like "ba ba ba ba" or "da da da da." He is now on the brink of learning his first words, for his parents respond to some of the syllable trains in his babbling. For example, when he says "da da da da," his mother may get his doll. She may also say "doll" as she hands it to him. This is an important moment. His babbling has controlled another person. He has also heard that person say a syllable that is very close to the sounds he is making. On another occasion his mother may say, "Do you want your doll?" as she hands him the toy. The child is likely to parrot her and say "da da da . . ." His mother's pleased smile again rewards him. A few more experiences like this and he will have learned to babble "da" whenever he wants his doll. He is now well on the road toward learning to talk. All he needs is time; time for added experiences, time to learn new words through hearing them, and time to master vocal control by hearing his own speech.

The control the ear exerts over speech is revealed differently by the adult. Habits of hearing become so fixed that an older person has trouble mastering the pronunciations of a new language. His ear fails to distinguish new patterns from the ones to which he is accustomed. Erroneous impressions thus serve as the person's guide in speaking the new language. He talks with a foreign accent. For example, many Latin Americans have no need in their native Spanish to distinguish b and v except at the beginning of words. They consequently do not always use b and v correctly when they speak English.

EFFECT OF HEARING LOSS ON SPEECH

Because it is natural for the ear to be the channel through which we learn to talk, a serious impairment in hearing will hinder a child's normal development of speech. Furthermore, because the ear serves as a guide to accurate control of the speech mechanism, degeneration of speech often follows hearing losses that occur later in life.

The most obvious example of the role played by hearing in acquisition of spoken language is furnished by the child who is born totally deaf. Unless special training is undertaken, of the kind described in Chapter 17, such a child never learns to talk. He grows up mute. His deafness closes for him the door through which he would normally acquire both knowledge of speech and control of the speech organs.

The child who hears low frequencies well but is insensitive to middle- and high-frequency tones faces a different problem. It is likely to be years before this child's defi-ciency is discovered. Because he can hear low frequencies, he reacts to many of the sounds in his world. People, seeing his response, reason that his hearing is normal. They fail to realize how distorted and imperfect are his impressions of sound. Confusion is this child's lot. He misses the acoustical elements that give speech its distinctive character. One outcome of this confusion is slow and uncertain development of his use of language. Moreover, the child incorporates in his own speech only the imperfect distinctions that he perceives in the speech of others. The result is a mushy and slurred pattern of talking that may border on the unintelligible.

Any substantial loss of hearing that exists at birth or occurs soon thereafter will hinder both language development and the establishment of adequate speech habits. Two factors are responsible. First, the hearing loss reduces sharply the number of listening experiences that the child has and thus slows up the process of learning to talk. Second, losses of certain types make it impossible for the child to distinguish some of the elements in speech. No child will learn to pronounce distinctions he does not hear, unless of course he has special guidance.

Speech defects may arise as the result of hearing losses that begin after childhood. If the ear can no longer serve as a monitor when one talks, slow degeneration of speech results. The sharpness and precision of enunciation disintegrate. The melodies of speech become monotonous. Intonations lose their life. The quality of the voice becomes rigid. Finally, control over the loudness of the voice suffers.

THE NATURE OF SPEECH

Speech may be considered from many points of view. It may be analyzed acoustically, relating the body's vibrating and resonating systems to the acoustical properties of the sounds of speech, namely frequency, intensity, and duration. Considered physiologically, the emphasis may be on interaction of muscles, cartilage, and bone, or on neurological activity such as excitation, transmission, integration, and responses of the body's nervous system. Viewed psychologically, speech is concerned with personality, self-expression, and such processes as motivation, attention, perception, recognition and memory. Speech also has a sociolinguistic base as the prime vehicle for symbolically expressing meaning through language and as an important medium through which humans interact among themselves. We can understand better the problems of speech which grow out of auditory impairment if we consider three primary factors that influence speech intelligibility. These are *articulation*, *voice*, and *rhythm*.

Articulation

The process of shaping the breath stream from the larynx out through the mouth to form the speech sounds of language is called articulation. The fundamental units of articulation that influence meaning are called *phonemes*. Phonemes are abstractions, somewhat like an averaging of those sounds that actually occur in connected speech. In the words *tea, cat, stay,* and *cattle* we recognize a recurring common sound represented by the letter "t." It is made slightly differently in each of the words but has some common distinctive features of manner and place of production.

Place of production of a sound refers to that part of the speech mechanism involved specifically in the production of the sound. Such structures as the lips, teeth, alveolar or gum ridge, the palate, the velum or soft palate, and the tongue articulate to obstruct and

thus change the acoustic characteristics of the flow of breath and voice passing through the oral cavity, the pharynx, and the nasal cavity.

Manner of production describes the way in which speech sounds are produced. Four classes of manner of speech sound production are *stops, fricatives, affricates,* and *resonants*. The production of stops, sometimes called plosives, is accomplished by interruption of the breath stream by a closure within the oral cavity. The stop action has two phases called the *implosion* (closure) and the *explosion* (release). Stop phonemes include /b/, /p/, /t/, /d/, /k/, and /g/. The formation of fricatives requires constriction of the breath stream with audible friction. Fricative sounds include /f/, /v/, /θ/ (thin), /ð/ (this), /s/, /z/, /ʃ/ (shoe), /ʒ/ (measure), /ʍ/ (white), and /h/. Many other speech sounds include some degree of frication in their production but are not dependent on friction for their perception. Affricates are sometimes called "stop-fricatives" because they combine a stop sound immediately followed by a fricative sound in the same syllable. During the stop portion of the affricate, the fricative position is anticipated by tongue movement so that the release of the stop produces the breath stream for production of the fricative portion of the affricate. Illustrative affricates are /tʃ/(chair), /dʒ/ (jam), /ks/ (box), and /kʍ/ (queen). Resonant sounds depend primarily on alterations of voice resonance for their recognition. Resonant consonants include the nasals /m/, /n/, and /ŋ/ (thing), the glides /w/, and /j/ (yes), the lateral /l/, and the /r/. Consonants are conventionally classified by manner and place of production.

Vowels are also the result of resonance. They are relatively sustained and strong sounds. They are produced by initiating a tone in the voice box (larynx) and passing this tone through the mouth cavity, which is formed into a relatively open channel. Differences between vowels are achieved by shaping the mouth channel distinctively for each vowel. The tongue and the lips play a particularly important part in this shaping. Each vowel is actually a distinctive pattern of pure tones produced by the resonances of the various chambers of the mouth and nose. It is by means of this distinctive pattern that the listener identifies the vowel. Typical vowels (and their phonetic symbols) are those found in the following words: *seat* /i/, *sit* /ɪ/, *set* /ɛ/, *sat* /æ/, *saw* /ɔ/, *soot* /ʊ/, and *suit* /u/.

Diphthongs are blends of two vowels. They are produced by shifting the mouth channel from one vowel position to another while the sound continues. Acoustically, the tone initiated by the voice box is "resonated" as for a vowel, but in this instance the distinctive feature is the glide from the initial pattern of resonance to the final one. Typical diphthongs are those appearing in the following words: *boy* /ɔɪ/, *bay* /eɪ/, *bough* /aʊ/, and *buy* /aɪ/. An arrangement of consonants and vowels frequently used in teaching deaf children is shown in Figure 17-5.

The influence of adjoining sounds on individuals phonemes is called *coarticulation*. Coarticulation may affect both production and perception of speech. For example, the place of production of /k/ varies with the vowel that follows or precedes it. The point of elevation of the tongue for the /k/ phoneme is forward on the palate for the syllable /ki/ while it is farther back on the velum for /ku/. Vowels are similarly influenced by the consonants around them. Note for example the difference in duration of the vowel /i/ in the words *eat* and *ease* as the result of the difference in the consonant following and terminating the vowel. The transitional and durational cues present in coarticulation of running speech give the listener important perceptual information about adjoining phonemes.

Voice

Voice is produced by the actions of *respiration*, *phonation*, and *resonation*. These occur simultaneously and cooperatively to produce changes in pitch, quality, and loudness of the voice. Respiration is accomplished by a complex interaction of muscles of the thoracic and abdominal cavities. In normal breathing the relative durations of inhalation and exhalation are about the same. But when speaking, the duration of exhalation in a single respiratory cycle is about ten times as long as that of inhalation and may be as much as fifty times as long for practiced speakers. Since no more breath is used in speaking than in the exhalation of regular breathing, the extended duration of exhalation during speech reflects a remarkable economy in using the breath stream in order to produce and sustain connected speech. This economy is realized by the efficient and synergistic functioning of the respiratory muscles, the larynx, and articulators. The process of the larynx acting on the exhaled breath stream as it passes through the glottis to create voice is called *phonation*. During phonation the vocal folds follow this rhythmic cycle: closing of the glottis, increasing of air pressure beneath the glottis, bursting apart of the folds from the air pressure and emission of a puff of breath, and closing of the folds again under constant muscle tension and with decreased air pressure. Air pressure beneath the glottis increases and the cyclical pattern is repeated. The resulting periodic puffs of breath produce the sound of voice. The frequency of puffs of air from closing and opening of the glottis determine the *fundamental frequency* of the voice. Change in the fundamental frequency of voice is accomplished by complicated interaction of the tension, length and mass of the vocal folds, accompanied by changing the subglottal air pressure.

When there is a considerable increase in air pressure below the glottis, the vocal folds are forced farther apart during their close-open-close cycle. This increase in vocal-fold amplitude is accompanied by an increase in the amount of air emitted and thus an increase in the perceived loudness of the voice. In producing rhythmic closure of the glottis for the fundamental frequency the vocal folds set up secondary vibrations, which create overtones called *harmonics*. The harmonics of the voice are influenced by cavities of the vocal tract through which voice passes: the trachea, pharynx, oral cavity, and the nasal cavity. These cavities are set into vibration themselves by the flow of vibrating voice passing them. In vibrating they reinforce some harmonics of voice more than others, further modifying the voice. This process of modification is called *resonation*. The combination of fundamental voice frequency, *overtones of the vocal folds*, and characteristics of resonating cavities contribute to a complex of relations we refer to as *voice quality*. Most English speech sounds are made primarily with oral voice resonance, with the oral cavity open at the mouth and the velopharyngeal port closing off the nasal cavity at the pharynx. With nasal consonant /m/, /n/, and /ŋ/, the nasal cavity is opened and the oral cavity is closed by action of the lips or tongue.

Rhythm

Rhythm refers to the prosodic, temporal, or patterned features of speech, or sometimes as the "melody" of speech. These features are rhythmic because they recur in patterns. Rhythm is generated by changes in voice and articulation, and usually by a combination of the two. Changes in intensity, frequency, and duration combine to produce varying "time envelopes" that constitute the fundamental cues for perception of rhythm. For speech rhythm, the basic unit is the syllable. The essential features of speech rhythm are *accent, emphasis, intonation, phrasing,* and *rate. Accent* involves stress within a word of one syllable over another. It is produced primarily by increasing voice intensity and by making stressed syllables longer. It is fundamentally characteristic of English that every word of more than one syllable has a stressed syllable. Improper accent can hinder speech intelligibility. *Emphasis* is achieved by giving increased stress to a word in a phrase. Like accent, it is produced primarily by a combination of increased intensity and increased duration of syllables within the stressed word but may also be achieved by pauses surrounding words. Emphasis does not have a set pattern characteristic of the language as does accent, but is used to communicate speaker intent. *Intonation* is accomplished by changing pitches of syllables. Intonation patterns are described ·by the direction of pitch change, the degree of change, and by absolute pitch levels. Patterns of intonation are governed both by individual characteristics of talkers and by commonly used patterns comprised of many syllables to give listeners additional language information without using additional words. To signal the end of a declarative sentence, for example, we commonly use a falling pitch on the last word of the statement.

Phrasing, a continuous utterance bounded by silent intervals, ignores the boundaries of words and deals with syllable clusters. Phrasing helps understanding by organizing words into groups related to units of thought. Which words get linked and the varying durations of pauses are left to the speaker's judgment, although there are some conventions in the language. By increasing the duration of the pauses, the speaker takes into account the information absorption rate of his listener for different kinds of content and in differing listening environments. *Rate*, the number of syllables uttered per unit of time, is affected by both stress and phrasing patterns. Stressed syllables are typically longer in duration than unstressed ones. In phrasing, the quantity of units of speech decrease with the greater the number and duration of pauses. In conversational speech we average five to six syllables per second or about two hundred and seventy words per minute.

Nonauditory Cues

Another way to view speech production is to consider the direct information about speech that can be made available to the visual, tactile, and kinesthetic senses along with audition. These possibilities are no more forcefully illustrated than in the use to which they are put in the speech instruction of profoundly deaf children.

Visual Cues

Visual cues offer the deaf child his main approach to the experience of communication. He sees the facial activity that is the visible aspect of speech, notably articulation. By proper guidance he can be taught to attend to these facial activities as meaningful signals of the wishes and intentions of others. He can thus be started on the road to speechreading and mastery of language (see Chapter 13).

Tactile Cues

Through the sense of *touch*, the deaf child learns that the visible movements of speech are accompanied by a modulated flow of the breath and by vibration. Although he cannot hear the sounds produced as the breath is modulated by the larynx, tongue, and lips, the deaf child can be made aware of many tactile cues that will help him understand the nature of the process. For example, the skilled teacher places the child's hand in front of her mouth as she articulates plosive consonants such as /p/ or /b/. The child is trained to feel the momentary gust of air escaping from the mouth as the plosive is released. Similarly, a hand placed on the cheek receives vibratory sensations when vowels are produced. The nasal consonants produce agitation that can be felt on the nose, and all voiced sounds give rise to vibration that can be felt at the Adam's apple (larynx). These various tactile cues are among those used, not only to make the child aware of major phases in speech production but also to teach him to control his own speech mechanism. By alternately feeling the effects produced as the teacher speaks and then attempting to achieve the same effects with his own speech organs, the child learns techniques of sound production and enunciation.

Kinesthetic Cues

In the final analysis, the deaf child must control his speech primarily through the sensations he receives from effects occurring within his own body. These internal sensations are called *kinesthetic cues*. They are of various types, such as feelings of jaw movement, tongue movement, position of the lips, position of the soft palate, nasal vibrations, and laryngeal vibration. During the initial stages of training, the teacher may even manipulate the child's organs of speech so that they execute patterns of movement that the child must learn. The purpose is to get the child to feel the kinesthetic cues that characterize each movement. Furthermore, as the child is required to control his own speech through vision and touch, kinesthetic sensations will also occur. With the passing of time he learns to rely upon these kinesthetic sensations to tell him what he is doing. Thus whereas the person with normal hearing judges the adequacy of his speech by the way it sounds, the deaf child must base the same judgment on the way it feels.

SPEECH AND POSTLINGUAL HEARING LOSS

Speech production may deteriorate in a number of ways when serious hearing loss is sustained following the development of speech and language (postlingual). With sudden bilateral hearing loss, caused by such diseases as mumps or meningitis, speech is usually maintained intact for a short time and then begins to deteriorate rapidly, depending upon severity of the loss. With gradual loss, as in presbycusis or otosclerosis, speech deteriorates slowly as hearing loss progresses. Defects of articulation usually appear first. Distortion or omission is typical of speech sounds characterized by low intensity and high frequencies such as /s/, /ʃ/, /tʃ/, /f/, and /ɵ/. Consonants in the final position in words are particularly vulnerable to erosion. Abnormalities of voice quality, control of volume, and irregularities of speech rhythm may follow as hearing deteriorates.

CONSERVATION OF ADEQUATE SPEECH

As we have already pointed out, the occurrence of a substantial loss of hearing may cause deterioration in speech. Such a situation exists when the auditory impairment does not occur until after normal patterns of speech have been firmly established. Thus, it is a situation that affects only older children and adults. Furthermore, the deterioration in speech is neither instantaneous nor complete.

Speech Insurance

The facts just mentioned call for a special type of training based on the concept of *speech insurance*. Stated differently, the person we are discussing enters the ranks of the hearing-impaired with normal habits of speech. The main educational task is to teach him to *retain* these habits in order to conserve the skill he already has. *If training can be started soon enough after the hearing loss occurs, no deterioration in speech need result.* The technique is to give the person substitute channels for controlling his speech efforts, since his ear no longer serves as a fully effective monitor when he talks.

Only under two circumstances is it necessary to combine speech reeducation with the program of speech insurance. Sometimes the hearing loss has existed long enough so that deterioration in speech is evident, and sometimes the person has a speech defect that is independent of the hearing loss. In either event, faulty habits must be broken. They must be replaced by adequate habits, and at the same time the substitute channels of control must be learned.

When the hearing loss is complete (or nearly so), speech insurance must depend mainly on learning effective use of kinesthetic cues. To this end, the person with extreme loss must first become acquainted with the nature of the speech process. He must understand the activity that he wishes to control. He must learn to preserve the phonetic elements of speech by becoming fully aware of the kinesthetic distinctiveness of each element. Second, he must develop awareness of the bodily sensations associated with proper control of melody, quality, rhythm, and emphasis. In the third place, he must maintain physical alertness, facial expressiveness, and spontaneous gestures. Naturalness in speaking depends in part upon abandoning oneself to the act of communication.

It is of fundamental importance for the person to learn to maintain effective control of the loudness of his voice. A speaker ordinarily adjusts the loudness of his voice to the situation in which he is talking. In fact, the adjustment is so natural that few people even realize it takes place. The speaker has unconsciously learned to raise his voice when background noise is strong or when the listener is at a little distance. We find that our voices are tired after conversing while riding on the bus. Our efforts to talk over the din of traffic lead us unconsciously to shout, and a half hour of shouting tires the voice. By contrast, we unconsciously soften our voices in quiet surroundings. In other words, *we tend to maintain a favorable margin between the loudness of our speech and the background noise*. We thus achieve intelligibility without talking so that our listeners find our speech unpleasantly loud.

A person learns the proper balance between the loudness of his speech and his acoustic surrounding in the same way that he learns other features of acceptable speech —by the experience of hearing himself talk. Through his experience the ineffective levels of loudness are given up in favor of levels that result in successful communication.

A hearing loss disturbs the ability to adjust the level of one's voice to the needs of the moment. Two factors enter the picture. For one thing, the person with impaired hearing will miss much of the background noise. Thus, he has an imperfect gauge of the requirements of the moment. In the second place, the speaker with a hearing loss may receive a false impression of the loudness of his own voice. When the loss is of the sensorineural type, his own voice sounds faint. Such a person has a tendency to talk loudly, regardless of the surrounding circumstances. In doing so his voice reaches a level where it seems of normal loudness to him. The reverse effect occurs when the loss is of the conductive type. Here the speaker's voice is transmitted effectively to his own ear by bone conduction. His voice seems to him so much stronger than other sounds that he of-

ten softens it until the balance between his voice and the background noise is more to his satisfaction. Such a person tends to talk more faintly than he should, and as a consequence he is hard to understand.

Successful mastery of control of loudness is particularly difficult. However, two measures allow a reasonable solution to the difficulty. The person must first master the ability to talk at each of four or five general levels of loudness. He must learn to shift at will from one level to another. These levels, which are under kinesthetic control, must range from soft speech to very loud speech. Second, the person must study and classify typical sound environments. With the help of his instructor, he can learn what level of background noise he is most likely to encounter in each type of situation. He can then meet the requirements of loudness with reasonable success by speaking at the level (of the five he has learned) that is ordinarily demanded by the situation at hand. Furthermore, an alert talker will notice when his listeners are having difficulty responding to his speech and will raise his voice to the next level. He thus avoids relying rigidly on a set of rules in situations in which it happens that the rules do not apply.

PROBLEMS OF PARTIAL HEARING LOSS

When the hearing loss is partial, both the need for speech insurance and the techniques necessary to achieve it depend upon the degree and pattern of the hearing loss. The primary requisite is to retain, insofar as possible, control of speech by the ear. *Here a good hearing aid can be of great help*, since it may raise to a usable level many elements of the wearer's own speech that are inaudible to him without the instrument.

The task of speech conservation then divides itself into two phases. To the degree that components of speech remain inaudible even while the hearing aid is being worn, the person must be taught kinesthetic control of speech. Second, if some components that are made audible by the instrument are reproduced somewhat "unnaturally," he will require auditory training in interpreting his own speech. For example, when wearing a hearing aid, the person must learn to make allowances for changes in the way phonetic elements sound through his instrument. Otherwise, he may modify his articulation to satisfy his own unschooled ear and thus achieve an enunciation that is less effective for his listeners. Another example involves the loudness of speech. A peculiar situation often exists because the wearer's own voice seems extremely loud to him through the hearing aid. The balance between his own voice and the background noise is entirely different without the aid from what it is when he is using the instrument. This difference will work to his disadvantage unless he is taught to accept a balance that he does not particularly like but that is most acceptable to the listener.

Progressive Hearing Loss

Special considerations are required when the hearing loss has been diagnosed as one that is progressive. The auditory impairment may not at the moment be sufficient to endanger the patterns of speech. However, the future outlook may demand that a program of speech conservation be begun immediately. A full system of kinesthetic control over speech should be built while the patterns of speech are still good and while it is still easy for the person to understand instructions from the teacher. The person can thus be prepared to apply kinesthetic control when his hearing drops to the point where this control becomes necessary.

Training in the conservation of speech is best obtained from teachers or clinicians who have been specifically prepared for their type of work. They are to be found in schools offering special work for hearing-impaired children, in hearing and speech clinics, aural rehabilitation centers, and similar organizations. Children needing guidance in speech conservation can often get help through schools, and both adults and children have access to speech and hearing clinics.

Family and friends can help the person who is fighting the threat of speech deterioration. As with other problems the first step is to find a qualified teacher and enlist his participation. The second step is to cooperate fully with the teacher. The cooperation can be extensive since the person in training can profit from much drill at home. The student needs the help of either a relative or a friend. Following specific instructions from the teacher, this assistant, who must have both normal hearing and normal speech, serves as a monitor who corrects errors made by the student as he works on his drills. And finally, members of the student's immediate social circle can build favorable morale by taking a positive and sympathetic attitude toward his misfortune and toward his efforts.

Prelingual Hearing Loss

If hearing loss is present at birth or is acquired before normal speech and language have developed (prelingual), then speech comprehension and its production are drastically affected. Furthermore, hearing loss reduces the frequency of language listening experiences of the child. Consequently, the mechanical difficulties in speech production encountered by the prelingually hearing-impaired child is compounded by the deficiency of his knowledge of the phonologic, semantic, and structural features of language. He must know the right word, place it in the right order, and avoid syntactic error. Even if he is able to do all of this properly, his language may suffer from the impoverishment of variety. Therefore, the task for the prelingual hearing-impaired child is essentially one of *development* of spoken language rather than its conservation. And this is usually performed in the larger context of special education described in Chapter 17.

If all other conditions are equal, the attainment of spoken language by the prelingually hearing-impaired child is most likely determined by the degree and frequently the kind of his hearing loss and the extent to which this is recognized in providing amplification. Obviously, the greater the information about the features of speech perceivable over the auditory channel the greater is the probability that speech production will benefit accordingly. Figure 14-1 relates the degree of impairment to an estimate of the amount of information features of speech. In Chapters 12 and 17 we see the possibilities for developing and improving speech production through constructive use of residual hearing.

And some children, particularly the profoundly deaf, will also require intensive use of nonauditory channels to develop, improve, and maintain speech.

MAINTENANCE OF SPEECH

Whether a hearing loss occurs before or after speech and language development, the hearing-impaired adult will continue to need support for speech. In addition to direct help, the following suggestions may be helpful:

1. *Constant usage:* There is no substitute for continual use of speech in all situations, not only to practice self-correction but also to reinforce confidence in its value.

2. *Maximum use of amplification:* As we have stressed for children, the adult should maintain and use the best possible acoustical amplification. Hearing and hearing-aid evaluation should be carried out periodically by professionally qualified persons, and promising new hearing aids should be tried.

3. *Awareness of speaking situations:* A hearing-impaired person can help his naive listener in a number of ways. Among these are:

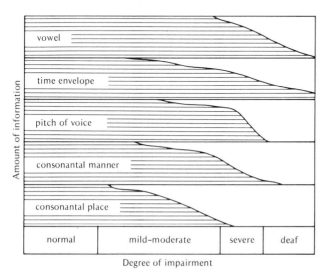

Figure 14-1   A gross composite estimate of the information features of speech related to severity of hearing loss. *(Courtesy of James D. Miller, Central Institute for the Deaf)*

(a) Helping the listener to speechread. In any stressful listening situation, whether because of ambient noise, competing messages, or deviant speech of a talker, the listener seeks supplementary visual cues. The hearing-impaired talker should place himself in a position so that his face is clearly visible.

(b) Helping the listener to hear. Develop sensitivity to the requirements of the acoustical situation frequently, but not always, detectable by a hearing aid. The masking effects of noise, of whatever origin, and the influence of distance from the listener should be understood. If it is necessary and practical, a quiet place should be sought for conversation.

4. *Preparing the listener:* The listener can be helped and even put at ease if at the outset he is given a sample of small talk such as "I'm glad to meet you," "How are you?" or "Good morning."

5. *A second chance:* When a listener does not understand speech, a hearing-impaired person should not assume that the listener understood *none* of what was said. He probably understood part but not enough to "put the pieces together" for complete understanding. The sentence should be repeated with *exactly* the words as first spoken. The listener will have a second chance to fill in what was first missed. Of course, if the listener does not understand the repeated sentence, the speaker must then change the wording and resort to intentional redundancy. Here is a situation where economy of verbalization should not apply.

6. *Another ear:* It is advisable for the hearing-impaired talker to develop a special relationship with a person with normal hearing who can act as a constructive and sympathetic critic of his speech. Care should be taken that the friend's judgment is not blunted by "getting used to" the speech. The "other ear" may, if desired, be a properly qualified professional who understands and is able to meet the distinctive speech needs of adult hearing-impaired speakers.

SUGGESTED READINGS AND REFERENCES

Denes, P. B., and E. N. Pinson. *The Speech Chain; the Physics and Biology of Spoken Language.* Baltimore: Williams & Wilkins Company, 1963.
   A popular but accurate treatment of our knowledge of communication by speech by workers at the Bell Telephone Laboratories.
Fairbanks, G. *Voice and Articulation Drillbook.* New York: Harper & Row, 1960.
Gray, G. W., and C. M. Wise. *The Bases of Speech,* 3d ed. New York: Harper & Row, 1959.
   Speech treated from the following bases: social, physical, physiological, neurological, phonetic, linguistic, psychological, genetic, and semantic.
House, A. S. (ed.). *Communicating by Language: The Speech Process.* Bethesda, Md.: U.S. Department of Health, Education and Welfare, National Institute of Child Health and Development, 1964.
   Report of a 1964 conference of investigators and clinicians at Princeton, N.J., dealing with the perception of speech, speech behavior, the structure of the linguistic code, development and deficits in language skills, produc-

tion of speech, disorders of speech production and perception, neural mechanisms and models, man-machine communication, and machine analogies of human communication.

Lieberman, P. Intonation, Perception, and Language, Monograph 38. Cambridge, Mass.: Massachusetts Institute of Technology Press, 1967.

Analysis of some linguistic aspects of intonation. Discusses in detail the breath group as both a physiological and linguistic event. Presents a theory of the development of intonation in the very young infant.

Malmberg, R. (ed.). Manual of Phonetics. Amsterdam, Holland: North-Holland Publishing Company, 1970.

A scientific and current treatment of phonetics.

Pickett, J. M. (ed.). "Proceedings of the Conference on Speech-Analyzing Aids for the Deaf, Hearing and Speech Center, Gallaudet College, Washington, D.C., 1967," Amer. Ann. Deaf, 113(2): 116–330 (1968).

This issue is devoted to the proceedings of a 1967 conference on speech-analyzing aids for the deaf. A substantial portion of the issue is concerned with the use of instruments to transmit information about speech to the hearing-impaired and aimed at the development and improvement of their speech.

Travis, L. E. (ed.). Handbook of Speech Pathology and Audiology. New York: Appleton-Century-Crofts, 1971.

A massive reference work of more than 1300 pages containing much fundamental information on speech production. The bibliographies are impressively extensive.

Winitz, H. Articulatory Acquisition and Behavior. New York: Appleton-Century-Crofts, 1969.

A book attempting to "bring articulation, as studied by the speech pathologist, within the mainstream of present-day psycholinguistic thought." Methods and models of descriptive linguistics, instrumental phonetics, and learning theory related to articulatory behavior and correction.

Zemlin, W. R. Speech and Hearing Science: Anatomy and Physiology. Champaign, Ill.: Stipes Publishing Company, 1964.

A good treatment of the fundamentals of the subjects of the title.

Rachel I. Mayberry, M.S.

15
Manual Communication

Everyone uses manual communication to some extent. We beckon people to us, wave them away, point to things we want, and illustrate the size of the fish we caught. Manual communication is simply sending information with our hands and arms and receiving information with our eyes. The manual communication used by hearing people to elaborate oral-language messages depends on environmental context for its information content. Thus it is a secondary information source. On the other hand, the manual communication used by many deaf individuals and educators of the deaf does not depend on environmental context for its information context. Thus it is a primary information source.

There are two categories of manual communication serving as a primary information source. The first category consists of manual communication that is independent of oral languages. We shall refer to this category as *sign languages*. The second category consists of manual communication that is derived from oral languages. We shall refer to this category as *sign systems*. Only after we understand the characteristics of sign languages and sign systems are we in a position to ask appropriate questions regarding the complex issues underlying the use of manual communication in education and rehabilitation of the deaf.

This chapter was completed while Ms. Mayberry was a graduate student in the School of Human Communication Disorders, McGill University, Montreal.

SIGN AND ORAL LANGUAGES

Sign languages are independent of oral languages in much the same way that one oral language may be independent of another. This independence is best illustrated by the major similarities between sign and oral languages. First of all, sign and oral languages are both the creation of human communities to meet their communicative needs. Second, both kinds of languages are acquired as first languages by the children of these communities. Third, both sign and oral languages are structured information codes. Their structure consists of three linguistic levels: (1) *phonetic* or *cheremic*—the pattern of the physical signal; (2) *syntactic*—the relationship of the symbols; and (3) *lexical-semantic*—the organization of the symbols' meanings. The fourth similarity is that translation from any sign or oral language into another sign or oral language requires varying degrees of reorganization at each linguistic level. Just as we are unable to translate literally from Hebrew into English, we also are unable to translate literally from American Sign Language into Chinese Sign Language or spoken French. Finally, like oral languages, sign languages form genetically related groups as a result of linguistic migration and evolution. There are greater structural likenesses within groups than between groups. For instance, Scandinavian oral languages are structurally closer to one another than they are to Semitic oral languages. Similarly, French sign languages are structurally closer to one another than they are to Asian sign languages.

There are, of course, major differences between oral and sign languages. Obviously, the primary difference is that oral languages are transmitted and received through the oral and auditory modalities—through the mouth and ears—whereas sign languages are transmitted and received through the manual and visual modalities—through the hands and eyes. The extent to which the transmission and reception modalities determine the linguistic structure and human use of language has probably been underestimated in the past. A second difference is that because sign languages evolve within oral-language environments, they are influenced by oral languages, whereas oral languages are never influenced by sign languages. Finally, the geographical boundaries of sign languages are not identical to those of oral languages. For example, users of American and British sign language experience great difficulty understanding one another, but their speaking counterparts do not.

AMERICAN SIGN LANGUAGE

The sign language about which we have the most information is American Sign Language (ASL; sometimes also known as Ameslan). ASL, one of a number of sign languages with ties to old French Sign Language, is used in both the United States and Canada. (French-Canadian Sign Language is also used in Quebec and a variation of British Sign Language is also used in Nova Scotia.) A general discussion of ASL should clarify the characteristics of sign languages in general.

Origin and Development

In 1760 the Abbé Charles Michel de l'Epée became interested in the instruction of deaf children and shortly thereafter established France's first school for the deaf, the National Institute for Deaf-Mutes. From Lane's translation of de l'Epée's documents (1976), it appears that many of de l'Epée's students came to his school with gestural systems of their own invention. Once gathered at the Institute, the students shared their gestural systems with one another, creating a common gestural system. De l'Epée and his successor, the Abbé Roch-Ambroise Sicard, observed and used these gestures as a basis for classroom instructions. This was the beginning of French Sign Language. (The students' gestural system bore little linguistic resemblance to spoken French; though both de l'Epée and Sicard were aware of this, they were unsuccessful in their attempts to alter the students' gestural communication into a form closer to spoken French.)

In 1816 Laurent Clerc, a deaf instructor at the Institute and one of Sicard's outstanding pupils, accompanied Thomas Gallaudet to the United States. French Sign Language was thus about 50 years old when Clerc taught it to Gallaudet and the teachers of the school Gallaudet established in Connecticut. French Sign Language undoubtedly had some influence on the gestural systems that were already in existence in the United States.

During the next century and a half or so, the young sign language continued to evolve until it became a complex sign language guided by the communicative and cultural needs of those who have used it. This is the sign language known as ASL. Today nearly 500,000 deaf individuals use ASL as a means of communication. It is only recently, however, that we have begun to learn very much about the structure of this language that is the fourth most commonly used—after English, Spanish, and Italian—in the United States (O'Rourke, 1975).

Cheremic Characteristics

Cheremes   In all sign languages the equivalent to the word is the sign. Signs are made with the dominant hand performing most of the work within the space in front of the body bounded by the top of the head and the bottom of the hands. It was William Stokoe who first recognized that every sign can be analyzed into at least three components: (1) the *place* on the body where the sign is made; (2) the *shape* of the hand or hands making the sign; (3) the *movement* of the hand or hands. Because these components are meaningless in themselves, yet integral to every sign, they are roughly analogous to the phonemes of oral languages. Stokoe labeled these components *cheremes* (kéreemz). Place cheremes are called *tabula* or *tab*. Handshape cheremes are called *designation* or *dez*. Movement cheremes are called *signation* or *sig*. Some recent investigators have concluded that the *orientation* of the hands is also a group of cheremes.

When we change a phoneme of a word, the word changes meaning, such as *pat* to *pet*. Likewise, changing a chereme of a sign alters the sign's meaning. (As is the case for phoneme changes, chereme changes may also result in nonsense.) For example, the sign *mother* consists of touching (sig) the thumb of an open hand (dez) to the chin (tab) with the palm facing to the left (orientation). If we change the tab chereme to the forehead, keeping all other cheremes the same, the sign becomes *father*. Using the cheremes for *father* but changing the sign chereme to a movement away from the forehead creates the sign *grandfather*. Changing the dez chereme of *grandfather* to a hand with the thumb tucked in results in the sign for *hello*. Finally, changing the orientation chereme of *hello* to the palm turned away from the face results in nonsense. Stokoe has proposed that all ASL signs are made from 55 cheremes: 12 tab, 19 dez, and 24 sig.

Like phonemes, cheremes can be further analyzed into distinctive features. Recent experiments by Lane, Boyes-Braem, and Bellugi have suggested that there are 11 distinctive features for ASL handshapes (dez). Undoubtedly distinctive features for places (tab), movements (sig), and orientations will also be found.

Cheremes in signs   Some further analogies

between cheremes and phonemes will help us understand what signs and signing are like. First, there are allowable and disallowable combinations of cheremes based on rules. These rules, in turn, may result from the perception and production characteristics of the visual and manual modalities. In English there are many phonetic combinations we recognize as possible words and others we recognize as impossible, such as /læz/ versus /lzæ/. A comparable example from ASL is a potential but nonexistent sign consisting of: dez—both hands in a closed fist with the little fingers extended; sig—touching; tab—the temples; orientation—palms out. Achieving the same combination of cheremes by crossing the arms is not a possible sign. Another useful analogy is that cheremes and signs, like phonemes and words, are not static, but subject to variation. Variation among signers is exactly like dialectal or individual differences among speakers. Variation of signs within sentences is the result of "motor preplanning"; that is, a sign's cheremes are modified depending on which signs precede and follow it, similar to the modifications producing the "gonna" and "lotsa" of spoken English. Incidentally, these variations, which frustrate the student of foreign oral languages, also frustrate the student of sign languages.

Suprasegmentals   As is the case for connected speech (see Chapter 14), sign-language discourse has prosodic or suprasegmental characteristics determined by the intent of the signer. The end of an idea or sentence is signaled by both the pause length and final resting place of the hands. This is in front of the stomach or chest for a declarative sentence and slightly higher with a longer pause for a question. The breadth of movement during signing is akin to the intensity dimension of speech: wide and high movement is like loud speech, whereas restricted and small movement is like whispering. The sharpness and speed of movement accompanied by varying facial expression provide intonation contours that affect the meaning of sentences, similar to the contrast between "*He* must leave" and "He must *leave.*"

Lexical-Semantic Characteristics

Vocabulary   It has been estimated that there are probably not more than 6000 signs in the ASL vocabulary. This relatively small store of signs, compared to the 600,000-word vocabulary of English, may make us wonder how ASL signers manage to communicate all the ideas of which English speakers are capable. The apparent disparity becomes less startling when we know that the typical English conversation involves a vocabulary of less than 3000 words. Most people who use ASL also use a backup system known as fingerspelling, which we shall discuss later. Fingerspelling allows the direct borrowing of any English word or of any foreign word that can be spelled with the Roman alphabet.

There are several reasons why ASL's vocabulary, which is growing, is not comparable to that of English. ASL is a very young language as far as languages go and does not have the multitude of historical-lexical inputs that English has enjoyed. Also, additions to the vocabulary of a language are often the result of direct borrowings from other languages, as "kindergarten" and "filet mignon" have come into English. For obvious reasons, sign languages probably borrow vocabulary more easily from one another than from oral languages. If this is the case, we need to remember that ASL has been relatively isolated from other sign languages.

When we make vocabulary comparisons between ASL and English we run the risk of thinking of ASL as a gestural cipher or writing system for English. Since ASL has no written form, we must talk about signs by using English words. However, just as the meanings of the words of one language are not equivalent to the meanings of the words of another language, the English words we use to translate ASL signs are often not precise meanings but close approximations. There are many ASL signs that are very difficult to translate into English. Bellugi and Klima have observed, for instance, that ASL vocabulary is rich with signs for "ways of looking" that do not have English equivalents, such as *to-look-away-in-disdain, to-do-a-double-take,* and *to-make-eyes-at-someone.*

Transparency Perhaps the effect transmission and reception modalities have on the structure of language (mentioned above) is clearest at the lexical-semantic level of ASL. In the past ASL has been characterized erroneously as iconic in nature or limited to concrete concepts. It is easy to see how ASL gives this impression. Many signs bear some visual resemblance to what they symbolize, such as the signs *house, book,* and *tree.* From this it follows that if a language can symbolize only what can be drawn in the air, then its ability to symbolize what cannot be seen is severely restricted. Actually, ASL's vocabulary includes numerous abstract concepts, which can be discussed as easily in ASL as in English. The deceptive aspect of ASL is that some signs for both concrete and abstract concepts convey visual clues or hints of their meanings. This is called *transparency.* Perhaps the characteristics of the manual and visual modalities make the transparency of sign languages more striking than the onomatopoeia of oral languages.

Evolution of signs If we were suddenly restricted to using our hands and eyes to communicate, we would try to imitate the shape or action of what we wanted to symbolize. This is what happens in the game of cha-

rades; the more accurate the imitation or drawing in the air, the more effective the communication. This is precisely the way in which many signs began. On a regular basis our elaborate imitation would be very time-consuming, cumbersome to produce, and fatiguing to watch. To circumvent these problems we would stylize and abbreviate our gestures. As a matter of fact, in 1872 Charles Darwin hypothesized that the words of oral languages and the signs of sign language evolve from an imitative to a stylized form due to the pressure to communicate rapidly.

Cheremic evolution By comparing the shapes of French and ASL signs from the early nineteenth century up through those of today, Frishberg has documented such an evolution. The shapes of signs move from an imitative to a more arbitrary form. This cheremic evolution is guided by *ease-of-perception* and *ease-of-production* principles. One-handed signs made below the neck evolve into two-handed signs with the hands reflecting one another in handshape. Since the sign receiver focuses on the sender's face, the area below the face is in peripheral vision. Two identical hands are easier to see, not to mention being easier to produce signs with. For the same reasons, signs that were once made to the side of the body are now made in the center of the body. Signs that formerly consisted of two movements have evolved into one-movement signs and are therefore easier to produce and less distracting to watch. Yet in some signs a trace of the original imitative form often persists, such as the shape of a house, the action of opening a book, or the form of a tree. It is these visual clues or *iconic traces* that give many signs their transparent quality.

Semantic evolution In the late nineteenth century Wilhelm Wundt observed another kind of sign evolution. Studying the signs of North American Indians and German deaf children, Wundt noticed that the meanings of signs evolved from concrete to abstract concepts and speculated that this might also be true for oral languages. For example, a sign might begin as referring to "mule." Later in time the meaning of the sign would be narrower, referring to "mule's head." Finally the meaning might refer to an attribute of mules in general—"stubbornness." Semantic evolution and cheremic evolution occur simultaneously.

Today the ASL sign *stubborn* is suggestive of a mule's ear. The sign's shape is stylized and conforms to the ease-of-perception and ease-of-production principles. However, a naive observer of the sign *stubborn* can usually select its meaning when given alternatives from which to choose, or will exclaim, "Of course!" when told the sign's meaning, and will even use the association of "mule" to help remember how to make and recognize the sign. The sign that is so reminiscent of a mule to the naive observer is a visual linguistic symbol for the concept "stubborn" to the ASL user, no different from the English speaker's acoustic linguistic symbol /stʌbɚn/. It is probably the transparency of both "concrete" and "abstract" signs that has led past observers to the mistaken conclusion that ASL is iconic in nature or limited to concrete concepts. Transparency is the unique result of language evolution in the visual and manual modalities and in no way diminishes ASL's communicative efficiency or topic range.

Syntactic Characteristics

Like the English speaker, the ASL signer constructs utterances according to syntactic rules and finds it difficult to explain these rules. If a foreign speaker should ask us how to construct the past tense in English, we would probably have to consult a grammar text in order to delineate the rules underlying our several examples. Linguists have only begun to unravel ASL syntax, so this is probably the linguistic level about which we know the least. However, modality effects clearly exert a strong influence on ASL syntax.

Time pressure Bellugi and Fischer have noted that signs generally take twice as long to produce as spoken words. Hands are considerably larger than tongues, and the distance from the waist to the head is much farther than that from the teeth to the middle of the palate. Nevertheless, Bellugi and Fischer have also found that ASL and English require the same amount of time in which to express ideas. It has been speculated that there might be some "presentation rate" at which the human mind best understands ideas communicated through language. This is a familiar phenomenon. Exceedingly fast or slow speech is difficult to comprehend. Since signs take longer to produce than spoken words, ASL needs to economize time. This is largely accomplished in two ways. First, ASL omits the redundant syntactic markers used in English. Second, ASL takes full advantage of the multidimensionality present in the visual and manual modalities.

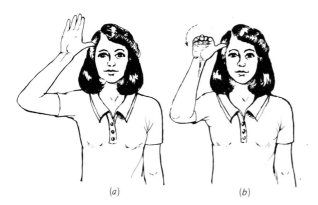

(a)   (b)

Figure 15-1 The ASL sign *stubborn.* Dez: open hand; tab: forehead; sig: thumb touches forehead, palm bends (*a* to *b*); orientation: palm out.

Omission A great many English syntactic markers are redundant. In the sentence, "A boy is eating," both the "a" and the lack of "-s" on "boy" indicate the singular. Both the auxiliary "is" and "-ing" indicate the present-progressive tense. One way to save time is to eliminate this redundancy. ASL does just that. There are no function words ("a," "the"), no verb "to be" ("The ball *is* blue" or "It *is* a girl"), and few auxiliary verbs ("She *has* eaten" or "We *were* going"). Thus the ASL translations for the above examples are: *boy eat, ball blue, it girl, she finish eat, we go.* Once again, because we use English words to talk about ASL syntax, we risk concluding that ASL syntax is a simplified copy of English. Although ASL saves time by omitting redundant syntactic markers, it also saves time by packing greater syntactic information into its signs than English does into its words. There is much more to ASL syntax than meets the eye on the printed page.

Multidimensionality

Pronouns ASL utterances are oriented with reference to the sender and receiver. ASL pronouns illustrate this nicely. Singular pronouns are indicated by a pointing handshape and movement. First person consists of the sender pointing to him or herself. Second person consists of pointing to the receiver. Third person consists of pointing either away to the side between the sender and receiver or to a point in space where the referent for the pronoun has been previously established. Plural pronouns are located in the same places and made with the same handshape, but a sweeping motion replaces the pointing movement. Possessive pronouns are made with an open handshape replacing the pointing handshape. ASL uses both a singular and plural "you," and does not differentiate between pronouns in the nominative and accusative cases ("I, he" versus "me, him").

Directional verbs A large class of ASL signs, called directional verbs, provides an excellent example of economizing time by optimum use of movement through space. The direction these verbs take always indicates subject and object, and depending upon the particular verb, indirect object and adverb or adjective. For example, the ASL verb *to-give-a-gift* consists of: dez—both hands' index fingers bent; tab—at midchest level; orientation—palms facing each other; sig—dependent on the relations expressed in the sentence. If the sender begins the sign to his or her side and sweeps toward him or herself, the English translation is "They give a gift to me." Here the English sentence requires six words. The ASL sentence expresses the same concepts and indicates the same syntactic relations through one sign. The sentences of both languages require about the same amount of time to produce. Next, the tense of this ASL sentence can be changed and an adjective added by altering the direction of movement. If the sender begins the sign *to-give-a-gift* at the receiver and moves it in an arc toward himself or herself one arm at a time, repeating this movement twice, the signer creates the ASL translations of "You (singular) are giving many gifts to me."

Another example using the above sign will illustrate the extraordinary information-packing power of directional verbs. The ASL translation of "I have already given gifts to the children," consists of two signs, *finish* + *to-give-a-gift : finish* (dez—open hands; tab—at the stomach; orientation—palms up; sig—palm up to palm down) + *to-give-a-gift* with the movement beginning at the sender and sweeping to the side at a level lower than the stomach. In this ASL sentence the auxiliary *finish* indicates the past-perfect tense ("have, -en") and the adverb ("already"). This movement's direction and scope indicate subject ("I"), verb ("give"), and direct object ("gift"). The indirect object ("children") is indicated by the movement *incorporating the place chereme* of the sign *child* (to the side below the waist) while *simultaneously pluralizing* it through the sweeping movement. Here the ASL sentence requires two signs in contrast to the eight words of the English sentence, a real saving of time.

Incorporation   Another ASL syntactic mechanism that capitalizes on multidimensionality to economize time is incorporation. Incorporation is the recombination of the cheremes of two or more signs into one sign and usually involves the meshing of a verb and direct object. For example, the ASL translation of "I hold the ball" is *me + hold-ball,* where the dez of *ball* replaces the dez of *hold,* resulting in one sign. Another example is the ASL translation of "The boy puts the cup up," which consists of two signs, *boy + put-cup-up.* The dez of *cup* and the tab of *up* replace the dez and tab of *put,* resulting in a single sign. Incorporation clearly follows rules; that is, some cheremes can replace others, whereas some cheremes cannot without distorting a sign or sentence beyond recognition. However, these rules have yet to be systematically formulated.

Sign order   Thus far we have discussed how directional verbs and incorporation of cheremes into one another indicate syntactic relations in ASL utterances. When neither directionality nor incorporations are used, the order of the signs in the utterance can convey syntactic relations, just as word order does in English. When a sentence's subject and object are *nonreversible,* any sign order is permissible. For example, the ASL translation of "The man starts the car" could be *man start car, car start man,* or *start car man.* When the subject and obejct are nonreversible, there is no potential confusion (cars do not start men). However, if the subject

and object are *reversible,* such as in "The girl kisses the boy," ASL usually follows a subject-verb-object order.

Previously we mentioned that sign languages are influenced by their oral-language environments. Current ASL sign order (when the subject and object are reversible) appears to be the result of English influence. Fischer studied ASL and French Sign Language texts of 100 years ago and discovered that ASL formerly followed a subject-object-verb order, which French Sign Language also used. She notes that ASL contains vestiges of its former sign order in some idioms, such as *shoes resole, water-turn-faucet* (object-verb order).

From our general discussion of ASL cheremic, lexical-semantic, and syntactic characteristics, it should be quite clear that ASL is not like English. It should be equally clear that many of the major differences between ASL and English result from modality effects. Hands and arms do not operate like oral mechanisms, and visual processes do not operate like auditory processes.

SIGN SYSTEMS

Deaf individuals live and work in oral-language environments. English-language skills are a prerequisite for successful interaction with the English-speaking community at large. Hence, teaching oral language has always been a central task for all educators of the deaf. Sign systems, as opposed to sign languages, are attemps by educators of the deaf to create manual-visual equivalents to oral languages in response to the central task of education of the deaf. The impetus for creating sign systems is based on the following reasoning: If deaf children could watch oral language as easily as hearing children listen to oral language, then they might learn it as readily. The reasoning seems logical, but the task is difficult. Everyone has a different approach to presenting English on the hands.

Fingerspelling

One way to present oral language on the hands is to create symbols for the letters of the alphabet and then "write in the air." Fingerspelling was probably the first sign system invented.[1] In the sixteenth century Pedro Ponce de Leon reputedly invented fingerspelling as a means of teaching Spanish to deaf children. In the eighteenth century Pereira and his outstanding deaf student Fontenay traveled to France and taught Spanish fingerspelling to the Abbé de l'Epée. De l'Epée modified the system, and Clerc and Gallaudet brought it to the United States. The resulting North American fingerspelling is one-handed, whereas British fingerspelling, which developed separately, is two-handed.

Fingerspelling seems to be the only sign system that has persisted through the ages. Today nearly all ASL signers use fingerspelling in conjunction with ASL as a means of directly borrowing from English words for which there is no sign. In other words, fingerspelling plays a supplemental role for deaf adults who sign—it is generally not used as a major means of communication among them. However, fingerspelling is still used as a means of teaching oral language. In the United States this is known as the *Rochester Method*, in which the teacher and students fingerspell English utterances letter for letter.

Manual English Systems

In the United States there are basically four sign systems designed to represent Eng-

[1] Fingerspelling is sometimes referred to as dactylology.

lish on the hands. Three of these are offshoots of an attempt begun in 1969 to systematically develop an English sign system. The original sign system was named *Seeing Essential English*. Disagreements concerning the rules of the system resulted in a second sign system named *Signing Exact English*. Further disagreements concerning the written form of the sign system resulted in *Linguistics of Visual English*. The fourth sign system, named *Signed English*, is not related to this group.

Seeing Essential English (SEE₁)   The first attempt to make a formal sign system based on both English and ASL was headed by David Anthony. SEE₁ has formal rules for altering the semantic boundaries of ASL signs so that they are equivalent to English words. When the semantic boundaries of an English word differ from those of a sign, those of the sign are extended or narrowed to those of the English word, resulting in one sign for every English word (represented in the vocabulary of this system). This change occurs when two of these three conditions apply: *same spelling, same sound, same meaning*. For example, the ASL meaning of the sign *ship* is limited to "boat." Because the "ship" of "friendship" is spelled and pronounced the same in both words, the SEE₁ translation is signed *friend + ship*. Another example is the SEE₁ sign for "right." In ASL there are three signs translated "right": *to-the-right, correct, all right* (similar to the French "à droite, bien correct, d'accord"). SEE₁ uses the ASL sign *to-the-right* in the phrases, "Turn right; we're right; everything's all right," because the word "right" is spelled and pronounced the same, meeting two of the three criteria. However, the SEE₁ sign for "all right" has a different sign because the English word is spelled differently and has a different meaning, not meeting two of the three criteria. SEE₁ also creates a great many new signs by replacing the dez of ASL signs with finger-spelling handshapes. For example, SEE₁ creates "yard" by replacing the dez of the ASL sign *box* with a Y handshape. Needless to say, SEE₁ signs in sentences often look rather strange to an ASL signer.

At the syntactic level, SEE₁ has devised signs for all English pronouns, and follows English word order. SEE₁ also has devised signs for all the syntactic markers we noted that ASL omits, such as "a, the," the verb "to be," auxiliary verbs, and subject-verb agreement.

Signing Exact English (SEE₂)   The second system was developed by Gustason, Pfetzing, and Zawalkow. SEE₂ is best characterized as an attempt to limit SEE₁ in order to prevent the system from becoming so distant from ASL that it is rendered unintelligible to ASL signers. SEE₂ rules for altering the meanings of ASL signs are identical to those of SEE₁, although not followed as rigorously for the above reason. SEE₂ signs for pronouns, auxiliary verbs, and subject-verb agreement are also identical to those of SEE₁. Of course, it too follows English word order.

Linguistics of Visual English (LOVE)   The third sign system was developed by Wampler. LOVE rules for altering ASL signs are identical to those of SEE₁ and SEE₂. However, LOVE's vocabulary is not as extensive as that of either of the first two systems. LOVE uses signs for pronouns, auxiliary verbs, and subject-verb agreement identical to those of SEE₁ and SEE₂. It also follows English word order. LOVE places somewhat greater emphasis on the spoken aspect of English than the other two systems in that the movements of signs are repeated, if necessary, to correspond to the number of syllables in the English word. LOVE is used less extensively than SEE₁ and SEE₂.

A distinguishing feature of these sign systems is their printed presentation. SEE₁ is written in a symbol system devised by Anthony. SEE₂ is presented in drawings. LOVE is written in a modified version of William Stokoe's symbol system devised for ASL.

Signed English   The sign system that goes by the name *Signed English* was created specifically for preschool children by a group at Gallaudet College. This system uses ASL signs without alteration. Rather than create signs for all English syntactic markers, this system creates signs for only those syntactic markers that have a high frequency of occurrence in the preschool child's language. It uses signs for English pronouns, subject-verb agreement, and a limited number of auxiliary verbs. It too follows English word order.

Additional Sign Systems

As we previously mentioned, everyone has a different approach to presenting English on the hands. Presently there appears to be a proliferation of informal or unpublished sign systems used to teach English to deaf children. In addition, educators in other countries are creating sign systems.

Informal sign systems   By "informal" sign systems we refer to the creation of sign systems for use within a specific school or geographical locale. For example, a particular school for the deaf might create a sign system by using ASL vocabulary without alteration, signing in English word order, and using sign markers for verb tenses and subject-verb agreement selected from among the manual English systems. Another school might use ASL vocabulary without alteration, signing in English word order, and fingerspelling all verb phrases and function words. Yet another school might use ASL vocabulary, altering the semantic boundaries following the rules specified by the manual English systems, and use manual English system tense markers for regular verbs while fingerspelling irregular verbs. In other words, the possible permutations and combinations of English and ASL elements are nearly infinite.

Sign systems in other countries

England   In England, a physical scientist named Richard Paget developed a sign system called *Systematic Sign Language*, which he hoped would be discarded when the deaf child had mastered English. Paget developed pantomimic signs for a basic English vocabulary of 850 words following the notion that every English word should have only one sign. He also devised signs for root words, suffixes, prefixes, verb inflections, and pronouns. The signs of the system are quite different from those of either ASL or manual English systems. Currently the system is being further developed and used experimentally with multiply handicapped deaf children.

Canada   In English-speaking parts of Canada, both manual English systems and informal sign systems are being used. In Quebec a sign system is being developed to present French on the hands. Since there are no published works on French-Canadian Sign Language, this system uses ASL signs in French word order, altering the dez of signs to correspond to French words if necessary. For example, the ASL sign for *church* uses a *C* dez; the French-sign system uses the same sign with an *E* dez to correspond to the French *église*. This French sign system also has devised signs for French pronouns, function words, and verb inflections.

ASL-English Pidgin

Before any of these specific sign systems were developed, ASL signers who also knew English frequently used (and continue to use) an ASL-English pidgin when communi-

cating in formal situations or with hearing and deaf individuals who are not fluent in ASL. A pidgin is a mixture of two languages where the vocabulary of one language (in this case ASL) is used with the syntax of another (in this case English). This type of ASL-English signing typically consists of using ASL signs in English word order and fingerspelling various English syntactic markers, such as "a, the, is," plurals, and verb inflections. The goal of using this ASL-English pidgin is usually to make communication easier for the person who is learning ASL as a second language, or to demonstrate a knowledge of English.

ASL-English Continuum

It should be obvious by now that although the distinctions between ASL and English are rather sharp, the distinctions among various sign systems are not. Perhaps an example will clarify how the manual English systems, informal systems, and ASL-English pidgin might vary. The sentence, "I didn't give any Christmas gifts to the teacher," might be signed in the ways shown in the table. As this example illustrates, the distinctions among sign systems are rather fine. In practice, the distinctions among sign systems and the ASL-English pidgin are very blurred, depending on who is signing to whom and for what purpose. Sign systems form a continuum between ASL and English. Fingerspelling English utterances would be closest to English in terms of orthography, followed by SEE$_1$. The ASL-English pidgin is closest to ASL, followed by *Signed English*. SEE$_2$ and LOVE would fall somewhere in the middle. An informal sign system would fall anywhere between the Rochester Method and ASL, depending on the rules and mechanisms involved. In everyday usage the terms *signed English, manual English, visual English,* and *siglish* do not refer to a specific sys-

Rochester Method	I D-I-D-N-'T G-I-V-E A-N-Y C-H-R-I-S-T-M-A-S G-I-F-T-S T-O T-H-E T-E-A-C-H-E-R = 39 fingerspelled letters
SEE₁	I DO+PAST+N'T GIVE AN+Y CHRIST+MAS GIFT+S TO THE TEACH+ER = 15 signs
SEE₂, LOVE	I DO+PAST+N'T GIVE AN+Y CHRISTMAS GIFT+S TO THE TEACH+ER = 14 signs
Signed English	I DO+PAST NOT GIVE ANY CHRISTMAS GIFT+S TO THE TEACH+ER = 13 signs
Informal Sign System	I D-I-D-N-'T G-I-V-E ANY CHRISTMAS GIFT+S TO T-H-E TEACH-ER = 8 signs + 12 fingerspelled letters
ASL-English Pidgin	ME NOT ANY CHRISTMAS TO-GIVE-A-GIFT T-H-E TEACH+PERSON = 7 signs + 3 fingerspelled letters
ASL	TEACH+PERSON NOT TO-GIVE-A-GIFT CHRISTMAS = 5 signs; *to-give-a-gift* is directional

tem. These terms are interchangeably used to refer to using ASL signs in English word order with or without additional devised signs or fingerspelling for English syntactic markers. Frequently such signing consists of a little bit of everything: ASL, fingerspelling, and signs for syntactic markers from all the systems we discussed. The purpose of signing in English, regardless of how it is accomplished, is always the same: to present English on the hands. The closer the signing comes to replicating English, the more complicated it becomes and the more it distorts ASL. Conversely, the more the signing maintains ASL integrity, the less like English it becomes.

The Sign Systems of de l'Epée, Sicard, Clerc, and Gallaudet

Frequently, twentieth-century sign systems are regarded as a completely new way of teaching oral language to deaf children. In fact, sign systems are as old as education of the deaf itself. Fingerspelling was probably the first sign system. As already noted, the second sign system was invented by de l'Epée, who used his students' signs in French word order and devised some additional signs for French syntactic markers. Sicard continued the system. When Gallaudet began his school in Connecticut, he and Clerc devised an English sign system patterned on the basic ideas of the French sign system. Although sign systems designed to represent *oral* language were used in the first schools for the deaf established in both France and the United States, these sign systems, as we know, did not become the manual communication of deaf individuals on an interpersonal basis. This is obvious in view of the fact that French Sign Language and ASL are very different from spoken French and English, respectively. Perhaps if we stop a moment to think about what history has to teach us, we can objectively discuss some of the complicated educational considerations underlying the use of sign systems in deaf education.

EDUCATIONAL CONSIDERATIONS

Since we do not know the structural details of de l'Epée, Sicard, Clerc, and Gallaudet's sign systems, how they were taught, or how they were used to teach oral language, we can only speculate about the reasons why these systems did not become the manual communication of deaf individuals on an interpersonal basis. However, these speculations should prove useful in discussing guidelines for both using sign systems and future research needs.

Why Sign Systems Might Not Succeed

There are three overlapping areas of sign system usage about which we can speculate in considering why oral-based systems did not last: (1) the sign system itself; (2) how the sign system is used; (3) transmission and reception modalities.

The sign system Perhaps the sign systems of these early pioneers did not really represent the oral language they were designed to symbolize. We clearly know a good deal more about oral-language structure now than was known in the eighteenth and nineteenth centuries, however incomplete our present knowledge is. It may be that the rules of the sign systems did not capture the regularities of oral-language rules or were incapable of dealing with the irregularities of oral language. Another possibility is that the rules of the sign systems were incomplete and specified only the simplest or most obvious of oral-language structures. There is the possibility that some of the rules were incorrect. In addition to potential syntactic nonequivalence between these sign systems and oral languages, perhaps there were semantic differences that caused problems. For example, if the systems used the students' signs without altering semantic boundaries and used these signs in oral-language word order, perhaps the result was a pidgin sign language unlike either the students' sign language or the dominant oral language. In effect, perhaps these sign systems resulted in

a third language that the students were required to master.

Use of the sign system Perhaps there were too few sign system models in the students' environment, that is, too few individuals who were fluent in the sign systems with whom the students regularly communicated. If only one or two teachers used the sign system, while everyone else (teachers, family, friends) did not, then the students' opportunities to learn the sign systems were severely restricted. The situation would have been compounded if the students only used the sign systems in the classroom and used their own sign language outside the classroom.

A related possibility is that there were few consistent sign-system utterances from which the students could induce rules. If the teachers were not highly fluent in the sign system or if there was little or no agreement among the teachers concerning the rules of the sign system, the result would be inconsistency in how utterances were signed. For example, it would be extremely difficult, if not impossible, to learn the gender of French nouns if some French speakers marked nouns for gender only part of the time, other French speakers never marked nouns for gender, and still others frequently marked masculine nouns as feminine, and vice versa.

Transmission and reception modalities Throughout this chapter we have emphasized the modality differences of oral and sign languages and noted how the visual and manual modalities appear to affect the structure of ASL. Perhaps the structure of early sign systems was not compatible with communication in the manual and visual modalities. For example, we now know that there are perception and production restraints that affect the shapes of signs. If these systems included signs that violated such restraints, then the signing would have become both awkward and time-consuming. Likewise, we now realize that signing a sign requires more time than speaking a word. The early sign systems may have required too many signs, hence too much time for effective communication. Finally, the sign systems may have placed too great a strain on the students' short-term memory capacity. By stringing signs together sequentially much like oral languages, the sign systems may have ignored the spatial-organizational features of visual memory and perception. In other words, the sign systems may have been too cumbersome for effective communication. Perhaps the pressures of the visual and manual modalities were most responsible for students selecting their sign language rather than their instructors' sign systems for interpersonal communication. Human communication flows because it has evolved to fit the transmission and reception modalities. We have no reason to believe that this is not also true for visual-manual communication.

Guidelines for Sign-System Use

Now we are in a position to discuss some guidelines for using sign systems. We cannot, however, pick and choose among sign systems. This very difficult and complicated task must be left to the individuals who decide to use a sign system; the choice will, of course, depend on the purposes and goals of sign system usage:

1. Whichever sign system is selected, it is probably most important that the individuals responsible for teaching it are consistent in their signing, especially of syntactic markers. Only chaos and confusion can result if consistency is not maintained.

2. The people who use the sign system should be as fluent as possible in their signing. Strangely, some individuals who are not fluent in sign systems tend either to invent signs on the spot for words for which they do not know the signs or fill the gap with a wave of the arms. Clearly, these makeshift expedients only contribute to inconsistency. Fingerspelling should be used as the backup system in such situations. For example, it is obviously easier to learn the word "democracy" if we see it fingerspelled a dozen times than if we see a dozen different gestures for the word.

3. There should probably be as many sign-system models in the environment as possible, which means that students' families as well as entire school faculties must make an effort to learn the selected sign system.

4. It is important always to be aware of the phonologic, syntactic, and semantic limitations of a sign system. When using a sign system there is a great temptation to think that we are "signing in English" and therefore can decrease our efforts to teach English. Sign systems are not English. They clearly do not have, for example, English phonology. There is no sign system that successfully represents the syntax of English, especially considering that we do not know what all the rules of English are.

5. It is important to be aware of current sign language research. An understanding of the cheremes of ASL can, for example, provide a guide for selecting, rejecting, or creating new signs or explain why the form of the sign of a sign system undergoes changes when it is used in conversation. Such knowledge can also be used to evaluate alternative sign-system mechanisms for a given syntactic structure in English. In other words, knowledge of current sign language research allows us to make wiser choices.

Research Needs

There has been a small explosion of interest in greatly needed sign language research over the past five years as compared with such interest in the past. Successful sign language research requires the cooperative effort of workers in fields ranging from anthropology to zoosemiotics. Psychologists and linguists in particular are beginning to realize that sign language research can help shed some light on issues germane to their fields of study. Although this increased interest in sign language is both encouraging and exciting to witness, it is disheartening to see some researchers shy away from questions involving sign systems and their educational implications. It is equally disheartening to see clinicians and educators ignore the questions and investigations of researchers. In questions regarding sign language and sign systems, clinicians, educators, and researchers have much more in common than they might imagine.

There are many questions regarding language learning that need to be answered. For example, what is the course of sign language acquisition and how does it compare with oral-language acquisition? How does sign-system acquisition compare with both sign- and oral-language acquisition? Do the stages of bimodal bilingual language acquisition correspond to those of unimodal bilingual language acquisition? Does early acquisition of a manual-visual language facilitate later learning of an oral-aural language? Does the critical age hypothesis also hold true for manual-visual language acquisition? Answers to these questions would uncover valuable information for individuals interested in the language acquisition process and in teaching sign languages and sign systems.

Many questions in second-language learning and bilingualism address themselves to both research and education. For example, is there a collection or set of skills, attitudes, or motivations that correlate with and are predictive of second-language learning of sign language? How does this collection of attributes and skills compare with those for second-oral-language learning? What is the most effective means of teaching adults sign languages and sign systems and are these methods similar to those for teaching oral language? Are there individuals who cannot obtain proficiency in sign language? If so, why? Is it easier to learn a second sign language than it is to learn a second oral language, and if so, why? Answers to these questions would enable us to teach sign languages and systems to teachers of the deaf much more effectively and efficiently.

Clearly there are very important linguistic questions that need to be asked and answered. One important question that comes immediately to mind is the degree to which the phonological or suprasegmental level of oral language is tied to the syntactic and semantic levels. In other words, if the suprasegmental aspects of spoken language are removed or severely distorted, what is the effect on the organization of the remainder of the message? Although this may appear to be a rather esoteric question, the answer applies directly to signing and talking at the same time. When we simultaneously speak and sign, how much do we distort the visual and auditory portions of the message? Does it make a difference? If so, what is that difference?

There are innumerable questions to be asked and answered regarding our ability to receive and handle information and the effect modalities have on this ability. These questions are directly applicable to the simultaneous use of sign and spoken language. Is it possible to pay attention to an auditory and visual message at the same time? Does the visual modality dominate the auditory modality when competing messages arrive simultaneously? Is this affected by whether we have normal or impaired hearing? How many visual stimuli can we attend to at one time? Through research investigation aimed at answering such questions, we might discover, for example, that sign and oral languages are best taught separately. The answers to these and to the inevitable additional questions to which they lead are pertinent to basic understanding and to constructive applications of manual modes of communication.

REHABILITATION CONSIDERATIONS

The implications and ramifications of using sign language and sign systems in rehabilitation and counseling work with deaf clients are an important and complicated topic, but well beyond the scope of this chapter. However, any professional who comes into contact with deaf adults who sign and who are in need of professional services should know about the *Registry of Interpreters for the Deaf.* RID is an organization whose main purpose is to ensure quality interpretation for deaf individuals in need of such services. RID carries out an evaluation and certification program for individuals who wish to become interpreters, promotes the acceptance of interpreting as a paid profession, and publishes a *Directory of Interpreters for the Deaf,* which is a listing of interpreters' names, addresses, and certification level. The various levels of interpreting certifications are as follows:

1. *Expressive translating:* An individual with this certification is able to interpret spoken English into the ASL-English pidgin (and, depending on the individual, into a sign system).
2. *Expressive interpreting:* An individual with this certification is able to interpret spoken English into ASL, the ASL-English pidgin (and perhaps a sign system).
3. *Reverse skills:* An individual with this certification is able to interpret ASL, the ASL-English pidgin (and perhaps a sign system), into spoken English.
4. *Comprehensive skills:* An individual with this certification is able to interpret in all the above situations.
5. *Legal specialist certificate:* An individual with this certification holds a comprehensive skills certificate and has completed a special training course enabling him or her to interpret in a variety of legal situations.

SUGGESTED READINGS AND REFERENCES

Anthony, D. *Seeing Essential English,* Anaheim, Calif.: Educational Services Division, Anaheim Union High School District, 1971.

Bellugi, U., and E. Klima. "The Roots of Language in the Sign Talk of the Deaf," *Psychol. Today,* 61–76 (June, 1972).
A brief introduction to ASL and its interest to psycholinguistics.

———, and S. Fischer. "A Comparison of Sign Language and Spoken Language," *Cognition,* 1:173–200 (1972).
The results of a study examining the amount of time ASL and spoken English require to send messages and includes a description of ASL syntactic devices which save time.

———, E. Klima, and P. Siple. "Remembering in Signs," *Cognition,* 3:93–125 (1975).

The results of ASL short-term memory experiments demonstrating that cheremes function for ASL signers like phonemes function for English speakers.

Bornstein, H. "A Description of Some Current Sign Systems Designed to Represent English," *Amer. Ann. Deaf,* 118:454–463 (1973).

——, "Signed English, a Manual Approach," *J. Speech Hearing Dis.* 39:330–343 (1974).

Darwin, C. *The Expression of the Emotions in Man and Animals.* Chicago: The University of Chicago Press, 1965.

Directory of Registered Interpreters for the Deaf. Registry of Interpreters for the Deaf, P. O. Box 1339, Washington, D.C. 20013.

Fischer, S. "Sign Language and Linguistic Universals," in *Acts du Colloque Franco-Allemand de Grammaire Transformationelle,* Vol. II, C. Roher and N. Ruwet (eds.). Tübingen: Max Niemeyer Verlag (1974).

Examines the linguistic universals hypothesized to exist for all languages and concludes that ASL meets each universal except auditory patterning.

——, "Influences on Word-Order Change in American Sign Language," in *Word Order and Word Order Change,* C. Li (ed.). Austin: University of Texas Press, 1975.

Frishberg, N. "Arbitrariness and Iconicity: Historical Change in American Sign Language," *Language,* 51:676–719 (1975).

Describes ASL cheremic evolution and the perception and production pressures that guide it.

Gustason, G., D. Pfetzing, and E. Zawalkow. *Signing Exact English.* Silver Spring, Md.: Modern Signs Press, 1972.

——, and J. Woodward (eds.). *Recent Developments in Manual English.* Papers presented at a special institute sponsored by the Department of Education Graduate School, Gallaudet College, Washington, D.C. 1973.

Papers by the authors of SEE$_1$, SEE$_2$, LOVE, and Signed English, each briefly describing their sign system and the philosophy behind it; introduced by a linguist's view of sign systems. (Available through the Gallaudet College Bookstore.)

Lane, H. "The Great Sign Controversy," in *The Wild Boy of Aveyron.* Cambridge: Harvard University Press, 1976.

Provides translations and commentaries on selected writings of de l'Epée, Sicard, and Itard concerning manual education in education of the deaf.

——, P. Boyes-Braem, and U. Bellugi. "Preliminaries to a Distinctive Feature Analysis of Handshapes in American Sign Language," *Cognitive Psychology,* 8:263–289 (1976).

O'Rourke, T. J., T. Medina, A. Thames, and D. Sullivan. "National Association of the Deaf Communicative Skills Program," *Programs for the Handicapped,* 75 (No. 2). Washington, D.C.: Office for Handicapped Individuals, Department of Health, Education and Welfare. (April 15, 1975)

A report of research done in connection with proposed federal legislation to include deaf persons in the Bilingual Courts Act.

Schlesinger, H., and K. Meadow. *Sound and Sign.* Berkeley: University of California Press, 1972.

Presents some results of a preschool project using a sign system with deaf children.

Sign Language Studies. Silver Spring, Md.: Linstok Press.

This journal is edited by William Stokoe and publishes articles on manual communication and sign-language research.

Siple, P. (ed.) *Understanding Language through Sign Language Research.* New York: Academic Press, in press.

A collection of sign language research papers presented at the Conference on Sign Languages and Neurolinguistics held in Rochester, N.Y., in September 1976. The papers cover such topics as ASL chereology, creolization, linguistic dating of ASL, laterality, and processing of ASL.

Stokoe, W., D. Casterline, and C. Croneberg. *A Dictionary of American Sign Language on Linguistic Principles.* Washington, D.C.: Gallaudet College Press, 1965. (Reissued 1976, Silver Spring, Md.: Linstock Press.)

An outline of ASL vocabulary up to 1965 with an explanation of cheremes and presentation of a symbol system for ASL. The reissue contains sociolinguistic articles and a useful bibliography of ASL research.

————. *Semiotics and Human Sign Languages. Approaches to Semiotics,* Vol. 21, T. Sebeok (ed.). The Hague: Mouton, 1972.

A discussion of semiotic and linguistic approaches to sign language research.

Wilbur, R. "Linguistics of Manual Languages and Manual Systems," in *Communication Assessment and Intervention Strategies,* L. Lloyd (ed.). Baltimore: University Park Press, 1976.

A detailed linguistic description of ASL and sign systems with an extensive bibliography.

Wundt, W. *The Language of Gestures. Approaches to Semiotics,* Vol. 6, T. Sebeok (ed.). The Hague: Mouton, 1973.

A translation of Wundt's classic ponderings on ethnic gestures, and the sign languages of Cistercian monks, North American Indians, and German deaf children.

Part V
EDUCATION

S. Richard Silverman, Ph.D.

16

From Aristotle to Bell— and Beyond

THE EARLY PERIOD

The evolution of the present social point of view toward deafness has been marked by a growing recognition of its problems and by an increasing collective effort to do something practical toward their solution. We need go no further than the pages of this book for a forceful illustration of the variety of talents that are now cooperating in the attack. The removal of professional barriers, which now permits the physician, the researcher, the educator, the sociologist, the psychologist, the physicist, the psychiatrist, the industrial engineer, the audiologist, parents, laymen and, very significantly, hearing-impaired persons themselves to work together with mutual understanding, is one of the most promising developments of recent years. It forecasts a progressively broader and more intelligent base of social awareness of the entire question.

The development of an increasingly enlightened social attitude toward deafness, however, is no exception to the general rule that man's struggle toward enlightenment is slow, faltering, and, in many instances, haphazard. This development might be traced in the history of the education of the deaf, but only fragmentary bits of information are available prior to the sixteenth century. Some of the bits are indirect and inferred, and it is difficult to trace any complete structure of systematic thought.

In the pre-Christian era, however, Aristotle and, later, Pliny the Elder observed that there was some relationship between congenital deafness and dumbness, but neither one elaborated on the relationship. It is still questionable whether Aristotle assumed a common organic basis for deafness and dumbness, but he placed strong emphasis on sound (speech) as the primary vehicle for conveying thought and therefore as the chief medium for education. Aristotle presumably believed that since the deaf could neither give utterance to speech nor comprehend it from others, they were relatively incapable of instruction, and furthermore that the deaf were less capable of instruction than the blind. At any rate, Aristotle made no clear statement that dumbness is a consequence of deafness (of the congenital type) and that speech is an acquired skill whose patterns are learned through the ear. Of course, hearing is the normal channel through which speech is most readily perceived and consequently imitated. Note the stress on the *normal* channel for we have also learned that it is possible for the deaf to acquire speech through touch, sight, and the sense of movement. Many deaf people receive information through the use of manual alphabets and the language of signs.

The idea that deafness and muteness depend on a common organic abnormality and the idea that the deaf were poor educational prospects persisted through medieval times. It is probable that the derogatory use of "dumbness" in our modern slang, suggesting an inferior intellect, has its roots in the supposed mental incapacity of the deaf. And it was inevitable that the notion of the limited mental capacity of the deaf should exercise a powerful influence on their legal and civil status. Roman law classified the deaf and dumb with the mentally incompetent, and the Justinian Code (sixth century A.D.) excluded the deaf and dumb from the rights (entering into contracts, and so on) and obligations (witnessing in a court of law) of citizenship. In justice to Justinian's Code, it must be said that a sharp differentiation was made between deaf-mutes and those whose deafness was acquired and who had learned

spoken and written language. Although the Code did not prohibit marriage for the deaf, its influence later caused medieval law to deny to the congenitally deaf and dumb the highly cherished right of primogeniture.

Although information concerning the attitude of religious institutions toward deafness during this early period is comparatively meager, fragments of evidence from church literature indicate that the church shared the prevailing notions of the times. Mosaic Law, through its Code of Holiness in the sixth century B.C., exhorted the faithful not to curse the deaf since their deafness was presumably willed by the Lord. In the second century B.C. the rabbis of the Talmud classified the deaf with fools and children. Although the rabbis were perfectly correct in calling attention to individual differences, their pronouncements reflect an inadequate understanding of deafness. We do note, however, in Isaiah 35, the prophecy that "...the ears of the deaf shall be unstopped ... and the tongue of the dumb sing."

Similarly, the Christian Church looked with disdain on the intellectual capabilities of the deaf, although it did permit marriage by a ceremony conducted in the language of signs. We perceive a glimmer of enlightenment, however, in Bede's references (about the seventh century A.D.) to the feat of Bishop John of York in teaching a deaf-and-dumb youth to speak intelligibly. This accomplishment, however, is chronicled in the nature of a miracle, and the educational method is left to our imaginations. Nevertheless, the mere recording of the incident is a first, admittedly feeble, attempt (conscious or otherwise) to dispel the fog of misunderstanding in which deafness was enshrouded.

RECOGNITION OF POTENTIAL FOR EDUCATION OF THE DEAF

It was not until the middle of the sixteenth century that the mists began to lift. At that time an intellectually versatile Italian physician, Girolamo Cardano de Padua, in referring to the work of Rudolphus Agricola of Groningen proposed a set of principles that promised a more hopeful educational, and hence social, outlook for the deaf. He stated, in essence, that the deaf could be taught to comprehend written symbols or combinations of symbols by associating them with the object or picture of the object they were intended to represent. To this day, the association of meaningful language with experience is the keystone of techniques for teaching the deaf. The significance of Cardano's contribution lies not so much in his statement of basic principles of teaching as in his implicit rejection of the notion that the

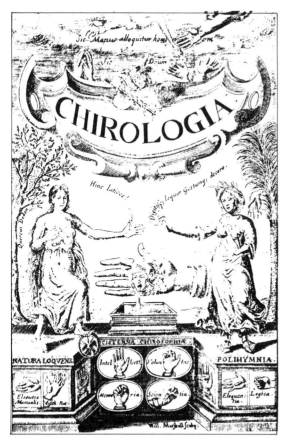

Figure 16-1 Frontispiece of *Chirologia* ("hand speech") *or Natural Language of the Hand* by John Bulwer, 1644.

Philocophus:
OR,
THE DEAFE
AND
Dumbe Mans Friend.
EXHIBITING THE
Philosophicall verity of that subtile Art, which may inable one with an *observant Eie*, to *Heare* what any man speaks by the moving of his lips.
UPON THE SAME
Ground, with the advantage of an Historicall Exemplification, apparently proving, That a Man borne Deafe and Dumbe, may be taught to *Heare* the sound of *words* with his *Eie*, & thence learne to speake with his Tongue.

By *I. B.* firnamed the *Chirosopher*.

Sic canimus Surdis ——

London, Printed for *Humphrey Moseley*, and are to be sold at his shop in Pauls Church-yard 1648.

Figure 16-2 Title page of *Philocophus* ("lover of the deaf"), first book on lipreading in English, by John Bulwer, 1648.

deaf cannot be educated and consequently are doomed to social inadequacy. It would not be too extravagant to attribute to Cardano the concept of an educational Magna Carta for the deaf.

Cardano's pronouncements initiated a series of serious, although sporadic, attempts to implement his principles. It is reasonable to credit these heartening developments in part also to the liberation of humanistic forces by the Renaissance and to the subsequent popularization of education in the vernacular induced by the Reformation. As early as 1555 we find instruction of deaf children of the nobility carried on by a Spanish monk, Pedro Ponce de Leon, in a convent in Valladolid. It was in Spain, too, that the first book exclusively on the deaf, by Juan Pablo Bonet, appeared in 1620. Bonet's pupils were taught articulation and language, supplemented by a manual alphabet and the language of signs. Other works in many tongues dealing with the education and intellectual and spiritual status of the deaf appeared soon after. John Bulwer, John Wallis,

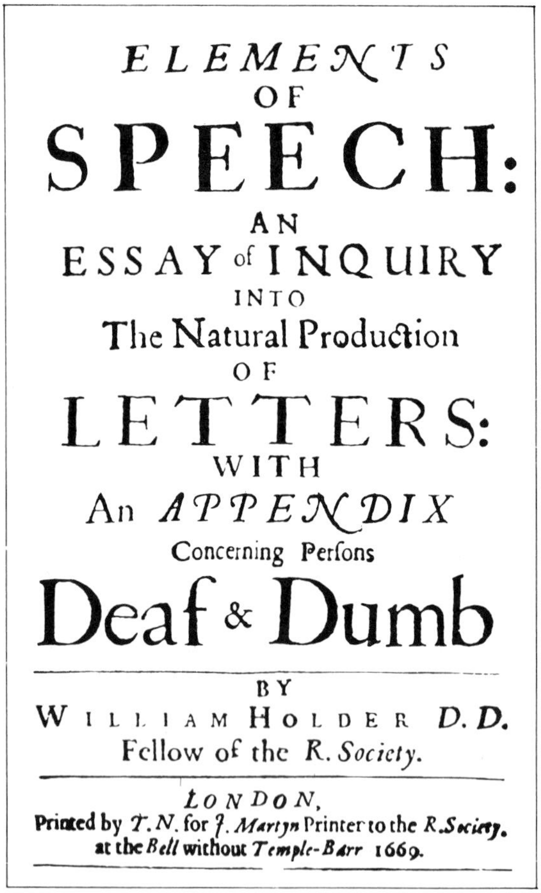

ELEMENTS
OF
SPEECH:
AN
ESSAY of **INQUIRY**
INTO
The Natural Production
OF
LETTERS:
WITH
An *APPENDIX*
Concerning Perſons
Deaf & Dumb
BY
W I L L I A M H O L D E R *D. D.*
Fellow of the *R. Society.*
LONDON,
Printed by *T. N.* for *J. Martyn* Printer to the *R. Society.*
at the *Bell* without *Temple-Barr* 1669.

Figure 16-3 Title page of *Elements of Speech* by William Holder, 1669.

DIDASCALOCOPHUS
Or
The Deaf and Dumb mans Tutor.
To which is added
A Diſcourſe of the Nature and number of Double Conſonants: Both which Tracts being the firſt (for what the Author knows) that have been publiſhed upon either of the Subjects.

By *GEO. DALGARNO.*

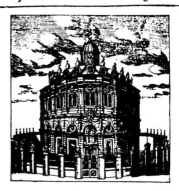

Printed at the T H E A T E R in O X F O R D,
Anno Dom. 1680.

Figure 16-4 Title page of *Didascalocophus* ("teacher of the deaf") by George Dalgarno, 1680.

William Holder, and George Dalgarno carried on the work in the British Isles; Jan Baptiste van Helmont and John Conrad Amman, in Holland; Saint Francis de Sales, in Switzerland; Ernaud and Pereire, in France; and Otto Lasius and Arnoldi (among a host of others), in Germany.

In contrast to Aristotle's views comparing the intellectual capabilities of the deaf and blind, the beginning of enlightenment is best typified by a quotation from Dalgarno's *Didascalocophus*, published at Oxford in 1680:

Taking it for granted, That Deaf People are equal, in the faculties of apprehension, and memory, not only to the Blind; but even to those that have all their senses: and having formerly shewn; that these faculties can as easily receive, and retain, the Images of things by the conveiance of Figures, thro the Eye, as of Sounds thro the ear: It will follow, That the Deaf man is, not only as capable, but also as soon capable of Instruction in Letters, as the blind man. And if we compare them, as to their intrinsick powers, has the advantage of him too; insomuch as he has a more distinct and perfect perception, of external Objects, then the other. . . . I conceive, there might be successful addresses made to a Dumb child, even in his cradle. . . .

Note the emphasis on equality with others, the suggestion that the deaf could be taught even in early childhood, and an implicit plea for what we now call early detection and identification.

Two individuals, however, tower above all others in their contributions to advancing the cause of the deaf in the latter part of the eighteenth century—the Abbé Charles Michel de l'Epée in France and Samuel Heinicke in Germany. De l'Epée found a fruitful outlet for his religious emotions, as many clergymen have since his time, in promoting the well-being of the deaf through education. It is to his everlasting credit that he founded the first public school for the deaf in 1775 in Paris. Heinicke, his contemporary in Germany, founded the first public school for the deaf in Germany. It was the first recognized by any government.

De l'Epée and Heinicke disagreed about the merits of signs and "oralism" as methods of instruction, de l'Epée favoring signs and Heinicke writing prolifically on the advantages of speech and of speechreading. So widespread was the influence of these two men that the pattern of their controversy was repeated later and indeed still persists in many countries, including the United States. Our purpose here, however, is not to evaluate the merits of their contentions but to stress their extremely important contributions to the liberalization of the social point of view toward deafness. By the end of the eighteenth century it had been convincingly demonstrated that the deaf were capable of instruction, and it was also clearly recognized that it was the moral and legal obligation of society to see that instruction was provided, even though the development of free public schools was slow. Such recognition was indeed a landmark of social progress.

THE RISE OF EDUCATION AND SOCIAL AWARENESS IN THE UNITED STATES

The moral and intellectual advancement of the social attitude toward deafness in Europe naturally exerted its influence in the United States. Although there had been scattered instances of instruction of the deaf, of attempts to found permanent schools, and of mention of the deaf in the literature, it was not until 1817 that the first permanent public school for the deaf in the United States was founded, at Hartford, Connecticut. The establishment of this school was given its chief impetus by a young divinity student, Thomas Hopkins Gallaudet, who was sent abroad by a group of citizens to observe European methods in the education of the deaf. On visiting England he was disappointed in the help he received from the Braidwoods, who were said to be obtaining good results using the oral approach to deaf children. It appears that the Braidwoods, British educators of the deaf, were secretive about their methods.

Gallaudet therefore crossed the Channel to France and enlisted the services of Laurent Clerc, a French teacher of the deaf trained in the manual approach of de l'Epée, whom he succeeded in bringing to Hartford. Incidentally, Clerc, who was introduced to Gallaudet by the Abbé Roch-Ambroise Sicard, de l'Epée's successor, was deaf himself and hence was the first deaf teacher of the deaf in the United States. The school at Hartford, called the American Asylum for the Education and Instruction of the Deaf and Dumb (now known as the American School for the Deaf), had to depend upon private funds for support, but in a relatively short time public assistance was made available. It was the forerunner of the great system of state-supported schools for the deaf that we have in the United States today. Later in the nineteenth century and early in the twentieth century outstanding private and denominational schools were also established that became notable for their encouragement of an oral emphasis in instruction.

Thanks to the indefatigable efforts of a few pioneers, the great vision of universality of educational opportunity for the deaf has been transformed into reality. These trailblazers included Thomas Hopkins Gallaudet, for whom the federally sponsored college for the deaf in Washington, D.C., is named; Edward Miner Gallaudet, who carried on his father's work; Sarah Fuller, who promoted the day school for the deaf; Alexander Graham Bell and his father, Melville, who among other accomplishments elevated speech to the status of a science; Caroline Yale, who implemented many of the Bells' principles; and Max A. Goldstein, founder of the Central Institute for the Deaf, who drove home the needs of the deaf to the medical profession and who developed methods for training residual hearing. The ever-expanding opportunities for the deaf in publicly supported residential and day schools and in parochial and private institutions attest the wisdom and influence of these workers in the cause of the deaf. It is because of their foresight and energy that no deaf child need be denied an opportunity for education.

The happy combination of talents brought to bear on the problem of increasing the op-

portunities for the deaf is best epitomized in the person of Alexander Graham Bell. He established the Volta Bureau to disseminate information on deafness and he opened new vistas in the teaching of speech to the deaf; and, of course, his invention of the telephone laid a firm foundation for the electrical transmission of sound. The writers of this book, consciously or otherwise, take inspiration and stimulation from his sympathetic understanding, his spirit of incisive inquiry, and his inventive genius. It was fitting that 1947 (the date of the first edition of this book), the hundredth anniversary of the birth of Alexander Graham Bell, should witness the emergence of the art and science of audiology, which in broad terms seeks the answer to the question, "How can we do a better job for the deaf and the hard-of-hearing?" There is no doubt that Bell's inspiration is still with us as we seek more and better answers to this basic question.

As the schools for the deaf became more widespread and adequate, it was inevitable that the social point of view toward deafness should become proportionately more enlightened. The alumni of these schools were beginning to demonstrate how seriously the deaf had previously been underestimated. They have taken the initiative in promoting broad and intensive studies now under way dealing with the psychiatric and vocational needs of the deaf. The schools themselves are tending to become purely educational institutions, subject to boards of education and not to administrators of almshouses or to penal authorities.

Society now understands that the deaf not only can be educated but also can, with proper guidance and assistance, become economically and socially productive men and women. Agencies for vocational rehabilitation and guidance, emphasizing special training for adults in cooperation with schools and industry, have been established to facilitate the economic and social adjustment not only of the deaf but of the hard-of-hearing as well. And paralleling the enlarging educational and economic opportunities for the deaf, the unnecessary legal restrictions upon them have gradually been removed.

The progressive development of the education of the deaf reflected the popularization and liberalization of general education, particularly with respect to the spread of opportunity for education, the improvement of teacher training, and the application of better teaching techniques. The process has also worked in reverse. Educators of the hearing have consciously or otherwise borrowed from teachers of the deaf, especially the principle of "learning by doing." It is heartening to note also that recognized universities are increasingly introducing curricula dealing with the educational, linguistic, psychological, sociological, and physiological problems of deafness.

GOVERNMENT RESPONSE TO PROBLEMS OF HEARING IMPAIRMENT

Perhaps the most tangible and significant expression of national concern for the hearing-impaired is the recent enactment of federal legislation aimed at improving and expanding the preparation of professional personnel, stimulating research, and fostering extended services.

Undoubtedly, this response was stimulated by the substantial prevalence of hearing disorders in all segments of the population. In a Public Health Service monograph on *Human Communication and Its Disorders* (NINDS Monograph No. 10, 1970) the main points on prevalence of hearing disorders are summarized as follows:

1. There are approximately 236,000 deaf individuals of all ages and both sexes in the United States today.

2. Approximately 6,000,000 Americans have partial hearing impairments of handicapping degree that are bilateral.

3. An additional 2,500,000 or so have significant unilateral losses.

4. Among school-age children there are about 52,000 in schools and classes for the deaf, about 100,000 more requiring intensive special management, and some 250,000 more who are auditorily handicapped to an important degree in the school environment.

5. About 700,000 persons suffer a combination of at least some degree of handicapping hearing deficit and some degree of handicapping visual problem.

6. Handicapping hearing losses are particularly prevalent in the older age group and here they are more often frequently combined with visual disabilities.

7. No reliable general data are available on the prevalence of hearing losses by cause, on the distribution or the patterns of losses, or on the incidence of dysacusis.

The major portion of the federal effort is concentrated in the Department of Health, Education and Welfare, which administers these programs through the Social and Rehabilitation Services Administration, the National Institutes of Health, and the Office of Education.

A number of specific enactments and projects are worthy of mention to illustrate the growing commitment of the federal government to hearing-impaired children and adults. In October 1965, acting on a recommendation contained in a report to the Department of Health, Education and Welfare entitled *Education of the Deaf*, Congress established the National Advisory Committee on the Education of the Deaf, setting forth its functions as follows:

1. To stimulate the development of a system for periodic gathering of information to

make it possible to assess progress and identify problems in the education of the deaf

2. To identify emerging needs and suggest innovations that promise to improve the educational prospects of deaf individuals

3. To suggest promising areas of inquiry to guide the federal government's research effort in the education of the deaf

4. To advise the Secretary on desirable emphases and priorities among programs

One of the first tasks accomplished by the Committee was the sponsorship and execution of a National Conference on the Education of the Deaf in April 1967. The committee has now been absorbed into the National Advisory Committee on the Handicapped, whose charge with respect to all handicaps includes the original mission of NACED.

The nation is concerned with the increasing number of young people who enter the labor market without any marketable skills or with skills that are marginal at best. The technological revolution that goes on unabated and at a rapidly increasing pace is drastically reducing the employment opportunities for those with marginal or obsolescent skills. Realism compels us to recognize that in any economy those persons with severely disordered communication find their economic opportunities limited. Aware that burgeoning technology compounds our problem and underlines our responsibility, Congress in 1965 enacted legislation establishing a National Technical Institute for the Deaf to provide for a residential postsecondary technical education facility that would prepare deaf young adults for successful employment. In December 1966 the Secretary of Health, Education and Welfare entered into an agreement with the Rochester Institute of Technology, Rochester, New York, to establish and operate the Institute on its campus, thus making available to deaf students a broad modern range of educational opportunities comparable to those available to hearing students in the technical fields (see Chapter 18). Of course, the federal government continues to sponsor Gallaudet College, which provides a liberal arts curriculum.

To focus attention on the needs of all handicapped children, Congress in November 1966 amended the monumental Elementary and Secondary Education Act of 1965 to establish a Bureau of Education for the Handicapped within the Office of Education to encourage and support professional training, research, improved demonstration of services, and the dissemination of information. A measure of the impact of federal support is the increase of badly needed trained teachers of hearing-impaired children. Similar increases in professional workers in audiology and speech pathology, and vocational counseling have resulted from training programs in the Social and Rehabilitation Services Administration and the United States Public Health Service.

Support by the National Institute of Neurological and Communicative Disorders and Stroke for the preparation of investigators has attracted many promising young trainees. In the course of time they should increase our understanding of the biomedical and psychoacoustic aspects of deafness on which advances in diagnosis and treatment undoubtedly depend.

In recent years, stimulated by judicial decisions in favor of maximum opportunities for the education of handicapped children, Congress has passed legislation that requires handicapped children to be educated in the least restrictive alternative settings. This and other legislation places an obligation on local school districts to provide, to the maximum extent appropriate, that handicapped children should be educated with children who are not handicapped. These are some of the important features of the Education for All Handicapped Children Act of 1975, which includes generously funded federal authorizations.

The needs of elderly persons, too, have been recognized by federal legislators. For example, The Older Americans Act Amendments (1975) authorize projects to inform hearing-impaired elderly persons about hearing loss and the availability of pertinent services. The act encourages increasing the supply of clinical services and, implicitly, of personnel concentrating on the requirements of older people.

Other agencies of the federal government have become involved in one way or another with the problems of deafness. A look back to the time of the first edition of this book (1947) reminds us that as much as anything the military audiology program during World War II laid the groundwork for audiology as we know it today. An estimated 15,000 servicemen received help for their hearing impairments in military centers established specifically for their needs. These "aural rehabilitation services" were available at Deshon (Pennsylvania), Borden (Oklahoma), and Hoff Army General (California) Hospitals for the Army and at the United States Naval Hospital in Philadelphia for the Navy. Services consisted of thorough diagnosis, medical treatment where indicated, speechreading, hearing aid selection, auditory training, and vocational and psychiatric counseling. On returning to civilian life military personnel who had worked in these programs applied the experience gained in them to the establishment of comprehensive services, to the development of academic and professional curricula for preparation of professionals, and to stimulation of basic and applied research. The Veterans Administration has continued the policy of comprehensive services to its clients and has fostered substantial training and research efforts.

The prevention and amelioration of hearing impairment have not escaped the atten-tion of government agencies exhorted to respond to the rising tides of "consumerism" and "environmentalism." Of intense current interest to all concerned with hearing impairment is the activity of the Federal Trade Commission, directed by Congress to develop trade regulation rules designed to govern the distribution and sale of hearing aids. Following its conventional pattern of hearings, interviews, and its own investigation, the Commission has proposed rules dealing with such matters as advertising, buyers' right to cancel a purchase, and medical and/ or audiological clearance before purchase. The Food and Drug Administration has recommended that rules for "professional and patient labeling" of hearing aids having to do with instructions for use and maintenance, effects of environmental conditions (humidity, temperature), and technical data of the kind discussed in Chapter 10 be included in a User Instruction Brochure and based on a proposed American National Standard Specification of Hearing Aid Characteristics. Currently, much of this is in the proposal stage and has yet to clear another round of public hearings.

As we have seen in Chapter 5, the Occupational Safety and Health Act (1970) and the Noise Control Act (1972) are concerned with protection from industrial noise of the "public health and welfare." OSHA is administered by the Department of Labor through the National Institute for Occupational Safety and Health and the Noise Control Act by the Environmental Protection Agency. Careful consideration of these and similar legislative measures suggests two distinct classes of problem. One of these is the technical requirement of accurate and appropriate measurement of conditions and their effects. This lies within the province of the qualified professional, whether audiologist, acoustical engineer, otologist, or industrial physician. The other class of problem relates to what in the modern managerial idiom we call cost benefits. In a sense a condition is safe if its risks are judged to be acceptable. Acceptability as it is expressed in legislation results from a kind of algebraic sum of many judgements that are primarily social and economic in nature. The professional defines the risks, the "public" judges whether they are worth taking.

A number of government agencies, including the Armed Forces and the Military, have joined in support of the National Research Council Committee on Hearing Bioacoustics and Biomechanics (CHABA). Any of the supporting agencies requiring advice on a particular question related to hearing or deafness may request such advice from CHABA. The conventional procedure is for CHABA to convene a working group of experts in the area in question, which then reports its findings through CHABA to the requesting agency. Among the requests dealt with during the first half of the 1970s were directions for research to improve hearing aids and services for the hearing-impaired, guidelines for a training course in noise survey techniques, research facilities in audition within the Armed Forces, and a compensation formula for hearing loss.

Another encouraging development fostered by federal support is the establishment of temporal bone banks in various laboratories to correlate histopathology of cases of deafness with prescribed information ob-tained during the life of the subject. Perhaps the large number of cases of deafness labeled "cause unknown" will be reduced because of these investigations.

Increased organized activities on the national and international scene by academic, professional, philanthropic, and lay groups is further evidence of the growing interest in the hearing-impaired. This is revealed, for example, in the "Annual Directory of Services" of the *American Annals of the Deaf.*

Although mankind has traveled a long, tortuous road from the pre-Christian era in evolving an enlightened understanding of the social problems of deafness, there is still a long road ahead. A large number of people still look upon the deaf and hard-of-hearing as queer, dependent, and sometimes ridiculous. We are all familiar with the cheap humor of which they are often the target. Since their handicap is not as visible as those of the blind and crippled, hearing-impaired persons often find themselves in embarrassing and humiliating situations because others do not understand their special problems. Their answer to such misunderstanding is to continue their social and economic achievements as self-respecting and productive individuals. Enlightened legislative action, therefore, does not aim for special privileges for them, but strives to provide opportunity, *without social or economic discrimination,* for them to help themselves.

SUGGESTED READINGS AND REFERENCES

Altshuler, K. Z. (ed.). *Education of the Deaf: The Challenge and the Charge.* Washington: U.S. Government Printing Office, 1967.

A report of a National Conference on Education of the Deaf arranged by the National Advisory Committee on the Education of the Deaf at the request of the Secretary of the Department of Health, Education and Welfare of the United States in April 1967. The conference brought together educators, audiologists, physicians, legislators, psychologists, social workers, leaders of the deaf community, deaf students, and others to discuss the needs of deaf persons. The conference was organized around the special needs of particular age groups, 0 to 5, 6 to 16, 17 to 22, and 22 plus. Recommendations for action to meet these needs are contained in the report.

Bender, R. E. *The Conquest of Deafness.* Cleveland: Press of Western Reserve University, 1960.

A recent historical treatment.

Békésy, G. von, and W. A. Rosenblith. "The Early History of Hearing—Observations and Theories," *J. Acoust. Soc. Amer.*, 20:727–748 (1948).

Author's summary: "The debris of broken systems and exploded dogmas form a great mound, a Mount Testaccio of the shards and remnants of old vessels which once held human beliefs. If you take the trouble to climb to the top of it, you will widen your horizon, and in these days of specialized knowledge your horizon is not likely to be any too wide." Oliver Wendell Holmes, 1882.

Boatner, M. T. *Voice of the Deaf: A Biography of Edward Miner Gallaudet,* Washington, D.C.: Public Affairs Press, 1959.

A sympathetic treatment of the life of the man associated with the founding and nurturing of Gallaudet College. Chapter 13 is particularly interesting because it discusses Gallaudet's relations with Alexander Graham Bell.

Bruce, R. V. *Bell: Alexander Graham Bell and the Conquest of Solitude.* Boston: Little, Brown & Company, 1973.

A definitive scholarly biography of Alexander Graham Bell, emphasizing and documenting his commitment to help for deaf persons.

Carhart, R. (ed.). *Human Communication and its Disorders: An Overview,* NINDS Monograph No. 10. U.S. Department of Health, Education and Welfare. Bethesda, Md.: Public Health Service, National Institutes of Health, 1970.

A report prepared by the Subcommittee on Human Communication and its Disorders, National Advisory Neurological Diseases and Stroke Council. A comprehensive report containing contributions from a substantial representation of the scientific and professional community addressed to definition of the extent of the field of human communication and its disorders, to review of the present status of research, and to an outline of unresolved problems and unmet needs, including recommendations for solutions.

Farrar, A. *Arnold's Education of the Deaf,* 2d ed. Derby, England: Francis Carter, 1923.

An account by a British author focused on the evolution of the education of the deaf from its European beginnings prior to the twentieth century.

Frisina, R. (ed.). "A Bicentennial Monograph on Hearing Impairment: Trends in the U.S.A.," *Volta Rev.* 78:1–148 (1976).

A collection of 18 brief essays on many facets of deafness.

Garnett, C. B. Jr. *The Exchange of Letters Between Samuel Heinicke and Abbé Charles Michel de l'Epée.* New York: The Vantage Press, 1968.

Author's summary: A monograph on the oralist and manualist methods of instructing the deaf in the eighteenth century, including the reproduction in English of the salient portions of each letter.

Goldstein, M. A. *Problems of the Deaf.* St. Louis: The Laryngoscope Press, 1933.
  Essentially a collection of essays on topics pertinent to deafness, including an excellent historical chapter.

Meyers, L. J. *The Law and the Deaf,* rev. ed. Washington, D.C.: U.S. Department of Health, Education and Welfare, 1971.
  A comprehensive treatment on how the law relates to the hearing-impaired.

Oyer, H. J. (ed.). *Communication for the Hearing Handicapped: An International Perspective.* Baltimore: University Park Press, 1976.
  An international view of philosophies, programs, methods, and research presented by professionals from 14 different countries.

Schein, J. D., and M. T. Delk. *The Deaf Population of the United States.* Silver Spring, Md.: National Association of the Deaf, 1974.
  A national study of the numbers and characteristics of deaf people.

Tower, D. B. (ed.-in-chief). *Human Communication and its Disorders,* Vol. 3. New York: Raven Press, 1975.
  One volume of a three-volume work commemorating the twenty-fifth anniversary of the National Institute of Neurological and Communicative Disorders and Stroke. An excellent compendium of scientific papers by recognized investigators dealing with hearing, speech, and central processes. A more than representative sampling of the kinds of problems that have attracted able scientists and of the methods they are using to address them.

Trudeau, E. (ed.) *Digest of State and Federal Laws: Education of Handicapped Children.* Arlington, Va.: The Council for Exceptional Children, 1971.

S. Richard Silverman, Ph.D.
Helen S. Lane, Ph.D.
Donald R. Calvert, Ph.D.

17

Early and Elementary Education

DEFINITIONS

A great deal of unnecessary confusion among the laity and well-intentioned professional workers alike has surrounded the precise definition and classification of hearing-impaired children and unfortunately has frequently obfuscated discussions of their problems. The confusion seems to grow out of the differences in frameworks of reference to which classification and nomenclature are related. For example, some workers classify the child who develops speech and language prior to onset of deafness as "hard of hearing" even though he may not be able to hear pure tones or speech at any intensity. This child, it is argued, unlike the congenitally profoundly deaf child who has not acquired speech naturally, behaves as a hard-of-hearing child in that his speech is relatively natural or "normal," and therefore he should be classified as "hard of hearing." It is obvious that an imprecise educational standard has guided the labeling if not the definition of the child. If, however, we consider the same child from a purely physiological standpoint, it is grossly misleading to term him "hard of hearing" when for all practical purposes he hears nothing at all.

The situation is complicated further by the use of terms that suggest not only physiological, communication, and educational factors but also gradations of hearing loss and time of onset. To this category belong such terms as *deaf and dumb, mute, deaf-mute, semideaf, semimute, deafened,* and others. These terms are of little value from the physiological, communicative, or educational points of view, and it would be well to eliminate them from general usage.

For purposes of this chapter we need to define the child in terms of his educational and psychological potential. A useful point of departure is a set of general definitions recommended by a special committee of the Conference of Executives of American Schools for the Deaf:

Hearing Impairment. A generic term indicating disability which may range in severity from mild to profound: it includes the subsets of *deaf* and *hard-of-hearing.*

A *deaf* person is one whose hearing disability precludes successful processing of linguistic information through audition, with or without a hearing aid.

A *hard-of-hearing* person is one who, generally with the use of a hearing aid, has residual hearing sufficient to enable successful processing of linguistic information through audition.

We can elaborate these definitions by describing the hearing-impaired child in terms of his ability to understand speech, his ability to progress in school, and the extent to which these abilities are affected by his hearing loss. In making generalizations about the significance of various degrees of hearing impairment we shall assume that the hearing loss occurred before the child acquired speech and learned to use language. Obviously, if speech and language are acquired before the hearing loss occurs, the handicap imposed by the loss is much less severe. Hearing-impaired children may be usefully divided into five classes, depending on their hearing levels for speech. (These levels may be estimated quite accurately, as pointed out

in Chapter 4, by averaging the hearing levels for pure tones at 500, 1000, and 2000 Hz. All levels are ANSI.) Table 17-1 delineates the classes and the particular needs of their members.[1]

The distinction between hard-of-hearing children and those whom we have termed deaf is not always entirely clear. The reason is that individual children may differ greatly in the use they are able to make of the remainder of their hearing. It is not simply a matter of hearing level for speech but also of such different factors as the age of onset, the severity and the type of hearing loss, the intelligence of the child, the amount of training the child has had, the age at which the training was begun, and the child's auditory and language environment. As we have learned from experience with "culturally disadvantaged" children who hear, an impoverished language environment retards development of skills of communication, a condition that is difficult to remedy when the optimum time for acquisition has been passed. It is a matter also of the attitude of parents and their degree of understanding of the significance of the hearing impairment.

Even within the broad group of the hard-of-hearing there is a wide range of the ability to make use of hearing for communication by speech. As we have seen in Chapter 9, the relatively mild hearing losses with hearing levels for speech of less than 40 dB cause only a little handicap, except perhaps for

[1] The hearing levels that mark the divisions of these classes are substantially the same as those given in Chapter 9. It will be noted that a hearing level of 90 rather than 100 dB is here chosen as the level dividing the fifth from the fourth class. This choice agrees well with a more recent definition of "100 percent hearing impairment" for medicolegal purposes and is discussed in Chapter 9. The scale given by the Committee on Hearing also subdivides what is here the first class into "normal" and "near normal." For the purposes of the present chapter, however, we have grouped all of these children together because they are all likely to "get along" in school and to have normal speech.

faint speech or for hearing at a distance. At the other extreme, with hearing levels for speech of 70 dB or thereabouts, and particularly if the hearing loss is congenital or of early onset, the child may require painstaking instruction to learn to "hear" adequately, even with a hearing aid, and to understand and use language. Furthermore, as we have seen in Chapter 4, the impairment of hearing is often not merely a loss of sensitivity, which may be overcome by amplification, but it may involve also a loss of ability to discriminate among certain sounds. Such a failure of discrimination is common when there is a great loss of sensitivity for the high frequencies.

Just as there are gradations in the usefulness of hearing, so are there gradations in the quality and intelligibility of the speech of hard-of-hearing children. Many hard-of-hearing children speak so well that the lay observer notices no abnormality, whereas the speech of the severely impaired may be almost unintelligible to those unaccustomed to this type of speech.

Many investigators have sought to define the relations of these various factors of hearing impairment: intelligence, personality, emotional stability, social behavior, and the like. Our best generalization from their studies is that it is impossible to draw a *single* composite picture of the hard-of-hearing child. There is too much variation, both in the severity of the hearing impairment and in many other pertinent factors. The personality structure of a child with hearing impairment is determined by many factors other than his difficulty in hearing.

Some object vigorously to the restricting influence of the definitions and classifications of impaired hearing contained in the definitions of the Conference of Executives. They maintain that the continuing increase of fundamental clinical and therapeutic audiological knowledge precludes any "static

categorization." For example, study of the thresholds of tolerance for speech and for pure tones has suggested that there is a useful portion of the auditory area even beyond the range of conventional audiometry. Some individuals who have heretofore been termed "totally deaf" as a result of audiometric tests may be reached by auditory stimulation using proper amplification. And it may prove to be more relevant to classify the person with a physical disability on some psychological scale of behavior that expresses how he lives with his disability.

We are aware that delimiting definitions are hazardous, and we recognize that each child's capabilities must be assessed individually by the best methods available to us so that we are not constrained by the need to classify. Nevertheless, we need some orientation to the kinds of children we are writing about in order that we may discuss them in general terms.

For convenience of exposition those children in classes 1, 2, and 3 (see Table 17-1) will be labeled *hard of hearing;* those in Classes 4 and 5 will be labeled *deaf.* We shall treat them separately.

HARD-OF-HEARING CHILDREN

Magnitude of the Problem

If we examine the results of mass testing surveys among schoolchildren, we find a range from 2 to 21 percent reported as having defective hearing. This great variability in reports of hearing impairment is undoubtedly due to differences in definitions of hearing impairment, in techniques, apparatus, and conditions of testing, and in the socioeconomic status and climate of the communities in which the surveys were carried out.

Our best estimate, supported by an extensive detailed study of Pittsburgh schoolchil-

TABLE 17-1
HEARING LEVELS FOR SPEECH AND EDUCATIONAL RECOMMENDATIONS

Class	Hearing Level for Speech	Educational Recommendation
1	*30 dB or better* These children may have difficulty in hearing faint or distant speech but are likely to "get along" in school and to have normal speech.	Children should be given the benefit of favorable seating in regular classrooms and may be assisted by special instruction in speechreading.
2	*30–55 dB* These children usually understand conversational speech at a distance of 3 to 5 feet without great difficulty. They may have some defects in the articulation of their own speech, and they may have difficulty in hearing adequately in school if the talker's voice is faint or if his face is not visible to them.	Children should wear hearing aids and be given training in their use. They should be taught speechreading and also be given the benefit of speech correction and conservation of speech. They should also have the advantage of favorable seating in classrooms.
3	*55–70 dB* These children understand conversational speech only if it is loud, and they have considerable difficulty in group and classroom discussions. Their language and especially their vocabularies may be limited, and abnormalities of articulation and voice production are obvious.	Hearing aids and auditory training, special training in speech, and special language work are all essential. With such assistance and with favorable seating, some children can continue in regular classes. Others may derive more benefit from special classes.
4	*70–90 dB* These children may hear the sound of a loud voice about 1 foot from the ear, and they may identify some environmental noises and may distinguish vowels, but even with hearing aids they have difficulty with consonants. The quality of their voices is not entirely normal, and they must be taught both speech and language. Many, but not all, children in this class should be considered "deaf" for educational purposes until or unless the combination of an adequate hearing aid and sufficient auditory training makes them only "hard of hearing."	Children should be taught by means of educational procedures for the deaf child, with special emphasis on speech, on auditory training, and on language. After a period of such instruction it is possible that these children may enter classes in regular schools.
5	*90 dB or worse* These children are deaf, even though they may hear some very loud sounds. They never can rely on the auditory channel as a primary avenue of communication. Their speech and their language must both be developed through careful and extensive training.	These children require special educational procedures described in this chapter. Some of them, however, eventually enter high schools for the hearing.

dren, is that 5 percent of school-age children have hearing levels, in one ear at least, outside the range of normal and that one to two of every ten in this group require special educational attention. (These figures do not include children in special schools for the deaf.) The others are likely to respond to medical care, or their hearing loss is not apt to reach the handicapping stage. All should be assessed for possible "learning disabilities." Table 17-2 shows the Pittsburgh findings according to class of handicap. (Although the Pittsburgh classifications do not coincide exactly with our own as shown in Table 17-1, they do not alter our basic point.) Of course, account should be taken of children below school age. Our judgment is that the statistics would be the same for them.

Significance of the Problem

The problem of the hard-of-hearing child is one of serious social significance. Specifically, the community should feel a concern for the unfortunate financial and social effects of the retardation in school of children whose handicap has been neglected or not recognized. Obviously, the repetition of grades is costly, and, in the long run, it is only a grossly superficial remedy that leaves the root of the problem quite untouched.

To those public school authorities and taxpayers who view with alarm the financial outlay necessary for a really constructive program for the hard-of-hearing child, we may point out that the saving resulting from avoidance of repetition of grades offsets a large part of the cost of the program. In addition, we must reckon the cost of truancy and various forms of antisocial behavior that characterize the child who becomes bored with the schoolwork in which it is so difficult for him to participate.

In the smaller community of the schoolroom itself the teacher is often not aware that the learning or behavior difficulty of a hard-of-hearing child is due to his impaired hearing and not to lack of mental ability or to some fault in her methods of teaching. For example, Goetzinger and his co-workers (1964), in studying children with as good a hearing level as 30 to 45 dB, found that the hearing-impaired children had poorer auditory discrimination and more errors of articulation than children with normal hearing. Furthermore, the incidence of comments from teachers stressing poor work habits, poor attitudes, and emotional variability was

TABLE 17-2
IMPAIRED HEARING IN THE PITTSBURGH STUDY POPULATION

	Class of Handicap				
	A	B	C	D	E and F
Impairment[a] (Ages 5 to 10 years, inclusive)	Not more than 25 dB	26–40 dB	41–55 dB	56–70 dB	More than 70 dB
Number (total 4062)	3996	36	19	9	2
Percentage	98.3	0.9	0.5	0.2	0.05
				← 0.3 % →	
		← 1.7 % →			

[a] Impairment refers to the average hearing-threshold level for 500, 1000, and 2000 Hz. The original ASA-1951 categories have been translated to equivalent ANSI categories (see Chapter 9).

much higher for the children with even mild hearing loss. Failure to understand the basic cause of the child's difficulties frequently leads to fruitless remedial measures that are time-consuming for both the child and his classmates. And when by good fortune the teacher recognizes the child's hearing impairment, his lack of special training and information and the requirements of other children in the room make quite impossible any adequate solution to the child's particular problem.

In the narrower confines of the family circle, too, the hard-of-hearing child presents a problem that requires sympathetic understanding. Apparent inattention to the spoken word is often interpreted as sheer naughtiness. The misdirected punishment often results in tensions within the family that would be avoided if the parents were only aware of their child's handicap. Furthermore, repetition of grades in school delays the day when the child can become a self-supporting individual. In many families the prolonged dependence is a serious problem.

The desirability of identifying hearing losses early by various methods of screening audiometry and individual hearing tests, as well as the possibility of conserving hearing by proper diagnosis and by treatment of the medical conditions that are so disclosed, has been discussed in Chapter 6. In detecting hearing losses in children, informal procedures and simple intelligent observation can be of great value. Both teachers and parents should be informed of the clues in a child's behavior that suggest the possibility of a hearing loss. The symptoms include inattention, frequent requests for repetition of spoken words, cupping the hand to the ear, cocking the head, difficulty in copying dictation, indifference to music, abnormalities of speech, reluctance to participate in activities that require oral communication (such as dramatics), failure to follow oral directions, daydreaming, and poor scholarship. Not to be overlooked are truancy, lying, stealing, extreme introversion, and other forms of atypical behavior that frequently serve as compensations for the child who feels socially inadequate and wishes to attract attention to himself. Of course, such behavior may also depend on a host of other conditions. We merely note that the possibility of hearing impairment as a cause should not be overlooked by teachers or laymen. Medical indications, such as earache, bad tonsils, frequent colds, and so on, have already been discussed in Chapter 6.

Educational Needs

The educational needs of the hard-of-hearing child as shown in Table 17-1 are different from those of the deaf child, discussed later. The hard-of-hearing child can learn to talk, to understand speech, and to learn language by more nearly "natural" means and by relying primarily on his hearing. Furthermore, if his difficulties are recognized and if he is given proper assistance, his needs may well be met in a special class for the hard-of-hearing within the public school system or even in the regular classroom itself. The assignment to a particular class will depend on both his hearing level and the availability of special help. The aim should be to educate him with children with normal hearing whenever this is practicable.

In Chapters 12, 13, and 14 we were acquainted with principles and techniques of auditory training, speechreading, speech development, and conservation of speech that are suitable for hard-of-hearing children. Special help in these aids to communication may be available through a special class, a resource teacher or a community speech and hearing center.

Guidance

Certainly we must not overlook the need for psychological, educational, and vocational guidance, which should avert or eliminate the atypical forms of behavior that may characterize the hard-of-hearing child. He must be made to understand that speechreading lessons and his hearing aid are as necessary as geography, arithmetic, or any other school activity. In fact, they may be more so. He should be particularly encouraged to join in extracurricular and community activities, such as scouting, athletics, Hi-Y, 4-H, church functions, and other wholesome pastimes of youth. Success in any of these activities should do much to avert extreme introversion and preoccupation with the impairment of hearing.

Of course, extreme cases should be referred for psychiatric study. Career plans for the child should take into account the existence of hearing impairment. Obviously we would not suggest preparation for any calling that demands a high degree of accuracy in oral communication. We are too well aware of the psychological distress that inevitably accompanies a trying occupational situation. Bookkeeping, for example, would be preferable to stenography. On the other hand, career guidance should stress the child's assets and not his liabilities. There are many occupations at all levels in which hearing impairment is not a barrier to success.

Throughout our discussion we have implied—and it is well now to stress—that although the welfare of the hard-of-hearing child should be entrusted to specially trained personnel, all remedial measures should be carried out within the framework of the regular school and health system. It is psychologically and educationally desirable for the child to associate with children who

hear normally. True, he must be segregated for speechreading lessons and auditory training, but these activities should be considered part of his school program. In fact, we suggest that academic credit be given for participation in such classes, since, for the hard-of-hearing child, they involve the development of communication skills as important as composition or public speaking. They should be so recognized and integrated with the curriculum. When the child is convinced that he is a person with a particular need that has been recognized, he has hurdled the chief obstacle to his eventual adjustment.

In summary, the management of hard-of-hearing children requires:

1. Public information about hearing impairment
2. Case finding through appropriate screening and identifying programs in hospitals, clinics for babies, and schools
3. Complete medical diagnosis of hearing difficulties
4. Appropriate medical and surgical treatment
5. Thorough assessment of hearing after all indicated medical and surgical procedures have been completed, with particular attention to educational needs
6. Special educational measures that include auditory training, speechreading, speech correction and conservation of speech, vocational planning, and psychological guidance

DEAF CHILDREN

Goals of Education of the Deaf

Deaf children are more likely to be identified earlier in life and with greater confidence than hard-of-hearing children because their difficulty in reception of auditory signals is much more obvious. Nevertheless, the task of educating deaf children is much more complex, and consequently it gives rise to conflicting and divergent points of view as to how it is best accomplished. Obviously, how we go about educating deaf children is related to the goals we have set for them, and these goals are in turn determined by what we consider to be the overall educational, psychological, and social potential of deaf persons. In other words, some of the sharp differences of opinion concerning the most desirable arrangements and methods for the education of deaf children really have their roots in fundamental differences of opinion on the long-range outlook for these children. This outlook may be determined, among other considerations, by our own value system, by our experience with postschool accommodation and adjustment of deaf persons, by our own education and indoctrination, by our professional training, by our relation to deaf persons, or by some combination of these.

The overwhelming amount of literature on the subject (a bibliography would probably exceed 2000 titles), ranging from school papers and convention resolutions to lengthy sections of books, reveals an intense polemicism. Of course, there are many shades of opinion, but stated views and observed practices suggest what we may term three "schools of thought." We are aware that we may be indulging in caricature and that "it all depends on the individual child," but we believe that a sorting out of views is desirable if we are to understand the rationale for particular views of the education of deaf children.

One group appears to stress the limitations, especially the social limitations, of deafness. It is concerned about the exclusion of the deaf from certain types of desirable employment, the effect on the deaf of insurance practices and legislation, the implication of what amounts to minority group status in certain educational and social contexts, the impact of isolation from other deaf people, the difficult if not impossible task for some of learning speech and speechreading, and the misunderstanding of the general public concerning the abilities and aspirations of the deaf. This group would suit the method of communication to the child; its view is best summarized by the following statement:

The aim of the education of the deaf child should be to make him a well-integrated, happy deaf individual, and not a pale imitation of a hearing person. Let us aim to produce happy, well-adjusted deaf *individuals,* each different from the other, each with his own personality. If a child cannot learn to read lips well or cannot speak well, it is far better to encourage additional modes of expression and communication, writing and gesturing, than to make him feel ashamed and frustrated because he cannot acquire the very difficult art of speech and lipreading. Our aim must be a well-balanced, happy *deaf* person and not an imitation of a hearing one.

The educational program should be geared to the production of contented members of a deaf community (see Chapter 20), secure in its sanctions, its modes of communication, and its opportunities for social expression.

A second group emphasizes the immense potentialities of the deaf, as yet untapped, particularly for education and for participation in a world of hearing people. It stresses the importance of early education and the great possibilities of auditory training, and it is apt to emphasize the objective of "normalization." In essence there is "one world" in which the deaf person must function, and that is a world of hearing and speaking people. The adherents of this view reject the validity of the "deaf community" concept for deaf people and strive toward their complete assimilation in the world of the hearing.

A third school of thought points to the record of economic, academic, and social achievement of deaf persons *among both the deaf and the hearing* as a strong, tangible justification for the belief that forward-looking, proper, and early fundamental training enables the deaf child to make the fullest use of his capabilities. Yet it is apparent, at least in our present state of knowledge, that there are situations in which the deaf will always be marginal, and our approach to them should be influenced accordingly. Realism urges us to spare parents and the child himself the psychological distress of failure to achieve the "normalcy" that was set up as an attainable goal.

To sum up succinctly, the first group says there are two distinct worlds, the deaf and the hearing. They communicate very little and only when necessary, and the deaf may not be too concerned with devaluation of their group. The second says there is only the world of the hearing, and deaf people must adjust to it through integration. For the third group the two worlds overlap. Some deaf people penetrate the majority culture more than others, perhaps because of their education, their native ability, their skill in oral communication, emotional makeup, their families, or for other reasons. These factors require more study in order that the knowledge we gain may enable us to set goals more rationally.

The prevalent attitudes influence not only the means of communication in and out of the classroom and the content and nature of the curriculum, but they have a direct bearing on the organizational and administrative education arrangements, day or residential, integrated or segregated, that we make for deaf children and on the important and essential practice of guiding and counseling parents.

A reasonable guiding principle in our present state of knowledge is to reject the notion that deaf persons are an undifferentiated, monolithic mass and to avoid the stereotyping to which it gives rise. Deaf persons differ among themselves, as do the hearing, and therefore there should be a reasonable and carefully thought-out range of educational options available to them. After all, this is the essence of our entire culture, and we achieve its aspirations to the extent that we increase the opportunities for people to be themselves.

This point of view has recently been reinforced by a resolution adopted by the Council on Education of the Deaf, which is composed of representatives appointed by constituent organizations professionally involved in the education of the deaf. The resolution follows:

Be it resolved that the Council on Education of the Deaf (CED) hereby signifies its commitment to the initiation, expansion, and improvement of educational options in order to serve every hearing-impaired child of school age, in recognition of the right of every deaf or hard-of-hearing child of school age to have an appropriate individualized educational program including such aspects as: (1) the educational setting, ranging from partial or full-time regular classroom placement to partial or full-time educational programs offered in special classes in public/private day schools or public/private residential schools; (2) the method of instruction and instructional strategies which shall be employed during the school day; (3) the need for continuing monitoring, assessment, and modification/extension of each school-age child's program, including method of instruction and educational setting as his/her changing personal, social, and instructional needs dictate.

At any rate, until more facts are available to fill the gaps now occupied by opinion, a rational attitude points to the recognition that deafness imposes certain unavoidable limitations that must be accepted. At the same time, proper education in its broadest sense strives to relate the deaf person to the world about him in a psychologically satisfying way.

THE EDUCATION OF THE DEAF

We now turn to consideration of what we judge to be a "proper education." It is both convenient and logical to organize our discussion around the following topics:

1. The communication controversy
2. Organization of the education of the deaf
3. The rise of the preschool movement
4. Psychological and educational assessment of deaf children
    (a) Intelligence
    (b) Educational achievement
    (c) Personality
    (d) Language development and concepts
5. The skills of communication
    (a) Speech
    (b) Auditory training
    (c) Speechreading
    (d) Language
6. Curriculum development in schools for the deaf
7. Problems of parents

The Communication Controversy

Common to all methods or general strategies of early "management" or education is the premise, as we shall emphasize later in this chapter, that the early years are optimal for establishing the foundation for the child's acquisition of communication and his emotional or "affective" maturation. And, what happens then is more than likely

to determine the course of his subsequent formal education, particularly its setting, its relative emphasis on certain modes of communication, the preparation of its teachers and its explicit goals.

For our purposes it is useful to present some general features of two current, essentially differing approaches that curiously enough rest on the same basic premise of the importance of the early years. One of these is what we call the *Auditory Global Method.* The principal features of this "method" are that the primary, though not always exclusive, channel for speech and language development is auditory and that the input is fluent, connected speech. The terms "auditory-oral," "aural-oral," "acoupedic," "natural," and "unisensory" are conventional synonyms for the same fundamental method, or they designate variations within the same general framework. The method stresses maximum use of the auditory channel, however much its sensitivity is reduced (see Chapter 12). The more enthusiastic among its followers say "There is no such thing as a totally deaf child" and "Every remnant of hearing is usable for developing oral communication," which incidentally is an explicit goal, the attainment of which is crucial for the most desirable development of the child. Even if one disagrees with this rather extreme position on the potential usefulness of residual hearing, the data on the hearing status of children in our schools reported by the Center for Demographic Studies at Gallaudet College (1972–1973) do point to a substantial number of children with residual hearing that, if cultivated, would facilitate their development of useful everyday oral communication. The data indicate that 45 percent of hearing-impaired children are reported to have hearing levels of 84 dB or less in the three speech frequencies. Incidentally, if the frequency 250 Hz had been included in the calculation and a cutoff established at 90 dB the number of children with hearing significant for speech and language acquisition would be much greater. It is essential, for best results, that a communicating environment positively responsive to a child's oral communication be developed and maintained. The emphasis in the method on connected speech with its prosodic and suprasegmental cues recognizes that the child with abnormal hearing not only imitates what he hears but formulates inductively the rules of spoken language. However, the restricted auditory sensitivity of the hearing-impaired child reduces the redundancy and the linguistic cues of the language available to him. Nevertheless, it is argued, there may still be sufficient auditory and visual cues to facilitate inductive acquisition of the rules of speech and language. If all requirements of the method are satisfied, practical oral speech and language competence should be acquired, thus paving the way for the child's integration or "mainstreaming" in schools for hearing children with all the advantages for subsequent economic and social self-realization. The impressive number of hearing-impaired persons who have achieved these goals is inspiring and should, so the reasoning goes, influence our aspirations accordingly. *Nevertheless, we need to anticipate realistically that the Auditory Global Method will not be attainable, for whatever reason, for all children.* Even if the major focus of a program for an individual child is oral competence and our goal is maximal exploitation of the opportunities of the world of the hearing, alternate methods or modifications need to be considered—for example, those that stress multisensory stimulation, described in the pages that follow, deliberate development of and drill on speech sounds and their combinations, smaller units of speech input, and more structured language instruction. The point is that we need to know if, when, and how we should intervene to change a general strategy that may have seemed promising at the outset.

Another "method" that proceeds from the premise of the importance of early education is probably best subsumed under the rubric *Total Communication.* The primary feature of this approach is that all modes of communication are recommended from the beginning. Its advocates reject the exclusion of manual forms of communication described in Chapter 15. They stress that sole reliance on residual hearing and speechreading for communication results in ambiguous or deficient communication (or none at all), which in turn retards cognitive development. Furthermore, poor communication between parent and young child may lay the groundwork for emotional difficulties. Continuing experience, it is maintained, confirms the reality and the necessity of an active "deaf community," which can attract deaf adults who find security in its sanctions, its modes of communication, its opportunities for social expression, and its organized advocacy of causes beneficial to deaf persons (see Chapter 20). Therefore, this aim is to be preferred to a goal of "integration" into "hearing society." And it is most likely to be attained by the Total Communication approach instituted as early as possible. As of now there appears to be no universal agreement on what constitutes Total Communication. The proportionality of fingerspelling to signs (or their omission entirely, as in the "Rochester method"), the choice of a language-gesture or a concept-gesture relation and its effect on language learning, the probability that the prosodic features of speech so important for optimum use of residual hearing are blurred when speech and manual forms are presented simultaneously, and the effect of selective reinforcement of one mode over another are among the many open questions. More fundamental questions pertain to processing of sign language, its "grammar" and its relation to spoken language—not to mention its acquisition by "nonnative" signers, such as parents and teachers.

To exhaust all of the key unanswered questions about any approach or to formulate any of them precisely is obviously beyond the scope of this text. The controversy is by no means settled, but it is encouraging that numerous investigations are under way to study not only the linguistic, conceptual, intellectual, and economic effects of modes of communication for deaf persons but also their influence on such features of personality as emotional maturity and self-identity. Because there is universal agreement among educators of the deaf that every deaf child should be given an opportunity to communicate by speech, our attention in this chapter is directed at the essential elements that comprise this opportunity.

Organization of the Education of the Deaf

Perhaps the most significant fact about the education of the deaf in the United States is that it is universally available to all deaf children of school age. Of course, the quality of education may vary, but it is important that no child need be denied an opportunity for it. Where are these opportunities available?

Of 52,485 children enrolled in schools for the deaf in the academic year 1975–1976 a total of 19,120 attended public residential schools for the deaf. These schools, open to qualified children without charge, are supported either directly or indirectly by state tax funds. Most of the public residential schools are supported by legislative appropriation and hence come under the control of state authorities. The educational services of the remaining schools of this kind are purchased by the states on a per diem or per capita basis and are controlled by their own boards. Examples of the first group are the Indiana and Illinois schools for the deaf; in the second group we find such schools as the Lexington (New York) and the Clarke (Massachusetts) schools for the deaf.

Other tax-supported institutions for the deaf are public day schools and classes. A school is usually large enough to be a separate entity; for example, A. G. Bell School, in Cleveland. Day classes are usually groups within a larger school unit, and there may be as few as one in a school or as many as ten; for example, in Pomona, California. In the 1975–1976 school year 7024 children were being educated in public day schools, and 22,132 were in public day classes. The trend of the past decade toward increasing the number of deaf children educated in nonresidential settings reflects the growing emphasis on "mainstreaming" and education of all handicapped children in their own school districts. The remaining children were being educated in private schools, such as Lutheran School (Detroit) and Central Institute for the Deaf (St. Louis). Such schools may be either day or residential, or a combination of the two. There were 822 children in schools and classes for the multiply handicapped. The number of children in each class ranges generally from five to ten. Some deaf children have been absorbed into classes for the hearing. Deaf individuals attend high schools and colleges for the hearing. Most public residential schools provide education at the secondary level, and higher education exclusively for the deaf is available at Gallaudet College, Washington, D.C. Technical postsecondary education is provided at the National Technical Institute for the Deaf, which is an integral part of a larger technical institute for the hearing, the Rochester Institute of Technology, Rochester, New York. Other opportunities for postsecondary education are discussed in Chapter 18. (Statistical data are from the Directory of Programs and Services issue of the *American Annals of the Deaf*, April 1976.)

Until we have more evidence to support

the point of view of either the day or the residential school, we must study each child's situation thoroughly to determine what educational placement is likely to be most fruitful for him. This points up the crucial need for early identification, diagnosis, and careful assessment. In addition to information about a child's hearing, among the significant points to be considered are the etiology of the deafness, the child's age at its onset, his physical development, his behavioral development, his social maturity, his home environment, and the insight of his parents.

The Rise of the Preschool Movement

The encouraging progress in the assessment of hearing of young children has stressed the value of preschool programs for deaf children. The period from birth to age 5 is particularly vital for the learning and overall development of children, whether hearing or deaf. The importance of early auditory experience is now recognized, and hearing aids are being recommended with greater confidence than previously. It is worthy of mention that the extent to which auditory stimulation is combined with specific modes of visual communication such as speechreading, gesture, and fingerspelling varies and is the subject of much critical discussion.

Indirect evidence from neurophysiology suggests that there is an optimal early period of life when the nervous system is still plastic and sensory experience exerts an important influence on its development. Psycholinguists, too, point to an optimal period for the acquisition of language, particularly the induction of rules underlying its phonologic, syntactic, and semantic features. Since the young deaf child is denied many of the normal experiences that lead to better socialization, it is all the more important that he be given help and opportunity for his best development as early in life as possible. This

means not just a sensible program for developing the skills of communication that so greatly contribute to socialization, but also a regimen that removes where possible the barrier that tends to isolate the deaf child from the world about him, from the world of his home, his parents, his sisters and brothers, and from other children. Formal and informal intercommunications (by whatever means) tend to lessen the child's feeling of apartness and hence make him feel wanted and significant.

The child is thus motivated to communicate, and it is the task of the parent and the teacher to show him the usefulness of speech as a tool of communication. "The situations," according to the prominent British educators of the deaf, Professor and the late Mrs. Ewing, "do not happen enough by themselves; they must be anticipated and contrived frequently and deliberately" by all who are in close contact with the child. Although it is not generally mandatory for tax-supported schools to provide preschool classes for deaf children, the need is beginning to be recognized. A major funding priority of the Bureau for the Education of the Handicapped is "early education."

In discussing the young deaf child it is appropriate to mention the increasing amount of information and guidance available for parents of deaf children. Although here and there an effort may be misguided, the proliferation of parent institutes and clinics and of correspondence courses, reading lists, and literary output is one of the most constructive and forward-looking developments in the education of the deaf.

For parents of very young deaf children there are now correspondence courses that offer guidance, practical suggestions, and information concerning the home care of the child before the nursery school years. Probably the first such correspondence course was established by the Wright Oral School in New York City, but the best known at the

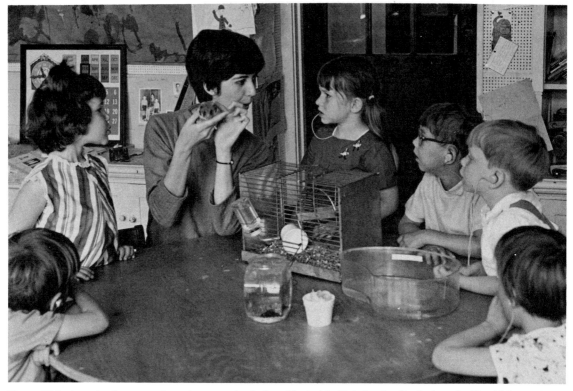

Figure 17-1 Learning from experience in a preschool class. *(Central Institute for the Deaf; photo by Harold Ferman)*

present time is operated by the John Tracy Clinic in Los Angeles. Intelligent and cooperative parents have found these courses most helpful in giving them specific step-by-step procedures in beginning stages and a good psychological approach to the deaf child. Other procedures include the development of visual discrimination by matching colors and pictures and the comparison of objects varying in size and shape, practice in discriminating odors and tastes, exercise in the imitation of bodily movements, and the use of materials that will aid the child in better muscular coordination. Training of this type is continued in the nursery school on a more extensive and advanced scale. Such a correspondence course is particularly useful for those who are too remote to obtain information and advice in person from one

of the well-established schools for the deaf. Children instructed by the parents who have followed a correspondence course of this type are better prepared to benefit immediately from a nursery school.

In general there appear to be no universally accepted specific aims or procedures in guiding parents of very young children. The emphases vary. For some the primary aim is to create realistic "acceptance" of the child's condition, and counseling is weighted toward psychotherapy. For others the emphasis is on conveying information in order to create an understanding of sensory deprivation and its effect on the total development of the child in general and of his communication deficit in particular. There is a growing and encouraging trend toward carrying on parent "training" in homes and homelike settings, sometimes called demonstration homes, where, by demonstration and practice, parents learn to contrive and take advantage of natural situations in the home to sharpen perceptions and foster communication.

Of great interest to educators of deaf children is the knowledge likely to be gained from the programs of early education such as Head Start directed at "culturally disadvantaged" children. Here too, vigorous schools of thought appear to be taking shape. On the one hand, there are those who would emphasize "cognitive" approaches that stimulate intellectual functioning. In its extreme form it has been labeled the "pressure-cooker" view, which aims to compensate for the lack of opportunity for perceptual development. Others would stress the child's social and emotional growth without too much "structured" teaching.

Most of these commendable efforts in orientation and guidance have been directed at parents of children of preschool age. This is natural, since the initial shock of the discovery of deafness must be intelligently cushioned, and crucial and immediate decisions must be made about the child's future. Even though we are discussing here children of preschool age, it should be realized that the placement of a child in a satisfactory educational situation in no way decreases the need for the guidance of parents. This was forcefully driven home to us in a survey made of the parents of present and former pupils at Central Institute for the Deaf. Parents of teenagers and young adults wanted an opportunity to share information and experiences about such problems as choices of career, marriage with the deaf or the hearing, the genetics of deafness, and the choice of companions for the deaf. In short, social adjustment is just as much a problem for the deaf youth as it is for the preschool child, and it is important that parent institutes and clinics concerned with their problems be fostered as well.

Whatever evidence exists for the value of particular procedures and programs of parent counseling is meager and is generally anecdotal or based on studies (frequently retrospective) of children's records. It will be helpful, for the programs we undertake, to evaluate all of the following: *genetic counseling* (see Chapter 4) for deaf married couples and parents of deaf children; the use of the *high-risk register* (see Chapter 8); the *adaptations* necessary because of differences in the intelligence, motivation, and education of parents; the *emotional needs* of parents; the *special training* necessary for those who counsel parents; and the implications of the concept of *optimal periods* in development.

Psychological and Educational Assessment of Deaf Children

Intelligence Measures of the mental ability of deaf children are important in decisions concerning educational placement, instructional groupings, readiness for continuing education in classes for hearing children, and vocational and academic guidance.

What is intelligence? How we define it determines the confidence with which we measure the intelligence of the deaf child. If it is the ability to carry on abstract thinking and to use abstract symbols in the solution of problems, as defined by Terman, we are testing in an area requiring verbal behavior. In fact, Terman considered the size of vocabulary to be the best single indicator of intelligence. Selection of mental tests that satisfy this definition would lead to the conclusions that deaf children are either mentally retarded *or* that their ability cannot be measured. However, if intelligence is defined as the aggregate or global capacity of the indi-

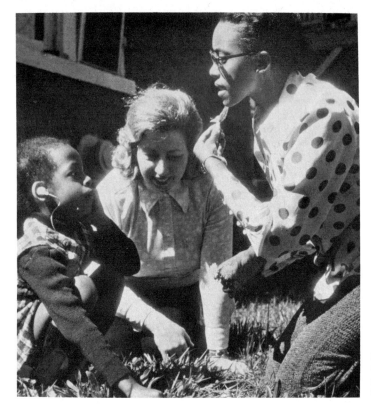

Figure 17-2 Instructing a parent to take advantage of everyday opportunities to encourage communication. *(Central Institute for the Deaf; photo by Ken Nicolai)*

vidual to act purposefully, to think rationally, and to deal effectively with his environment (Wechsler), then nonverbal tests can yield an estimate of mental ability.

The need for measures of mental ability of the deaf child preceded the development of intelligence scales. In 1889, at what is now the Lexington School for the Deaf, Greenberger used colored picture books and blocks as a part of the procedure for admission of children to the school. Observation of facial expression and behavior with "test materials" enabled him to weed out the mentally subnormal child.

Pintner and Paterson (1917) attempted to apply the Binet-Simon scale to a population of deaf children and concluded that difficulties in the use of the scale occurred due to the lack of comprehension, the lack of environmental experience, and "the peculiar psychology" of the deaf child.

Pintner and his associates were pioneers in the psychological testing of the deaf. They attempted to use and modify existing tests developed for hearing children and finally constructed a performance test, a Non-Language Scale for group testing, and an Educational Scale for the deaf (1917). The results of a national survey reported by Reamer (1921) led to the conclusion that deaf children were mentally retarded (2 to 3 years) and educationally retarded (4 to 5 years or 3½ grades). These conclusions were accepted by many educators before 1930.

With the realization that a child with a hearing impairment must learn to understand language and to communicate came the recognition that a test of mental ability must measure what the child is capable of learning. This required the selection of tests that were nonverbal in administration and response. Pantomime instructions were standardized, and gestures were substituted for such verbal instruction as "Watch me carefully and do as I do" or "Put the blocks in the box quickly."

Test batteries in use included the Randall's Island Performance Series, the Ontario School Ability Examination, the Grace Arthur Point Scale, the Goodenough Draw-a-Man Test, the Hiskey-Nebraska Test of Learning Ability, the Leiter International Scale of Intelligence, and the performance sections of Wechsler tests. These tests were administered to hearing populations, and their validity was determined by comparison with verbal tests. When the performance tests were administered to the deaf, results indicated a normal distribution of intelligence test scores.

The psychometrist using these tests needs to be skilled in getting rapport quickly, in stressing the importance of speed in some tests that are timed, in observing carefully

the attention of the child, and in accurately recording significant behavior as well as test scores. Many performance test batteries use the same test items, and the test-retest reliability of some of these items is questionable. Therefore, the psychometrist must be alert to the child's familiarity with a test and be prepared to substitute other test batteries. It is especially important in clinical evaluation to avoid duplication of tests, since many parents take deaf children to clinics throughout the United States to get additional opinions and diagnoses.

Recent emphasis has been placed on qualitative instead of quantitative differences in the mental ability of the deaf compared with that of the hearing. There is a tendency to view intelligence on a continuum of concrete-abstract. According to Myklebust (1964), when one type of sensory experience is missing, it alters the integration and function of others. Experience for the child is constituted differently, and the world of perception, conception, imagination, and thought has a new configuration. Oléron (1950) has suggested that conventional tests

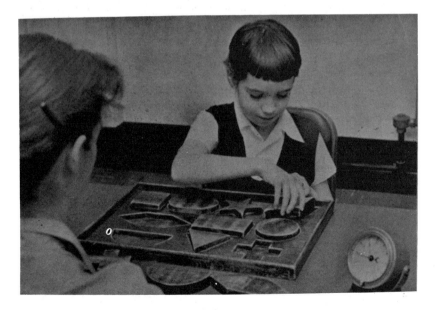

Figure 17-3 A form board is used to test mental ability. *(Central Institute for the Deaf)*

have not served our purposes and that we need fresh approaches to study difficulties in perceptual analysis and organization, abstract thinking, and concept formation. An attempt in this direction is the Snijders-Ooman Non-Verbal Scale (SONS) (1959), used in Europe, which is designed to include nonverbal items requiring conceptual thinking with a minimum of items requiring speed of performance.

Several investigators suggest that the low predictive value of IQ scores on performance tests as indicators of future academic achievement is evidence that the performance test is inadequate as a measure of the kind of intelligence needed to succeed academically or perhaps is evidence that educators have failed to produce academic achievement commensurate with intelligence.

The Hiskey-Nebraska Test of Learning Aptitude has been revised (1966), extending the age limits to which it is applicable. Tests have been added, but it is still scored as a learning quotient (LQ), indicating its use to predict learning skills based on observations in classrooms for the deaf. Birch and Birch (1951) used the Leiter International Performance Scale and the Goodenough Draw-a-Man, together with other test batteries, to predict which children will present serious teaching problems in speechreading, oral expression, and reading. On these two tests the children with learning problems test significantly lower than on the other test batteries.

The performance portion of the Wechsler Intelligence Scales has become one of the widely used tests to measure the intelligence of the deaf. All of the scales are constructed to have a verbal and a performance section with scores expressed in a verbal quotient, a performance quotient, and a full-scale quotient. It is assumed that in a normal population the mean of differences between the verbal and performance quotients is zero, with a normal distribution of differences. Therefore, psychometrists testing the deaf give only the performance portion and report a score on a test that is meaningful to educators and psychologists. The verbal portion may be significant as an index of readiness of the deaf child to be integrated into classes for the hearing. When the deaf child achieves a verbal quotient within normal limits, he should be able to cope with the language of the school curriculum for the hearing.

Early identification of deafness and parent-infant programs have created a need for tests from infancy to 3 years of age. Developmental scales such as the Gesell norms and the Vineland Social Maturity Scale serve as guides to which the teacher can supplement her observations of behavior. The Smith Non-Verbal Performance Scale constructed by Dr. Althena Smith (1967) at the Tracy Clinic is a behavior scale to be used to estimate levels of development with items (graded in difficulty) that present a broad clinical picture in children from 2 to 4 years of age. Studies of scores on developmental scales compared with later tests of intelligence on the same children indicate that later mental performance cannot be predicted from infant tests.

Testing the multiply handicapped deaf presents additional problems. There are no reliable measures for deaf children with poor motor coordination. Tests of speed are not fair, and tests requiring precision of coordination are frustrating. The psychometrist can only estimate ability, and this must be confirmed by a trial period of teaching.

Deaf children with learning difficulties frequently show a wide range of abilities in the test items. Scores on tests involving memory span are apt to be lower than on other tests in the battery. The distribution and pattern of test scores in a battery of tests become significant in class placement that takes into account the individual differences of deaf children.

Educational achievement Educational progress is generally measured by scores on achievement tests, generally administered at regular intervals, preferably annually, from the time the child reaches the equivalent of the second grade until he is prepared to leave the school for the deaf. These tests measure reading, arithmetic, social studies, science, language, spelling, and study skills. There is no need for special tests for the deaf to measure educational attainment in terms of grade and age equivalents. The value of these tests is to compare the educational level of the deaf child with national norms for the hearing. However, Wrightstone, Aranow, and Moskowitz (1963) have developed reading-test norms for the deaf using the revision of the Metropolitan Achievement Test, Elementary Reading Test 2. These norms enable educators to compare groups of deaf children.

There has been great concern about the gap between mental ability and educational level of deaf children from the time of the studies of Pintner in the 1920s to the present date. Hall (1929) and Fusfeld (1935) reported the educational test level of students entering Gallaudet to be a mean grade equivalent ranging from 9.2 in 1929 to 10.0 in 1932.

The average grade equivalents on the Stanford Achievement Test of deaf children over 16 years of age leaving school programs were tabulated by Boatner (1965) and can be summarized as follows:

	Total N	Diplomas	Certificates
Residential schools	1145	8.2	5.3
Day, private, denominational schools	132	7.3	5.0

These statistics, however, fail to include deaf children prepared to leave special schools before the age of 16. The Babbidge report (1965), citing the median grade average of 920 students who left residential schools in the 1963–1964 school year, revealed that at no age was a median seventh grade achievement attained.

Some deaf children are prepared to enter schools for the hearing in the lower elementary grades or at the high school level. The educational quotient for these children based on standardized tests usually indicates educational retardation, or that it takes deaf children a longer time to achieve the academic requirements of the hearing schools. Lane (1976) reported an achievement test grade equivalent of 4.4 for 142 deaf children who integrated into hearing classes early and of 8.0 for 189 who graduated from the eighth grade, but the median educational quotients were 87.9 and 85.1 respectively, a retardation of approximately two years.

It is important to emphasize that mean or median scores on a test battery do not give a meaningful measure of the child's achievement. Deaf children do not score equally well on all tests. Poorest scores are found in reading tests (paragraph meaning and word meaning) and in arithmetic reasoning or problem solving. Best scores are recorded in arithmetic computation and spelling. A pretest of reading is recommended as a quick screening measure to select children who are ready for a battery of achievement tests. A reading pretest was used in a national survey, by the office of Demographic Studies at Gallaudet College (1971), of academic achievement of schools for the deaf in the United States to determine the grade level of the Stanford Achievement Series to be used. Approximately 17,000 deaf children ranging in age from 6 to 21+ were tested. The Primary Batteries (grades 1–3) were administered to 70.6 percent of the population tested, the Intermediate Batteries (grades 4–

6) to 25.1 percent, and only 4.3 percent were ready for the Advanced Battery (grades 7–9). Both the Spelling Test and the Word Study Skills Test are dictated in the Primary Tests, and the Word Study Skills for the Intermediate Battery I. Because dictated tests are not valid for the deaf, grade scores on the total test were not reported.

Wrightstone, Aranow, and Moskowitz (1963) reported that deaf children between the ages of 10 and 16 gain only 8 months in reading skills. Lane and Baker (1974), however, showed an improvement of 2.5 grades for a comparable age range in a study of five consecutive achievement tests given over a four-year period and a mean reading grade equivalent of 6.2 for 92 students who graduated from the eighth grade. The rate of progress was slower, but it was steady and had not reached an asymptote at grade 6.

The deaf child generally does not learn at the same rate as the hearing child. With the need to master new vocabulary and language, it takes about two or more years to achieve second grade level and an additional one and a half to two years to complete third grade. This plateau in learning may be discouraging, but it is not the fault of the child or teacher. It can be attributed to the time necessary to build a foundation for future progress.

Personality   Results from personality tests of deaf children are meager and contradictory and are obviously complicated by language difficulties. Information has been obtained from three types of tests: (1) behavior rating scales and questionnaires with the parent, houseparent, or teacher as informant, for example, the Vineland Social Maturity Scale or the Haggerty-Olson-Wickman Behavior Rating Scale; (2) questionnaires answered by deaf children, for example, the Rogers Test of Personality Adjustment, revised for the deaf by Brunschwig, or the California Test of Personality; (3) projective techniques such as the Rorschach Ink Blot Test, the Draw-a-Person Test, the Make-a-Picture Story Test (MAPS), or the Hand Test.

All of the questionnaires contain items that are of questionable validity for use with the deaf because they require communication skills and normal hearing. When these items are eliminated, ratings indicate that the deaf have more emotional problems and less maturity. When a child fills in the questionnaire, the problems of reading comprehension, interpretation of qualifying vocabulary (such as "usually" or "sometimes"), and imagination influence his responses. In a study of the California Test of Personality as a tool for measurement, Vegely and Elliott (1968) found that items that were not understood presented semantic rather than syntactic problems. It was hypothesized that even after revision of items and test norms, deaf children would continue to show poorer adjustment.

Using the Rorschach Test, Levine (1956) found confirmatory evidence of mental "underdevelopment" and that personality development is closely linked to language development. Myklebust (1964) reported emotional immaturity with more emotional stress, conflict, and frustration for deaf children enrolled in day classes and more isolation for those in residential schools. On the Draw-a-Person Test used in his study, the deaf child showed perceptual distortions regarding himself and projected these to others. Hess (1969) has developed a nonverbal modification of the MAPS test for children 8, 9, and 10 years old. In a preliminary report the deaf differed from the adjusted and emotionally disturbed by showing faster and more impulsive reactions to new situations but with indication of adequate involvement. There was evidence of more expansive fantasy life, superficial personal attachment, and depressive emotional tone. The Hand

Test devised by Wagner (1962) was applied to three linguistically divergent groups of young deaf adults by Levine and Wagner (1974). The exceptional group—with reading ability at the high school or college level and average or higher intelligence and oral communication skills—had test scores that looked like those of the hearing with a slight trace of withdrawal. The typical group of high school students in a residential school had a reading grade of 6.9, normal intelligence, and both oral and manual communication. They had more in common with hearing high school students than differences. The illiterate group—with a mean reading grade of 2.4, intelligence ranging from dull normal to average, and poor communication skills—was not a happy group. They substituted quantity for quality of response and had a negative evaluation of self.

Levine and Wagner concluded that the deaf must be prepared with the communicative wherewithal to engage in the total scope of human communication. They must be supplied with all opportunities for enculturation, for this represents unity with society. The surest means to this end is linguistic capability, especially the ability to read.

Personality tests are valuable tools in counseling the deaf because they may reveal problems that the counselors did not suspect. They are essential in the vocational counseling program because they aid in assessing the ability of the deaf person to adjust to society. There does not seem to be a "personality of the deaf" but rather individual differences that are significant in teaching and guidance and more often than not are related to the linguistic ability of the deaf.

Tests of manual dexterity, motor coordination, mechanical aptitude, and spatial relations are pertinent to the type of work recommended in vocational training. As is the case with personality tests, aptitude and special interest tests are dependent on linguistic competence.

Language development and concepts We know that language is fundamental for hearing-impaired children. A satisfactory description of language is essential for an improved understanding of how language is learned and consequently of how it should be taught. Investigators and teachers have not been satisfied by vague and frequently misleading assertions about deaf children being "2 to 5 years retarded" or about their having typical "deaf language." They have used such measures as sentence length and complexity, the frequency of occurrence of certain parts of speech and certain orders of words, the extent of vocabulary, so-called type-token ratios (the relation between the number of *different* words and *total* words in a sample of language), and subordination and abstractions. They have also used the methods of structural linguistics to analyze the functional and lexical features of the spoken and written language of deaf children. This is one of many possible leads to better descriptions of language and to improved techniques of teaching vocabulary, syntactical patterns, and the semantic rules that relate words or sentences to things or events, not to mention the subtle and little-understood interweaving of the learning of language and the forming of concepts.

Psycholinguists are suggesting descriptive methods that enlighten us on how a child comprehends and manipulates language, particularly syntax. It has been suggested that children have a general capacity to acquire syntax, and this may be thought of as an inborn set of predispositions to develop a complex grammar from small amounts of information. The implications of this view for language instruction for deaf children are being explored.

How, if at all, language competence is related to concept formation in deaf children is still an open question. The situation is complicated by generalizing about rather select groups of deaf children, who are taught by one "method" or another and educated in different environments, day or residential, manual or oral, or combinations of these. In general the tasks presented to deaf children in studies of their ability to "conceptualize" have been weighted heavily in the direction of categorization. The studies show that deaf children can categorize "concrete" material as well as hearing children can but do less well in categorizing verbally. The tasks have been quite simple, and higher mental processes seem not to have been investigated. Throughout there is an assumption that verbal performance is equated with linguistic competence, but it may be reasonable to suggest that a sign or gesture, though not verbal, may have linguistic attributes.

In any event, a helpful way for parents and teachers to think of language development, suggested by A. A. Simmons-Martin, is shown in Figure 17-4.

The Skills of Communication

It is obvious that the skills of *speaking*, of *understanding* speech (speechreading and "hearing"), and of *language* are interrelated in their development. For convenience, however, and without slighting the interrelations, we shall consider separately the following topics (treated generally in Chapters 12, 13, and 14):

Skills
reading, writing,
spelling, composing

Mature language
involved syntax and reflection
vocabulary of 5000 +

Connected language
simple structure—requests
and questions

Larger expressive units
prepositional phrase
participial phrase

Limited expressive language
naming—adjectives
few verbs

Imitations
actions including mouthing
sounds including speech

Free comprehension
concepts
connected language

Situational comprehension
concrete items
visible actions

Awareness
concepts
vocabulary

Exposure

Figure 17-4 Some steps in language development. *(Courtesy of A. A. Simmons-Martin, Central Institute for the Deaf)*

Speech Studies of the speech of deaf children have, by and large, dealt with differences between the speech of the deaf and of subjects with normal hearing. By a technique of kymographic recording, the late Dr. C. V. Hudgins, at Clarke School for the Deaf (1937), found the following abnormalities in the speech of the deaf: slow and labored speech, usually accompanied by high chest pressure with the expenditure of excessive amounts of breath; prolonged vowels with consequent distortion; abnormalities of rhythm; excessive nasality of both vowels and consonants; and imperfect joining of consonants, with the consequent addition of superfluous syllables between abutting pairs.

We gain a substantial insight into the speech of the deaf from the investigation of Dr. Hudgins and F. C. Numbers (1942), who departed from the usual approach of comparing the speech of the deaf with that of the hearing and studied the relation between errors of articulation and rhythm and the intelligibility of the speech of deaf schoolchildren. Sentences spoken by deaf children were recorded and then were analyzed by a group of auditors. They found two general types of error: errors of articulation involving both consonants and vowels and errors of rhythm.

Consonant errors were classified into seven general types, as follows: failure to distinguish between voiced and unvoiced consonants, consonant substitutions, excessive nasality, malarticulation of compound consonants, malarticulation of abutting consonants, omission of arresting consonants, and omission of releasing consonants.

The vowel errors were vowel substitutions, malarticulation of diphthongs, diphthongization of vowels, neutralization of vowels, and nasalization of vowels.

In general, our experimental and empirical evidence indicates that the deaf child who lacks an adequate auditory monitor is likely to develop, at least under present methods of instruction, a breathy, nasalized vocal quality, abnormal temporal and intonational patterns, and some surprisingly consistent "errors" of articulation. These observations do not imply that deaf children cannot be taught to speak intelligibly. Many do. The observations do, however, show where there is the greatest opportunity to improve our methods of teaching speech to deaf children.

Fundamental attitude As far as we can determine, all educators of the deaf endorse the proposition that all deaf children shall have an opportunity to learn to speak. But the implementation of this notion in everyday practice reveals fundamental differences in attitudes.

For some educators, speech is a subject to be taught like a foreign language to those who can "benefit" from it. Practice and atmosphere are not aimed at vitalizing speech for the child. Rather, speech is viewed as an eminently desirable but not essential skill. For others (including ourselves), a corollary to the proposition of universality of opportunity to learn speech is inescapable: Speech is a basic means of communication and hence is a vital mechanism of adjustment to the communicating world about us. Therefore, we set the stage for speech *everywhere* —in the home, on the playground, in the schoolroom—from the moment we learn that a child is deaf, so that speech eventually will become meaningful, significant, and purposeful for him at all times. We believe that parents, counselors, teachers, and all others who are responsible for the child's development should share this attitude. Only constant practice and actual use of speech will develop fully the deaf child's latent ability to communicate by speech. The absence of a "living speech environment" may account for some of the so-called "oral failures" in schools for the deaf.

The multisensory approach Obviously the teacher must use all available sensory channels for teaching speech to a deaf child: the visual, the auditory, the tactile, and the kinesthetic.

When we consider the use to which we put *the visual system* in teaching speech, we tend to think primarily of speechreading. The child learns to watch with purpose the movements of the lips and the expressions of the faces of those about him and to imitate, however imperfectly, these movements in attempts to express himself. This really is the initial technique with deaf infants. Other well-known uses of vision include systems of orthography, color codes that differentiate the manner of production of phonetic elements, fingerspelling, models and diagrams that show position and movement of the mechanisms of speech, and acoustic translators of various sorts that display speech patterns visually and can carry information to the eye about time, frequency, and intensity. Now under consideration in some schools is the system of "cued speech" that aims to improve the acquisition of speech and its production. It is a system of communication in which phoneme, syllable, or word is identified from lip movements with the aid of 12 cues supplied by the hands.

We know that the literature, even of the nineteenth century (Urbantschitsch, 1897), mentioned the desirability of using *the auditory system* to aid in teaching speech to the deaf. Today we are better able to exploit this possibility because of the development of modern, wearable—and also group—hearing aids designed to deliver speech to the auditory area that the child still possesses. For the kind of child whom we are here discussing the auditory area is greatly restricted, but, as we have seen in Chapter 12, even a limited perception of stress patterns can help a child to achieve better rhythmic and voice quality and to better understand speech. (See Figure 14-1.)

The tactile or vibratory sense is most commonly used by placing the child's fingertips or hands in contact with his own or the teacher's face or head during speech or during phonation. We have mentioned that some techniques use sounding boards, including pianos, and diaphragms that are caused to vibrate by speech and music. Of increasing interest are studies to determine the value of instruments capable of delivering vibrotactually contrasting distinctive features of speech sounds to the skin, for example, nasal and nonnasal. Their value in development and improvement of speech is yet to be demonstrated, although there is some indication that they may aid speechreading.

The kinesthetic sense is used in "getting the feel" of certain articulatory and vocal movements and in tongue and lip exercises. Some teachers employ rhythmic gross-muscle movements to reinforce kinesthetically the utterance of connected speech and of suitable nonsense syllables.

Many techniques to teach speech to the deaf are in common use. One reason for their variety is the wide difference of opinion concerning the relative emphasis that should be placed on each sensory pathway. As we have seen in Chapter 12, some believe that speech is better learned if attention is concentrated on one sense at a time and the others are deliberately excluded. The other view favors mutual reinforcement of the senses and a coordinated sensory input. In support of the latter view, it has been shown that a small fragment of hearing may be trained to supplement vision usefully in a visual-auditory presentation. In other words, the eye and the ear together perceive speech better than either one alone. Hence, it is argued, the bisensory approach is likely to produce better speech. The counterargument is that, at least in the early stages, speechreading should be excluded from auditory training because the speechreading is likely to divert the child from full use of his hearing. Shutting the eyes of the child while he is learning to differentiate vibrations has also been suggested.

In applying techniques, it is desirable for the teacher to analyze the speech skill he is trying to cultivate and to select the combination of sensory channels best suited to stimulate the child. For example, the perception of the phonetic element *p* is best accomplished through vision reinforced by feeling, and vowel differentiation is greatly aided by a combination of auditory, visual, and tactile stimulation. In a sense the teacher is the primary sensory aid. In the classroom he is an ever-present interacting aid, shaping his own immediate input to the child in response to his speech behavior. The teacher decides when and whether to intervene in order to reinforce, correct, or improve speech, not to mention his important role in its development. In doing so, he has to make a choice of channel and mode to communicate to the child. Should he use the child's ears, his eyes, his skin, or some combination of these? Should he speak louder? Should he show the child the placement of his tongue? Should he have him feel the stream of air characteristic of a fricative consonant? His decision will depend on the particular circumstances, based of course on his knowledge of the child, as described earlier in this chapter. Our point is that he exploit the possibilities inherent in his own person in communicating information about speech. Table 17-3 shows the features of speech that can be "aided" by the teacher, along with other sources of sensory input.

Discriminating use of sensory aids, whether of a teacher's own person, common classroom devices, or elegant electronic instruments, demands a continuing concern for their value. Does the aid deliver what is intended? Will something simpler do just as well? Does the result justify the expenditure of time, energy, and money? Will apparent initial motivation wear off? Is there evidence that it carries over to extramural speech situations? It is important to note that any

"hard" evidence that exists for the value of engineered visual and tactile sensory aids is based on short-term data from laboratory contexts. It is incumbent upon investigators to carry on evaluations in the classroom and in everyday speech situations. Here is a splendid opportunity for teachers and investigators to collaborate effectively in pursuit of a common goal. As much as anything, the deliberations of recent conferences on speech-analyzing aids, sensory training aids, and sensory capabilities of hearing-impaired children point emphatically to this need.

Systems of orthography Students of speech are aware of the irrationality of our symbols for discrete units of speech. The letters of our alphabet bear no consistent relation to the sounds they represent. Furthermore, most of our symbols represent more than one sound, and most of our sounds are represented by more than one symbol. This situation has led teachers of the deaf to devise systems of orthography that carry more information about speech units than do the unrelated letters of the alphabet.

The Bells created their system of *visible speech* in 1894. In this system consonants are represented by four fundamental curves that relate to the "articulators," that is, to the back of the tongue, the top of the tongue, the point of the tongue, and the lips. The insertion of a short "voice" line in the bow of the curve changes a voiceless consonant to a voiced consonant. For example, ꝯ (which is k) becomes ꝯ (which is g). There is also a system for modifying the fundamental symbols to represent the vowels. This system is described in the Bells' book, entitled *The Mechanism of Speech* (1906).

The Northampton charts, originated at Clarke School for the Deaf and popular with many teachers of the deaf, are arranged to give more phonetic significance to letters of the English alphabet. The charts do this by arranging the symbols in columns and rows according to the method of production of the

TABLE 17-3.
DIGEST OF SENSORY AIDS APPLIED TO THE PRIMARY FACTORS OF SPEECH

Primary Factors of Speech	Teacher's Sensory Aids	Common Classroom Devices	Sample Electronic Equipment[a]
VOICE			
Loudness	Intensity of acoustic signal (A)[b]	Balloon on teacher/child face (T)	Light activated by microphone (V)
	Intensity of vibration on skin (T)	Musical instruments (A) (T)	Tactual vocoder (T)
Pitch	Frequency of vibration on skin (T)	Musical instruments (A) (T)	Pitch meter or indicator (V)
	Vertical movement of larynx (T) (V)		
Nasal-Nonnasal	Place of vibration on skin (T)		Nasal indicator (V)
Quality	Display of muscle tension and relaxation (T) (V)		
ARTICULATION			
Manner of Production			
Voicing	Vibration on skin (T)		Tactual vocoder (T)
Breath	Breath on skin (T)		
Force of Articulation	Exaggerated Force (V) (T)	Feather, flame, paper strip (V)	
Place of Articulation	Model as static display (V)	Diagram, model, mirror (V)	Vowel Indicator (oscilloscope) (V)
			Spectrograph (V)
	Model exaggeration (V)		
Acoustic Features			
Intensity			"S" meter (V)
Frequency		Written symbol codes (V)	Spectrograph (V)
Duration	Gesture (duration) (V)		
Dynamics of Coarticulation	Model as slow motion (V)		
	Manipulate speech mechanism (K)		
RHYTHM			
Rate	Model (A)		
	Gesture (V)		
Stress (accent, emphasis)	Model (A) (V) (T)	Written symbol codes (V)	Light activated by microphone (V)
	Pressure on hand (T)	Musical instrument (A)(T)	
Intonation	Model	Written symbol codes (V)	Pitch level meter (V)
		Musical instrument (A)	VU meter
Phrasing		Musical instrument rhythm (A) (T)	

[a] The hearing aid, which applies to all features of speech, is treated in Chapter 10.
[b] (A) = auditory; (V) = visual, (T) = tactile, (K) = kinesthetic senses.

Consonant sounds

h—

wh   w—

p   b   m

t   d   n   l   r—

k   g[1]   ng
ck
c

f   v
ph

th[1]   th[2]

s[1]   z
c(e)   s[2]
c(i)
c(y)

sh   zh   y—

ch   j   x = ks   qu = kwh
tch   g[2]—
          —ge
          dge

Vowel sounds

oo[1]   oo[2]   o—e   aw   —o—
(r) u—e   oa   au
(r) ew   —o[2]   o(r)
                    ow

ee   —i—   a—e   —e—   —a—
—e   —y   ai   ea[2]
ea[1]   ay
e—e

          a(r)   —u—   ur
                    —a   er
                              ir

a—e   i—e   o—e   ou   oi   u—e
ai   igh   oa   ow[1]   oy   ew
ay   —y   —o[2]
                    ow

Figure 17-5 *The Northampton Consonant Chart.* In the consonant chart the left-hand column is occupied by the English breath consonants; the second column, by the voiced forms of the same sounds; the third, by the nasal sounds. The horizontal arrangement classifies these sounds according to formation. A dash following a letter indicates that the sound is initial in a word or syllable.

The Northampton Vowel Chart. In the vowel chart the upper line contains the back round vowels (those modified chiefly by the back of the tongue and the rounded aperture of the lips). The second line contains the front vowels (those modified chiefly by the front of the tongue). Remaining vowels are in the third line. The lowest line contains all the diphthongal sounds. Although $\bar{a}$ and $\bar{o}$ appear in the rows to which their radical (long component) parts belong, they are repeated here because their compound nature makes them diphthongs also.

An attempt it also made in these charts to teach the simple rules of pronunciation. For illustration, a-e (representing a) when contrasted with -a- (representing ă), is easily made intelligible by the introduction of the same consonants in both sets of blanks: rate, rat; hate, hat, and so on. Children will not find diacritical marks over the words in their books or in other material, but if they are familiar with the principles of pronunciation represented here, they will know that final e modifies the sound of the vowel preceding it, making a, ā; e, ē; i, ī; o, ō. The secondary spellings under each sound generally indicate frequently occurring variations for those sounds. Numbers above the sounds differentiate pronunciations for similar spellings. In this way words are made to pronounce themselves to the eye of the child. Eventually, the children learn the diacritical marks of the dictionary. *(Adapted from Caroline A. Yale, Formation and Development of English Elementary Sounds. Northampton, Mass.: Gazette Printing Company, 1925)* sounds (see Figure 17-5). Thus the consonants p, b, and m are in the same row because the lips are initially shut in the production of all three. They are in different columns because p is voiceless, b is voiced, and m is nasal. This arrangement shows the differences and similarities among sounds. The multiplicity of letters and combinations of letters that represent the same sound are handled by arranging secondary spellings under the primary symbol, which is the one that occurs most frequently in the English usage. Thus a-e is the primary symbol for the dipthong in "cake." Here the dash represents any consonant. A secondary spelling under a-e is ay, as in "say."

The diacritical system used in our dictionaries assumes familiarity with the pronunciation of common key words. Where one letter may represent more than one sound, a differentiating symbol is used; thus e as in "be" is ē, and e as in "bed" is ĕ.

Phoneticians and linguists generally use the *International Phonetic Alphabet*, which has a single standard symbol for each sound and adds new symbols to the Roman alphabet to provide the necessary extra symbols.

Dr. A. Zaliouk, late Director of the Institute for the Deaf (in Haifa, Israel), devised a *visual-tactile system of phonetic symbolization* for teaching speech to the deaf. This uses two categories of symbols, static and dynamic. The static symbols represent the hard palate, the tongue, the teeth, and the lips, all of which participate in various "articulatory positions." The dynamic symbols indicate movement.

There have been other attempts, too numerous to mention, that have sought through shorthand or other means to convey phonetic information by a logical and consistent system of symbols. An ideal system of orthography would convey information on how to articulate, use the ordinary alphabet, be within the grasp of children, and be free of ambiguities. Obviously these criteria are

in conflict, and some compromises must be made. For example, if we were looking primarily for symbols to convey information on how to articulate, we would probably choose the system of Bell or of Zaliouk. The Northampton charts, with their secondary spellings, represent the letters and combinations of letters used most frequently in the English language, and hence should show how to pronounce the written word. On the other hand, because there are so many secondary spellings and exceptions, the learned combinations may be confusing out of the context of the chart. The diacritical markings of the dictionary are obviously useful, but everyday printed English does not carry these marks. One of the drawbacks of the International Phonetic Alphabet is that some of its symbols are not letters of our alphabet. Some teachers prefer to start children with the Northampton charts and then to teach the diacritical marks when children reach the appropriate academic level. These comments on the various systems are by no means exhaustive, but they may be useful as a guide in choosing a system of phonetic symbolization, or they may discourage use of any formally contrived system.

Developing speech Since the prelingually deaf child will develop little or no speech without specific training and stimulation, the earlier this can begin the better. This training should involve his family, of course. Given the encouraging trend toward early identification and assessment of hearing-impaired children, instruction to develop speech for them is likely to begin before they reach age 5. The variety of sensory capacities, learning and physical abilities, home environments, motivations and experiences encountered among young children suggests that the teacher has access to an array of alternative approaches to systematic instruction. In this section we mention three current "methods" of developing speech that, although they overlap, are discrete and distinctive enough to merit separate treatment. Elsewhere (Calvert and Silverman, 1975) we have called these the "Auditory Global," "Multisensory Syllable Unit," and "Association Phoneme Unit" methods. They constitute a gradient of instructional requirements concentrating primarily on the degree of teacher control and direction, the unit of speech input to and production by the child, the extent of purposeful drilling, and the relative emphasis on particular sensory channels or combinations of them to transmit information about speech and its feedback.

The principal features of the *Auditory Global Method* are that the primary, though not always exclusive, channel for speech development is auditory and that the input is fluent, connected speech. The central characteristics of the method are as follows:

1. *Maximum Emphasis on Use of Hearing.* The undergirding premise of the Auditory Global Method is that the most useful way to achieve intelligible speech is input of spoken language to the child's auditory channel, however much its sensitivity is reduced. Cultivation of the child's hearing requires the early use of amplification as soon as the child's hearing loss has been identified, periodic reexamination of hearing, selection of an optimum amplification system with special emphasis on feedback of speech, periodic examination of the hearing aid to determine that it is in proper operating order, and constant use of amplification in an advantageous acoustical environment.

2. *Comprehensive Intervention.* Although systematic and coordinated auditory stimulation is the central focus of the Auditory Global Method, it achieves its full potential only if the intervention is timely, broad, comprehensive, and generally individualized. For this method, appreciably more than other methods, the "classroom" is the child's total environment. Teacher control and direction stress at all times the opportunities for acquisition of speech by abundant auditory experience. At the core of comprehensive intervention is the development and maintenance of a milieu positively responsive to the child's speech output. Responsiveness is especially important to the hearing-impaired child because reduced or absent feedback limits the appreciation of his own voice.

3. *Emphasis on Connected Speech.* Connected speech input to the child is not left to chance. The best acoustic amplification and comprehensive intervention may be ineffective unless the amount, nature and direction of stimuli are taken into account. Increased speech input to the child should begin at a very early age, even though there is no apparent sign from the child that he is understanding what is said. The overall amount of connected speech input should be increased over that which would normally be available to a child without impaired hearing. He should, of course, be exposed to the "small talk" and courtesy phrases which we use daily. If it can be arranged, the deaf child should have language and speech input from nonimpaired children his own age. Situations should be arranged to stimulate the child to associate spoken language with observation and action. The natural rhythm of connected spoken language gives the child the opportunity to hear a model of the important patterns of speech and to imitate them.

As the Auditory Global Method continues in the child's school experience, it may begin to emphasize specific auditory training, precision of articulation, selective reinforcement of appropriate speech utterances, and association of an orthographic system with speech.

The *Multisensory Syllable Unit Method* is popularly considered to be the "traditional" method of teaching speech to deaf children. Its value has been historically demonstrated by the substantial number of those who have achieved impressive functional speech. Of course, the Multisensory Syllable Unit Method has much in common with the Auditory Global Method, but its more distinctive characteristics are as follows:

1. *Multisensory Stimulation for Speech.* The visual, tactile, kinesthetic, and auditory senses are used selectively and discriminatingly for speech development. Unlike the emphasis in the Auditory Global Method, the auditory system—though used since it contributes particularly to patterning and voice quality—is not likely to make a major contribution to the development of articulation. As we have said, in developing articulation the teacher makes use of the prominent "sensory" possibilities of sounds and their combinations, whether they are visual, tactile, kinesthetic, or auditory.

2. *Focus on the Development of Speech Sounds.* This method assumes that speech will *not* develop merely from the child's hearing and seeing connected speech in the course of conversation, however natural or planned. The production of individual sounds and their combinations, as well as speech rhythm, must be learned by focused instruction. Speech sounds will be introduced a few at a time and in a predetermined order. The rate and sequence with which new sounds are introduced are governed by the child's progress toward mastery of the sounds in combinations. Stimulation for production suggests a progression that derives from the principle that "natural" speech development is the preferred, but frequently not the sufficient, basis for speech instruction. The teacher may move from planned stimulation hoping for the child's imitation of his pattern, to demonstration of the place and/or manner of production of speech sounds and finally, if necessary, manipulation of the student's speech mechanism for production. In studies of the development of sounds in young children with normal hearing it has been shown that by the tenth month practically all of the different sounds have appeared. Yet it is curious that even though a child may have produced *l* and *r* during his infantile babbling, he frequently cannot, at the age of 2 or 3, produce these sounds correctly in English words. Apparently he finds it difficult to use the

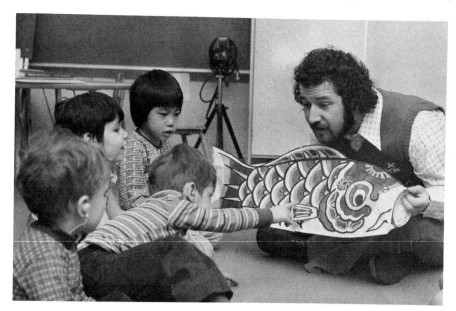

Figure 17-6 Auditory and visual experiences are associated. *(Central Institute for the Deaf; photo by Ken Nicolai)*

phonetic elements of his babbling as the phonemes of his language. This relearning comes about by biologic maturation, perceptive development, both auditory and kinesthetic, and, in the case of the deaf child, by the use of whatever sensory channels are available.

3. *The Syllable as the Basic Unit for Speech Instruction.* This method assumes that extensive use of units smaller than the longer sequence of connected speed is fundamental to instruction. Of course, individual sounds may be corrected, but they should not be considered learned until they are articulated properly in the kinds of syllables in which they are likely to occur. The syllable is sufficient for coarticulation of phonemes and yet is small enough to allow for accuracy of articulation by not placing too great a demand on motor memory. Furthermore, it is the irreducible unit of speech that communicates voice quality, inflection, and stress. The babbled syllable and the building of connected rhythmic speech from syllabic units are used in many methods for the development of speech. Development of patterns of connected speech proceeds from the simple to the complex and is approached deductively from general rules applied to specifically structured practice and drills.

The *Association Phoneme Unit Method* was motivated by the need to devise an alternative for those children who were not learning to talk by the methods previously described. It has its origins in the ideas and experience of Mildred McGinnis at Central Institute for the Deaf and was intended for those whose hearing impairment was overlaid by conditions that would render conventional procedures unsuitable to the achievement of oral communication. The more distinctive characteristics of the Association Phoneme Unit Method are as follows:

1. *Speech Production Is Associated with Other Language Modalities.* The Association Phoneme Unit Method is based on the idea that speech perception is influenced by speech production. We tend to hear the speech of others as we produce it. The child is taught to produce each sound very precisely, thus developing a strong motor pattern that should be easy for him to remember. He learns to associate most of the speech he sees and hears with the patterns he has produced. No formal speechreading, listening, or reading is attempted in the Association Phoneme Unit Method except for words the child can say. When a child produces a sound correctly, it is immediately associated with a written symbol, speechreading, and the speech sound produced by the teacher. Writing is always associated with oral production.

2. *The Phoneme Is the Basic Unit for Speech Instruction.* The precise articulation of a single phoneme in isolation enhances the memory for the motor acts associated with it and its combinations. Drills blend consonant and vowel sounds, leading to the articulation of a word. Even after words are begun, the child continues to practice the phoneme separately and blended in syllables, to individual words, to sentences and questions.

3. *Speech Development Progresses in Small Increments.* From mastery of his first phoneme the child develops speech in small units, progressing from the simple to the complex. A reasonable number of individual phonemes are developed before blending of consonants and vowels is attempted. When the child can blend with some confidence, two or more phonemes are combined into single-syllable words. When a number of words are mastered, the child is ready to put a few together into simple sentences. The child is given opportunity for success at each level before going on to the next. For the child who has experienced failure and discouragement by other methods, the expe-

rience of success is especially to be stressed.

The *initial* method of choice among those mentioned should be appropriate for very young children (even infants) whenever they are identified, should give maximum opportunity for each child to develop his hearing ability regardless of early estimates of the nature and degree of hearing loss, should allow for an opportunity to identify other disabilities that might affect speech improvement, and should provide sufficient experience for assessing progress in speech. These conditions are probably best satisfied by the Auditory Global Method.

Evaluation of speech Frequent critical evaluation of the *intelligibility* of the speech of hearing-impaired children is important as a guide to modifying existing methods of teaching. Evaluations can be made periodically during the school career of a deaf child, during which he is exposed to formal training in speech by one method or another. Other long-range procedures could be designed to discover how intelligible the speech of deaf pupils continues to be after they have graduated from schools for the deaf.

A child's improvement in speech intelligibility may be evaluated by periodic tests, but the available tests are not as objective or as valid as our corresponding tests of many other skills or of a child's mastery of subject matter. In one popular procedure a child reads a selection, and auditors indicate the extent to which the selection has been understood. Or carefully selected word samples are read and scored by the auditors. In a sense the tests determine the extent to which the deviant talker imposes a loss of discrimination for speech on a normal listener. Although this may yield a limited but fairly reasonable appraisal of the mechanics of the child's speech, it does not simulate the pattern of usual oral exchange that takes place without benefit of a printed or written visual aid. What is being evaluated is a form of *oral reading* and not speech in broad social terms. The translation of the child's *own* thoughts into intelligible speech is an ability neglected by this type of evaluation.

The use of memorized material without visual aid is subject to similar criticism since the thoughts expressed usually are not the child's own; if they are, they still have been memorized. This furnishes the child an advantage he does not have in a normal social situation. The interview, in which the child is stimulated to talk freely, may yield a fairly accurate appraisal of speech if it is conducted skillfully. Very often in an interview, however, the child may correctly anticipate the question; furthermore, the technique fails to appraise the child's ability to initiate speech. The use of speech recordings for periodic evaluation has considerable value. However, the limitations of printed or memorized selections and of the question-and-answer type of sample should be kept in mind. Of course, it would help to capture for study the casual conversation of children. We should be cautious about the inferences we make that relate tests of talker intelligibility to social usefulness of speech. The two are not always linearly related. Attitudes of talker and listener having to do with confidence, encouragement, frustration, and motivation all play their role in the use a deaf person makes of his speech.

The outcomes of speech teaching that are most important in the long run are those that reveal the extent to which the benefits of the child's training in speech persist after he has left school. Unfortunately, we have no satisfactory evidence in this area, and the information that comes to us is frequently biased and invariably anecdotal. Good follow-up studies are a task that zealous oralists might profitably undertake.

Future investigations of the speech of deaf children should be greatly stimulated by the availability of improved tools and methods for the study of speech as an acoustical (spectrographic) and motor (myographic) event. Techniques are at hand for analyzing and synthesizing speech, for displaying it visibly and tactually and for repackaging it by selective filtering, frequency transposition, temporal expansion and compression (see Chapter 10). Our understanding of the physiological mechanisms of speech is being enriched by the techniques of high-speed photography of the larynx during phonation and of X-ray views of the articulators in action. Helpful, too, is our study of speech that is deviant because of structural pathologies, such as cleft palate, vocal nodules, absent or partially removed larynx, or deficient innervation of speech musculature, as in cerebral palsy.

Our discussion of teaching speech to the deaf suggests the following guides to practice:

1. An environment should be created or maintained for the child in which speech is experienced as a vitally significant and successful means of communication.
2. Spontaneity of speech should be encouraged, but formal instruction is necessary at the appropriate stage in a child's development. Good speech in deaf children does not come of itself.
3. The proper combination of the visual, auditory, tactile, and kinesthetic pathways should be exploited early, rationally, and vigorously.
4. A functional system of visual phonetic aids is helpful.
5. Judicious correction of poor articulation, including individual phonetic elements, and of undesirable rhythm and voice quality is necessary. The acceptance of poor speech encourages its use. The teacher is the accurate monitor of the child's speech, and he must let him know how he can improve it.
6. Periodic and long-range evaluations of the social effectiveness of the speech of the deaf, even though informal, are useful for both diagnosis and educational planning.

Auditory training The great advance in electroacoustic instrumentation of the past three decades, both for testing hearing and for amplifying sound, has generated a sustained and substantial interest in auditory training. We must remind ourselves that in this section we are concerned with children who have a severely restricted auditory area. The auditory area that remains to them, if any, lies at high sound-pressure levels near the threshold of pain (see Chapter 2). These levels can be reached for communication only by means of powerful, well-designed hearing aids. Both group hearing aids and individual hearing aids have been described in Chapter 10. There we have pointed out the necessity for proper limitation of acoustic output and the advantages and limitations of compression amplification in "packaging" speech for effective delivery to the child's restricted auditory area. Our understanding of the reception of speech has been aided greatly by the contributions of information theory and by our knowledge of pertinent acoustical properties of speech. Information theory concerns itself with the predictability of elements in communication or, in other words, guessing what comes next based on probabilities of occurrence of a phoneme, a word or a phrase according to the particular structure of a language. What is important for the hearing-impaired is that we now know that much can be "guessed" in the absence of parts of a message. The cuing that may be possible with a small amount of residual hearing, properly amplified, may be greater than heretofore supposed.

The presence of low-frequency hearing in many children has stimulated various schemes of signal processing that re-form the speech signal to improve its perceptibility.

In general, speech-compression systems of one sort or another are being tried that reduce the bandwidth much as is done in transmission by radio and telephone. For many children, listening over such systems requires that a new language be learned.

Several objectives of auditory training are within the reach of deaf children. They are as follows:

1. *Improvement in Speech Perception.* Deaf children are not likely to achieve much auditory discrimination for speech, certainly not enough to understand ordinary language through hearing alone. However, they can be taught to appreciate temporal patterns of speech and to improve their control of the intensity and in many instances the pitch of their voices. Refined appreciation of phrasing and stress patterns may be expected to improve the child's ability to attain the "rhythmic grouping" that can contribute greatly to the intelligibility of his own speech. Auditory training appears to improve speech perception, particularly when it is combined with speechreading. Failure of improvement in communication by speech after a regimen of auditory training may often be due to the fact that the training was not begun early enough. It should begin in the first year of life.

2. *Improvement in Language Skills.* Although there is no definitive experimental evidence that auditory training improves language skills, it seems likely that the information carried by stressing and phrasing, not easily discerned by speechreading, adds to the meaning and significance of connected language. Vocabulary, particularly words with auditory associations, may be enriched. For example, if a child reads "The baby cried," the word "cried," which has auditory connotations, has limited meaning for him even though he is able to draw a line between it and the word "baby" in his workbook and he has seen a picture of a baby cry-

ing. On the other hand, a recording of the cry of a baby played over an amplifying system, even though not perceived precisely, should enrich the meaning of the word "cry."

3. *Improvement in Psychological Coupling to the Hearing World.* Again, convincing experimental evidence is lacking. Nevertheless, consider the deaf child at a ball game. A thrilling play is made on the diamond that evokes a spontaneous outburst of yelling from the crowd. The child sees the hands clap and wave, the spectators rise from their seats, the mouths open, but he has not caught the full emotional impact of the moment because its basic richness lies in the yelling of the crowd and the accompanying noises. This is an auditory experience. If the child could perceive just the presence of these noises, however distorted, through a hearing aid, he would share more richly in the group experience. Not to be overlooked are the aesthetic appreciations that may result from auditory exposure to the rhythm of music. Many deaf children who have been trained to appreciate rhythmic cadences seem to enjoy dancing and eurythmics.

Although it is likely that the future will reveal additional and greater values of auditory training, our statements of objectives within reach suggest that we must be cautious of the extravagant claims sometimes made for the use of hearing aids by deaf children, particularly the claim that if they are equipped from infancy with a hearing aid, they do not need special education.

Despite the unsolved problems that are still with us, there is no longer any question about the usefulness of the auditory system in the education of deaf children. In Chapter 12, Dr. Erber and Dr. Hirsh have described the fundamentals of auditory training for children. Out of our experience grow the following guides for practice in auditory training:

1. Most deaf children have a small but

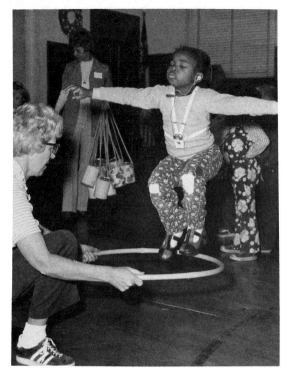

Figure 17-7 Rhythmic exercises accompanied by spoken cadences. *(Central Institute for the Deaf; photo by Peter Ferman)*

useful portion of the auditory area that lies above the range of usual audiometry. Consequently, many children who have been termed "totally deaf" as a result of audiometric tests actually can hear properly amplified sound. Audiograms may not tell the whole story of a child's ability to appreciate speech by his hearing. Formal auditory training is essential, however, to teach the deaf child to make use of this remnant of hearing. The hearing aid alone is not enough.

2. Auditory training appears to be more effective, through mutual reinforcement, when hearing is combined with vision and/or touch. There are times when hearing alone is used to teach a child to concentrate on specified information-bearing cues.

3. The techniques of auditory training

should be geared to a child's auditory capabilities. This requires frequent assessment of his hearing.

4. Auditory training, even without a hearing aid, should be begun as soon as it is determined that a child is deaf.

5. Formal instruction can make hearing aids more acceptable to children by giving them experiences that are meaningful. Such instruction should teach children to discriminate, even though grossly, various environmental sounds, and, within the limits of their hearing, teach them to understand speech by hearing.

6. Informally and wherever practicable, the child should have the benefit of amplified sound, either by a group hearing aid or a wearable one, in all of his classroom work, at home, and also at play.

7. Children should be taught as early as possible the use, the management, and the care of their own hearing aids.

Speechreading As we have said repeatedly, children with normal hearing learn oral language primarily by hearing, which is complemented by other sensory experience. The sounds are later associated with the visual symbols, that is, the movements of the talker's face, that partly represent language. This is speechreading (see Chapter 13). The deaf child is denied the possibility of learning this by association with auditory language, and is forced to learn his visual speechreading language directly. The extent to which he is able to do this may depend upon a number of factors, some of which are exceedingly complex and difficult to analyze. One group of factors concerns the speaker. These include his distance and position and direction from the speechreader and how well his face is illuminated. They include the character of his speech, his precision of articulation, how fast he talks, the mobility of his face, and the familiarity of the speechreader with the particular speaker. Then there are factors concerning the language material, such as the vocabulary and the language structure. Finally, there is the speechreader himself: his vision, his intelligence, his general information, and his ability to synthesize from contextual clues, to recognize discrete units of speech, to associate his own "feel" for speech with the speech he sees on the face, and the fundamental structure of his personality, which may determine his attitude toward speechreading.

Speechreading is further complicated by the ambiguities that result from hidden movements, such as h and k, from homophonous words (words that look alike on the lips, such as "smell" and "spell"), and from the difficulty of appreciating patterns of stress, intonation, and phrasing.

Numerous attempts have been made to assess the role of these factors in speechreading to diagnose difficulties, to evaluate progress and methods of instruction, and to predict performance.

Among the possible factors that may be related to skill in speechreading and have been investigated are intelligence, reading ability, perceptual and synthetic ability, motivation, and rhythmic skills. These studies have led to no generalizations in which we have confidence. One of the major problems in studying these relations is the adequacy of tests of speechreading. The test constructors are faced with formidable variables that are unique to the population to be tested. Among these are the degree and kind of hearing loss, the time of onset of impaired hearing, the language ability of the subjects, and the standardization of the test material itself, particularly of the manner of its presentation. There is also the difficulty of establishing norms for a heterogeneous population. Furthermore, the validation of the tests appears to rely solely on ratings by teachers. This introduces new problems.

Instruction in speechreading for deaf children is usually not a thing apart. In the beginning, even before the child enters school, he is encouraged to watch the face of the talker. The deaf child is not as aware as the hearing child that he can get information, in its broadest sense, by watching the movements of the face. When formal instruction is begun, the child is taught to associate movement of the lips, jaws, and tongue with objects, feelings, and actions. The objective here is not merely the enlargement of speechreading vocabulary but cultivation of the idea that watching the face of the talker is useful. Finally, speechreading pervades every act of speech perception by the child and becomes an increasingly useful tool of communication as it is practiced in purposeful situations.

The inadequacy of our formal tools for assessment of the ability to speechread need not deter us from suggesting the following guides to practice in developing this valuable skill in deaf children:

1. An atmosphere of oral communication should be encouraged. Speechreading must be shown to serve a purpose.
2. Even if the child is not expected to understand every word of a spoken message, he should be talked to, and he should be encouraged to take advantage of situational clues.
3. Speechreading should be reinforced by other sensory clues whenever practicable.

Language In our discussion of the skills of communication to this point we have, in a sense, considered the development of the skills of talking and "listening," namely, speech, auditory training, and speechreading. We now turn to the message itself, the stuff of communication. This is language. The "ear-to-voice link" is essential for talking and listening. It is the basis of a child's attachment of meaning, in speaking, in writing, in listening, and in reading, to words and combinations of words. The absence of hearing is catastrophic for the "natural" but complex development of association of language with experience.

It is the task of the teacher, nevertheless, to develop language in deaf children, although they do not have full use of the sensory channel that is considered essential for the growth of language. In the performance of this task he needs to be aware of the unique problems created by the absence of hearing or by the severe distortions of auditory verbal experience. Among the major problems for the child are vocabulary, multiple meanings of words, the verbalization of abstractions, and the complexity of the structure of language.

Vocabulary It is difficult to determine when a child really "knows" a word. Does he have it in his spoken, his written, his reading, his listening, or his seeing vocabulary? The different kinds of vocabulary account for differences in the estimates of the functional vocabulary of children. At any rate, hearing children "know" hundreds of words even at age 2 and 3. Compare this with zero words that a deaf child without any language experience is likely to know when he enters school even at the age of 3 or more frequently at 5.

Multiple meanings Single words in our language may have many meanings that are eventually clarified for hearing children, chiefly by the repeated auditory experience that is denied the deaf child. An average of almost four meanings per recurring word was found by count in twelve commonly used arithmetic textbooks. For example, the word "over" could mean "above" (the number over 5 is the quotient); "across" (over the Arctic Ocean); "again" (do your work over); "at an end" (the show is over); "more than" (over half the children); "besides" (left over); "during" (over a period of two years); "present" (turn the meeting over to); "on the other side" (turn the card "over"); "by means of" (over the radio).

Verbalization of abstractions Of course, hearing children and, for that matter, adults may experience difficulty in attaching words to abstract concepts, but the deaf child is in particular need of formal and informal but nonetheless deliberate instruction in the meaning of such relatively simple abstractions as *hope* and *want*.

Complexity of structure By the age of 5 the spoken sentence of the average child has reached five words in length. For the superior child it is about ten words long. This increase in length is inevitably accompanied by the use of complex syntactical relations that clarify and enrich meaning. These involve such grammatical concepts as pronouns, connectives, tense, person, and word order, as well as relations among clauses and among phrases of various sorts. If the hearing child reaches these levels of complexity at the age of 5, we are again struck by the extent of the language gap between the deaf and the hearing. It was found by the Heiders at Clarke School (1940), after their thorough comparison of sentence structure in the written compositions of deaf and hearing children, that the "whole picture indicates a simpler style [for the deaf] involving relatively rigid unrelated language units which follow each other with little overlapping structure or meaning."

S. P. Quigley and his coworkers at the University of Illinois (1977) have investigated in depth the development of syntactic structure in deaf students. They found, as others have, some frequently occurring difficulties, particularly in verb systems (*Jim have sick* for *Jim is sick*), complementation (*John goes to fishing*), and relativization (*John saw the boy who the boy kicked the ball*). The deaf children performed somewhat better, but still below the hearing children, in negation, question formation, and conjunctions. The degree to which these characteristics of the studied samples are a product of instructional methods or are in some way the result of learning difficulties imposed by deafness is still an open question.

In general, the deaf appear to be comparatively deficient in the flexible manipulation of our language in order to make the best use of it as a tool of communication. This may be due to their educational retardation; or it may be due to the methods of teaching language, or, in addition to these, to the idea suggested by the Heiders that "the difference between the deaf and the hearing cannot be fully expressed in quantitative terms as the degree of retardation" and "that they represent differences not merely of skill in the use of language forms but in the whole thought structure." Subsequent studies by and large confirm these generalizations.

Methods of instruction in language   Methods of instruction of the deaf in language can be divided conveniently into two major approaches: the natural method, sometimes known as the synthetic, informal, or mother method; and the grammatical method, sometimes referred to as the logical, systematic, formal, analytical, or artificial method.

Historically, the grammatical method preceded the natural method. It was based on the notion that after memorization of classifications of words and their conjugations and declensions, they could be used as building blocks for connected language. This approach evolved into a multiplicity of "systems" that were created primarily to provide a systematic set of visible symbols to guide deaf children in the use of language. We shall briefly describe three of the more popular ones.

The Barry Five-Slate System   The assumption underlying this system, developed by Katherine E. Barry (1899) at the Colorado School for the Deaf, is that ability to analyze

the relations among parts of sentences is necessary to the "clear thinking" essential to an understanding of language. Five slates or columns are visible on the walls of the schoolroom. The subject of a sentence goes on the first slate, the verb on the second, the object of the verb on the third, the preposition on the fourth, and the object of the preposition on the fifth. Children then learn the rationale of the verbalization of their actions according to the visual aid afforded by the slates. This system, many believe, tends to stultify idiomatic expression and actually may result in ungrammatical, stilted language.

Wing's Symbols   This system, devised in 1883 by George Wing of the Minnesota School for the Deaf, is based on a set of symbols, mostly numbers and letters, representing the functions of different parts of speech in a sentence. These symbols are placed over the word, phrase, or clause in order to demonstrate the form, function, and position of the parts of a sentence, rather than just to illustrate parts of speech. For example, 1 stands for the noun, 2 for a possessive, and 0 for the object. Advocates of the system believe that it is of great value as a corrective tool throughout the child's career and that it encourages correct grammatical usage.

The Fitzgerald Key   This system, first published in 1926, was developed by Edith Fitzgerald (1949), a congenitally deaf person, when she was head teacher at the Virginia School. Ms. Fitzgerald advocated developing "natural" language but thought that this could be aided by developing the child's power of reasoning, judgment, and discrimination about language. This is accomplished by a set of key words and symbols related to language that was developed as it was needed by the children. There are six symbols, one each for verbs, infinitives, present participles, connectives, pronouns, and adjectives. For example, the symbol for a verb is =. Among the advantages of the method are its comprehensiveness, its flexibility, and the possibilities for self-correction.

The basic feature of the grammatical systems is the emphasis on getting the child to *analyze* functional relations among discrete units of language and, by repetition and visual aids, to impart to him an understanding of language principles or linguistic "rules," including the way in which the arrangement of words affects the meaning of a sentence. Methods that combine an analysis of the structure of language, a key system, and expanding "kernel" sentences or patterns are also in use.

One of the early advocates of the *natural method* was Greenberger, previously mentioned. He believed that language was best learned by supplying it to children in the situations in which they had need for it. Practice was geared to actual and natural situa-

tions. A leading advocate of this approach was the late Dr. Mildred Groht, who suggested that prior to the time a language principle is to be introduced formally it should be used in natural situations through speechreading and writing. It is then drilled on in various ways that are interesting and purposeful for the child. In essence, the teacher creates situations that provide many and varied contacts with the principles of language. The method is claimed to be more consistent with the laws of learning of language by hearing children than is a formal, analytical method.

Stepped-up investigation of normal language development is an allied field that has had an impact on the thinking, if not on the instructional practices, in language. Evidence of application and results are not at hand, probably because of the recency of

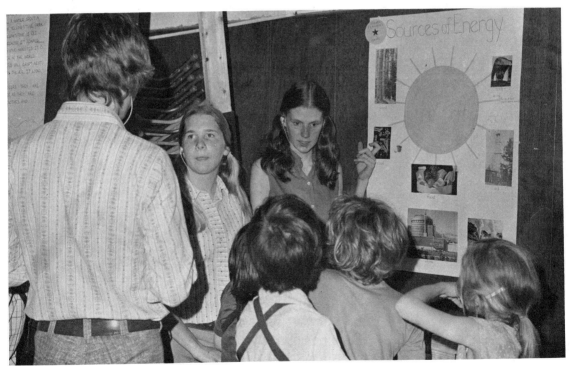

Figure 17-8 A science class of deaf children using the combined auditory and visual approach. *(Central Institute for the Deaf)*

findings, the issues related to them, and the undetermined significance they may have for language acquisition and instruction of deaf children. For example, in the approach of generative grammar, language is characterized by acquisition of increasingly complex rules that approximate the rules of adult language. How a child accomplishes this is not clear but it has been suggested that frequent parental expansion of a child's telegraphic speech may be fundamental. It appears from this that language learning is accomplished by imitation of adult structures with appropriate and timely reinforcement and in its more extreme form, as in the case of language-delayed children, by a programmed "behavior modification" approach. On the other hand, there is evidence that children respond to the imitation task in a manner more or less consistent with their present level of grammatical rules and that listening to increasingly complex utterances is a basis for the rules that govern the child's language production. These approaches may not be mutually exclusive, and the emphasis on one or the other may depend on the child's language development at a given time.

The rigorous generative grammar approach is questioned by some who find that the same two-word utterance may be employed in a variety of contextual situations so as to have a variety of meanings to a child. For example, "baby water" may mean "the baby is in the water," "the baby spilled the water," "the baby wants water," and so on. We need certainly to be concerned with the "semantic rules" that relate words or sentences to things and events. Concurrent with this notion and perhaps stimulated by it are studies on what we referred to as the "subtle interweaving of language and thought." These studies argue that cognitive development both precedes and enables language development. The aim here is to extract the child's cognitive understanding underlying language performance and to specify the nonlinguistic strategies that determine the child's response to linguistic tasks. The possibility that cognitive strategies are universal in the sense that there are linguistic universals is a hypothesis meriting consideration.

Possible applications to the education of deaf children of research in the development of language in hearing children should command our serious and earnest attention. It is conceivable that these findings may influence, among other things, our modes of communication, the timing, sequencing and structuring of language input, our concepts of "correctness" of language production at various levels in a child's development, our assessment of language competence and achievement, and how we integrate language teaching with the all-important skill of reading.

Until we gain more insight into how the deaf child conceptualizes, the teacher of language will need to use all the knowledge and ingenuity at his command to combine the best features of a grammatical method with the obvious excellent possibilities of the natural method. He will use such commonly accepted techniques as general conversation, composition, news items, trips, action work, topical essays, experience stories, letters, and descriptions of places, events, and persons. The child's progress in acquiring language will be governed only by the extent to which the teacher uses his own ingenuity, flexibility, and knowledge of how children grow and develop. Perhaps he may find some help in the following guides to practice:

1. Language teaching should be related to significant and meaningful experiences of children.
2. Language should constantly be made to serve a purpose for the child.

3. All sensory channels should be used to teach language.

4. Teachers need to be alert to the ideas that are developing in children so that they may provide the children with language with which to express them.

5. Children need many varied contacts with the same language in order to make it theirs.

6. Many children need formal, systematic aids to the acquisition of language. Many shun language when they feel insecure in its use.

7. Schools and homes should create an atmosphere in which language is used and books are read regularly.

Curriculum Development in Schools for the Deaf

In general the curricula of schools for the deaf resemble those in schools for the hearing, with appropriate adaptations for difficulties of verbal communication. However, the growing national concern for improving education of all children at all levels has expressed itself primarily in focusing attention, energy, and abundant resources on curricular revision and reform. Stimulated by these efforts, educators of the deaf are seeking ways to improve the performance of their schools. Efforts in curriculum development have centered around considerations of goals, processes, and materials, and their dissemination, implementation, and evaluation.

Goals   An obvious first question in goal setting is: Who sets them? Shall it be school administrators, teachers, parents, deaf adults, mature students, psychologists, social scientists, humanists, employers, psychiatrists, specialists in particular disciplines, funding agencies, or some combination of these? We

appear to be a long way from examining on a rational basis the contributions that these and other elements have to make to our formulation of goals. For example, what can students of mental health tell us about the wisdom of such long-range goals as complete integration of the deaf person into the world of the hearing, on the one hand, or production of contented members of a subgroup, on the other? Certainly the grand design of the educational experience we arrange for our children would be crucially influenced, if not fundamentally determined, by what we think about this issue.

Another question pertinent to goal setting is: How shall they be stated? Shall they be outlines of "content," like "how a plant grows"; shall they be skills like reading, writing, and so on, or behavioral objectives like identifying, describing, distinguishing, naming, stating, and applying a rule? Shall they go beyond the cognitive and apply to total human functioning? What schemes are possible to bring these categories into some reasonable relationship?

Attainability is still another important aspect of goal setting. What is ideal and what are the realistic constraints imposed upon us by the limitations of deafness, by physical facilities, by financial needs, by geography, by the distressing unavailability of enough able and motivated teachers, and by the changing technological and social scene?

Processes and materials   Given a set of goals for a learner it is now the task of the technologists, be they "media specialists," discipline experts, educational psychologists, or just plain teachers (in combination or individually), to develop processes and materials to attain the goals. Here we must be careful that the materials do not determine the goals and processes. All too frequently a kind of Parkinsonian principle operates. Goals are developed to use the materials available to attain them, often to the exclusion of more desirable goals.

The impressive array of processes and the increasing abundance of materials underline the growing importance of the educational technologists. The range and kinds of learning and teaching processes that are now or are soon likely to be available to us are indeed imposing. They include tutoring, small group discussions, lectures, laboratory demonstrations, individual programmed instruction, textbooks, slides, tapes, films, instructional television, and computer-aided instruction. The contemplation of these possibilities for curriculum improvement is as intriguing as the questions posed by them are formidable.

To assist in the dissemination and implementation of improved materials the Office of Education of the Department of Health, Education and Welfare is supporting the development of regional centers for instruc-

tional materials for special education. In addition, courses dealing with curricula in teacher education programs are being updated and elaborated. Yet there are subtle questions related to dissemination and implementation. For example, one of the appealing attributes of outstanding teachers of deaf children has been their spontaneity, their ability to sense an opportunity for learning by a child, and their skill in exploiting the situation. In disseminating and stressing prepared materials are we likely to create a dependence on them that will stultify spontaneity and imagination? The textbook is a classic example of prepared materials (antedating modern technology). There are few among us who do not have grim recollections of teachers who "taught from the book." Nevertheless, we need not face a forced choice. Our deliberations on curriculum improvement point toward the preparation of professional "disseminators" whose

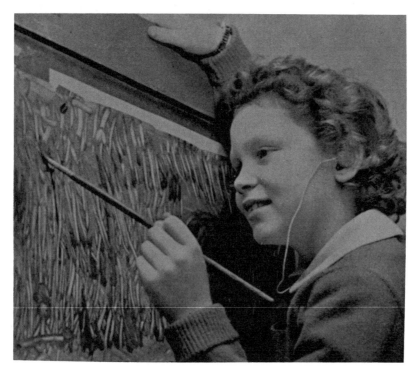

Figure 17-9 Art is an excellent medium of expression for deaf children. *(Central Institute for the Deaf)*

performance reflects an understanding of the learning problems of deaf children and how, for better or worse, they are taught.

Evaluation In his summary of the 1967 National Conference on the Education of the Deaf, the chairman said:

A nagging concern was the problem of evaluation, whether it be of curriculum, of a method of communication, teaching or guidance, or of a system of organization and administration. Common sense requires that the effectiveness of any procedure, or change therein, be tested by the most objective investigations we can devise, so that substantive grounds are established for eliminating, amending or modifying our arrangements and practices. In education this is devilishly difficult to accomplish. Many of the outcomes we seek resist satisfactory measurement, and some results must await the passage of years before an attempt at evaluation is even appropriate. Nevertheless, the conference time and time again pointed to evaluation as a crucial issue demanding more concentrated attention.

We may ask: what needs to be evaluated? Dyer, in speaking of all schools, expresses a sobering thought:

The extraordinary fact is, however, that in spite of mountains of data that have been piled up from teachers' reports, tests, questionnaires and demographic records of all kinds, we still have only very hazy and superficial notions of what the effects of school experience really are.

Of course, we have academic achievement tests, which incidentally may have an undue influence on our goals and frequently are not too pertinent at certain levels to our particular problems in the education of deaf children. But little is done to evaluate the effective and social outcomes of school experience. A teacher may be doing an excellent job of teaching reading as measured by a reading test, but has he also taught some

children to despise reading? Do we tend to evaluate only that for which we have tests, and do we accommodate assumptions to requirements of technique rather than to reality? Who shall do the evaluating? Should it be members of the closed system we call "the school"? (That is, should it be the teachers, the administrators, the school psychologists, all of whom conventionally evaluate their own product?) How about parent evaluations? Or extramural individuals or groups? Or employers of deaf persons? Or deaf persons themselves?

Ours is a time of "rising expectations" nurtured by "great advances in technology" with its inevitable idolatry of evangelistic technologists and its comforting faith in equating change with improvement, newness with validity, gimmickry with innovation, and public relations with evaluation. Nevertheless, we must continue to probe for strategies for curriculum improvement, with the recognition that it is a complex and demanding task.

Problems of Parents

In concluding our discussion on deaf children it is fitting to return to the problems of parents.

When parents become aware that their child is deaf, their initial reaction is one of profound grief. It is a shock to hear that one's child is deaf and that it is hopeless to expect a restoration of his hearing. Unfortunately, some parents refuse far too long to face the fact squarely. They begin a pilgrimage from one physician to another, always hoping for a miracle and still not heeding advice about the necessity for special education. Instead, they may squander funds and waste valuable nursery school years grasping for any and every "cure" they read about, from airplane rides to surgery.

Other parents surround the deaf child

with an overwhelming, protective "love" as soon as deafness is recognized. They want to do everything for the child to compensate for his deprivation; they dress him, feed him, and amuse him, and shield him from contacts with other children. He is thereby deprived of opportunities for normal development, and his education is delayed.

Sooner or later all parents realize, as many do at the very first, that special education is necessary; but here they are naturally bewildered. "My child is deaf, but what do I do next?" Otologists, educators, audiologists, and psychologists can help the parent make the educational arrangements best suited to the child's needs. Children differ, schools differ, communities differ. No single answer is correct for all deaf children in all places. We have outlined some of the principles of education for the deaf child, but the actual choice of a particular school is often a difficult problem, particularly when, as often happens, the advice of "experts" conflict.

Finally, however, a school for the deaf child is selected, and now comes the "long pull" for the parents, the extended period of learning how to work most effectively with the school throughout their child's educational career. Parents are more apt to enter willingly on this third and important stage of their evolving attitude if they realize that their earlier grief and bewilderment have been recognized, sympathetically understood, and met with kind, clear, but not too insistent, counsel. Here a heavy responsibility lies on the school: first, to recognize the nature of the strong emotions that surround the relationship of the parents with their deaf child; second, to develop home cooperation by sending constructive and informative reports and by encouraging the parents to make frequent visits to the classroom.

Parents must seize upon every opportunity at home for the child to emphasize and apply what he has learned at school. They can assist materially in developing and correcting the child's speech, in enriching his vocabulary, and in translating his experience into meaningful language. If the child is at a residential school, contacts with home should be maintained by letters and photographs. News from home is very essential to the deaf child's happiness. Reports from the teachers and at least an annual visit keep the parents informed concerning the child's progress.

As the deaf child reaches adolescence, his basic needs are the same as those of other children. He must soon be ready to earn money, to make decisions, to associate with the opposite sex, and to compete with the hearing. The schools and the home must prepare the deaf child for this broader environment.

Teachers, parents, and school executives must again cooperate in the selection of a school for further education or for vocational training after the boy or girl is graduated from the school for the deaf. Once more, many variables affect the decision: the age of the child, his intelligence, his ability to communicate, his academic record, his interests and skills, the schools available to him, and the vocational opportunities in his community. Parents should also make a sincere effort to help the deaf child make friends in his home community.

When the parents are able to observe the fruits of their long labors, they experience the comforting satisfaction of knowing that their efforts, augmenting those of the school, have played a tremendously significant role in the happy adjustment of their child. And on the part of the school, no Pollyanna philosophy but an attitude of realistic undertanding of the parents' problem has facilitated the arduously long process of adjustment. Parents should not overlook their debt to the teachers whose wisdom, patience, and understanding have made possible the deaf child's development and growth.

SUGGESTED READINGS AND REFERENCES

American Annals of the Deaf.

> *Each year the April issue of this periodical is a statistical compilation of information about the hearing-impaired. It also contains a directory of personnel and services.*

Babbidge, H. D. *Education of the Deaf: A Report to the Secretary of Health, Education, and Welfare by his Advisory Committee on the Education of the Deaf.* Washington, D.C.: U.S. Department of Health, Education and Welfare, 1965.

> *An assessment of the status and needs of the education of the deaf from preschool through adult levels. Recommendations for involvement of the federal government are included.*

Barry, K. E. *The Five Slate System: A System of Objective Language Teaching.* Philadelphia: Sherman, 1899.

Birch, J., and J. Birch. "The Leiter International Performance Scale as an Aid in the Psychological Study of Deaf Children." *Amer. Ann. Deaf,* 96:502–512 (1951).

Boatner, E. B., E. R. Stuckless, and D. F. Moores. *Occupational Status of the Young Adult Deaf of New England and Demand for a Regional Technical-Vocational Training Center.* West Hartford, Conn.: American School for the Deaf, 1964.

> *An investigation of the achievement of young deaf adults and an analysis of their needs.*

———. "The Need of a Realistic Approach to the Education of the Deaf." Paper presented at the Convention of the California Association of Parents and Teachers of Deaf and Hard-of-Hearing Children and the California Association of the Deaf, November 1965.

Bolton, B. *Psychology of Deafness for Rehabilitation Counselors.* Baltimore: University Park Press, 1976.

> *Discussion of intellectual, personality, social, and vocational development; academic achievement; early intervention.*

Calvert, D. R., and S. R. Silverman. *Speech and Deafness: A Text for Learning and Teaching.* Washington, D.C.: Alexander Graham Bell Association for the Deaf, 1975.

> *A guide for teaching speech to hearing-impaired children. Discusses current approaches for speech teaching and recommendations for selecting among them.*

Connor, L. E. (ed.). *Speech for the Deaf Child: Knowledge and Use.* Washington, D.C.: Alexander Graham Bell Association for the Deaf, 1971.

> *A monograph addressed to teachers and allied workers interested in speech for the deaf. Includes sections on speech science, speech development and disorders, speech teaching, and organizational patterns.*

Cornett, R. O., "Cued Speech," in *International Symposium on Speech Communication Ability and Profound Deafness,* G. Fant (ed.). Washington, D.C.: Alexander Graham Bell Association for the Deaf, 1970, pp. 214–222.

Craig, W. N., and H. W. Barkuloo (eds.). *Psychologists to Deaf Children: A Developing Perspective.* Pittsburgh: University of Pittsburgh, 1968.

Report of a meeting of psychologists who have to do with deaf children. Contains contributions on functions of school psychologists, predictive and evaluative measures, psychiatric and counseling services, and research findings and tasks.

Davis, H. (ed.). "The Young Deaf Child: Identification and Management," *Acta Otolaryng. (Stockholm), Supplement 206 (1965).*

Report of a 1964 conference of American, Canadian, and European specialists, held in Toronto, Canada, dealing with the high-risk register, prevention of deafness in very young children, identification, definitive tests of hearing of young children, differential diagnosis, medical and nonmedical management, parent training, biology of sensory deprivation, use of amplification, development of language, and improvements in electroacoustic instrumentation.

Dodd, B. The Phonological Systems of Deaf Children. *J. Speech Hearing Dis.,* 41:185–198 (1976).

Doehring, D. G. "Reading Theories and Hearing Impairment," in *Hearing and Davis,* S. K. Hirsh, D. H. Eldredge, I. J. Hirsh, and S. R. Silverman (eds.) St. Louis: Washington University Press, 1976, pp. 313–321.

Eagles, E. L., W. G. Hardy, and F. I. Catlin. *Human Communication: The Public Health Aspects of Hearing, Language, and Speech Disorders,* Public Health Service Publication No. 1754. Washington, D.C.: U.S. Government Printing Office, 1968.

A concise (28-page) document from the National Institute of Neurological Diseases and Blindness dealing with definitions, prevalence, effects, prevention, and management of children with communicative disorders. There are also sections on services and goals for adults and essentials for community health programs.

———, S. M. Wishik, L. G. Doerfler, W. Melnick, and H. S. Levine. *Hearing Sensitivity and Related Factors in Children.* St. Louis: Laryngoscope, 1963.

A detailed audiologic and otologic study of about 5000 Pittsburgh school-children.

Elliott, L. "Research on the Language Acquisition of Hearing-Impaired Children," in *Hearing and Davis,* S. K. Hirsh, D. H. Eldredge, I. J. Hirsh, S. R. Silverman (eds.) St. Louis: Washington University Press, 1976, pp. 301–312.

Fitzgerald, E. *Straight Language for the Deaf.* Washington, D.C.: Gallaudet College Bookstore, 1949.

Furth, H. G. *Thinking Without Language: Psychological Implications of Deafness.* New York: The Free Press, 1966.

Fusfeld, I. "Suggestions for the Use of Standardized Tests at Gallaudet College." *Amer. Ann. Deaf,* 80:384–391 (1935).

Gallaudet College, Office of Demographic Studies. *1971 Academic Achievement Test Performance of Hearing-Impaired Children in the United States.* Series D, No. 9, August 1972. Washington, D.C.: Gallaudet College.

Galloway, J. H. "The Rochester Method," in *Report of the Proceedings of the International Congress on the Education of the Deaf and of the Forty-First Meeting of the Convention of American Instructors of the Deaf.* U.S. Document No. 106. Washington, D.C.: U.S. Government Printing Office, 1964, pp. 440–444.

> *An exposition of the Rochester Method by a former superintendent of the Rochester School for the Deaf.*

Goetzinger, C. P., C. Harrison, and C. J. Baer. "Small Perceptive Hearing Loss: Its Effect on School Age Children," *Volta Rev.,* 66:124–132 (1964).

———, and G. O. Proud. "The Impact of Hearing Impairment upon the Psychological Development of Children." *J. Aud. Res.,* Supplement 4 (1975).

> *An excellent monograph summary of research on the subject. Includes a comprehensive catalog of psychological tests that are appropriate for use with hearing-impaired children and adults.*

Groht, M. *Natural Language for Deaf Children.* Washington, D.C.: Volta Bureau, 1958.

> *Exposition of the "natural method" of teaching language to deaf children by a prominent teacher.*

Hall, P. "Results of Recent Tests at Gallaudet College." *Amer. Ann. Deaf,* 74:389–395 (1929).

Harris, G. M. *Language for the Preschool Deaf Child.* New York: Grune & Stratton, 1971.

> *Structured sequential instructional activities for preschool deaf children.*

Heider, F. K., and G. M. Heider. "A Comparison of Sentence Structure of Deaf and Hearing Children," in *Psychological Monographs,* No. 232, Studies in the Psychology of the Deaf. Columbus: American Psychological Association, 1940, pp. 42–103.

> *An investigation that analyzes the differences in structural features of language between deaf and hearing children.*

Hess, D. W. "Evaluation of the Young Deaf Adult." *J. Rehab. Deaf,* 3:6–21 (1969).

Hiskey, M. *Hiskey-Nebraska Test of Learning Aptitude.* Lincoln, Neb.: Union College Press, 1966.

Hudgins, C. V., and F. C. Numbers. "An Investigation of Intelligibility of Speech of the Deaf," *Genet. Psychol. Monogr.,* 25:289–392 (1942).

> *An analysis of errors of articulation and temporal patterns in the speech of deaf children.*

Illinois Commission on Children. *A Comprehensive Plan for Hearing-Impaired Children in Illinois.* Springfield: Illinois Commission on Children, 1968.

> *A forward-looking plan for the statewide organization and administration of the management of hearing-impaired children.*

Kohl, H. R. *Language and Education of the Deaf.* New York: Center for Urban Education, 1966.

> *A critique of the education and achievement of profoundly deaf individuals in contemporary American society emphasizing the "relative failure" of*

oral teaching and advocating the teaching of sign language, with oral language taught as a second language.

Kopp, H. (ed.). "Curriculum: Cognition and Content," *Volta Rev.,* 70 (September 1968).

The entire September 1968 issue of the Volta Review *is devoted to curriculum in schools for the deaf. Included are a formulation of issues, contributions on instruction in natural and social sciences, mathematics, language, art, health education, and pertinent features of learning theory. Educational media are also discussed.*

Lack, A. *The Teaching of Language to Deaf Children.* London: Oxford University Press, 1955.

Systematic step-by-step procedures for teaching language to deaf children. Contains many specific suggestions for correlating spoken and written language.

Lane, H. S. "The Profoundly Deaf: Has Oral Education Succeeded?" *Volta Rev.,* 78:329–340 (1976).

———, and D. Baker, "Reading Achievement of the Deaf: Another Look." *Volta Rev.* 76:279–291 (1974).

Levine, E. *Psychology of Deafness—Techniques for Appraisal for Rehabilitation.* New York: Columbia University Press, 1960.

A good reference on tests used by educators and rehabilitation counselors.

———, and E. Wagner. "Personality Patterns of Deaf Persons: An Interpretation Based on the Hand Test," *Percept. Motor Skills,* 39:1167–1236 (1974).

A comprehensive review of studies of the personality of deaf persons.

Levitt, H., and P. W. Nye (eds.). *Proceedings of the Conference on Sensory Training Aids for the Hearing Impaired.* Washington, D.C., 1971.

A conference of engineers, speech scientists, electroacousticians, psychoacousticians, and educators of the deaf.

Ling, D. "Recent Developments Affecting the Education of Hearing-Impaired Children." *Public Health Rev.,* 4:117–152 (1975).

———. *Speech and the Hearing Impaired Child: Theory and Practice.* Washington: Alexander Graham Bell Association for the Deaf, 1976.

A systematic approach involving broad sequential stages in teaching speech to hearing-impaired children. Stresses scientific studies of speech perception applied to instruction.

McGinnis, M. *Aphasic Children: Identification and Education by the Association Method.* Washington, D.C.: Alexander Graham Bell Association for the Deaf, 1963.

A practical approach to instruction of hearing- and language-handicapped children who have difficulty in learning.

Morkovin, B. V. "Language in the General Development of the Preschool Deaf Child: A Review of Research in the Soviet Union," *ASHA Monogr.,* 10:195–199 (1968).

Myklebust, H. R. *The Psychology of Deafness,* 2nd ed. New York: Grune & Stratton, 1964.

Studies of psychological abilities of deaf children.

Northern, J. L., and M. P. Downs. *Hearing in Children*. Baltimore: Williams & Wilkins Company, 1974.

Centers on pediatric audiology with emphasis on etiology and assessment.

Oléron, P. V. "A Study of the Intelligence of the Deaf," *Amer. Ann. Deaf*, 95:178–185 (1950).

Pintner, R., and D. Paterson. "Psychological Tests of Deaf Children," *Volta Rev.* 19:661–667 (1917).

Quigley, S. P. *The Influence of Fingerspelling on the Development of Language, Communication and Educational Achievement in Deaf Children*. Urbana, Ill.: Institute for Research on Exceptional Children, 1969.

As the title indicates, this work describes fingerspelling investigations in public residential schools for the deaf.

————, W. C. Jenné, and S. B. Phillips. *Deaf Students in Colleges and Universities*. Washington, D.C.: Alexander Graham Bell Association for the Deaf, 1968.

A study of the factors related to success of deaf students in colleges and universities, the problems encountered by them, and suggestions for improving their opportunities and performance.

————, D. J. Power, and M. W. Steinkamp. "The Language Structure of Deaf Children," *Volta Rev.* 79:85–92 (1977).

A brief synthesis of a series of investigations on comprehension and production of syntactic structures by deaf children.

Reamer, J. C. "Mental and Educational Measurement of the Deaf." *Psychol. Rev. Monogr.* 29 (3):1–130 (1921).

Summary of early psychological test results of Pintner and associates.

Smith, A. "Psychological Testing of the Preschool Deaf Child," *Proceedings of the International Congress on Education of the Deaf*, 1:162–181 (1967).

Smith, F., and G. A. Miller (eds.). *The Genesis of Language: A Psycholinguistic Approach*. Cambridge, Mass.: The M.I.T. Press, 1967.

Proceedings of a conference on language development in children. The aim of the conference was to "direct attention to the stages in the acquisition of grammar and phonology by children and to whatever biological and clinical evidence we have concerning the child's innate capacity for this acquisition."

Snijders, J., and N. Ooman. *Nonverbal Intelligence Tests for Deaf and Hearing Subjects*. Groningen, Netherlands: J. B. Wolters, 1959.

Stark, R. E. (ed). *Sensory Capabilities of Hearing-Impaired Children*. Baltimore: University Park Press, 1974.

Proceedings of a workshop of speech and hearing scientists and workers on speech of hearing-impaired children, dealing with the needs and capabilities of children for whom auditory and nonauditory aids were being designed. The topics included sensory capabilities, perceptual and cognitive strategies, and language processing.

Stepp, R. E. (project director). "Symposium on Research and Utilization of Educational Media for Teaching the Hearing Impaired," *Amer. Ann. Deaf*, 110:508–620 (1965).

Report of a national conference at the University of Nebraska dealing with the use of media in the instruction of deaf children.

Stokoe, W. C., D. C. Casterline, and C. G. Croneberg. *A Dictionary of American Sign Language on Linguistic Principles.* Washington, D.C.: Gallaudet College Press, 1965.

Tervoort, B. T., and A. J. Verberk, *Developmental Features of Visual Communication.* New York: North-Holland Publishing Company, 1975.

Report of an investigation of linguistic features of communication of deaf children based on filmed observations. Esoteric (the children's own system) and exoteric (the system being taught) systems of communication are compared.

Urbantschitsch, V. *Des Exercises dans la Surdi-mutité et dans la Surdité Acquise,* translated by L. Egger. Paris: A. Maloine, 1897.

One of the first expositions of the possibilities and methods of auditory training.

Vegely, A., and L. L. Elliott. "Applicability of a Standardized Personality Test to a Hearing Impaired Population," *Amer. Ann. Deaf,* 113:858–868 (1968).

Whetnall, E. and D. B. Fry. *The Deaf Child.* London: William Heinemann Ltd., 1964.

An exposition of the development of communication in deaf children emphasizing an early auditory approach.

Wing, G. (original author). *An Exposition of Wing's Symbols in Their Relation to the Teaching of Language.* Faribault, Minn.: Minnesota School for the Deaf, 1938.

Withrow, F. B., and C. J. Nygren. *Language, Materials, and Curriculum Management for the Handicapped Learner.* Columbus, Ohio: Charles E. Merrill Publishing Company, 1976.

Emphasizes application of specially designed curricular materials to language development. Chapter 3 describes a "generative linguistic" model for language instruction for deaf children.

Wrightstone, J. W., M. S. Aranow, and S. Moskowitz. "Developing Reading Norms for Deaf Children." *Amer. Ann. Deaf,* 108:311–316 (1963).

Yale, C. A. *Formation and Development of Elementary English Sounds.* Northampton, Mass.: Gazette Printing Company, 1925.

A description and principles of the Northampton charts.

Zaliouk, A. "A Visual-Tactile System of Phonetical Symbolization," *J. Speech Hearing Dis.,* 19:190–207 (1954).

Robert Frisina, Ph.D.

18

Postsecondary Education

POSTSECONDARY EDUCATION IN THE UNITED STATES

Postsecondary education is a significant American enterprise by virtue of its size and pervasiveness. Its "product" is knowledge of all kinds. Throughout its existence in the United States postsecondary education has expanded from serving a restricted elite population to serving the broadest-based population of any like "industry" in the country. As defined in *Financing Postsecondary Education in the United States* (1973),

Postsecondary education currently consists of formal instruction, research, public service, and other learning opportunities offered by educational institutions that primarily serve persons who have completed secondary education or who are beyond the compulsory school attendance age and that are accredited by agencies officially recognized for that purpose by the U.S. Office of Education or are otherwise eligible to participate in federal programs.

This definition includes six categories of institutions: research universities, comprehensive colleges, liberal arts colleges, two-year (community or junior) colleges, specialty schools (in fields such as law, medicine, art, music, and engineering), and noncollegiate institutions (such as flight, cosmetology, and hospital schools). Each of these types has evolved over the years and in sum they have come to satisfy a variety of clientele and purposes.

The Beginnings

In 1636 Harvard College was established as the first college of the colonies. It was private, serving only the elite of the time by means of a classical curriculum intended to prepare young men for law, medicine, education, and the clergy. It was not until 1805, when South Carolina established the first tax-supported college, that our pluralistic system of private and public higher education began.

The egalitarian movement, along with a number of other factors, led to the passage of the Morrill (Land Grant) Act in 1862, which gave rise to a third type of institution, the comprehensive college. The Morrill Act represents the most significant piece of educational legislation passed in the three-century history of higher education in America; it contributed to the following developments:

Women's postsecondary education was advanced.

The "separate but equal" doctrine that fostered the black college movement was established.

Land grant colleges brought higher education to a broader segment of the population.

Military training was offered for the first time in regular colleges.

Technical-vocational education, with particular emphasis upon engineering and agriculture, was begun.

Land grant colleges provided many states with the campuses for state universities.

Secondary education was influenced greatly since entrance to these new institutions required that background.

Between 1890 and 1930, high schools doubled their enrollment every ten years.

Two years after the passage of the Morrill Act, both Gallaudet College for the Deaf and Howard University for blacks were established in Washington, D.C., with direct federal support. For the first time, the special requirements of deaf persons' postsecondary education were recognized. The influence of the German university, with its orientation to scholarship and research as legitimate functions of higher education, eventually led to the opening in 1876 of the Johns Hopkins University as the first research-oriented university in the United States.

In 1944 returning war veterans were greeted with the Servicemen's Readjustment Act (G.I. Bill) and in 1947 nearly 1,150,000 entered higher education under its auspices. Existing colleges grew and new colleges were established to accommodate them. Veterans continued to enter colleges after World War II, the Korean conflict, and Vietnam. Moreover, the post-World War II "baby boom" resulted in a significantly higher percentage of high school graduates choosing to enter college during the 1960s.

In many ways World War II represented the coalescence of cumulated scientific knowledge and new technologies. Research became an important national priority, federal funds for its conduct came to higher education, and further expansion of existing research institutions resulted.

New initiatives in federal and state legislation gave higher education more new clients to serve. Older students entered for the first time or returned to classrooms, minority groups (blacks and Mexican-Americans) were encouraged to participate in higher education, enrollment of women expanded, and the disadvantaged were beginning to be served.

The growth in two-year colleges far outstripped that of other colleges and universities during the 1960s. While the numbers of all institutions grew 2.6 percent during the decade of the sixties, two-year colleges grew by 61 percent. Correspondingly, the number of students in community colleges grew more rapidly than those in all other colleges and universities. The total increase for all colleges and universities was 122 percent, whereas two-year colleges increased their enrollment by 279 percent.

All in all, from 1944 to 1976 the expansion of access and choice for a broad cross section of U.S. citizens was phenomenal. The approximate increase in total enrollment was 560 percent! Higher education at present serves more than 10 million students; this is in contrast to 1.5 million in 1940, 2.6 million in 1950, 3.2 million in 1960, and 7.1 million in 1970. The number of postsecondary institutions serving these students exceeds 3000.

The Emerging Learning Society

Movement toward a "learning society," much in evidence in our country today, was greatly stimulated in 1936 when the Center for Continuation Study at the University of Minnesota was opened. This signaled the beginning of the move beyond extension work to a more general emphasis on continuing education. For example, in 1974 one-third of all postsecondary students were over 25 years of age; one million or approximately 10 percent were over 35 years of age; two-thirds of all part-time students were over 25 years of age. These are indications that a "learning society," albeit incomplete, is growing in the United States. The need for continuing one's education beyond the traditional high school or college age is becoming of increasing importance from a personal as well as a socioeconomic perspective.

These milestones and observations regarding postsecondary education in the United States constitute the framework for understanding the opportunities available to deaf students and the distinctive challenges confronting the education of deaf children and youth in order for them to be able to take advantage of these opportunities.

INDUSTRIALIZATION, THE WORK FORCE, AND POSTSECONDARY EDUCATION

In economic terms it is the condition of the extractive (mining, fishing, forestry, agriculture), manufacturing, and service industries that determine whether or not a society is able to support industrialization. In highly developed countries such as the United States, the full occupational ramifications lead to as many as 20,000 different occupational titles.

In order to specify the challenges of preparing deaf people at the postsecondary level, some understanding of the employment circumstances of our industrialized nation can be helpful. Let us consider first the broad employment picture of the general population, and second, the patterns of the adult deaf presently in the work force.

Characteristics of the Work Force

Numbers in the work force The total number of people in the U.S. work force in 1976 exceeded 86 million, one-third of whom were women. The number of women in the work force has steadily increased over the past decades, and this increase is expected to continue.

Age distribution Currently the fastest growing age group in the work force includes those individuals 25 to 35 years of age. Seventy-five percent of these persons have completed at least four years of high school education. Since continuing education serves many purposes but relates particularly to enhancement of employment status, it is significant that one-third of all postsecondary students are over 24 years of age.

Education levels in employment Employment rates have consistently favored those with more education more than those with less.

For example, within the 18–34-year age range those with less than a high school education have been shown to suffer unemployment rates twice that of high school graduates, and nearly three times that of persons with postsecondary education experience. Employment percentage rates for those with postsecondary education, and particularly those who have completed a two- or four-year study program, consistently range in the mid- to high 90s. In general the amount of education each person receives has been increasing. In 1900, only 6 percent of 17-year-olds graduated from high school. By 1970, this figure had increased to 75 percent, and 50 percent of these went on to college.

Where most people work It has become apparent that as a nation begins moving toward industrialization, the goods-producing sector of the economy employs the greatest number of people. In a fully industrialized society, the service-producing industries gradually overtake the manufacturing sector as a place of employment. For example, extrapolation from U.S. Bureau of Census reports indicates that workers have distributed themselves among the extractive, manufacturing, and service industries as seen in Table 18-1.

Service industries include such areas as transportation and public utilities, trade, finance, government, education, insurance, and real estate. The realities of a service-dominated economy should be of great interest for those concerned with education and communication in deaf children and youth because of the heavy reliance in these activities on telecommunication, linguistic fluency, and personal/social sophistication.

Among the fastest growing occupational groups in our country is the professional and technical group. The need for service workers is increasing, whereas mechanization in agriculture is decreasing the need for farm workers. This view is reflected in the occupations entered by the 1975 graduates of the National Technical Institute for the Deaf. Of 35 graduates, 24 entered service occupations, 10 entered manufacturing, and only one went into extractive and agricultural work. These observations emphasize the need for more formal education, training, and linguistic development associated with employment as scientists, engineers, skilled craftsmen, technicians, managers, and other professionals.

Characteristics of the Labor Force Among Deaf Adults

A comprehensive assessment of the occupational status of deaf adults in the United States was completed in 1972 (Schein and Delk, 1974). Compared with hearing persons, deaf adults primarily were found to be earning salaries and wages in private industry; this seemed to be at the expense of their not being self-employed or in government service.

Although the rate of employment was found to be essentially the same for the deaf as the general population, there were differences in occupations. Nontrained operators and craftsmen make up the principal occupations of the deaf. They are seriously underrepresented in the professional and technical, managerial, entrepreneurial, clerical, sales, and service occupations. Deaf persons

TABLE 18-1
PERCENTAGE DISTRIBUTION OF WORKERS IN
MAJOR ECONOMIC SECTORS: U.S.A.

Year	Extractive and Agriculture	Manufacturing	Services
1900	38	34	28
1920	30	39	31
1940	25	34	41
1960	11	39	50
1970	5	36	59

are overrepresented among farm workers and nonfarm laborers. The general picture suggests that specialized training and education of a more advanced level than heretofore is necessary for future generations of deaf adults. Such opportunities are becoming available. We shall consider them next.

POSTSECONDARY OPPORTUNITIES FOR DEAF PERSONS

The Early Years

In 1864 the concept of a special college gave to the deaf an opportunity for postsecondary education in the liberal arts. Equally significant was the realization that a deaf person, when given appropriate learning opportunities, could in fact succeed at the college level. In addition to the more than 6000 who have graduated from Gallaudet since its inception, a few hundred others have succeeded with limited or no help at regular colleges and universities. It was not until the 1960s that the college-going rate of deaf persons was examined. The concern was undoubtedly stimulated by the situation of deaf persons caught in a changing work force that clearly required education and skills beyond those accomplished by most deaf youngsters at the termination of their secondary experience. Analysis revealed that low levels of academic achievement greatly reduced the chances for access to regular colleges and universities by any except a very few. Their number far exceeded the number of comparable graduates from hearing high schools. This led to the recognition that the occupational choices in an industrialized nation were unfairly and unreasonably limited for deaf persons. The employment statistics and educational outcomes at the secondary level underlined the need to provide more diverse education and training opportunities for them.

Recent Developments

Promising contributions of the emerging field of audiology to education of the hearing-impaired from preschool through secondary school encouraged professionals, the adult deaf community, parents, and other interested lay and government groups to seek more diverse opportunities for deaf students at the postsecondary level. These groups were aware of the significant educational shortfalls that would confront any serious efforts to develop and to execute such new endeavors. Among the problems were these:

1. There was a general concern that many deaf students exiting from secondary programs were as ill-prepared for further academic work at the postsecondary level as they were for employment. This meant that any new constructive efforts would demand close working relationships with the secondary school systems throughout the nation. Bridging the academic gap between requirements for entrance to regular postsecondary institutions and the average levels of academic attainment by deaf students completing secondary schools was viewed as an extraordinary challenge.

2. There was general recognition of the problems of communication between teachers and students in learning situations. Note that the question here is not one of method but one of communication. Individual differences would require diagnosis and evaluation in order to prescribe educational activities that would succeed, that is, diagnosis and evaluation not only of content but also of style and format.

3. It was known that the extra-academic capabilities—that is, the personal-social competencies at the point of entry to postsecondary environments—were often less than optimum. The same was true of communications. In marked contrast to the hear-

ing student, whose competencies can be reasonably assumed, a great deal (as we have seen in Chapter 17 in terms of fundamental skills and knowledge) must be taught to deaf students. Concern for survival in the postsecondary environment was paramount and required some creative approaches and adaptations to existing conditions.

It was somewhat ironic that in 1965 the U.S. postsecondary education network was at the midpoint of the greatest ten-year growth period in its history, yet remarkably little effort, if any, was made to accommodate it to the special needs of deaf citizens. This reality led to the establishment in 1965 by a public law of National Technical Institute for the Deaf (NTID), a complementary institution to Gallaudet College. NTID was organized as a national center with these aims:

Technical education and training of deaf youth and adults in order to prepare them for successful employment and community participation

Preparation of professional personnel to serve the deaf nationally

Conduct of applied research into deafness

NTID was a unique and significant endeavor in that it was to be established and operated within an existing college or university setting. Further, in its eventual placement at Rochester Institute of Technology, it represented an amalgam of private with public legal entities, college with federal fiscal policies, non-profit with federal governance, and local with national geographic orientations. The model being proposed, if indeed one were to be developed, could serve as a prototype for other efforts elsewhere. In the ten years following NTID's establishment nearly 40 all-hearing schools have opened their doors to deaf and hearing-impaired students. Although it is relatively new and perhaps somewhat tenuous, a network of educational opportunities is beginning to emerge in the United States, as is the case nowhere else in the world. Let us next examine this network in greater detail.

A GUIDE TO COLLEGE/CAREER PROGRAMS FOR DEAF STUDENTS

Following the establishment of NTID a five-year research and demonstration project, begun in 1968, was conducted at Del-

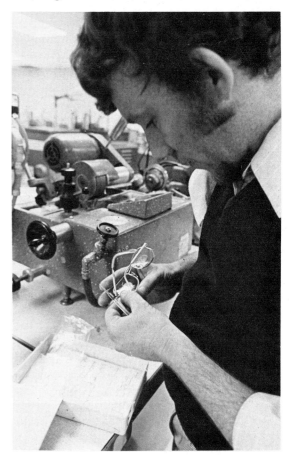

Figure 18-1 The optical finishing technology program at National Technical Institute for the Deaf prepares students to work as technicians in optical firms throughout the country.

gado Community College (New Orleans), Seattle Community College, and St. Paul (Minnesota) Technical Vocational Institute. The purpose of the project, jointly sponsored by the U.S. Office of Education and the Vocational Rehabilitation Administration, was to determine the feasibility of incorporating deaf students into regular community college programs. In 1972 this writer encouraged a meeting of representatives from these three programs and others in existence (with enrollments of 50 or more students) at that time to consider ways to improve the quality of the programs. That effort resulted in a publication *A Guide to College/Career Programs for Deaf Students* edited by Dr. E. Ross Stuckless and Dr. Gilbert L. Delgado and produced jointly by NTID and Gallaudet in 1973. Updated and revised in September 1975, it is broadly distributed and provides a data base for discussing characteristics of programs presently in existence. The reader is referred to revised editions as they are produced for specific details of each program.

Existing Programs

Numbers of programs During the 1974–1975 academic year, 41 postsecondary institutions reported serving 10 or more students. In addition to the two national programs, NTID and Gallaudet, 39 programs in 23 states were identified. The educational environments in which these 41 programs are placed include seven university and four-year colleges, 26 community colleges, seven vocational/technical institutes, and one rehabilitation center. The university and four-year colleges offer graduate as well as undergraduate programs. Some community colleges emphasize technical and vocational education, and others emphasize liberal arts. Several of the community college programs offer a two- or three-year associate degree

program that prepares students to enter four-year colleges as juniors or seniors.

Organization Each of the 41 reporting schools satisfied the following criteria:

It has either a full-time director specifically for the deaf program or a part-time director who devotes at least 50 percent of his time to the program for deaf students.

It has a minimum of 10 full-time deaf students enrolled.

It accepts students directly from high school.

It is part of an accredited postsecondary program.

Since these requirements determine inclusion in a book related to programs, individual students attending regular colleges and universities and "on their own" would be in addition to the 1766 students attending the 41 programs meeting these criteria.

Enrollment The number of deaf students in settings other than the 41 cited above is not known. Individual students have been identified, and an estimate of the total might be about 50. In toto, the round-figure size of the deaf population enrolled in postsecondary education facilities is approximately 3000. This is at least three times the number being served eight years ago. Enrollment during the 1974–1975 academic year was distributed among the 41 educational settings as follows:

1524 in the two national programs, NTID and Gallaudet

207 in the other five universities and colleges

701 in the 26 community colleges

319 in the seven vocational technical institutes

15 in the one rehabilitation center setting

Program graduates The number of students graduating in 1975 from this network of postsecondary programs was 512. These graduates earned 190 certificates/diplomas, 108 associate degrees, 169 baccalaureate degrees, and 45 advanced degrees. These attainments recognize the accomplishments of many capable and dedicated parents and teachers throughout the lifetime of these students and, most important, the persistence of the students themselves. The range of earned credentials calls attention to the heterogeneity of the group. These data suggest, too, an impressive variety of interests, ability, and performance.

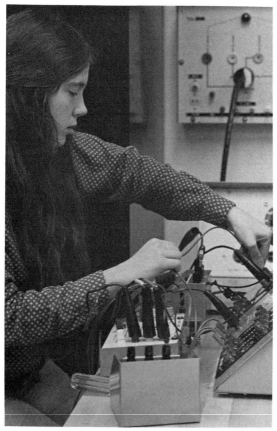

Figure 18-2 The electromechanical technology program at National Technical Institute for the Deaf offers students hands-on experience in electrical and mechanical systems.

Functions of postsecondary education The functions of postsecondary institutions in a democratic society include educational, cultural, and socioeconomic elements. The *educational functions* address themselves to higher flexibility and autonomy of mind, an inquiring attitude, and acquisition of knowledge necessary for participation in a rapidly changing world. These functions are implied in virtually all curricula, but especially in general studies courses, which unfortunately may be viewed with skepticism by students and faculty in career-oriented programs.

The *cultural functions* relate to the appreciation of the history and the rich cultural heritage of humankind. Art exhibitions, theatre performances, musical offerings, special lectures, and other such activities constitute a special part of the informal academic program of any university and college. Although extra effort is required to assure participation of deaf students, the rewards are high.

The *socioeconomic functions* of postsecondary education are well known, but they particularly bear emphasis since they influence the extent to which deaf students have the opportunity to get "into the thick of things" or stand idly by on the sidelines as mere spectators. Reluctance to exploit special talents vigorously in the marketplace of work lead to self-devaluation and underemployment. Appropriate credentialing procedures attesting to the deaf person's demonstration of competence should ease this situation.

Special Services

Students attending special programs are generally selected on the basis of their needing some assistance beyond that regularly offered to students in postsecondary education. The services likely to be considered for use are listed below. (The percentage in parentheses indicates the proportion of the 41 programs reporting the availability of the specific service to students.)

Special classes for deaf students (54 percent)
These classes range from remedial instruction in English, mathematics, or science to courses that emphasize verbal skills such as the humanities and social sciences.

Interpreters in regular classes (98 percent)
Virtually all interpreting is done in the simultaneous mode (speech and manual communication) and is variously successful, depending among other factors on the subject matter, the students' language backgrounds and familiarity with the subject matter, the physical conditions of the environment, and the skills of the interpreter. Interpreting spontaneous discussions in large-group functions is a circumstance where simultaneous reception is invaluable.

Tutoring services (93 percent)
Tutoring is a service much used by those attending regular classes. Research on the process is concerned with the amount of tutoring time versus class time, use of peer versus professional tutors, and the characteristics of tutors. The extent of tutorial need varies with a student's ability to deal with course-related printed material, the nature of the learning situation, and the instructor's understanding of the student.

Notetaking services (85 percent)
A special notetaking book that has been developed is widely used in many of these programs. The book incorporates a copying process that reproduces the notes for immediate use by more than one student. Volunteer versus paid peer notetakers, peer versus other paid notetakers, and a variety of notetaking styles and procedures are under study.

Vocational development services (93 percent)
Virtually all students are in need of career evaluation counseling. The concept of education leading to careers is not well understood or practiced in many school systems at the secondary level. A variety of career sampling approaches are being used at the postsecondary level. It appears that academic, career, and personal counseling needs of students are difficult to separate, and these require personnel who are in rare supply.

Manual communication training for deaf students (85 percent)
The extent of this training relates to the nature of the student population, the communication practices of the school, and the expectations of the staff and faculty.

Manual communication training of instructors (71 percent)
Enthusiasm for training in manual communication on the part of regular faculty members is not universal. Understanding deaf students involves more than the mechanics of communication, but manual communication often does have appeal to the uninitiated. To maintain initial interest is a major task of the special staff. Institutionalizing the teaching of deaf students is an extremely challenging task for any support group since it involves attitudes, vested interests, and competing priorities. It has been argued by some that the solution to the "handicap" of deafness (other than prevention) mainly has to do with the attitudes of the majority group, that is, hearing society. Interesting more hearing people, particularly general educators, in interacting with deaf people seems a reasonable first step in testing this hypothesis and thereby setting an example for the rest of society.

Personal counseling services (100 percent)
All programs reportedly have available on

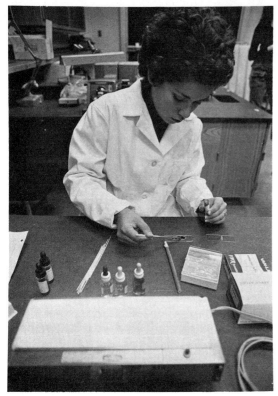

Figure 18-3 The medical laboratory technology program at National Technical Institute for the Deaf gives students opportunities to perform actual hospital tests in a simulated hospital laboratory.

their staffs personnel professionally trained in counseling and skilled in communication techniques as well. To reiterate, the triad of career, personal, and academic counseling is an important part of any program, particularly where career selection and job placement are major concerns of the program. Much of the substance of counseling could be reduced by more aggressive programming in the personal/social areas prior to high school graduation. Parents and educators working together are crucial to any significantly improved personal/social levels of accomplishment in groups of deaf youngsters.

Social/cultural activities (76 percent) Expansion of cultural interests could benefit vir-

tually all of the students enrolled. Development of self-esteem and of social competency are closely allied with social/cultural activities. Moreover, the understanding, enjoyment, and preservation of our varied cultural heritages are fundamental to the concept of a democratic society. Care must be taken to assure a balance between specialty requirements and the liberal arts. This can be accomplished when continuing sensitivity to the multifunction of postsecondary institutions is maintained.

Vocational placement services (80 percent) The process of successful placement of graduates is somewhat analogous to encouraging regular colleges and universities to be concerned about deaf students. Since deafness is outside the realm of most employers' daily experiences, systematic and sustained communication with those in business and industry and in other prospective employment contexts is required. New audiences with whom little or no contact has occurred need to be cultivated on behalf of potential employees. Employment prospects for educated and trained deaf graduates is excellent. Systematic approaches to job finding and job placement have proved to be very effective, with percentage rates of placement in the mid- and high 90s. Regional and national employment seminars have proved to be very useful in acquainting national corporations with the capabilities of educated deaf people. Moreover, legislation mandating the recruitment and accommodation of handicapped workers is an incentive to employers.

Speech and hearing services (46 percent) There is little doubt that much remedial or useful potential of residual hearing still goes unattended. Clearly 90 percent of all deaf graduates from secondary schools have some hearing that is potentially useful in the perception and expression of speech. Unfortunately, this has not always been recognized or exploited. Hearing-aid selection and usage are likely to be less than adequate in a third to a half of any postsecondary group of deaf students upon entry. When their value is realized, speechreading and speech, at least in one's major area of study, can be improved in most students. Success in motivating students is best demonstrated in the success of their peers and the feedback from graduates who have gone on and learned the importance of spontaneous communication in the work environment. Public speaking, parliamentary procedures, acting, and debating are other types of activities related to speech and hearing services that can benefit all students who choose to participate.

Supervised housing (32 percent)   Residential campus housing can be viewed as an obstacle to progress or it can be made into an educational opportunity. Crosstalk between deaf and hearing persons can be a significant part of the educational process, and within this framework living and dining arrangements can be helpful. This potential educational benefit should not be overlooked for its value in the social/cultural as well as in the personal development domains. Sociological perspectives on the concept of "handicap" suggest that a regular college setting may be a valued source for mutual understanding that benefits both groups.

This section has highlighted some of the special services likely to be useful in helping students to grow and to guide themselves through the educational experience and into the world of work. Fundamentally, students must "learn to learn" if they are to achieve technical competence, personal and social growth, and linguistic ability. The essential aim is independence. The special services, when effectively practiced, are a key to its attainment. Careful studies, which fortunately are under way, are imperative so that mean-

ingful changes for improvement can be made.

Career Areas of Study

The existing network of postsecondary programs offers an abundant choice of career areas. These opportunities range from skilled trades through doctoral-level work and are inclusive of all major occupational clusters. The U.S. Office of Education career clusters applied to the 1974–1975 enrolled students suggests the following areas in which deaf students now participate: agriculture, business, communication and media, construction, consumer and homemaking education, environmental and natural resources, fine arts and humanities, health, hospitality and recreation, manufacturing, marketing and distribution, product services, public services, and transportation. The specific courses of study are those regularly offered for hearing students in vocational/technical institutions, community colleges, and university and four-year colleges.

Special Observations

Career selection   What is true of hearing students is equally so in the case of young deaf people embarking on careers requiring postsecondary education. First, each has limited knowledge of the number and variety of work opportunities. Second, misconceptions abound concerning the career environments available for each occupational title or specialty. A frequent impression is that given practitioners, be they engineers, accountants, draftsmen, medical technologists or other, work in one preconceived place. In reality, more than one environment exists for each trade, technology, or profession. People educated and trained in a specific field can in fact practice that specialty in a variety of settings. An accountant, for example, can be in private practice or the construction sector or the agricultural sector or virtually any profit, nonprofit, or governmental enterprise.

Remedial work in career selection is provided in the postsecondary environment but frequently at a cost of an extended period of study beyond the basic curricula associated with a given field of study. The magnitude of this problem is such that virtually every program makes some allowance for it and expects to be involved in this process in some formal or informal manner.

Student profiles The students attending university and four-year colleges, community colleges, and vocational/technical programs overlap to a considerable extent in their basic characteristics. At the point of admissions, group average differences are likely to emerge among populations entering the three types of institutions, but considerable overlap is also very likely. Hearing loss and general communication skills would not likely differ between one program and another. Except as prerequisites would screen students out of any particular program of study, intellectual ability on the average might be a little higher in the university and four-year college students. There is some indication that in two cases out of three, graduates of residential schools select Gallaudet and Technical Vocational Institute rather than other institutions. On the other hand, slightly more than 50 percent of NTID students come from regular high schools where support services have been made available. The network is relatively new and not fully tested. The outcomes of graduates as evaluated in future census studies will gradually reflect the usefulness of these activities and programs.

Survival skills in college Students tend to come with limitations in the ability to solve problems and to make informed choices and decisions. This is, of course, common among hearing students but appears often enough among entering deaf students that efforts to assist are built into some programs. As they pursue the matter of career selection and embark upon their academic programs, they confront the problem of clarification of values related to work. Once again we find that this is not unique to deaf students but is part of a larger societal trend. An important current field of study is concerned with the existing divisions in our lives, namely work, education, and leisure. Our lives have been segmented into one-third education (youth), one-third work (adulthood), and one-third retirement and leisure (old age). But, the work ethic has moved from one of saving to not as precise as they once were, and their lifetime integration is being increasingly sought. Work sabbaticals are being tried in some European industries and will be watched with great interest. Essentially, the work ethic has moved from one of saving to one of consumption, and more recently to one of self-gratification. These conflicting values to which hearing and deaf young people of college-going age are exposed need to be dealt with accordingly. The difficulty is compounded by the need to achieve realistic self-appraisal relating to career selection.

Instruction and communication The extent to which "learning" and "problem-solving styles" of deaf students differ from those of hearing students, if they differ at all, is still an open question. How the almost complete dependence on vision affects learning, and consequently instructional practices, is a fundamental question. This involves an understanding of "visual processing" and the relative emphases to be placed on the combination of speech and the variety of manual systems, media, and the printed page. In conventional learning contexts such as large group lectures, seminar/discussions in small groups, and individual and group laboratory, shop, and studio activity, these modes of communication are being evaluated with respect to recurrent problems. Among these are accuracy, efficiency, and rate of transmission of information, interstudent exchange, and dependency on classmates and tutoring.

Successful participation in a highly industrialized community requires a marketable skill. The "infrastructure" for industrialization requires significant numbers of technical and service professionals in industry, business, education, government, health, and labor. The need for skilled workers, managers, and professionals advances with increased levels of industrialization. Educational achievement levels among deaf children must be improved in order to enable them to compete successfully in the world of work. In the training of deaf students, science and mathematics, the humanities, and social sciences all have their important place.

Language and vocabulary requirements increase and change continuously in a dynamic environment caused by technological developments. Exploitation of those modes of communication most appropriate to each child is of prime importance for purposes of educational advancement, personal and social adjustment, and job mobility. The case for a postsecondary education of deaf people is very clear, and the case for lifelong learning is emerging.

SUGGESTED READINGS AND REFERENCES

"Establishing Goals: General Education," in *Higher Education for American Democracy,* Report of the President's Advisory Commission on Education. Washington, D.C.: U.S. Government Printing Office, 1947.

Financing Postsecondary Education in the United States, Report of the National Commission on the Financing of Postsecondary Education. Washington, D.C.: U.S. Government Printing Office, 1973.

Rawlings, B. W., R. J. Trybus, G. L. Delgado, and E. R. Stuckless. *A Guide to College/Career Programs for Deaf Students,* revised 1975 edition. Washington, D.C.: Gallaudet College and the National Technical Institute for the Deaf, September 1975.

Quigley, S. P., W. C. Jenné, and S. B. Phillips. *Deaf Students in Colleges and Universities.* Washington, D.C.: Alexander Graham Bell Association for the Deaf, 1968.

Schein, J. D., and M. T. Delk, Jr. *The Deaf Population of the United States.* Silver Spring, Md.: National Association of the Deaf, 1974.

Part VI

PSYCHOSOCIAL ASPECTS OF DEAFNESS

Donald A. Ramsdell, Ph.D.

19

The Psychology of the Hard-of-Hearing and the Deafened Adult

Anyone who has closely observed an adult soon after he has lost his hearing has noted that he becomes discouraged and struggles with feelings of depression. Sometimes he even becomes suspicious of friends and family. In order to understand the psychology of the deaf, it is necessary to understand why this personality change occurs and why it does not occur with equal severity in children who are born deaf or in those who become blind.

That loss of hearing does tend to result in this peculiar and serious personality change has long been known, but the reason for the change is not obvious. The depression is usually more serious than we should expect from the loss of easy two-way communication, particularly if we recall that the adult has already learned to talk, to read, and to write before the onset of deafness. Nor is the depression prevented by prompt instruction in speechreading, although this assistance to communication is both desirable and helpful.

A study of the reactions of soldiers who lost their hearing in World War II has shown that the loss of communication is not the deaf person's only or most serious loss. Deafness produces a psychological impairment more basic and more severe than the difficulty in communication. The characteristic depression is caused by this more subtle impairment. Recognition and understanding of the cause are necessary if the depression is to be overcome and not attributed, as is so often the case, to a character weakness in the deafened. Fortunately, an understanding of the psychological factors involved is, in itself, a powerful means of overcoming the depression.

This chapter is written in the hope that it will help those adults who have suffered permanent impairment of hearing to understand the psychological problems involved and thereby overcome their depressive reactions, and that it will provide the families of the deafened with a clearer insight into the difficulties that deafness entails so that they, too, can help.

Before the person with normal hearing can attempt to understand the problem of deafness, he must make a conscious effort to imagine what it is like to become suddenly and totally deaf, cut off in a world of silence from the familiar sounds of everyday living. Most of us take normal hearing completely for granted because we hear without conscious effort. We do not even have to open an "earlid" in order to listen, nor do we have an "earlid" to close if we wish to experience for a moment what deafness is like.

One way to gain some idea of the deaf person's experience is to imagine what it would be like to start home in a silent world after your day's work. The outside door makes no noise as you close it after you and step out on the sidewalk. A heavy rain is falling silently. Five o'clock traffic is jamming the street; people are crowding past you, but you hear no sound. Newsboys in front of the building are arguing angrily over something, but you can only see the exaggerated movement of their lips as they shout at each other. Cars suddenly swerve to the curb and stop. Everyone turns to look behind you, startled by a sound that you have not heard. An ambulance rushes silently past. Everything moves with the unreality of pantomime. When you reach home, you see your family's smiles of greeting, you see their lips move, but the rich experience of hearing the tone and rhythm of their familiar voices is lost.

They, too, are like actors on a silent stage. If you can imagine such a silent world, you know something of how the deaf man feels, in close visual contact with his family and his surroundings but forced to substitute sight for hearing.

The loss of any sense organ imposes limitations, but the nature and severity of those limitations depend upon the particular sense organ affected. The most obvious limitation of the deaf person is that he cannot hear the spoken word. He may partially compensate, to be sure, by learning speechreading and, if he has sufficient residual hearing, by using a hearing aid. But if he depends on speechreading, he is definitely limited to clearly visible conversation directed to him. The deaf person's participation in the feelings and observations of others is restricted to those who deliberately address him. Without the full range of normal hearing, he misses the little asides that add immeasurably to the savor and zest of general conversation. He also misses the snatches of talk normally overheard as we ride the subway or bus or walk on a crowded street. Until these casual contacts are lost, it is impossible to realize how enormously they contribute to the feeling of group participation. The social handicap to communication with those around him therefore remains for the deaf person, even though it may seem to be partially overcome by speechreading or by the use of a hearing aid.

Because a blind person must also substitute one sense for another, blindness and deafness are popularly classed together. What we fail to realize is that the psychological effects of deafness are fundamentally different from those of blindness. The similarity between the two impairments is superficial, and the tendency to evaluate the effects of deafness in the terms used for blindness has retarded an understanding of the psychology of the deafened.

THE THREE PSYCHOLOGICAL LEVELS OF HEARING

To understand the psychological changes that accompany the loss of hearing, it is necessary first to comprehend how normal hearing operates. In order to make the explanation as simple as possible, we shall discuss normal hearing as though it occurred on three levels:

1. On the social level, as we all realize, hearing is used to comprehend language. Words are symbols for objects around us and for activities. The word "tree" symbolizes the tree growing in the yard; the word "gallop" symbolizes the rapid gait of a horse. Since language is symbolic in its nature, we shall call this level of auditory function the *symbolic* level.

2. Sound also serves as a direct sign or signal of events to which we make constant adjustments in daily living. At this level it is not the word "bee" (which is a symbol for the actual bee itself), but the sound of its angry buzz that makes us jump. We stop our car not because someone says "policeman" (the symbol for the officer) but because we hear the shrill sound of his whistle. This level of auditory function we shall call the *signal*, or *warning*, level.

3. Finally, and most basically, sound serves neither as symbol nor as warning but simply as *the auditory background* of all daily living. At this level we react to such sounds as the tick of a clock, the distant roar of traffic, vague echoes of people moving in other rooms in the house, without being aware that we do hear them. These incidental noises maintain our feeling of being part of a living world and contribute to our own sense of being alive. We are not conscious of the important role that these background sounds play in our comfortable merging of ourselves with the life around us because we are not aware that we hear them. Nor is the deaf person aware that he has lost these sounds; he only knows that *he feels as if the world were dead*. The real importance of this third level of hearing is the creation of a *background of feeling*, which the psychologist calls an "affective tone."

It was the constant reiteration, by hard-of-hearing patients at Deshon Army Hospital, of the statement that the world seemed dead that led to the investigation of this third level of hearing and of the psychological effect of its loss upon the deaf. This third level has not generally been recognized, although it is psychologically the most fundamental of the auditory functions. It relates us to the world at a very primitive level, somewhere below the level of clear consciousness and perception. The loss of this feeling of relationship with the world is the major cause of the well-recognized feeling of "deadness" and also of the depression that permeates the suddenly deafened and, to a lesser degree, those in whom deafness develops gradually. This level of hearing we shall designate as the *primitive* level.

The concept of levels of hearing has been chosen as the organizing principle of this chapter because this approach allows us to isolate and discuss the diverse but related auditory processes, together with their special implications for the deaf. "Hearing" is, of course, a combination of all these processes. At any given moment all are going on simultaneously. We hear on all the three levels at once. We hear the symbols of language, the signal of the ringing of the telephone, and we react to the background of sounds, which we do not consciously discriminate and of which we are not aware. These diverse processes, however, vary independently, sometimes with a predominance of one, sometimes of another, but there is usually an interweaving contribution from each in the total pattern of hearing.

We shall begin our analysis of the psychological problems of the deaf at the most basic, least objective, and least structured level (the *primitive* level) and then explain the other two levels in the order of their objectivity—second, the *warning* level, and third, the *symbolic* level. Although such an approach may seem to be working backward, the reverse is true. Impairment or loss at the primitive "affective" level is most fundamentally and intimately connected with the emotional difficulties of the deaf.

Hearing at the Primitive Level

At the primitive level of hearing we react to the changing background sounds of the world around us *without being aware that we hear them.* This primitive function of hearing relates us to a world that is constantly in change, but it relates us to it in such a way that we are not conscious of the relationship or of the feeling it establishes of being part of our environment.

When we are at a concert listening to someone sing, we are not aware of the constantly changing pattern of sounds from the audience around us, the little noises of body movement, of breathing, of creaking seats, because our attention is on the singer. We are, however, reacting to these background sounds without realizing it. This constant reaction establishes in us states of feeling that are the foundation for our conscious experiences, a foundation that gives us the conviction that the world in which we live is also alive and moving. This process is a difficult one to describe, yet one so fundamental to an understanding of the primitive level of hearing that it must be labored in order to be made clear.

While we are focusing our attention on the singer at the concert, we do not consciously hear the background sounds from the audience or from the city outside. At any given moment, however, one of these background sounds may vary and attract our attention.

The woman beside us may change the rhythm of her breathing by coughing. A horn on a car outside may become stuck and blow until we are aware of it. But the moment we become aware of such a background sound, it is no longer on the primitive level. As soon as we identify a sound, give it "thing" character, we are hearing on one of the other levels.

The most distinctive feature of these background sounds is that they are constantly changing because the world around us is in a state of constant activity. In the natural world there is constant motion: the wind blows; rain falls; animals move. In the mechanical world the same constant motion occurs. The pattern of environmental sound from this continued activity changes with each moment and with the different times of day.

In the human body there is also constant change and activity. Even in our deepest sleep we breathe, we digest our food, our hearts beat, and the brain continues its activity. We have then two patterns of change always in motion, the pattern of environmental change in the world around us and the pattern of change in the human body. By far the most efficient and indispensable mechanism for "coupling" the constant activity of the human organism to nature's activity is the primitive function of hearing.

We as living organisms are not and can never be completely independent of our environment. We live in our environment in different degrees of security, and since the security is never complete, we must maintain a readiness to react, to withdraw, or to approach as need arises. The primitive function of hearing maintains this readiness to react by keeping us constantly informed of events about us that do not make enough noise to challenge our attention. *The feeling state established by the primitive function of hearing is therefore characterized by this readiness to react as well as by the comfort-*

able sense of being part of a living, active world.

We must remember that this "coupling" of the individual with the world is not a conscious process. It is even less conscious than beating time to martial music without realizing that our feet are moving. That this "coupling" does exist, that it establishes an unconscious feeling of aliveness in us, is demonstrated by the overwhelming feeling of deadness in the deafened. It is possible to maintain some degree of coupling with the environment through other senses than hearing, but none of the others is so effective—as the characteristic depression of the deaf indicates.

The Depression of the Deaf

Observation of hundreds of patients has convinced this author that the answer to their persistent question, "Why do I feel so depressed, so caught in a dead world?" is to be found in the destruction of the sound coupling that connects the individual at an unconscious level with the aliveness and activity of the world. Undoubtedly the loss of conversation makes the deaf person feel isolated from those around him, but the basic emotional upset is caused by the loss of hearing at the primitive level.

The depressive reaction is much the same whether the impairment in hearing has been sudden or gradual. Soldier patients who had suddenly become deaf were, however, so bewildered by their unexpected depression that they attempted to describe it. All of them were conscious of an undefined feeling of loss. Many of them felt vaguely sad and insecure. One of them stated that it was almost impossible to believe in the passage of time since he couldn't hear a clock tick. Several fell asleep every time they turned off the hearing aids that brought them some sound from the world around them. Even those who faced the practical difficulties of deafness in a realistic manner still suffered from the same undefined but permeating depression.

One reason for the overwhelming nature of the depression is that, until it is pointed out to him, *the deafened person is not aware of the loss he has suffered* at the primitive level of hearing or of its effect on his feeling state. He is unaware of the loss because he is unaware that there is such a thing as this primitive level of hearing in the first place. Frequently, he attributes his depression to a lack of character, and often he feels that if he were man enough, he could shake it off. Bewilderment and self-accusation heighten the burden he has to bear.

An extremely important step toward relieving the characteristic depression is taken when the deaf person realizes the reason for his emotional state. The realization itself makes his depression more objective and thereby makes it possible for him to cope with it without bewilderment or self-blame. As long as he is blind to its cause, he suffers from the same vague feelings of discomfort that characterize the early stages of a disease before the symptoms have yet developed clearly. Diagnosis does not instantly remove a disease, but it makes the proper treatment possible. Similarly, knowing the cause of depression does not remove it, but fortunately *the mere understanding of the reason for a feeling state does much psychologically to relieve its intensity.*

The nature of the impairment of deafness at the primitive level and its consequent loss of coupling involve the deaf in a double threat. We have just described the aspect of experience in which its chief characteristic was that of feeling. But hearing at this low level also operates as a signal. It not only gives a quality of life to the present; it also serves as an indicator of what is to come. Even these undifferentiated feelings contain some reference to the future and serve to orient us unconsciously to meet it. They maintain in us a readiness to react to our environment. Without this orientation we suffer from a vague sense of insecurity, which may be described in the words of a patient who said, "When I went deaf I lost my way of acting."

If the impairment of hearing is severe, the loss of the primitive hearing sense and its effect upon "feeling tone" are permanent and absolute unless a hearing aid can bring *some* sound from the outer world. When compensation for the loss in the primitive function is the objective, it is not essential that the hearing aid transmit sounds in their true character or speech that is intelligible, since the basic function operates with undifferentiated sounds. From a psychological point of view the use of a hearing aid is advisable even when it only serves to couple the individual to a world of sound patterns.

A type of compensation for severe loss in the primitive function has been developed independently and unconsciously by many recently deafened individuals. They substitute continuous muscular movement for the missing sensation of movement in the world. This continuous muscular activity is an overcompensation for the loss of those involuntary shifts in muscular tension that are the normal response to sounds heard at the primitive level. It is a good idea to make this muscular activity purposeful by keeping busy at something. Practical suggestions made later in the chapter will help the deaf person to substitute a satisfying activity for purposeless movement, such as pacing the floor.

Sounds as Signs and Warnings

So far, major emphasis has been placed on the hearing of background sounds. Obviously, however, hearing at a higher level plays an even more important part in biological adjustment and survival. At this level, sound serves as a sign or signal and conveys factual knowledge about objects and activities within the range of hearing: there is a fan operating; someone is washing dishes; someone is coming up the stairs. Many of our adjustments are initiated by sounds of low intensity, that is, sounds that arise at a distance. The horn of the approaching car warns us far enough in advance to avoid an accident. The eye can see distant objects, but hearing has the advantage of being able to warn us of approaching events that are not directly in our line of vision. Because sound waves can bend around corners and travel through darkness, the ear can warn us of many things that we cannot see. A lack of hearing leaves us uninformed of events outside the visual field. At a given moment we can see only a *fraction* of what it is possible to observe, whereas we can receive *all* the possible sound signals simultaneously and without interruption, except, of course, as one sound may drown out another. A pedestrian cannot watch at the same time the car approaching him from the right and the truck approaching him from the left, but he can *hear* them simultaneously.

Hearing informs us of the events taking place around us, and it can also tell us something about the direction from which a sound comes. We can thus locate the event in which we are interested. Not only do we need advance notice that a car is approaching, but we need to know from what direction it is bearing down on us. Localization of the source is most accurate in the horizontal plane when we distinguish right from left. Discrimination is less accurate between front and back and still less accurate between up and down. Both ears are needed to perceive the direction from which sound comes, but in locating the source of a sound we are helped greatly by many additional clues and associations. The nature of the noise often restricts the number of possible directions from which it may come. An airplane in flight, for example, is always above, but a car is on the ground. If you know in which direction the nearby river lies, you will never be confused as to whether the sound of a boat whistle is coming from in front of or behind you, although you might be completely uncertain about the direction of a pure musical tone of unknown source.

The only noticeable handicap imposed by deafness in one ear is in the localization of the sources of sounds. For hearing language and background noises, one ear is almost as good as two. The person with one-sided deafness does not, however, suffer a complete loss of localization, since, as we have just mentioned, the principal cues for distance and some of the cues for direction do not depend on binaural hearing. The accuracy of localization depends largely on the recognition of the type of noise and its possible source. This substitute procedure, however, is not always accurate or quick enough in an emergency. The person with one-sided deafness is still liable to the right-left confusion that rarely occurs in a person with two normal ears.

Compensation for loss of hearing is easier at this warning level where sound is a sign or a signal than it is at the primitive level. Loss at this utilitarian level does not cause so basic an emotional upset. It does result in a feeling of insecurity because we are not able to hear warning signals or are uncertain of their source. Practical readjustments can be learned to help the individual meet the everyday demands of his environment. When the capacity to locate moving objects by their sounds is reduced or inadequate, a trained visual awareness will compensate to a considerable degree. A careful study of the conditions to be expected in certain situations, such as crossing a busy street, will give a feeling of security that approaches that of the hearing person.

Aesthetic Experience

In addition to its function as signal or warning for biological survival, hearing contributes at the second level to our aesthetic experience. We listen to music and the sounds of nature for the pleasure that we derive from the sounds themselves. All people do not possess an equal need for this type of aesthetic auditory experience, nor do they suffer equally from the loss of the aesthetic experience of sound.

Just as there are differences in the degree of need, so there are differences in the kind of experiences sought. Some of us need visual, others need auditory, and others (apparently) do not need any aesthetic experience at all. If the loss of hearing occurs in someone with a pronounced aesthetic need in the auditory field, the absence of musical experience is felt as an impoverishment, and the lack is interpreted unconsciously as a lack in one's self.

In individuals with a pronounced aesthetic auditory need, this lack sometimes assumes acute proportions. A musician of this author's acquaintance who had a severe impairment declared that she would gladly sacrifice a year of her life if she could only once hear a symphony again. Such acute need is unusual, however, and occurs most often in those who have reinforced their natural auditory need by an occupation in the field of music.

Probably those who satisfy an aesthetic auditory need through the varied and multitudinous sounds of nature outnumber those who have found the answer to their need in music. The sounds of nature are available to everyone, whereas music is not. The sound of the sea, the singing of birds, the patter of rain furnish many people aesthetic experiences as poignant as those received through music. The silence of the natural world deadens it for them and superimposes upon the self the same lack felt by music lovers.

A hearing aid for those with some residual hearing, or even the vibratory sense by which the totally deaf can appreciate the rhythm of music, may enable a person with an auditory aesthetic need to capture enough of the desired sounds and rhythms to stimulate his imagination to recreate familiar and beloved auditory images either from music or from the natural world and thus satisfy his need in part.

Sounds as Symbols

Animals as well as humans depend on sound for warning; they also recognize the meaning of particular sounds, such as the trickle of water, the snapping of twigs, or the call of a mate. Humans, however, can use ordered sounds as symbols for things not immediately present and even for abstract ideas. The use of sound as language sets human society apart as unique and different from animal societies. By the use of spoken language, a human's sphere of influencing and being influenced is enormously increased and made more complex.

Hearing in its symbolic, linguistic function enriches human life in *three* ways: (1) Language makes possible the communication of experiences through a medium that is flexible and manifold almost to the degree to which experience itself is complex. (2) Language clarifies and organizes our thoughts by supplying a grammatical, syntactical, and logical framework and thus makes possible our higher-order knowledge. (3) In the growing child, language serves to formalize and to bind those social prohibitions and permissions that make up the moral code. The *voice* of conscience, not a forbidding *glance*, directs our moral behavior.

Loss of hearing does not impair each of these three functions to an equal degree. The degree of hearing loss and the time of its on-set are important in determining the effect of the impairment on the personality. The adult who suffers a sudden and severe hearing loss is plunged into a world where sensory deficits form his principal handicap. The organizing of thought and the formulation of moral permissions and prohibitions have already been established; once established, they continue even with total deafness. The framework for higher-order knowledge and the moral code are not affected.

A New Significance

This chapter has been preserved almost exactly as it was written by Dr. Ramsdell in a Veterans Administration Hospital at the close of World War II. His opportunity for the observation of suddenly deafened young adults during the war was a rare one, and he used it with excellent insight. His recognition of the three stages of utilization of hearing and particularly the importance of the "feeling of oneness with an active environment" was a major advance in our understanding of the deprivation and isolation of the deafened adult.

For many years this concept attracted little attention, but recently it has acquired a new significance because the restoration of a sense of contact with the environment is apparently the most important benefit yielded by the "cochlear implant." This new prosthetic device and its limitations are discussed in Chapters 4 and 6. In its present single-channel form it does not provide understanding of speech, but it does "make the world seem alive," and to some extent it provides auditory warning signals. Some subjects who have received the implant have been eloquent in their gratitude for this benefit, in spite of their frustration in efforts to understand speech. The positive psychological benefits have provided the incentive and justification for continuing efforts to improve both the surgical and the electroacoustic features of the implant in the hope of extending its potentialities.

Congenital Deafness

So far we have considered only the problems of the adult who either suddenly or gradually loses his hearing. The psychological effects of deafness are somewhat different in the child who is born deaf or who becomes deaf before he has learned the structure of language. His failure to learn to talk spontaneously or to be able to communicate any but the simplest ideas without intensive and special training has been considered in Chapter 17. Fortunately, the greater difficulties in relation to communication are partly offset by a less devastating effect of the absence of the primitive auditory function. The child who has never established auditory "coupling" with the ongoingness of the world is not depressed by the absence of this coupling as the adult is by the loss of it. Nor has the child developed through training and experience any urgent aesthetic needs of an auditory nature. And once communication has been established, whether by visual reading, speechreading, the manual alphabet, or the language of signs, the deaf child is able to formulate successfully in nonauditory terms the structure for his thoughts and for his moral code.

PRACTICAL SUGGESTIONS

Hearing loss presents obvious problems at the language level even for an adult. Unless the hearing loss is very mild, situations involving spoken language as a means of communication are difficult and remain difficult. *The first step toward surmounting the difficulty is to admit it frankly and realistically.* Much of the tension of social situations is eased for the deafened as well as for others if the impairment is regarded as factually and objectively as the need for glasses. Society accepts glasses for impaired vision and will accept with equal readiness the wearing of a hearing aid and also the need for face-to-face conversation to facilitate speechreading by those whose impairment is too severe for a hearing aid.

A few simple suggestions will help those with hearing loss to master practical situations that must be met. The complexity of even such a simple transaction as buying a railroad ticket may be great. Here the experience of those who have most successfully surmounted such difficulties has taught them to study the situation, to anticipate the difficulties that may arise, and to attempt by so doing to avoid confusion. If you wish to buy a railroad ticket from Columbus to Cincinnati, for example, you should if possible consult a timetable in which the three alternate routes are listed before asking for your ticket. You will then be familiar with the names of railroad lines and train schedules so that you can more easily recognize the words used in answer to your questions. Such advance knowledge makes it possible for you to ask pertinent questions and reduces the chance of your getting on the wrong train. A hearing aid in this situation is valuable, not only as an amplifier but also, if visible, as a sign and reminder of impairment. It relieves the wearer of the need to mention his handicap frequently and signifies to strangers that his difficulty in the situation depends on a physical and not an intellectual defect.

When a conversation is primarily the exchange of experiences with friends, no bluff at all should be attempted. The handicap should be frankly admitted so that the strain of keeping up with the conversation may be eased. An effort should be made, however, to participate whenever possible, and an attitude of dependence should be avoided. Here, as in the simple transaction of buying a ticket, a careful analysis of social patterns will provide a useful repertoire of anticipations that will facilitate in advance the adjustment to the inevitable difficulties of a social situation.

Social situations are not infinitely variable. There are no more patterns to learn than exist, for example, on a checkerboard. A mastery of social amenities is helpful and can be acquired without inducing a feeling of submission or dependency. Viewed realistically, the anticipation of the demands of a situation can become a competitive game.

Many who are deaf believe it important to be able to hear in order to make new friends. If the deaf who hold this belief would distinguish between friendship and casual acquaintance, they would realize that although friendship is undeniably carried on through the senses, it does not follow that the loss or impairment of only one of them destroys, makes impossible, or even lessens the depth of such a relation. The deaf person is in no way handicapped in the exchange of warm and affectionate experiences if he has developed the requisite deep sensibilities.

There are many situations in which none of us need or use our hearing. In such instances when communication is unnecessary, the practical if not the emotional problems of the hearing and of the hard-of-hearing or deafened person are almost the same. For instance, all of us must face the problem of occupying leisure hours. For the hearing and for the deaf alike, idle time passes slowly, but occupied time passes quickly. The only difference in the problem for the two is that the hard-of-hearing or deafened person is more apt to fill his leisure hours with self-pity than with the chitchat of causal companions by which others may attempt to cover up a poor capacity for solitude.

Recreation should find a central place in the life of those suffering from hearing loss. They should habitually fill their leisure hours with some creative activity or avocation. If they do, they will soon realize that each person has his own individual and unique pattern of life and that it is worthwhile to find some definite interests and objectives as an outlet for this individuality. Since activity in a chosen field invariably leads to a relationship with others who share the same interests, those with hearing loss should make a careful survey of their interests and capabilities and discover the mechanical, artistic, or creative sphere in which they can express themselves. Those with mechanical ability can profitably spend their spare time repairing radios, electrical appliances, or watches. They can learn to refinish and upholster furniture or to rebuild antiques. An interest in furniture might lead eventually to cabinetmaking. A frequent approach to the artistic field is through model making. Models of airplanes, ships, houses, or trains may be made for personal pleasure alone or, if the individual develops sufficient skill, for the commercial market. Those with an interest in botany, biology, or medicine can apply their knowledge making models for classroom study. In the creative sphere, painting, writing, and modeling or sculpturing offer natural outlets. The amount of talent possessed is not important. If the individual is interested in one of these forms of creative work, he should try it as a means of personal expression and for the pleasure it brings. By identifying himself with a group interested in the same avocation, he may in part compensate for being unable to feel himself an intimate part of as large a social group as he could before hearing loss narrowed his conversational circle.

The experience of one man who developed a successful business from spare-time activity illustrates the professional possibilities of many avocations. Having time on his hands, he began by helping his mother, who was secretary of a large club, address the notices that she had to send out to its members. Friends of hers learned of his assistance and gave him letters to address for organizations with which they were connected. Requests for his aid increased. Today he runs a mailing and letter service that employs two assistants.

Interest in the problems of deafness, and assisting those who are similarly afflicted, is a common and very effective and useful form of social activity for the hard-of-hearing, provided that it does not turn into a form of mutual self-pity. Even better, if it can be achieved, is participation in more general social interests that do not depend on the handicap and do not make life and thoughts revolve about and continually emphasize it. More effort and skill may be required, but the most successful adjustment is the one that overrides and submerges the handicap in normal activity centering outside one's self.

Feelings of Suspicion

There is an additional reason why it is psychologically healthful for the deaf to make a decided effort to center their interests and activities outside themselves. Even in many persons with normal hearing there is a tendency to feel that conversation interrupted on their entrance into a room must have been about them or that half-heard remarks were critical and unfriendly. *Deafness accentuates this tendency and may make an oversensitive person unduly suspicious of hostility in those around him.* A word of explanation and warning is needed about such so-called *paranoid* reactions. Since the term "paranoid" is often used, perhaps erroneously, to characterize this hypersensitivity of the deaf, a simple explanation of the term is needed.

Not all persons can accept criticism without being hurt. It is possible for a friend to criticize your suit without implying any criticism of you. We all have a tendency, however, to interpret any criticism of something that is "mine" as a criticism of "me." If the tendency is strong, the person is described as sensitive. It is easy to imagine a person so sensitive that he is suspicious and anticipates that others are being critical of him. When the suspicion, reflecting a basic insecurity, is developed to this point, we speak of "paranoid reactions."

The tendency toward paranoid reactions exists to some degree in nearly all of us, but it is generally kept under control. Since control is lessened when a person is depressed, sensitiveness and suspicion are more easily aroused. *Deafness seems to be a powerful stimulus to any latent paranoid trend in the personality,* possibly because of the invariable association between depression and deafness.

We frequently observe that deaf people often think that conversations that they cannot hear are about them. They may often go so far as to think that derogatory remarks are being directed toward them in tones too low for them to hear. This is a typical "paranoid trend." Deafness alone, however, or even the insecurity that deafness may bring, is not enough to produce a paranoid trend. The person who becomes suspicious has a life pattern of placing his own insecurity in center stage and is preoccupied with the fear that others may see the lack he feels. *A person secure in his own emotional life will develop no paranoid trends even when deafened.* The frequency of such paranoid trends shows, however, how many persons feel insecure in their social relations. Deafness may not be the fundamental cause of the trends, but it waters the seeds and encourages them to grow.

The conquest of this morbid symptom reduces to the problem of attaining a mature point of view that is centered outside one's self. If one has developed a genuine interest in other people and in outside activities, statements not heard will be interpreted as objective statements of fact, not as remarks about one's self.

The Objective Attitude

The explanation of the psychology of hearing given in this chapter and the effect of impairment at the different levels have been realistically presented. There is no disguising the fact that anyone who becomes deaf or hard of hearing experiences an almost catastrophic loss when he must adjust himself to a completely or partially silent world. Only after he has faced this fact honestly and objectively can he determine the extent to which compensation is possible. An objective attitude furnishes the only sound basis upon which to build a readjustment.

Psychologically speaking, no permanent adjustment is possible until the individual realizes that the cause of his depressive state lies in the loss of the primitive function and until he faces the practical difficulties imposed by the loss at the two higher levels. Since depression and the feeling of deadness are the most destructive psychological effects of hearing impairment, it is fortunate that *the major step in recovering from these emotional states lies in a clear understanding of their cause.*

The suggestions made to facilitate mastery of the practical difficulties are by no means exhaustive. Each individual will work out his own, in accordance with the demands of his particular environment and his own personality and abilities.

The person with severe hearing loss will save himself much pain if he will realize that, although the difficulties imposed by deafness are now receiving recognition, he must not expect the general public to understand the problems of adjustment that are involved. Although this indifference is cruel, it does require him to develop a usefully independent and objective attitude toward his handicap.

SUGGESTED READINGS AND REFERENCES

Canfield, N. *Hearing: A Handbook for Laymen.* New York: Doubleday & Company, 1959.
An otologist talks to hard-of-hearing laymen.
Meyerson, L. "Somatopsychological Significance of Impaired Hearing," Chapter 5 in *Adjustment to Physical Handicap and Illness: A Survey of the Social Psychology of Physique and Disability,* R. G. Barker (ed.). New York: Social Science Research Council, 1953.

Jerome D. Schein, Ph.D.

20

The Deaf Community

Deaf persons usually experience their disability most keenly when they interact with persons who can hear. Communication is awkward. The deaf person has difficulty understanding because he or she cannot hear, and the hearing person has difficulty because the deaf person's speech may be flawed or absent. The result is frequently mutual withdrawal. Even worse, society generally treats deaf persons with barely disguised hostility or patient condescension. The former is due to the frustrated communication and the latter to the deaf person's appearance of intellectual deficit. Our culture has become heavily audio-dependent, placing deaf people at a severe disadvantage. To counter the disadvantage, the deaf community has evolved.

In the United States, deaf people have customs, morals, and institutions which differ from those of the larger society. These differences have led some to characterize the smaller, parallel society as a "subculture." The terminology is unfortunate. The prefix "sub" in this context may mean "beneath," implying inferiority. We prefer to speak of the *deaf community*—a grouping of persons who have a common characteristic, loss of hearing. The deaf community consists mostly of deaf people who communicate fluently in sign language and who share a wide variety of interests. Along with these shared traits have grown organizations, mores, and literature which are special to deaf people. Existing within and in continuous relation with the larger communities of the United States, the deaf community naturally adopts much of them; thus it is not in all respects unique. Often its general practices and institutions are adapted so subtly as not at first to appear different. Yet, taken as a whole, the deaf community emerges as a distinctive social entity, marked by the satisfaction deaf people usually find in company with each other.

The deaf community provides a fascinating example of the human capacity for adaptation. Study of its structure also affords an excellent means of understanding the negative social impact of deafness and the potential for overcoming it.

CHARACTERISTICS OF THE DEAF COMMUNITY

Size of the Deaf Community

Relevant to the psychology and sociology of deafness is the minority status of deaf persons. Their condition—inability to hear and understand speech through the ear alone[1]—is relatively infrequent, affecting about eight of every 1000 persons in the United States. Furthermore, persons who lost, or never had, their hearing before adulthood make up only 0.2 percent of the population.

The point in life at which deafness begins matters greatly in determining its social consequences. Those whose deafness occurred before 19 years of age tend to be relatively homogeneous with respect to their status in the deaf community. This group has been termed *prevocationally deaf.* Prevocationally deaf persons primarily tend to associate with other prevocationally deaf persons; those deafened in adulthood, however, share this affiliative tendency to a much lesser degree. As a rule, the earlier the age at onset, the greater the probability of association with other deaf persons. The deaf community, then, consists mostly of prevocationally deaf persons, who number about 410,000 in the United States—a small minority of the total population. Being relatively

[1] For a discussion of the definition of hearing impairment and the term "deaf," see pp. 433–436. The definition used here is taken from the National Census of the Deaf Population (Schein and Delk, 1974.)

very small, the deaf community can be easily ignored by the majority. At the same time, the tendencies toward homogeneity within the deaf community are increased by its comparatively small membership.

In the rest of this chapter, the term *deaf* refers to those whose loss occurred prevocationally. Any exceptions are duly noted.

Location of the Deaf Community

Sociologists generally include geographical proximity as a component of the definition of "community." Here we do not. Even when physically dispersed, deaf people find commonality of interests, language, and identification. The deaf community's boundaries lie outside of city and county lines; its purlieus are conceptual, not concrete. Deaf people relate to each other across great distances. National meetings draw sizable proportions of the deaf population; local conclaves can attract virtually the entire body of deaf adults from a wide radius. Deaf friendships and associations persist despite substantial geographical separation and limited access to telecommunications. The deaf community, therefore, extends across the United States, encompassing deaf adults in virtually every city in every state.

Communication in the Deaf Community

The lingua franca of deaf people is sign language. Until recently, linguists did not accept sign language as a true language. Rather it was considered to be merely a means of "writing English in the air." Scholars now recognize Ameslan (an acronym derived from *A*merican *S*ign *Lan*guage) as a distinct language, having a unique syntax as well as a distinct vocabulary. (See Chapter 15.)

Ameslan is seldom taught to deaf children in school. Indeed, for many years, deaf children were often forbidden to sign in class-rooms. Sign language, therefore, has been preserved by passing it along from deaf person to deaf person, a primitive situation not encouraging linguistic purity. Ameslan dialects are common, dictionaries are few, and published grammars are nonexistent. Nonetheless, signing remains the dominant means of communication between prevocationally deaf adults. Most deaf persons do, of course, use other means of communication: speaking, lipreading, listening to amplified speech, writing, and reading. But the method that sets them apart is manual communication—the use of sign language and finger-spelling to exchange thoughts and feelings with each other.

Family Background

Most deaf people had parents who could hear. More than 90 percent of prevocationally deaf adults come from families all of whose members had normal hearing. These parents who lack experience with deafness often react badly to the child's audiological diagnosis, rejecting the child along with the knowledge of his disability. Later the family cannot itself provide satisfactory role models for the deaf adolescent. In other words, the typical family with a deaf child does not adequately fulfill its role in the socialization process assigned to it by our culture.

By contrast, as investigations in the last two decades have shown, deaf children of deaf parents are more successful, both in school and in adulthood, than deaf children of normally hearing parents. The reasons for this generalization may be found in the earlier acceptance by deaf parents of deafness in their children, coupled with fewer delays and false starts in dealing with the problems. More effective communication between deaf parents and deaf child also plays a role in accelerating intellectual development. Plan-

ning for adolescence and adulthood is apt to be more realistic—less depressed by the child's handicap and more optimistic about the child's potential than is usually true of unsophisticated parents.

Education

There is no written evidence of a deaf community in the United States before the founding of the first permanent public school for deaf children in 1817. In any case, within the following two decades an organization of deaf adults was established. The conventional school, then, may be thought of as the deaf community's seedbed.

The formal instruction of deaf people is discussed elsewhere (see Chapter 17). At this point we are concerned only with the social aspects of education. For most deaf persons, the school affords their first contacts with other deaf individuals. It is the setting in which deaf persons learn how others like themselves cope with loss of hearing. They meet deaf peers with whom they form life-long associations and from whom they learn the mores, the language, and the adaptive behaviors that distinguish deaf people as a social group.

Deaf adolescents and adults do not enter postsecondary education as frequently as persons in the general population. Figure 20-1, which shows the number of students attending colleges and universities in proportion to all students in school, graphically exhibits this difference. (The diagram compares the deaf and general populations on an equal footing.) Early in the present century, as shown, deaf students entered higher education at a rate nearly equal to that of the general population. By 1950, the discrepancy had grown to nearly seven times; that is, attendance in higher education was nearly seven times greater for the general than for the deaf population. The discrep-

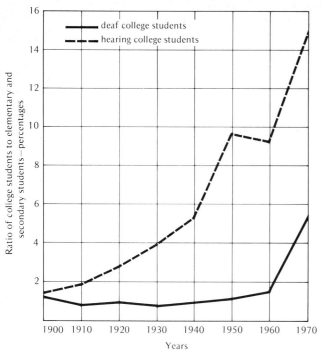

Figure 20-1 Deaf and hearing college students compared in relation to total elementary and secondary enrollments in the United States, 1900–1970. (The deaf students in 1900–1960 are those in Gallaudet College only.) *(Schein and Delk, The Deaf Population of the United States, 1974; by permission)*

ancy in rates has been markedly reduced in the last two decades, but it remains distressingly high. Deaf students enter higher education about one third as often as their peers in the general population.

Though most deaf students have attended Gallaudet College for their higher education, some have gone to other schools. Founded in 1864, Gallaudet College, the only liberal arts college in the world exclusively for deaf undergraduates, has held a commanding position as a source of leadership in the deaf community. To broaden the range of educational choices, Congress in 1965 established the National Technical Institute for the Deaf (NTID). This institution provides additional opportunities for deaf students to prepare for

employment, especially in technical and professional fields (see Chapters 16 and 18). Deaf students who successfully graduated from other universities before 1960 usually have done so without special assistance. Presently, however, a number of institutions have established programs for deaf college students that include interpreting, tutoring, and counseling (see Chapter 18). As these programs attract more deaf students, some changes may be anticipated in the character of the leadership of the deaf community that are likely to bring an increasing breadth of experiences and aspirations to it. This increasing breadth should invigorate the deaf community, strengthening its coping ability.

Marriage

Continuing a trend noted repeatedly over the last half century, deaf adults marry less frequently than their general-population age peers. The proportion of single, never-married adults is nearly three times greater in the deaf than in the general population.

Deaf persons also differ from the general population in age at first marriage. Deaf persons, on the average, marry later in life than persons in general. Once married, however, deaf persons have nearly an equal probability of maintaining the marriage. The proportions of the deaf and the general populations who are divorced have become almost identical: 3.6 percent for the general population, 3.8 percent for the deaf population.

When deaf adults marry, they most often marry other deaf adults. The earlier in childhood hearing is lost, the more likely that the spouse will also be deaf. Only 12 percent of prevocationally deaf males and 14 percent of females have married normally hearing persons. Some evidence has been found of greater stability in marriages between deaf persons than between deaf and nondeaf partners. The prevailing tendency to choose a deaf spouse, in many instances, connotes maturity; in others, it merely reflects the workings of propinquity.

Deaf women have fewer children than the average for the general population. This lower fertility rate is related to the mother's age at onset of deafness: born-deaf women bear proportionally fewer children than do those with later onsets of deafness (see Table 20-1). A self-imposed eugenics practice may be operating or other personal and economic factors may account for this reduced rate of reproduction. In any event, even if all her offspring were deaf, the average deaf woman does not alone bear sufficient children at a sufficient rate to maintain prevocational deafness in the population.

The majority of offspring of marriages having at least one prevocationally deaf parent are normally hearing: 88 percent overall. However, the rate for deafness in children differs significantly between marriages in which one partner is deaf and the other unafflicted—7.5 percent—and those in which both are congenitally deaf—18.6 percent. Nonetheless, for the group as a whole, the a priori expectation on the birth of a child to deaf parents is that the child's hearing will be normal.

TABLE 20-1
MEDIAN NUMBER OF CHILDREN EVER BORN TO DEAF FEMALES, 18 TO 64 YEARS OF AGE, BY AGE AT ONSET OF DEAFNESS: UNITED STATES, 1972

Age of Onset of Deafness	Median Number of Children Ever Born
All ages at onset	1.0
Born deaf	0.4
Birth to 1 year	0.9
1 to 3 years	1.2
3 to 5 years	1.8
5 to 18 years	2.3

Source: Schein and Delk (1974).

It is reassuring to note, therefore, that deaf parents are also successful in raising their normally hearing children. Many sons and daughters of deaf parents have become eminent entertainers, lawyers, physicians, educators. Their parents have been ingenious in anticipating and overcoming problems associated with deafness. The children, in turn, have often sought careers in education and rehabilitation serving deaf people. For the sake of society as a whole, as well as for the benefit of the deaf community, a thorough investigation should be undertaken of the factors that contribute to deaf persons becoming good parents.

Occupational Status

Deaf adults enter the labor force at a rate somewhat higher than that for the general population: 83 percent for the deaf and 80 percent for the general population. In 1972, deaf workers suffered less unemployment than workers in general. Deaf males had an unemployment rate of 2.9 percent versus 4.9 percent for the country as a whole. The trend was reversed, however, for females: 10.2 percent of deaf females were unemployed compared to the overall population rate of 6.6 percent. Furthermore, nonwhite deaf persons, male and female, did worse in the labor market than nonwhite persons generally. Table 20-2 summarizes these latest data. What has happened to deaf workers in the recent economic decline remains unstudied. Specialists in deafness have expressed grave concern that economic depression would more adversely affect deaf persons than others. We do not know if their fears have been realized.

General employment-unemployment statistics tell only a small part of the labor-force story. In what industries are deaf persons employed? Every industry employs some deaf workers. The heaviest concentrations

TABLE 20-2
PERCENTAGE DISTRIBUTION OF DEAF AND GENERAL POPULATIONS 16 TO 64 YEARS OF AGE IN LABOR FORCE, BY SEX AND RACE: UNITED STATES, 1972

| | Labor Force Status | | | | Employment Status | | | |
| | In | | Not In | | Employed | | Unemployed | |
Sex and Race	Deaf	Gen'l	Deaf	Gen'l	Deaf	Gen'l	Deaf	Gen'l
Male	82.7	79.7	17.3	20.3	97.1	95.1	2.9	4.9
White	83.9	79.6	16.1	20.4	97.8	95.5	2.2	4.5
Nonwhite	71.8	73.7	28.2	26.3	89.6	91.1	10.4	8.9
Female	49.4	43.9	50.6	56.1	89.8	93.4	10.2	6.6
White	49.6	43.2	50.4	56.8	90.5	94.1	9.5	5.9
Nonwhite	47.7	48.7	52.3	51.3	83.5	88.7	16.5	11.3

Source: Schein and Delk (1974).

are in manufacturing of both durable (16.7 percent) and nondurable goods (29.7 percent). The lowest rates are for mining (0.3 percent) and entertainment and recreation services (0.4 percent).

Nearly 80 percent of employed deaf persons work for private companies; only about 2 percent have their own businesses. Of the remainder, about 16 percent of deaf workers hold government jobs or work for their families (2 percent).

What occupational positions do deaf persons fill? Table 20-3 shows proportions of employed deaf persons in each of the categories used by the U.S. Bureau of the Census to classify occupations. Disappointingly few

TABLE 20-3
PERCENTAGE DISTRIBUTION OF EMPLOYED DEAF VERSUS GENERAL POPULATION, ADULTS (16 TO 64 YEARS OF AGE), BY PRINCIPAL OCCUPATION: UNITED STATES, 1972

| | Percentage of Population | |
Principal Occupation	Deaf	General
All occupations	100.0	100.0
Professional and technical	8.8	14.2
Managers and administrators (nonfarm)	1.4	11.0
Sales	0.5	6.4
Clerical	15.0	16.9
Craftsmen	21.3	12.7
Operatives, nontransit and transit	35.9	16.2
Laborers (nonfarm)	6.2	5.0
Farmers, farm managers, and farm laborers	1.6	4.0
Service workers	9.2	13.5
Private household workers	0.2	—

Source: Schein and Delk (1974).

deaf persons are employed in professional and technical careers. A comparatively high proportion have manufacturing jobs (non-transit operatives). But the important point is that some deaf persons are in every category of employment. This fact provides a strong antidote to vocational stereotyping, a condition afflicting many handicapped persons. Deaf persons have succeeded and continue to succeed in a broad range of occupations. Disproportionate numbers may enter one or another occupation or industry at a given time, but this occurs because of factors other than the abilities of deaf workers. Deaf people not unreasonably seek employment where other deaf people work. They desire companionship at work as at play. Also, they encounter less prejudice in plants that have deaf employees. Employer resistance to hiring deaf people drops after they demonstrate satisfactory performance, thus encouraging the employer to hire more deaf persons.

Counselors and job-placement personnel frequently recommend that the deaf client train and apply for positions in industries that are familiar to them as being receptive, rather than developing new opportunities. This tendency to follow the easiest path in job placement becomes cumulatively harmful to deaf people as the labor market shifts. By 1980, for example, the number of positions open to service workers will be greatly increased, while blue-collar jobs will be sharply decreased. The largest proportion of employment will be in white-collar jobs. Compare these Bureau of Labor Statistics projections to the current occupational distribution of the deaf labor force and the reason for concern about the next decade is obvious, as is the necessity for encouraging deaf future workers to shift their vocational sights and set them on positions not previously held by many, if any, deaf persons.

A related problem is underemployment. Underemployment remains a somewhat vague concept, so it presents measurement problems. Yet it has intuitive appeal—most people understand what it means. Though the precise extent is not known, deaf workers appear to suffer underemployment with disproportionate frequency as compared to the general population. They remain in entry jobs for years after others who entered at the same time are promoted; they fail to obtain employment commensurate with their education and experience. Future vocational rehabilitation strategies should be directed toward eliminating underemployment as well as unemployment.

Economic Status

Deafness imposes a severe penalty on the purse. Median personal income reported by deaf adults in 1971 fell far below national averages. The deaf adult earned only 72 percent as much as the average adult in the general population: $5915 versus $8188. Note that this finding held despite the higher overall labor-force participation and lower unemployment of deaf adults. The previous references to underemployment seem particularly relevant to explaining this poor economic performance. Some members of the deaf community do earn excellent salaries or derive substantial dividends from investments or both. Nevertheless, compared to the nation as a whole, the deaf community does not receive a share of the wealth corresponding to its economic contributions.

Members of the deaf community also find themselves at a disadvantage as consumers in the marketplace. Because of their communication problems, deaf people find shopping difficult. Their access to information is reduced, as is their ability to negotiate at the point of purchase.

Despite these obvious economic penalties of deafness, the U.S. Congress has not granted to deaf people the extra income-tax exemption given blind people. The matter has been discussed from time to time, but this curious omission in federal law persists. (Actually, in earlier years, leaders of the deaf community opposed such an exemption; see page 522.)

Organizations

Organizations of deaf people The desire of deaf persons to affiliate with each other finds formal expression in numerous national, state, and local organizations. Almost every state has an association of deaf persons. These, in turn, form the National Association of the Deaf (NAD). Now approaching its centennial, NAD is the first national organization of physically handicapped persons in the United States. It owns its headquarters, an office building in a suburb of Washington, D.C., from which it coordinates its member associations' social events, directs research on aspects of deafness, manages a nationwide program to teach sign language, and distributes special appliances for deaf users and literature about deafness aggregating a million dollars in annual sales. The federal government recognizes NAD as the principal advocate for deaf citizens. For the majority of deaf persons, NAD provides the organizational center of their lives.

The American Athletic Assocation of the Deaf (AAAD) serves many of the physical and recreational needs of deaf persons. It sponsors all kinds of athletic events: skiing, basketball, track and field, etc. AAAD awards trophies to winning football and basketball teams from residential schools. It manages a Hall of Fame for deaf sportsmen and sportswomen. It conducts regional and national annual basketball tournaments. It joins with 30 or more nations in the quadrennial World Games for the Deaf, also called ''The Deaf Olympics.''

In 1901, a group of deaf leaders incorporated the National Fraternal Society of the Deaf. Their purpose was to provide economical insurance, something deaf persons found difficult, if not impossible, to obtain from commercial sources. The Frat, as it is lovingly known, has grown rapidly; it now holds $7 million in assets to cover $13 million insurance in force and has 13,000 members and 126 lodges (local chapters). In addition to its insurance business, it plays a part in the social lives of deaf people. The Frat also encourages charitable activities by matching its lodges' contributions and offers academic scholarships to its members and their children.

Diverse in other ways, these organizations share characteristics in addition to their national scope: they were founded by and for deaf people, are presently managed by deaf people, and use sign language in the conduct of their internal affairs. There are other organizations of deaf people; for example, the American Professional Society of the Deaf, the Oral Deaf Adult Society, and others. They serve specialized groups within the deaf community, broadening the opportunities for satisfying relationships and outlets for civic drive. The Junior National Association of the Deaf, a branch of NAD, and the National Association of Homes for the Aged Deaf serve constituencies at opposite ends of the age continuum. Most of the larger and many of the smaller religious denominations are represented by national groups; for example, Christian Deaf Fellowship, National Congress of the Jewish Deaf, Catholic Deaf Association. Together, these organizations fulfill almost every variation in deaf persons' affiliative needs.

Organizations for deaf people No national charitable organization has ever solicited the general public on behalf of deaf persons. Organizations for deaf persons have either been concerned with education or with other professional affairs. The oldest groups are the Conference of Executives of American Schools for the Deaf and the Convention of American Instructors of the Deaf. Their interests are obvious from their names. The Alexander Graham Bell Association for the Deaf, Inc., almost as old as the Conference and the Convention, also concerns itself with the education of deaf children, particularly with the teaching of speech and speechreading and the use of residual hearing. Professional Rehabilitation Workers with the Adult Deaf is, by contrast, only recently founded (1966) and focuses its activities on vocational rehabilitation. Another newcomer is the Registry of Interpreters for the Deaf, established to improve the quality of manual interpretation—the bridge between hearing and deaf worlds.

These organizations have deaf members, though they are in the minority; organizational control rests with normally hearing persons. Meetings are usually interpreted manually for the benefit of deaf persons, but speech, not sign language, is the principal medium of communication. Relations between organizations *of* deaf persons and organizations *for* them have no central point of coordination. The Council of Organizations Serving the Deaf has not succeeded in bringing them together, though relations among the various groups are, for the most part, cordial.

Religion

The early history of services for deaf persons primarily involves religious workers. Almost every church group makes some effort to minister to deaf persons. Frequently, these efforts take the form of missions. Occasionally, religious groups have ordained deaf persons as ministers; the Episcopal Church probably leads in this. Some churches have separate services for deaf congregants. A few churches provide sign language interpretation of regular services.

The little research available indicates that deaf persons participate in religious activities about as often as their normally hearing peers. But the extent to which they find this participation satisfying is not known. Nor do we have an explanation for the somewhat greater tendency toward atheism, agnosticism, and absence of religious interest among deaf than general-population adults. Deaf persons do join every religious denomination, but not necessarily in proportion to expectations based on their parents' preferences nor on their numbers in the population.

In deaf marriages, cross-religious pairings occur in about one third of the marriages. Jewish and Catholic males most frequently marry females from other religious groups. Deaf females tend to marry males with the same religious preference: Protestants 85 percent, Catholics 73 percent, Jews 90 percent. Of course, the tendency of most deaf persons to seek a deaf mate reduced the weight given to religious background, especially when age and education are also considered. Nonetheless, religion is a factor in selection of spouse in a majority of deaf marriages. Whether this consonance of religious preference reflects socioeconomic background and related factors or a church-based spirituality remains moot. That religion plays a role in deaf adults' social lives, however, seems beyond dispute, even though its nature is not well understood.

Delinquent Behavior

The deaf community gives every appearance of being as law-abiding as or more so than the general population. Unfortunately, crime statistics rarely include hearing impairment among their parameters, so highly precise data are lacking on the relation of deafness to juvenile and adult delinquency. The difficulties deaf persons face in court have been well documented. Since their disability sets them apart, deaf people involved, or suspected of involvement, in crimes would be likely to attract the attention of the news media. The absence of knowledge about deaf persons' criminality, therefore, supports the contention that it is low.

Automobile driving provides abundant opportunities for delinquency. Yet deaf drivers have better records than drivers in general. The best-controlled study of deaf drivers was conducted in the District of Columbia, 1960–1962. Almost every deaf driver in the Washington Metropolitan Area was located. Then a search was made by the D.C. Department of Motor Vehicles for all records of violations and accidents they might have had. The resulting statistics for deaf drivers were compared to the rates for all drivers in the area. Table 20-4 summarizes the findings.

Deaf drivers received summonses for moving violations at less than half the rate for all drivers over the three years. In the case of accident-related violations, drivers in general received almost four times more summonses than deaf drivers. Deaf drivers were involved in all accidents recorded in the period, regardless of violations, less than one third as often as their proportion in the population would predict. The results of this study confirm reports from other areas. They provide no justification for restricting driving privileges because of deafness.

In sum, in connection with delinquent behavior, both implicit and explicit evidence supports the contention that deaf people, as a group, earn high marks for citizenship.

Leisure-Time Activities

The picture of a deaf person spending lonely hours in isolated inactivity does not fit the majority in the deaf community. Leisure time is a busy time for deaf adults, despite being partially deprived of the enjoyment of most mass entertainment media.

Motion pictures and television programs usually require hearing to appreciate their content. As a counter to the loss of recreational movies, the federal government sponsors Captioned Films for the Deaf (CFD), located in the U.S. Office of Education, which subtitles popular films and distributes them without charge to deaf groups. A proposal is under review by the Federal Communications Commission to provide television-program captions that could be seen only with special equipment. In that way, viewers who had the converter could choose when they wished to see captions. Meanwhile, the

TABLE 20-4
ACCIDENT RATES AND VIOLATION RATES PER 1000 DEAF VERSUS 1000 GENERAL-POPULATION AUTOMOBILE DRIVERS: WASHINGTON, D.C., 1960–1962

Year	Accident Rates per 1000		Violation Rates per 1000	
	Deaf	General	Deaf	General
Three-year average	5.3	17.3	31.2	65.9
1960	7.1	16.9	31.8	64.8
1961	3.5	16.6	35.3	68.3
1962	5.3	18.5	26.5	64.7

Note: These figures include only violations involving accidents or improper driving.
Source: Schein (1968).

American Broadcasting Company makes available its half-hour evening news to the Public Broadcasting Service, which adds captions and rebroadcasts it about four hours later on weeknights. News programs and some public-affairs telecasts appear in sign language on a number of independent television stations. "Christopher Closeups," an interview program seen on more than 200 stations weekly, and occasional important public-events telecasts feature a sign language interpreter who appears in a corner of the screen. These various efforts improve deaf persons' access to mass media, but much more remains to be done.

The theater provides entertainment as well as a creative outlet for deaf talent. Amateur deaf groups have performed on stage for at least 100 years. Invariably the plays have been adaptations from the standard repertoire. Offstage readers speak the script for the benefit of the nondeaf audience, while actors sign the dialogue. The technique is equally effective with Greek classics, Shakespeare, modern drama, and musical comedies—all of which have been staged by one or another deaf company. Recently, a deaf theatrical literature has emerged, spurred by the major acting companies: the National Theatre of the Deaf and the drama departments at Gallaudet College and National Technical Institute for the Deaf.

A printed literature for deaf readers has grown substantially in recent years. The National Association of the Deaf publishes a widely distributed monthly magazine, *The Deaf American*, as does the Frat. The residential schools maintain extensive mailing lists for their publications. To encourage cooperation and improve their quality, the journals have their own organization, The Little Paper Family, which meets annually. Independent tabloids, like *Silent News*, feature material exclusively for and about the deaf community.

As is evident from the extensive support

given the American Athletic Association of the Deaf by deaf people, sporting events occupy a high place in the hierarchy of the deaf community's interests. The relatively nonverbal nature of most physical games opens them to enjoyment by deaf people, both as spectators and participants.

Social gatherings also assure deaf people ample recreational outlets. Alumni reunions attract large crowds of deaf people, many of whom did not attend the institutions but who come to the gatherings to visit friends. Organizational meetings provide the occasion for socializing. The importance of these face-to-face meetings stems from the inconvenience of telephoning. Attachments now enable typed messages to be transmitted via the telephone, but such devices are still expensive; in any case, typing slows message exchanges, while also eliminating the important nuances contributed by facial expressions.

The Deaf Personality

Generalizing about the influence of early deafness on personality, writers most often use the word *immature*. Deaf persons, it is said, exhibit a lack of regard for others, naivete, over-dependency, irresponsibility, tendency to act or react without adequate thought, and inflexibility in problem solving.

If indeed these terms apply to typical members of the deaf community, a logical next question would be: Are these behavioral tendencies the necessary consequences of deafness? Or do these aspects of immaturity arise from a breakdown in the socialization process due to parents' and teachers' failure to contribute the appropriate adult influences?

Much of the material on which generalizations about the deaf personality are based comes from studies of psychiatric patients. Other studies deal with children. Investigations of the personalities of psychiatrically normal deaf adults are rare. Even rarer is research conducted by persons highly skilled in communicating with deaf persons.

One way for researchers to avoid some of the earlier methodological pitfalls is to make comparisons within the deaf community. If deafness is the cause of the personality factors observed, then there should be little differences among those with similar degrees of hearing loss. In such a study, Harris (1976) compared the impulse control of deaf children whose parents were also deaf with the impulse control of deaf children whose parents had normal hearing. Harris reasoned that impulsivity arises from frustrated communication and that since deaf parents generally communicate readily with their deaf children, their children should show greater impulse control. That is, in fact, the result Harris obtained. Of course, he did not attribute this personality difference between the two groups of deaf children solely to the parents' ability to communicate, but it does appear to be a major factor. For our purposes, the study raises doubts about theories that hypothesize that personality is altered solely by prelingual lack of hearing ability. The alternative formulation that personality characteristics reflect upbringing seems more tenable. It is also more hopeful. If negative traits result from poor socialization practices, then altering the practices can eliminate the negative features.

Another view of the deaf community's personality generates the adjective *independent*. Considering the obstacles facing deaf people, the extensive facilities they have created for their own welfare are awesome. As noted above, deaf organizations provide recreation, insurance, and political action. Outside of work, the deaf community maintains independent social activities. This is not to say that deaf people do not participate in affairs of the larger society, but rather that

the deaf community offers additional avocational options.

Few people outside the deaf community are aware that deaf people lobbied *against* being granted the extra income-tax exemption Congress awarded blind people in 1946. The record for that Congressional session shows that the president of the National Association of the Deaf testified in opposition to the extra exemption for the deaf, largely on the grounds that they did not wish to be singled out for special treatment. Today, many deaf people disagree with that extremely independent position. The point remains that that position was at one time taken by the deaf community's leadership.

Deaf people have also been characterized as passive, overaccepting. In recent years, the deaf community, like other minority groups, has become more politically active. The movement of the headquarters of the National Association of the Deaf to Washington, D.C., signaled a vigorous approach to the federal agencies on behalf of projects important to deaf people. A somewhat less energetic movement can be discerned within the states. For the most part, however, deaf political action has been less militant than that of other minority groups. It has largely taken the form of well-reasoned appeals to administrators and legislators for equity and justice.

Identifying traits that characterize groups can be useful in assessing progress and in planning educational and rehabilitation strategies. However, average tendencies of a group should not obscure individual differences. Furthermore, when circumstances change, the prevailing tendencies may change.

What constitutes a "deaf personality," then, depends on many things, including the observers' points of view. Those dealing in psychopathology will see it in the deaf community; those concerned with successful adaptation will observe that. In any case, the character of the deaf community—as of any community—defies simplistic summation. A valid portrait of the deaf personality must clearly emphasize its complexity and modifiability.

DYNAMICS OF THE DEAF COMMUNITY

The observations to this point describe the deaf community as it is now, with only a few historical references to illustrate its dynamic character. The nature of the deaf community has changed repeatedly in response to variations in conditions around it and to differences in its membership.

Many other changes undoubtedly lie ahead. For example, we anticipate positive effects from the federal legislation forbidding discrimination against physically handicapped persons and from court rulings granting deaf people the right to interpreters throughout the legal process. State vocational rehabilitation agencies have begun to increase allocations for deaf clients. Innovations in telecommunications should benefit deaf people, as might other technological advances yet to be introduced. The implementation of P.L. 94–142 ("Education for All Handicapped Children Act") promises educational opportunities for deaf children who have been overlooked. Similar increases in provisions for postsecondary and continuing education will benefit deaf adolescents and adults.

Not all portents are easily read. The deaf population has grown, doubling its proportion of the total population in the last 40 years. Still, the relative presence of deafness in the total is minuscule. A greater change is appearing within the deaf population—the balance of adventitiously to congenitally deaf persons has shifted radically: a greater portion of the deaf population is now congenitally deaf. Furthermore, disabilities in addition to deafness are present in an increasing proportion of deaf persons. How these changes in the characteristics of the deaf population will affect its social structure is not clear.

The changes in the nature of the deaf population are happening along with external events that may offset them. For example, educators, in theory, favor placing deaf children in schools with normally hearing children ("mainstreaming"). If this strategy becomes common and residential schools cease to be a major factor in deaf students' education, will the deaf community be markedly altered? Over the past decades the proportion of deaf children educated in day schools has increased. (See Chapter 17.) A corresponding influence on the deaf community's functioning has not been perceptible, but it is early for the effect of this educational change to be apparent.

Another consideration is public opinion. Attempts to acquaint the general public with deafness and to overcome its negative stereotypes are gaining ground. Public opinion, however, can be fickle. Will the appreciation of deaf people continue to grow? The answer obviously contains important consequences for the social and economic lives of deaf persons.

SUGGESTED READINGS AND REFERENCES

Best, H. *Deafness and the Deaf in the United States.* New York: Macmillan, 1943.
A compendium of statistics and miscellaneous information.

Brill, R. G. *The Education of the Deaf.* Washington, D.C.: Gallaudet College Press, 1974.
Presents information about administrative, organizational, and professional matters.

Harris, R. I. *The Relationship of Impulse Control to Parent Hearing Status, Manual Communication, and Academic Achievement in Deaf Children.* Doctoral dissertation, Department of Psychology, New York University, 1976.

Mindel, E. D., and M. Vernon. *They Grow in Silence.* Silver Spring, Md.: National Association of the Deaf, 1971.
Focuses on the deaf child's family life.

Rainer, J. D., K. Z. Altshuler, F. J. Kallmann, and W. E. Deming (eds.). *Family and Mental Health Problems in a Deaf Population.* New York: New York State Psychiatric Institute, 1963.
An extensive survey of the deaf population in New York State.

Schein, J. D. *The Deaf Community.* Washington, D.C.: Gallaudet College Press, 1968.
A survey of the metropolitan Washington, D.C., deaf population.

———, and M. T. Delk. *The Deaf Population of the United States.* Silver Spring, Md.: National Association of the Deaf, 1974.
A report of the National Census of the Deaf Population.

Schlesinger, H. S., and K. P. Meadow. *Sound and Sign.* Berkeley: University of California Press, 1972.
A developmental view of the born-deaf person.

Appendix
Tests of Hearing

In this appendix are presented several collections of words or sentences that are widely used as tests of hearing. Some of them are also useful for auditory training and as test material in the selection of hearing aids.

The principles of the tests that employ these words and sentences are explained in Chapter 7, and their use in the selection of hearing aids is discussed in Chapter 11. It is pointed out in Chapter 7, for example, that a "discrimination score" obtained with monosyllabic word lists has a totally different meaning from a "hearing level for speech" measured with the two-syllable word lists. The principles of the different types of test will not be discussed again, but a brief statement introduces each set of lists, telling something of their properties, how and where they were constructed, their general fields of usefulness, and whether they are available in recorded form.

Some of the shorter lists are given in full; others are represented only by samples, but by more generous samples than could properly be included in the text. It must be remembered, however, that word lists or sentences alone do not make a test of hearing. The loudness and clarity with which they are spoken and the acoustical conditions of the test are equally important. These lists are only the materials. As explained in Chapter 7, they must be correctly and intelligently used.

1. SPONDAIC WORDS (CID)

Auditory tests W-1 and W-2 were developed at Central Institute for the Deaf as modifications of Auditory Test No. 9 of the Psycho-Acoustic Laboratory of Harvard University. The test material is a list of 36 words, each composed of two syllables that are equally stressed (spondees). The words were chosen for familiarity and also for equal intelligibility when spoken at the same intensity as measured by the VU meter. Six different scramblings of the 36 words have been recorded.

Tests W-1 and W-2 are particularly suited to measuring the hearing threshold level for speech. In Test W-1 all of the spondaic words are recorded at the same intensity. The carrier phrase is recorded at a level 10 dB higher. A 1000-Hz calibration tone is also recorded at this level. In W-2 the intensity of the words descends systematically by 3 dB for each successive group of three words. With this form of test it is necessary only to count the number of words repeated correctly. Each word correct lowers the threshold level by 1 dB.

Phonographic recordings of these tests may be purchased from the Technisonic Studios, Inc., 1201 South Brentwood Blvd., Richmond Heights, Missouri 63117. These tests are described in an article entitled "C.I.D. Auditory Tests W-1 and W-2," by R. W. Benson, H. Davis, C. E. Harrison, I. J. Hirsh, E. G. Reynolds, and S. R. Silverman, in *Journal of the Acoustical Society of America*, 23:719 (1951), and, in more detail, in "Development of Materials for Speech Audiometry," by I. J. Hirsh, H. Davis, S. R. Silverman, E. G. Reynolds, E. Eldert, and R. W. Benson in *Journal of Speech and Hearing Disorders*, 17:321–337 (1952). (These tests were developed under contracts with the Office of Naval Research and the Veterans Administration.)

Tape recordings of test W-1 (7.5 inches per second on a 7-inch reel) are available from the Los Angeles Foundation of Otology at 2122 West Third Street, Los Angeles, California 90057. This recording is known as the "LAFO speech test tape." In addition to 35 W-1 spondee words in two arrangements and the calibration tone, each tape carries four W-22 PB word lists, described below, and a sample of "connected discourse" (Declaration of Independence). The talker is not the same as the CID talker, but the form of the tests and the word lists are the same, except for the omission of "airplane" from the LAFO version.

SPONDAIC WORDS: AUDITORY TESTS W-1 AND W-2

1. airplane	10. eardrum	19. iceberg	28. railroad
2. armchair	11. farewell	20. inkwell	29. schoolboy
3. baseball	12. grandson	21. mousetrap	30. sidewalk
4. birthday	13. greyhound	22. mushroom	31. stairway
5. cowboy	14. hardware	23. northwest	32. sunset
6. daybreak	15. headlight	24. oatmeal	33. toothbrush
7. doormat	16. horseshoe	25. padlock	34. whitewash
8. drawbridge	17. hotdog	26. pancake	35. woodwork
9. duckpond	18. hothouse	27. playground	36. workshop

2. PB (PHONETICALLY BALANCED) WORD LISTS

One of the 50-word phonetically balanced word lists prepared by the Psycho-Acoustic Laboratory is presented as a sample below. All 20 of the 50-word lists are given in the article by J. P. Egan entitled "Articulation Testing Methods" in *The Laryngoscope*, 58:955–991 (1948), and in American National Standard Method for Measurement of Monosyllabic Word Intelligibility, ANSI S3.2–1960 (R1971). Each list consists of 50 common English monosyllables. For articulation testing, the words should be arranged in different random order for each presentation. The special merits of these lists and the uses to which they may be put are described in Chapter 7. The words range in difficulty from quite intelligible to rather difficult.

Several of these lists, slightly modified, including PB-50—List 5, were recorded for experimental use at Central Institute for the Deaf. Rush Hughes was the talker. These recordings are unduly difficult, however, even for listeners with normal hearing, largely because of Hughes's particular manner of speaking; and the college-level vocabulary is not ideal for clinical use. Nevertheless the articulation scores obtained in the clinic with these recordings were made the basis of the Social Adequacy of Hearing Index (see Chapter 7). In spite of this historic interest the use of these recordings is not recommended.

CID Auditory Test W-22 is a set of recordings of phonetically balanced word lists that represent a more restricted and simpler vocabulary than the original Psycho-Acoustic Laboratory lists. (Four of the W-22 lists are on page 528.) The talker is Ira Hirsh. These recordings are considerably more intelligible than the earlier experimental Rush Hughes version. Test W-22 is described in detail, including the criteria for phonetic balance, in the article entitled "Development of Materials for Speech Audiometry" cited in Chapter 7.

CID Auditory Test W-22 and the Rush Hughes version of the PB-50 test can be obtained from Technisonic Studios, 1201 South Brentwood Blvd., Richmond Heights, Missouri 63117.

The LAFO speech test tape, described in the previous section, contains these same word lists spoken by a different talker. The address is Los Angeles Foundation for Otology, 2122 West Third Street, Los Angeles, California 90057.

PB-50—LIST 5

1. add	11. feed	21. love	31. rind	41. thud
2. bake	12. flap	22. mast	32. rode	42. trade
3. bathe	13. good	23. nose	33. roe	43. true
4. beck	14. Greek	24. odds	34. scare	44. tug
5. black	15. grudge	25. owls	35. shine	45. vase
6. bronze	16. high	26. pass	36. shove	46. watch
7. cheat	17. hill	27. pipe	37. shy	47. wink
8. choose	18. inch	28. puff	38. sick	48. wrath
9. curse	19. kid	29. punt	39. solve	49. yawn
10. drive	20. lend	30. rear	40. thick	50. zone

W-22 Word Lists

PB-50—LIST 1

1. ace	11. day	21. it	31. owl	41. toe
2. ache	12. deaf	22. jam	32. poor	42. true
3. an	13. earn (urn)	23. knees	33. ran	43. twins
4. as	14. east	24. law	34. see (sea)	44. yard
5. bathe	15. felt	25. low	35. she	45. up
6. bells	16. give	26. me	36. skin	46. us
7. carve	17. high	27. mew	37. stove	47. wet
8. chew	18. him	28. none (nun)	38. them	48. what
9. could	19. hunt	29. not (knot)	39. there (their)	49. wire
10. dad	20. isle (aisle)	30. or (oar)	40. thing	50. you (ewe)

PB-50—LIST 2

1. ail (ale)	11. dumb	21. ill	31. off	41. that
2. air (heir)	12. ease	22. jaw	32. one (won)	42. then
3. and	13. eat	23. key	33. own	43. thin
4. bin (been)	14. else	24. knee	34. pew	44. too (two, to)
5. by (buy)	15. flat	25. live (verb)	35. rooms	45. tree
6. cap	16. gave	26. move	36. send	46. way (weigh)
7. cars	17. ham	27. new (knew)	37. show	47. well
8. chest	18. hit	28. now	38. smart	48. with
9. die (dye)	19. hurt	29. oak	39. star	49. yore (your)
10. does	20. ice	30. odd	40. tare (tear)	50. young

PB-50—LIST 3

1. add (ad)	11. done (dun)	21. is	31. out	41. this
2. aim	12. dull	22. jar	32. owes	42. though
3. are	13. ears	23. king	33. pie	43. three
4. ate (eight)	14. end	24. knit	34. raw	44. tie
5. bill	15. farm	25. lie (lye)	35. say	45. use (yews)
6. book	16. glove	26. may	36. shove	46. we
7. camp	17. hand	27. nest	37. smooth	47. west
8. chair	18. have	28. no (know)	38. start	48. when
9. cute	19. he	29. oil	39. tan	49. wool
10. do	20. if	30. on	40. ten	50. year

PB-50—LIST 4

1. aid	11. clothes	21. his	31. ought (aught)	41. through
2. all (awl)	12. cook	22. in (inn)	32. our (hour)	42. tin
3. am	13. darn	23. jump	33. pale (pail)	43. toy
4. arm	14. dolls	24. leave	34. save	44. where
5. art	15. dust	25. men	35. shoe	45. who
6. at	16. ear	26. my	36. so (sew)	46. why
7. bee (be)	17. eyes (ayes)	27. near	37. stiff	47. will
8. bread (bred)	18. few	28. net	38. tea (tee)	48. wood (would)
9. can	19. go	29. nuts	39. then	49. yes
10. chin	20. hang	30. of	40. they	50. yet

PBF LIST 1

1. box	26. end
2. eyes	27. there
3. range	28. tone
4. soap	29. drive
5. pants	30. then
6. wheat	31. ford
7. rat	32. rag
8. prove	33. are
9. pan	34. guess
10. toe	35. pest
11. bad	36. bead
12. bar	37. such
13. frog	38. dish
14. this	39. heat
15. slip	40. hid
16. hurt	41. price
17. bite	42. pile
18. hose	43. net
19. rise	44. fork
20. farm	45. ride
21. smile	46. trade
22. crush	47. crash
23. rub	48. no
24. gift	49. not
25. is	50. plans

PBF LIST 2

1. niece	26. bill
2. fuse	27. bounce
3. tan	28. mad
4. bought	29. shoe
5. trash	30. our
6. rap	31. loose
7. vest	32. start
8. rib	33. boot
9. tongue	34. pump
10. cloud	35. wish
11. awe	36. five
12. shake	37. flood
13. charge	38. course
14. throb	39. tip
15. howl	40. grease
16. glass	41. log
17. else	42. hop
18. bean	43. night
19. them	44. arm
20. ways	45. job
21. hit	46. that
22. quart	47. smash
23. set	48. bud
24. did	49. nut
25. need	50. tank

PBF LIST 3

1. trip	26. jam
2. dig	27. why
3. check	28. dog
4. nest	29. may
5. town	30. whirl
6. fame	31. size
7. eight	32. thick
8. law	33. clown
9. take	34. class
10. far	35. fog
11. noise	36. air
12. dim	37. guard
13. tenth	38. sled
14. drop	39. flash
15. barge	40. oak
16. wedge	41. neck
17. vow	42. path
18. stood	43. horse
19. shout	44. cake
20. look	45. praise
21. leave	46. past
22. who	47. sad
23. fresh	48. laugh
24. please	49. deck
25. purse	50. late

PBF LIST 4

1. judge	26. tent
2. slap	27. earn
3. bee	28. gas
4. move	29. raise
5. meat	30. curse
6. thin	31. on
7. race	32. blonde
8. howl	33. rip
9. hog	34. fan
10. sour	35. food
11. hook	36. cod
12. aim	37. float
13. skid	38. frown
14. bus	39. pack
15. creak	40. hot
16. bush	41. beast
17. pipe	42. struck
18. pinch	43. bike
19. oils	44. badge
20. test	45. yes
21. cart	46. roe
22. fed	47. stitch
23. mat	48. touch
24. stars	49. mend
25. tick	50. new

3. FAMILIAR MONOSYLLABLES (PBF)

For testing young children and for subjects with restricted vocabularies we need lists of very familiar words. Exact phonetic balance is not important in this situation. Four lists of familiar monosyllables, approximately balanced phonetically, were developed at Clarke School for the Deaf by the late C. V. Hudgins. They are known as the PBF lists (page 529). They have not been recorded.

4. PHONEMICALLY BALANCED (CNC) LISTS

There are three rather distinct objectives of speech audiometry and its word lists: one is to assess the adequacy of the listener's hearing for social purposes; another is to analyze his auditory impairment for diagnostic purposes; and another is the analysis of normal speech from the linguistic point of view. Interest in this last objective has led to the study in detail of the phonetic and phonemic structure of English speech in general and of word lists that might be used as laboratory tools for the study of communication by speech. Several such lists have been prepared, and the new ways of using them are suitable for clinical use as well.

An analytical study by I. Lehiste and G. E. Peterson in the *Journal of the Acoustical Society of America,* 31:280–286 (1959) shows in detail the distribution of vowels, initial consonants, and final consonants in 10 of the original PB-50 lists and compares them with the corresponding distribution of the phonemes in the entire "corpus" of reasonably familiar English monosyllables that have the form consonant (C)–nucleus or "vowel part" (N)–consonant (C). The authors prepared 10 new CNC lists of 50 words each that match quite well the phonemic composition of the larger group. These authors distinguish between "phonetic," related to acoustics and physiology, and "phonemic," related to linguistics and the hearing of speech. Later they (G. E. Peterson and I. Lehiste) published a revision of their lists in the *Journal of Speech and Hearing Disorders,* 27:62–70 (1962). These lists provided a foundation for the Northwestern University Auditory Tests Nos. 4 and 6.

The Northwestern University Auditory Test No. 6 is the most carefully prepared and thoroughly studied set of CNC word lists so far published. There are four lists of consonant-nucleus-consonant words that have the phonemic balance of the Peterson-Lehiste lists and experimentally have high interlist equivalence and also test-retest reliability. The "articulation functions" (see Chapter 7) of a particular recording of these lists have been established for normal-hearing subjects and also for subjects with sensorineural hearing loss. For normal-hearing listeners the function rises linearly from about 8 percent correct at 4 dB below the speech-reception threshold (spondees 50 percent correct) to 75 percent correct at 8 dB above the SRT. The slope of this part of the curve is 5.6 percent per decibel. The function then bends horizontally to a plateau of 99 percent correct, attained at 32 dB above the SRT. The slope and the final plateau are both lower for subjects with sensorineural impairment.

The four lists of Test No. 6 are given in the table. The words that also appeared in the original PB-50 lists are marked with asterisks. The description of the lists appeared in a technical report of the USAF School of Aerospace Medicine (T. W. Tillman and R. Carhart, SAM-TR-66-55, in June 1966). The authors feel that this test is not merely a list of words but a particular recording of them. This test was developed strictly for research purposes and there is no expectation that the recorded version will be made available commercially.

CNC MONOSYLLABIC WORDS COMPRISING THE FOUR LISTS OF N.U. AUDITORY TEST NO. 6

List I		List II		List III		List IV	
bean*	met	bite	merge*	bar*	mouse	back*	mob
boat	mode*	book*	mill	base*	name	bath*	mood*
burn	moon	bought*	nice*	beg	note*	bone	near
chalk	nag*	calm	numb	cab*	pain	came	neat*
choice	page	chair	pad*	cause	pearl*	chain*	pass*
death*	pool	chief	pick*	chat*	phone	check*	peg*
dime*	puff*	dab*	pike	cheek	pole	dip*	perch*
door	rag*	dead*	rain	cool	rat*	dog*	red*
fall*	raid*	deep*	read*	date	ring	doll	ripe*
fat*	raise*	fail	room	ditch*	road*	fit*	rose*
gap	reach*	far*	rot*	dodge*	rush*	food	rough*
goose	sell*	gaze	said	five*	search	gas*	sail
hash*	shout*	gin*	shack*	germ	seize	get*	shirt
home	size*	goal	shawl	good*	shall	hall	should
hurl*	sub	hate*	soap*	gun*	sheep*	have*	sour*
jail	sure	haze	south*	half	soup	hole*	such*
jar	take	hush*	thought*	hire*	talk	join	tape
keen	third	juice	ton*	hit*	team	judge*	thumb*
king	tip*	keep	tool	jug*	tell*	kick*	time*
kite*	tough*	keg	turn*	late	thin*	kill*	tire*
knock	vine*	learn	voice	lid*	void*	lean	vote*
laud	week*	live	wag*	life*	walk*	lease	wash*
limb	which	loaf	white*	luck	when	long	wheat*
lot	whip	lore	witch	mess	wire*	lose	wife*
love*	yes*	match	young	mop*	youth*	make	yearn

*Also in original PB-50 lists.

5. MULTIPLE-CHOICE WORD LISTS

A multiple-choice word-intelligibility test was developed by Professor John W. Black of Ohio State University in collaboration with the United States Naval School of Aviation Medicine. It has been used extensively in tests of talkers speaking under various conditions of interest to military aviation. The talker is given a list of words to read. The listeners mark prepared blanks on which each word read by the talker appears as one of four rather similar possible choices. Twenty-four of these lists are published in the *Journal of Speech and Hearing Disorders*, 22:213 −235 (1957). The first of these lists is given on page 532 as a sample. The word in each group actually read by the talker is italicized.

6. THE RHYME TEST (Fairbanks)

A more precise test of *phonemic differentiation* known as the rhyme test was described by G. Fairbanks in the *Journal of the Acoustical Society of America*, 30:596−599 (1958). The test was designed to emphasize auditory-phonemic factors and to minimize linguistic factors. It somewhat resembles a multiple-choice word test, but instead it is of the completion type; and it also is oriented more to the study of speech communication than to the assessment of the listener or clinical diagnosis.

The stimulus words are drawn from a vocabulary of 250 common monosyllables consisting of 50 sets of 5 rhyming words each. One word from each set is read to the subject. On his response sheet are given the 50 stems, with a space in front of each where the subject enters one letter to complete the spelling of the word he believes he heard. The author imposed several constraints related to ambiguities of spelling and pronun-

ciation. The test is simple but rather limited in scope.

7. THE RHYME TEST (House et al.)

A modification of the Fairbanks rhyme test is described by A. S. House, C. E. Williams, M. H. L. Hecker, and K. D. Kryter in the *Journal of the Acoustical Society of America*, 37:158–166 (1965). These lists were modified slightly by A. S. House and N. Guttman but not published. The changes substituted new words for original ones that were objectionable and eliminated some repetitions. These changes are incorporated in the lists given here. The title includes the phrase "Consonantal Differentiation with a Closed-Response Set." The test was designed to be used in group-articulation testing of voice-communication systems.

The materials consist of six equivalent word lists in which no strict account is taken of word familiarity, of relative frequency of occurrence of sounds in the language, or of some of Fairbanks' constraints related to spelling. The listener's task is a multiple choice, not a completion task. The answer sheet provides a closed set of six alternatives. This procedure virtually eliminates learning time and also word-frequency effects. The lists are not phonetically or phonemically balanced, but they have reasonable phonemic similarity and contain representatives from the major classes of speech sounds. The words are nearly all of the consonant-vowel-consonant type.

Across the six lists the vowel in the nucleus is the same. In some sets the *final* consonant is the same; in others the *initial* consonant is the same. On the response sheet each set of six words is arranged in two lines of three words each and is enclosed in a rectangular box. The subject draws a line through one to indicate his choice.

groove	latter	nurse	wade
drew	ladder	first	waves
crew	*lattice*	birth	*wave*
grew	rabbit	*burst*	way
say	crash	named	*fine*
stay	crab	*name*	find
stayed	*craft*	main	sign
spade	crack	knave	kind
stung	modern	*last*	get
stun	moderate	lash	gap
sun	modesty	laugh	guess
stunned	*modest*	glass	guest
quench	forbade	gold	only
went	*pervade*	bowl	woman
whence	surveyed	cold	pullman
when	survey	*bold*	omen
pass	drunk	*vice*	swain
past	grunt	fight	*slain*
cast	brunt	mice	flame
task	runt	bite	plain
popular	busy	*chink*	pail
poplar	physics	kink	poor
hopper	*physic*	check	*polo*
opera	visit	chin	palace
immense	clearly	*intent*	
commence	weary	intend	
emit	quarry	content	
cement	*query*	intense	

	A	B	C	D	E	F
1	bat	bad	back	bass	ban	bath
2	bean	beach	beat	beam	bead	beak
3	bun	bus	but	buff	buck	bug
4	came	cape	cane	cake	cave	case
5	cut	cub	cuff	cup	cud	cuss
6	gig	dip	did	dim	dill	din
7	duck	dud	dull	dub	dug	dun
8	fill	fig	fin	fizz	fib	fit
9	hear	heath	heal	heave	heat	heap
10	kith	king	kid	kit	kiss	kill
11	late	lake	lay	lace	lane	lame
12	map	mat	math	man	mass	mad
13	page	pane	pace	pay	pale	pave
14	pass	pat	pang	pad	path	pan
15	peace	peas	peak	peal	peat	peach
16	pill	pick	pip	pig	pin	pit
17	pun	puff	pup	pug	putt	pub
18	rave	rake	race	rate	raze	ray
19	sake	sale	save	sane	safe	same
20	sad	sass	sag	sack	sap	sat
21	seep	seen	seethe	seed	seem	seek
22	sing	sit	sin	sip	sick	sill
23	sud	sum	sub	sun	sup	sung
24	tab	tan	tam	tang	tack	tap
25	teach	tear	tease	teal	team	teak
26	led	shed	red	bed	fed	wed
27	sold	told	hold	fold	gold	cold
28	dig	wig	big	rig	pig	fig
29	kick	lick	sick	pick	wick	tick
30	book	took	shook	cook	hook	look
31	hark	dark	mark	lark	park	bark
32	gale	male	tale	bale	sale	pale
33	peel	reel	feel	heel	keel	eel
34	will	hill	kill	till	fill	bill
35	foil	coil	boil	oil	toil	soil
36	fame	same	came	name	tame	game
37	ten	pen	den	hen	then	men
38	pin	sin	tin	win	din	fin
39	sun	nun	gun	fun	bun	run
40	rang	fang	gang	bang	sang	hang
41	dent	bent	went	tent	rent	sent
42	sip	rip	tip	dip	hip	lip
43	top	hop	pop	cop	mop	shop
44	meat	feat	heat	seat	beat	neat
45	kit	bit	fit	sit	wit	hit
46	hot	got	not	pot	lot	tot
47	nest	vest	west	test	best	rest
48	bust	just	rust	must	gust	dust
49	raw	paw	law	jaw	thaw	saw
50	way	may	say	gay	day	pay

The properties of these lists under conditions of various signal-to-noise ratios are given in some detail in the original article. The word lists appear on page 533.

8. QUESTION-ANSWER TYPE OF SENTENCE LISTS

The following sentences are the basis of Auditory Test No. 12, prepared by the Psycho-Acoustic Laboratory. The questions are relatively simple and can be answered by a single word. This feature makes them useful when a written test for use in group testing is desired. If only one subject is being tested, he may be allowed to repeat the entire sentence. This procedure allows him to concentrate more fully on his listening.

These sentences have been recorded phonographically in groups of four at successively lower intensities. In this form the test is useful for obtaining a *threshold* for speech. The threshold level determined by this test is normally about 4 dB above the threshold measured by the spondaic two-syllable words. This test, together with Test No. 9 (spondaic words), is described in detail in the article entitled "The Development of Recorded Auditory Tests for Measuring Hearing Loss for Speech," by C. V. Hudgins, J. E. Hawkins, J. E. Karlin, and S. S. Stevens, and published in *The Laryngoscope*, 47:57–89 (1947).

AUDITORY TEST NO. 12—LIST 1

Level	Answer	Question
0 dB	B	1. What letter comes between A and C?
	Yes	2. Do flies have wings?
	Monday	3. What day comes after Sunday?
−6 dB	3 or 4	4. How many colors are there in the American flag?
	11	5. What number comes after 10?
	Hammer	6. What tool do you drive nails with?
−12 dB	7	7. What number comes between 6 and 8?
	Yes	8. Are moths dangerous to clothing?
	February	9. What month comes after January?
−18 dB	5	10. How many pennies are there in a nickel?
	No	11. Is there a lot of water in the desert?
	Weak	12. What is the opposite of strong?
−24 dB	9	13. What number comes before 10?
	Bullets	14. Does a gun shoot flowers or bullets?
	Old	15. What is the opposite of new?
−30 dB	France	16. In what country is Paris?
	No	17. Do you climb mountains in a sailboat?
	X	18. What letter comes after W?
−36 dB	Tuesday	19. What day comes after Monday?
	Light	20. What is the opposite of dark?
	12	21. What number comes after 11?

AUDITORY TEST NO. 12—LIST 5

Level	Answer	Question
0 dB	Night	1. Which is darker, night or day?
	Pen	2. Do you write with a chair or a pen?
	E	3. What letter comes after D?
	Long, tall	4. What is the opposite of short?
−4 dB	Red	5. What is the color of blood?
	24	6. How many hours are there in a day?
	Pacific	7. What is the ocean west of the United States?
	Thursday	8. What day comes after Wednesday?
−8 dB	Tongue	9. What does a cat lick with?
	Cord, string	10. What do you tie a package with?
	Fish	11. Does a cat eat fish or straw?
	N	12. What is the first letter in "never"?
−12 dB	Bottom	13. What is the opposite of top?
	Hay	14. Does a cow eat hay or stones?
	Sour	15. Is a lemon sour or salty?
	20	16. What number comes between 19 and 21?
−16 dB	Ugly, homely	17. What is the opposite of pretty?
	White	18. What color is a ping-pong ball?
	13	19. What number comes between 12 and 14?
	Pacific	20. In what ocean is Pearl Harbor?
−20 dB	Thursday	21. What day comes before Friday?
	Glass	22. What are windows made of?
	Sun	23. What shines in the sky in the daytime?
	White	24. Is a polar bear white or green?
−24 dB	6	25. What number comes between 5 and 7?
	2	26. How many legs does a man have?
	60	27. How many seconds in a minute?
	No	28. Do fish swim in trees?

9. S-1 TYPE OF SENTENCE TEST

These lists of sentences were prepared at the Psycho-Acoustic Laboratory for testing sentence intelligibility. The listener writes down or repeats each sentence. Scoring is based only on the five italicized words in each sentence. One point is scored for each word heard correctly. In each sentence the five key words consist of four monosyllables and one disyllable. The vocabulary is fairly simple; nevertheless, the sentences tend to hold the attention of the listener. The lists are useful for practice in listening as well as for the elaborate articulation testing for which they were designed.

S-1 TYPE—LIST 1

1. The *birch canoe slid* on the *smooth planks.*
2. *Glue* the *sheet* to the *dark blue background.*
3. *It's easy* to *tell* the *depth* of a *well.*
4. These *days* a *chicken leg* is a *rare dish.*
5. *Rice* is *often served* in *round bowls.*
6. *John* is *just* a *dope* of *long standing.*

7. The *juice* of *lemons makes fine punch.*
8. The *chest* was *thrown* beside the *parked truck.*
9. The *hogs* were *fed chopped corn and garbage.*
10. A *cry* in the *night chills my marrow.*
11. *Blow high* or *low* but *follow* the *notes.*
12. *Four hours of steady work faced us.*
13. A *large size* in *stockings is hard to sell.*
14. *Many* are *taught to breathe through the nose.*
15. *Ten days leave is coming up.*
16. The *Frenchman* was *shot when* the *sun rose.*
17. The *rod* is *used to catch pink salmon.*
18. He *smoked a pipe until it burned his tongue.*
19. The *light flashed* the *message to* the *eyes of* the *watchers.*
20. The *source* of the *huge river* is the *clear spring.*

10. THE BTL SENTENCES

The Bell Telephone Laboratories sentences were for many years a standard tool for testing hearing and for testing the performance of instruments, such as telephone and radio. The original collection contains 49 lists of 50 sentences each. The questions are longer and more difficult in vocabulary than the Psycho-Acoustic Laboratory sentences, and for these reasons they are not satisfactory for clinical use. The scoring is a little less certain; and for many listeners, the difficulty may be in understanding or remembering rather than in correct hearing. A small sample from one list is given below.

1. What is meant by "A stitch in time saves nine"?
2. What is the first letter of your last name?
3. Why is there a spring in a window shade roller?
4. What is meant by the expression "during rush hours"?
5. How many judges make up the Supreme Court?
6. Why is it necessary to build foundations for houses?
7. Name the tool with which a burglar opens a window.
8. Of what benefit was the Red Cross to soldiers during the war?
9. What man is called the "Father of his country"?
10. What instrument do we use to drive nails into wood?

11. EVERYDAY SPEECH (CID)

A set of sentences has been prepared at Central Institute for the Deaf to represent "everyday American speech." The specifications for such a sample were laid down by a Working Group (chairman, Dr. Grant Fairbanks) of the Armed Forces-National Research Council Committee on Hearing and Bio-Acoustics. Some of the more important characteristics are as follows:

1. The vocabulary is appropriate to adults.
2. The words appear with high frequency in one or more of the well-known word counts of the English language.
3. Proper names and proper nouns are not used.
4. Common nonslang idioms and contractions are used freely.
5. Phonetic loading and "tongue-twisting" are avoided.
6. Redundancy is high.
7. The level of abstraction is low.
8. Grammatical structure varies freely.
9. Sentence length varies in the following proportion:

Two to four words	1
Five to nine words	2
Ten to twelve words	1

10. Sentence forms are in the following proportion:

Declarative	6
Rising interrogative	1
Imperative	2
Falling interrogative	1

The sentences have been recorded under contract with the Veterans Administration. The recordings are available from Recorded Publications Laboratory, 1100 State Street, Camden, New Jersey 08105.

No "test" has been developed from this material. It represents a sample of American speech of high face validity against which more specific tests of intelligibility or of "correct hearing" may be validated. In scoring the "correctness of hearing" of the new speech material, a system based on the correct repetition of 50 key words in each list of ten sentences has proved satisfactory.

The actual sentences, with the key words italicized, are as follows:

CID LIST A

1. *Walking's my favorite exercise.*
2. *Here's a nice quiet place to rest.*
3. *Our janitor sweeps the floors every night.*
4. *It would be much easier if eyeryone would help.*
5. *Good morning.*
6. *Open your window before you go to bed!*
7. *Do you think that she should stay out so late?*
8. *How do you feel about changing the time when we begin work?*
9. *Here we go.*
10. *Move out of the way!*

CID LIST B

1. *The water's too cold for swimming.*
2. *Why should I get up so early in the morning?*
3. *Here are your shoes.*
4. *It's raining.*
5. *Where are you going?*
6. *Come here when I call you!*
7. *Don't try to get out of it this time!*
8. *Should we let little children go to the movies by themselves?*
9. *There isn't enough paint to finish the room.*
10. *Do you want an egg for breakfast?*

CID LIST C

1. *Everybody should brush his teeth after meals.*
2. *Everything's all right.*
3. *Don't use up all the paper when you write your letter.*
4. *That's right.*

5. *People ought to see a doctor once a year.*
6. *Those windows are so dirty I can't see anything outside.*
7. *Pass the bread and butter please!*
8. *Don't forget to pay your bill before the first of the month.*
9. *Don't let the dog out of the house!*
10. *There's a good ballgame this afternoon.*

CID LIST D

1. *It's time to go.*
2. *If you don't want these old magazines, throw them out.*
3. *Do you want to wash up?*
4. *It's a real dark night so watch your driving.*
5. *I'll carry the package for you.*
6. *Did you forget to shut off the water?*
7. *Fishing in a mountain stream is my idea of a good time.*
8. *Fathers spend more time with their children than they used to.*
9. *Be careful not to break your glasses!*
10. *I'm sorry.*

CID LIST E

1. *You can catch the bus across the street.*
2. *Call her on the phone and tell her the news.*
3. *I'll catch up with you later.*
4. *I'll think it over.*
5. *I don't want to go to the movies tonight.*
6. *If your tooth hurts that much your ought to see a dentist.*
7. *Put that cookie back in the box!*
8. *Stop fooling around!*
9. *Time's up.*
10. *How do you spell your name?*

CID LIST F

1. *Music always cheers me up.*
2. *My brother's in town for a short while on business.*
3. *We live a few miles from the main road.*
4. *This suit needs to go to the cleaners.*
5. *They ate enough green apples to make them sick for a week.*
6. *Where have you been all this time?*
7. *Have you been working hard lately?*

8. There's *not enough room* in the *kitchen* for a *new table.*
9. *Where is he?*
10. *Look out!*

CID LIST G

1. I'll *see you right after lunch.*
2. *See you later.*
3. *White shoes are awful to keep clean.*
4. *Stand there and don't move until I tell you!*
5. *There's a big piece of cake left over from dinner.*
6. *Wait for me at the corner in front of the drugstore.*
7. *It's no trouble at all.*
8. *Hurry up!*
9. *The morning paper didn't say anything about rain this afternoon or tonight.*
10. *The phone call's for you.*

CID LIST H

1. *Believe me!*
2. *Let's get a cup of coffee.*
3. *Let's get out of here before it's too late.*
4. *I hate driving at night.*
5. *There was water in the cellar after that heavy rain yesterday.*
6. *She'll only be gone a few minutes.*
7. *How do you know?*
8. *Children like candy.*
9. *If we don't get rain soon, we'll have no grass.*
10. *They're not listed in the new phone book.*

CID LIST I

1. *Where can I find a place to park?*
2. *I like those big red apples we always get in the fall.*
3. *You'll get fat eating candy.*
4. *The show's over.*
5. *Why don't they paint their walls some other color?*
6. *What's new?*
7. *What are you hiding under your coat?*
8. *How come I should always be the one to go first?*
9. *I'll take sugar and cream in my coffee.*
10. *Wait just a minute!*

CID LIST J

1. *Breakfast is ready.*
2. *I don't know what's wrong with the car, but it won't start.*
3. *It sure takes a sharp knife to cut this meat.*
4. *I haven't read a newspaper since we bought a television set.*
5. *Weeds are spoiling the yard.*
6. *Call me a little later!*
7. *Do you have change for a five-dollar bill?*
8. *How are you?*
9. *I'd like some ice cream with my pie.*
10. *I don't think I'll have any dessert.*

Brief Glossary of Auditory Terms

Several terms or usages employed in this book, particularly in Chapters 3 through 10, are relatively new but are believed to be clarifications of, or improvements over, certain older usages. The following definitions (arranged in logical rather than alphabetical order) form a self-consistent system and are in agreement with current Acoustical Terminology, S1.1-1960 (R1971), and, to the best of our ability, with relevant authoritative statements by the Committee on Conservation of Hearing of the American Academy of Ophthalmology and Otolaryngology and the American Medical Association. The index should be consulted for terms not included in this list.

hearing impairment This is the most general term for malfunction of the auditory mechanism. It does not distinguish either the anatomical area primarily involved (central versus peripheral) or the functional nature of the impairment (sensitivity, frequency range, discrimination, sense of loudness or of pitch, recognition of meaning, and the like). In a medicolegal context "hearing impairment" implies a severity sufficient to "affect personal efficiency in the activities of daily living," specifically in respect to communication.

hearing handicap This term is a companion to "hearing impairment." It expresses the *result* of the impairment in terms of "personal efficiency in the activities of daily living." The basis of compensation is the degree of handicap (percentage handicap), not the extent of anatomical or physiological impairment. Such impairments are often too limited to produce a handicap in daily living.

disability of hearing This medicolegal term (sometimes misused for impairment or handicap) is avoided in this book because of its special connotation related to earning power. Impairment is only a contributing factor to disability.

Disability: actual or presumed inability to remain employed at full wages.

Impairment: a deviation or a change for the worse in structure or function, usually outside the range of normal.

Handicap: the disadvantage imposed by an impairment sufficient to affect one's personal efficiency in the activities of daily living.

normal-hearing persons   A normal-hearing person is one whose ears, on otological inspection, show no indications of present or past otological disease or anatomical deviation that might interfere with acoustic transmission, who has no history of past otological disease or abnormality, who has no hearing complaints, and who understands and cooperates in the tests of hearing that may be applied. Unless otherwise specified, normal-hearing persons are assumed to be of either sex and between 15 and 65 years of age. Many psychoacoustic relations have been established for such individuals, including threshold of sensitivity as a function of frequency; discrimination of loudness, of pitch, of words, and the like; as well as the relation of subjective loudness to physical intensity, and so on. For all quantitative tests of hearing a group of normal-hearing individuals shows a range of performance. The performance of the group is usually expressed as the mean or the median accompanied by some measure of the dispersion (scatter), such as the standard deviation.

actuarial hearing thresholds   The median threshold of sensitivity of normal-hearing persons varies as a function of many parameters of the stimulus, such as frequency, manner of listening (open acoustic field or under an earphone), the place and manner of measuring the sound-pressure level, and the psychoacoustic method employed in the test. These must all be specified. It also varies according to the age and sex of the individuals. "Actuarial hearing thresholds" are the average (median) expectations of hearing sensitivity for normal-hearing persons according to age and sex.

range of normal hearing   The scatter of actual determinations of hearing sensitivity of normal-hearing persons with respect to the median expectation for age and sex determines the range of normal hearing. The limit is sometimes taken as two standard deviations, sometimes as the 95th percentile.

normal threshold of hearing   *This term should be avoided because of its medical and medicolegal implications.* There is no single normal threshold of hearing; there are instead *various ranges of normal hearing* related to the various median actuarial hearing thresholds.

sound-pressure level (SPL)   This is the ratio, expressed in decibels, of the effective (root-mean-square) sound pressure of a particular tone or noise to a standard reference pressure that is the same for all frequencies and bandwidths. The usual reference pressure for airborne sound is 0.0002 dyne per square centimeter. This is also written as 2×10^{-4} microbar (μbar) or, in the International System of Units (SI), as 2×10^{-5} newton per square meter (N/m²) or 20 micropascals (20 μPa).

reference zero level for pure-tone audiometry   A single sound-pressure level is needed for each frequency and for each combination of earphone and coupler, to serve as the reference or zero level for the decibel scale of intensity of standard audiometers. A particular set of levels was recommended by the International Organization for Standardization (ISO) and has been adopted by the American National Standards Institute (ANSI) and by nearly all other countries that have national standards. The ISO-ANSI values are the weighted averages of 15 determinations in five countries of the median hearing thresholds of well-motivated normal-hearing young adults (18 to 30 years old), using comparable psychoacoustic methods. The ANSI reference levels for pure-tone audiometers do not, however, define or constitute a legal standard for normal hearing (see Chapter 9).

hearing level (HL) The ratio, expressed in decibels, of the sound-pressure level (produced by an audiometer meeting the ANSI specifications) to its reference zero level (ISO) at any particular setting of the frequency and intensity dials.

hearing-threshold level (for pure tones) (HTL) This is the ratio, expressed in decibels, of the threshold of an ear at a specified frequency to a standard reference zero level for pure-tone audiometers. Practically, it is the reading in decibels, on a standard audiometer, that corresponds to the listener's hearing threshold.

audiogram (threshold audiogram) An audiogram is a graph that shows hearing-threshold level as a function of frequency.

electric response audiometry (evoked-response audiometry) (ERA) Determination of the threshold of detection of any one of several electric responses of the auditory nervous system. (See Chapter 8.) The most useful varieties seem to be

Electrocochleogram (ECochG): based chiefly on the action potential of the auditory nerve.

Brain-stem response audiometry (BSRA, BER, and others): Based responses of the inferior colliculus and other neural structures in the brain stem.

Cortical ERA: based on either the primary (middle latency) cortical responses or the secondary (slow potential) cortical electric responses.

tympanogram A graph showing the relation of the acoustic impedance or admittance of the middle ear as a function of the atmospheric pressure in the external ear canal. (See Chapter 8.) This is a purely physical measurement of middle-ear function, but in association with it the threshold of the acoustic (stapedius) reflex is often determined as well.

speech-reception threshold (SRT) This term specifies the sound-pressure level, measured as described in Chapter 7, at which certain test words or sentences reach the threshold of intelligibility for a particular subject. The most commonly used material is a set of spondaic words, described in the Appendix, and the threshold of intelligibility is usually defined as 50 percent correct repetition of the words. Ambiguity is reduced if the value is given as sound-pressure level, that is, SPL.

reference level for speech audiometers The proposed (1976) ANSI draft of the revision of its standard for audiometers states that this reference level "shall be 12.5 dB above the 1 kHz standard reference sound-pressure level threshold as listed in Table 3." Table 3 lists the reference threshold levels for four different earphones, used with a 9-A coupler. For Telephonics TDH-49 with MX41/AR cushions this value is 7.5 dB re 20 μPa. The reference level for the speech threshold (with this earphone) is therefore 20 dB re 20 μPa.

hearing-threshold level for speech This is the ratio, expressed in decibels, of any individual's threshold (50 percent correct) for the spondaic words to the reference zero level for standard speech audiometers. (For the calculation of *percentage handicap of hearing*, which in principle depends on the individual's speech reception threshold, it is customary to use the average hearing-threshold level for the three pure tones, 500, 1000, and 2000 Hz, instead of a direct determination of the hearing threshold for speech; see Chapter 9.)

hearing loss This term has acquired three distinct meanings:

1. The symptom or condition of impaired hearing, particularly impairment of the sensitivity of hearing as tested by either pure tones or speech. For this meaning the terms "hearing loss" and "hypoacusis" are employed in this book.

2. The *hearing-threshold level* as defined above. This term should always be used instead of "hearing loss" when a numerical value in decibels is given. The set of standard reference levels employed (ANSI, ISO, ASA-1951, or other) must be specified.

3. A change for the worse in an individual's threshold of hearing. This meaning carries the connotation of disease, injury, or deterioration, as in the common phrase "to suffer a hearing loss." To avoid these connotations the term *threshold shift* is often employed. It is helpful to specify whether the threshold shift is *temporary* or *persistent*. The consistent use of the distinctive terms "hypoacusis," "hearing level," and "threshold shift" is particularly helpful and desirable in medicolegal contexts.

deafness (anacusis) Deafness is the traditional term for a severe or complete loss of auditory sensitivity. For adults it should only be used if the hearing-threshold level for speech, estimated as recommended above, is 93 dB (ISO) or worse. This implies a hearing loss sufficient to make auditory communication difficult or impossible without amplification. For children the cutoff level is often set as low as 70 dB for educational purposes, as explained in Chapter 17.

dysacusis Any impairment of hearing that is not primarily a loss of auditory sensitivity is called dysacusis. The cause of dysacusis may be a malfunction or injury of either the central nervous system, the auditory nerve, or the sense organ. Dysacusis is not relieved, like hypoacusis, by simple amplification of speech, and therefore is not measured in decibels. Among the many types of dysacusis are:

Discrimination loss for words, syllables, or phonemes

Reduced intelligibility for sentences

Auditory agnosia or *central auditory imperception*. This condition is explained in Chapter 4. It is also called "sensory aphasia," "receptive aphasia," "auditory aphasia," or "word deafness."

Phonemic regression. This is the symptom, found in the elderly, of loss of the ability to comprehend all of the words in a sentence, or even single words, spoken at normal tempo, in spite of relatively good sensitivity for pure tones or slow speech.

Recruitment. The recruitment of loudness (Fowler) is an abnormally rapid increase in subjective loudness as a function of sound-pressure level.

Binaural diplacusis. In this condition a single pure tone, presented alternately to the right and left ears, is judged to have a different pitch in each ear.

Monaural diplacusis. In this condition a single pure tone, presented monaurally, is heard as a group of tones, a noise, or both.

aphasia Aphasia is loss or impairment of the capacity to use words as symbols of ideas. The predominant defect may affect the ability to speak (*motor aphasia* or *expressive aphasia*), or the failure may be a lack of comprehension of the spoken word (*sensory aphasia* or *receptive aphasia*), or both. Receptive aphasia may be visual (*alexia*) as well as auditory.

dysmathia Dysmathia means "difficulty in

learning." It is contrasted with dysacusis, which means "difficulty in hearing." Dysmathia may occur in children with or without dysacusis or hypoacusis.

dyslogomathia Dyslogomathia means specifically *difficulty in learning language*. It is recommended as a more accurate substitute for "congenital aphasia" or "childhood aphasia" (see Chapter 4).

combined hearing impairment This term implies the combination of hypoacusis (a peripheral reduction of sensitivity) with a central dysacusis. This term is not applied to a combination of conductive and sensorineural hearing loss (mixed hearing loss).

air conduction Air conduction is the process by which sound is conducted to the inner ear through the air in the outer-ear canal as part of the pathway.

bone conduction Bone conduction is the process by which sound is conducted to the inner ear through the cranial bones.

air-bone gap The air-bone gap is the difference in decibels between the hearing-threshold levels for a particular frequency as determined by air conduction and by bone conduction.

conductive hearing loss A hearing impairment due to interference with the acoustic transmission of sound to the sense organ, usually in the outer or middle ear, is known as conductive hearing loss. The term "middle-ear hearing loss" is preferable to "conductive hearing loss" in most contexts because of the possibility of inefficient conduction of sound in the inner ear. In the past conductive hearing loss and middle-ear loss have been practically synonymous. In pure middle-ear conductive hearing loss the hearing-threshold levels measured by bone conduction are usually near normal, and the air-bone gaps are large, up to 60 dB.

sensorineural hearing loss The term implies a hearing impairment due to abnormality of the sense organ, the auditory nerve, or both. Some or all hearing-threshold levels by bone conduction are abnormal. With pure inner-ear hearing loss the air-bone gaps are small or absent.

mixed hearing loss A combination of conductive with sensorineural hearing loss, or a combination of middle-ear with inner-ear hearing loss, is known as mixed hearing loss. This term is restricted by custom to peripheral hearing losses.

INDEX OF NAMES

INDEX OF ORGANIZATIONS

INDEX OF SUBJECTS